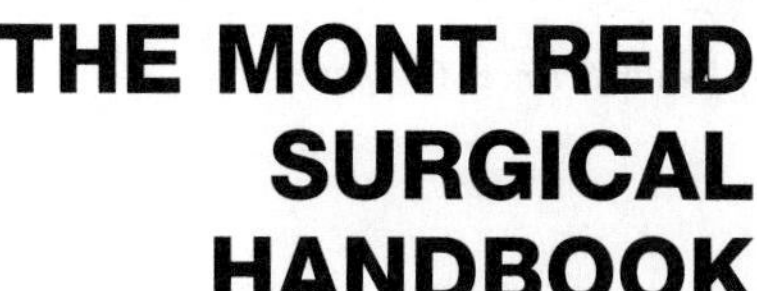

THE MONT REID SURGICAL HANDBOOK

a Mosby handbook

THE UNIVERSITY OF CINCINNATI RESIDENTS
From the Department of Surgery
University of Cincinnati, College of Medicine
Cincinnati, Ohio

FOURTH EDITION

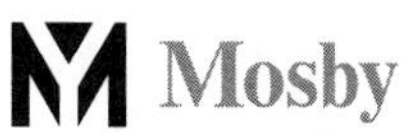

Mosby

A *Harcourt Health Sciences Company*
St. Louis Philadelphia London Sydney Toronto

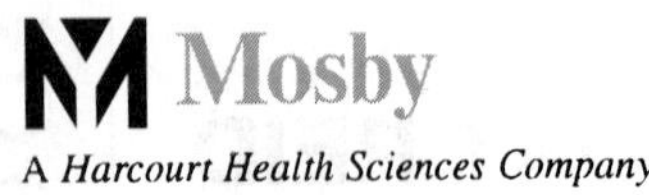

A *Harcourt Health Sciences Company*

Fourth Edition

Printed in the United States of America

Mosby, Inc.
11830 Westline Industrial Drive
St. Louis, MO 63146

Library of Congress Card Catalog Number 97-4039

01 / 9 8 7 6 5

Editor-in-Chief

Scott M. Berry, M.D.
Chief Resident, Department of Surgery,
University of Cincinnati, College of Medicine

Section Editors

Robert C. Bass, M.D.
Chief Resident, Department of Surgery,
University of Cincinnati, College of Medicine

Keith M. Heaton, M.D.
Chief Resident, Department of Surgery,
University of Cincinnati, College of Medicine

William James O'Brien, M.D.
Chief Resident, Department of Surgery,
University of Cincinnati, College of Medicine

Kevin J. Ose, M.D.
Chief Resident, Department of Surgery,
University of Cincinnati, College of Medicine

Stephen P. Povoski, M.D.
Chief Resident, Department of Surgery,
University of Cincinnati, College of Medicine

Contributors

Patricia A. Abello, M.D.
Senior Resident, Department of Surgery,
University of Cincinnati, College of Medicine

Stephen B. Archer, M.D.
Assistant Resident, Department of Surgery,
University of Cincinnati, College of Medicine

J. Kevin Bailey, M.D.
Assistant Resident, Department of Surgery,
University of Cincinnati, College of Medicine

Robert C. Bass, M.D.
Chief Resident, Department of Surgery,
University of Cincinnati, College of Medicine

Scott M. Berry, M.D.
Chief Resident, Department of Surgery,
University of Cincinnati, College of Medicine

Karl J. Bertram, M.D.
Assistant Resident, Department of Surgery,
University of Cincinnati, College of Medicine

David L. Brown, M.D.
Assistant Resident, Department of Surgery,
University of Cincinnati, College of Medicine

Rebecca L. Brown, M.D.
Senior Resident, Department of Surgery,
University of Cincinnati, College of Medicine

John Joseph Bruns, Jr, M.D.
Assistant Resident, Department of Surgery,
University of Cincinnati, College of Medicine

Robert J. Burnett, III, M.D.
Assistant Resident, Department of Surgery,
University of Cincinnati, College of Medicine

W. Bradley Craft, M.D.
Assistant Resident, Department of Surgery,
University of Cincinnati, College of Medicine

Robert A. Cusick, M.D.
Assistant Resident, Department of Surgery,
University of Cincinnati, College of Medicine

Carole Ebner, R.Ph.
Registered Pharmacist, Critical Care Pharmacy,
University Hospital, University of Cincinnati Medical Center

Martha A. Ferguson, M.D.
Assistant Resident, Department of Surgery,
University of Cincinnati, College of Medicine

Scott W. Gibson, M.D.
Assistant Resident, Department of Surgery,
University of Cincinnati, College of Medicine

Michael J. Goretsky, M.D.
Assistant Resident, Department of Surgery,
University of Cincinnati, College of Medicine

Keith M. Heaton, M.D.
Chief Resident, Department of Surgery,
University of Cincinnati, College of Medicine

Michael A. Helmrath, M.D.
Assistant Resident, Department of Surgery,
University of Cincinnati, College of Medicine

Scott C. Hobler, M.D.
Assistant Resident, Department of Surgery,
University of Cincinnati, College of Medicine

Robert E. Isemann, R.Ph.
Registered Pharmacist, Critical Care Pharmacy,
University Hospital, University of Cincinnati Medical Center

Michael D. Johns, J.D.
J.D. Candidate (1997), College of Law,
University of Cincinnati

Scott R. Johnson, M.D.
Assistant Resident, Department of Surgery,
University of Cincinnati, College of Medicine

Timothy D. Kane, M.D.
Assistant Resident, Department of Surgery,
University of Cincinnati, College of Medicine

Jeffrey Larson, M.D.
Resident, Department of Neurosurgery,
University of Cincinnati, College of Medicine

Susan E. MacLennan, M.D.
Assistant Resident, Department of Surgery,
University of Cincinnati, College of Medicine

Christopher S. Meyer, M.D.
Senior Resident, Department of Surgery,
University of Cincinnati, College of Medicine

Tory A. Meyer, M.D.
Assistant Resident, Department of Surgery,
University of Cincinnati, College of Medicine

Clyde I. Miyagawa, Pharm.D.
Clinical Pharmacy Specialist, Critical Care Pharmacy,
University Hospital, University of Cincinnati Medical Center

M. Ryan Moon, M.D.
Assistant Resident, Department of Surgery,
University of Cincinnati, College of Medicine

Francis Nazareno, M.D.
Resident, Department of Anesthesia,
University of Cincinnati, College of Medicine

Son Thanh Nguyen, M.D.
Assistant Resident, Department of Surgery,
University of Cincinnati, College of Medicine

William J. O'Brien, M.D.
Chief Resident, Department of Surgery,
University of Cincinnati, College of Medicine

Kevin J. Ose, M.D.
Chief Resident, Department of Surgery,
University of Cincinnati, College of Medicine

Alexander A. Parikh, M.D.
Assistant Resident, Department of Surgery,
University of Cincinnati, College of Medicine

Stephen P. Povoski, M.D.
Chief Resident, Department of Surgery,
University of Cincinnati, College of Medicine

David A. Rodeberg, M.D.
Senior Resident, Department of Surgery,
University of Cincinnati, College of Medicine

Michael B. Rousseau, M.D.
Chief Resident, Division of Urology,
University of Cincinnati, College of Medicine

David J. Shelley, M.D.
Assistant Resident, Department of Surgery,
University of Cincinnati, College of Medicine

Joel I. Sorger, M.D.
Junior Resident, Department of Orthopedic Surgery,
University of Cincinnati, College of Medicine

Gregory B. Strothman, M.D.
Senior Resident, Department of Surgery,
University of Cincinnati, College of Medicine

Khang N. Thai, M.D.
Assistant Resident, Department of Surgery,
University of Cincinnati, College of Medicine

Gregory M. Tiao, M.D.
Assistant Resident, Department of Surgery,
University of Cincinnati, College of Medicine

Betty J. Tsuei, M.D.
Senior Resident, Department of Surgery,
University of Cincinnati, College of Medicine

Leslie A. Wermeling, R.Ph.
Registered Pharmacist, Critical Care Pharmacy,
University Hospital, University of Cincinnati Medical Center

Arthur B. Williams, M.D.
Assistant Resident, Department of Surgery,
University of Cincinnati, College of Medicine

Foreword to the Fourth Edition

Four years have elapsed since the publication of *The Mont Reid Surgical Handbook,* Third Edition, and surgical practice has progressed significantly, making a fourth edition seemingly appropriate. The training program at the University of Cincinnati continues to occupy the core of the department with respect to our way of thinking as well as the various functions we serve. This textbook reflects the art and science of medicine and surgery at the University of Cincinnati Medical Center as exemplified by our residents. It is a tribute to the courage, intelligence, hard work, industry, and energy level of the surgical resident staff that is carefully selected, highly motivated, and above all an excellent and humanistic group. The expanding faculty's imprint is present in the protocols that have been established and the practices that currently go on at the University of Cincinnati; however, this volume appropriately represents the view of the residents being that the transmission of information from generation to generation has been not so much by the faculty, but by those we have trained.

This volume substantially reflects the important role of new technology in surgical practice, primarily videoscopic surgery, by including individual chapters on videoscopic surgery, laparoscopic cholecystectomy, appendectomy and herniorrhaphy, as well as advanced laparoscopic procedures. In addition, there has been a substantial effort to incorporate gynecological diseases, which will increasingly be seen by general surgeons. Thus, chapters focussing on gynecological malignancies, the management of abdominal pain in pregnancy, and gynecological causes of abdominal pain have also been added. The book is somewhat longer than its predecessors, but we believe that the added material is important enough to justify the length of the text.

Finally, the co-editors of this volume—Dr. Scott Berry, elected as Editor by his fellow chief residents; Robert C. Bass, M.D.; Keith M. Heaton, M.D.; William J. O'Brien, M.D.; Kevin J. Ose, M.D.; and Stephen P. Povoski, M.D.—have continued to impress me with their industry, excellence, and good humor in the face of adding this project to the myriad of other tasks in a difficult chief-residency year. And to their spouses, who have endured an additional sense of deprivation of an already busy chief resident, my salute for having borne with them during this difficult task.

Josef E. Fischer, M.D.
Christian R. Holmes Professor of Surgery
and Chairman of the Department of Surgery
University of Cincinnati Medical Center
Cincinnati, 1997

Foreword to the First Edition

Dr. Mont Reid was the second Christian R. Holmes Professor of Surgery at the University of Cincinnati College of Medicine. Trained at Johns Hopkins, he came to Cincinnati as the associate of Dr. George J. Heuer, the initial Christian R. Holmes Professor, in 1922, and became responsible for the teaching in the residency. He assumed the Chair in 1931 and died in 1943, a great tragedy for both the city and the University of Cincinnati College of Medicine. He was beloved by the residents and townspeople. A very learned, patient man, he was serious about surgery, surgical education, and surgical research. His papers on wound healing are still classics and can, to this day, be read with pride.

It was under Mont Reid that surgical residency first matured. In his memory, the new surgical suite built in 1948 was named the Mont Reid Pavillion. Part of the surgical suite is still operational in that building, as are the residents' living quarters. *The Mont Reid Handbook* is written by the surgical residents at the University of Cincinnati hospitals for residents and medical students and thus is appropriately named. It represents a compilation of the approach taken in our residency program, of which we are justifiably proud. The residency program as well as the Department reflect a basic science physiological approach to the science of surgery. Metabolism, infection, nutrition, and physiological responses to the above as well as the physiological basis for surgical and pre-surgical interventions form the basis of our residency program and presumably will form the basis of surgical practice into the twenty-first century. We hope that you will read it with profit and that you will use it as a basis for further study in the science of surgery.

Josef E. Fischer, M.D.
Christian R. Holmes Professor of Surgery
and Chairman of the Department of Surgery
University of Cincinnati Medical Center
Cincinnati, 1987

Preface to the Fourth Edition

The Mont Reid Surgical Handbook is a compilation of the practices of the surgical residents at the University of Cincinnati. Our practices are distinctly flavored by previous chief residents, who, in turn, were marked by the exacting nature and decisive leadership of our Chairman. This handbook is broad in scope and crosses many specialty boundaries. In doing so, it reflects our training program at the University of Cincinnati. We are decidedly proud of our classical general surgery training. *The Mont Reid Surgical Handbook* is entirely the work of the surgical residents in our program with the assistance of our resident colleagues in neurosurgery, plastics, urology, anesthesia, pharmacy, orthopedics, and law. The six chief surgical residents of 1996 serve as the editorial board. It is our hope that this work will be received in the spirit in which it is presented, not as an exhaustive text, but as a quick and portable reference to the most common problems encountered by practicing surgeons.

Scott M. Berry, M.D.
Editor-in-Chief

Preface to the First Edition

We can only instill principles, put the student in the right path, give him methods, teach him how to study, and early to discern between essentials and non-essentials.

Sir William Osler

The surgical residency training program at the University of Cincinnati Medical center dates back to 1922 when it was organized by Drs. George J. Heuer and Mont R. Reid, both students of Dr. William Halsted and graduates of the Johns Hopkins surgical training program. The training program was thus established in a strong Hopkins mode. When Dr. Heuer left to assume the chair at Cornell University, Mont Reid succeeded him as chairman. During Reid's tenure (1931-1943), the training program at what was then the Cincinnati General Hospital was brought to maturity. Since then, the training program has continued to grow and has maintained the tradition of excellence in academic and clinical surgery which was so strongly advocated by Dr. Reid and his successors.

The principal goal of the surgical residency training program at the University of Cincinnati today remains the development of exemplary academic and clinical surgeons. There also is a strong tradition of teaching by the senior residents of their junior colleagues as well as the medical students at the College of Medicine. Thus, the surgical house staff became very enthused when Year Book Medical Publishers asked us to consider writing a surgical handbook which would be analogous to the very successful pediatrics handbook, *The Harriet Lane Handbook* (now in its 11th edition). We readily accepted the challenge of writing a pocket "pearl book" which would provide pertinent, practical information to the students and residents in surgery. The six chief residents for 1985–1986 served as editors of this handbook and the contributors included the majority of the surgical house staff in consultation with other specialists who are involved in the direct care of surgical patients and the education of residents and medical students.

The information collected in this handbook is by no means exhaustive. We have attempted simply to provide a guide for the more efficient management of prevalent surgical problems, especially by those with limited experience. Therefore, this is not a substitute for a comprehensive textbook of surgery, but is rather a supplement which concentrates on those things that are important to medical students and junior residents on the wards, namely the initial management of common surgical conditions. Much of the information is influenced by the philosophies advocated by the residents and faculty at the University of Cincinnati and thus reflects a certain bias. In areas of controversy, however, we have also provided other views and useful references. The index has been liberally cross-referenced in order to provide a rapid and efficient means of locating information.

This handbook would not have been possible without the enthusiastic support and advice of our chairman, Dr. Josef E. Fischer, whose commitment to excellence in surgical training serves as an inspiration to all of his residents.

We also would like to acknowledge the invaluable advice provided by several of the faculty members of the Department of Surgery: Dr. Robert H. Bower, Dr. James M. Hurst, and Dr. Richard F. Kempczinski. The authors gratefully acknowledge the helpful input of Dr. Donald G. McQuarrie, Professor of Surgery at the University of Minnesota, for his review of each chapter in the handbook. Also we would like to thank Mr. Daniel J. Doody, Vice President, Editorial, Year Book Medical Publishers, for his patience and guidance in the conception and writing of this first edition of *The Mont Reid Handbook.*

None of this would have been possible were it not for the word processing expertise and herculean efforts of Mr. Steven E. Wiesner. His assistance in the typing and editing of the manuscript was invaluable.

Finally, this handbook is the result of the cumulative efforts of the surgical house staff at the University of Cincinnati as well as those residents who preceded us and taught us many of the principles that are advocated in this book. We wish to thank all of those who worked so diligently on this manuscript in order to make the first edition of *The Mont Reid Handbook* a reality.

Michael S. Nussbaum, M.D.
Editor-in-Chief
Cincinnati, 1987

Contents

PART I

Peri-Operative Care

1

Medical Record

Son Thanh Nguyen, M.D.

I. THE SURGICAL HISTORY AND PHYSICAL EXAMINATION

A. Meeting the patient.

1. ***Initial contact***—Gain his/her confidence and convey the assurance that help is available.
2. ***Put the patient at ease***—Be gentle and considerate, creating an atmosphere of sympathy, personal interest, and understanding. Be certain that the patient is as comfortable as possible and make yourself comfortable; demonstrate that you are *interested* and concerned about the patient.
3. ***Listen to your patient***—He/she is trying to tell you the diagnosis. Much can be learned by letting the patient "ramble" a little. Discrepancies and omissions in the history often are as much due to overstructuring and leading questions as to an unreliable patient.
4. ***Ensure the patient's privacy.***

B. History.

1. ***Chief complaint***—This should be in the patient's own words.
2. ***History of present illness (HPI).***
   a. *Pain*–A careful analysis of the nature of pain is an important feature of a surgical history. How did the pain begin? Was the onset rapid or gradual? What is the precise character of the pain? Does anything make it better? Worse? Is it constant or intermittent? Is anything else associated with the pain (eating, urination, bowel movement, exercise, etc.)?
   b. *Fever*–The onset of fever and cyclic patterns are important for excluding certain disease states.
   c. *Vomiting*–Inspect vomitus when possible. What did the patient vomit? What did it look like? How much? How often? Was the vomiting projectile? Was it associated with pain? The relationship between onset of abdominal pain and onset of vomiting will suggest level of obstruction.

d. *Change in bowel habits*–This common complaint is often of no significance. Any distinct change, however, toward intermittent constipation and diarrhea must lead one to suspect colon cancer or diverticular disease.

e. *Bleeding.*
   (1) A past history of bleeding is the best indicator of potential bleeding tendencies.
   (2) Any abnormal bleeding from any orifice must be evaluated carefully and should never be dismissed as being a result of some immediately obvious cause (e.g., hemorrhoids causing rectal bleeding).
   (3) Hematemesis or hematochezia–Character of blood helps differentiate between pathological states. Does it clot? Is it bright or dark red blood? Is it changed in any way? Coffee-ground vomitus is indicative of slow gastric bleeding; dark, tarry stool of upper GI bleeding.

f. *Trauma* –When a patient is subjected to trauma, the details surrounding the injury must be established as precisely as possible (see "Trauma").

g. *Medications*–Ask the patient what medications have been tried and whether the medications helped. It is very important to impress upon the patient that all medications tried must be related to the medical team, especially over-the-counter, herbal, diuretic, corticosteroid, and cardiac drugs. Indicate dose, route, frequency, and duration of usage.

3. ***Past medical history (PMH)***—Always obtain old records/reports. The past medical history is particularly important in assessing patients for potential anesthetic and peri-operative complications.
   a. Chronic illnesses–DM, HTN, MI, COPD, etc.
   b. Acute illness/hospitalizations–pneumonia, asthma attacks, DKA.
   c. Injuries/accidents–broken bones, trauma.
4. ***Past surgical history***—Again, obtain old records/operative reports.
   a. Type, date, and place (hospital) of surgery.
   b. Reason for the surgery–if known.
5. ***Allergies***—Specify drug reaction (i.e., rash, edema, stridor, anaphylaxis).
6. ***Social history***—Alcohol, tobacco, or other substance abuse–how much and how long.
7. ***Family history***—A significant number of surgical disorders are familial in nature (colonic polyposis, MEN syndromes, carcinoma of the breast, etc.).

C. Review of systems (ROS)—To make certain that important details of the history are not overlooked, this system review must be formalized and thorough. Note nutritional deficiencies, particularly acute fluid and electrolyte losses, recent weight loss, and anorexia. Record all pertinent positives and negatives.

D. Physical examination.

1. ***Put the patient at ease.***
2. ***Develop a system*** — The examiner must develop his/her own method of examining a patient in a detailed and orderly fashion in exactly the same sequence with each patient so that no step is omitted and no details excluded.
3. ***Assess the patient*** — Look at the patient prior to the "laying on of hands"; many clues to the diagnosis may be obtained. For example, a patient who is thrashing about and cannot seem to get comfortable may be suffering from renal or biliary colic. Very severe pain due to peritoneal inflammation or vascular disease usually forces the patient to restrict all movement as much as possible. Observe the patient's general physique, habitus, and affect. Carefully inspect the hands (many systemic disease may involve them, e.g., cirrhosis, hyperthyroidism, Raynaud's disease, pulmonary insufficiency, heart disease, nutritional disorders).
4. ***Inspection, auscultation, percussion, and palpation*** — Essential steps in evaluating both the normal and abnormal ("Look, listen, feel").
   a. Compare both sides of the body.
   b. Auscultation, particularly of the abdomen and peripheral vessels, is essential in evaluating surgical disorders.
   c. Palpation and percussion should be performed gently, carefully, and precisely.
5. ***Examination of the body orifices*** — Complete examination of the ears, mouth, eyes, rectum, and pelvis is an essential part of every complete examination.

E. Recap—After the history and physical, recap to the patient YOUR understanding of the patient's problems and/or findings. This will give the patient a chance to clarify/correct any misconceptions. Also, after the physical, new questions or clarifications of the history might be warranted.

F. Ancillary studies.

1. ***Objectives of laboratory examination.***
   a. Confirm suspected diagnosis.
   b. Screen for asymptomatic disease that may affect the surgical result.
   c. Screen for diseases that may contraindicate elective surgery or require treatment before surgery.
   d. Diagnose disorders that require surgery.
   e. Evaluate the nature and extent of metabolic or septic complications.
2. ***Routine laboratory tests*** — CBC, electrolyte profile, BUN, creatinine, PT, PTT, urinalysis, and electrocardiogram (patient over age 40 or with history of cardiac disease). Hepatic profile if there are known liver problems or hepatic surgery is planned.
3. ***Radiologic evaluation*** — A chest radiograph is indicated in most patients undergoing major surgery. Special radiographs

and studies are required in certain specific clinical situations. When sending a patient for a particular x-ray study, it is essential that the radiologist be provided with an adequate account of the patient's history and physical and your specific reason for ordering the study.

G. **Assessment and plan**—Following a thorough history and physical exam, one should be able to make a reasonable assessment of the patient's problem and form a differential diagnosis, construct a problem list, and develop a diagnostic and therapeutic plan.
   1. ***Problem list***—List in order of importance the particular problems identified in the history and physical examination.
   2. ***Assessment***—This is a concise and precise summary of the important data that are relevant to the patient's problem and that support the tentative conclusions and diagnosis.
   3. ***Plan***—List specific plans for further diagnostic evaluation and therapeutic measures.

H. **Emergency history and physical examination**—In cases of emergency, the routine history and physical must often be truncated and initial efforts directed toward resuscitating the patient. The history may be limited to a single sentence or may be obtained from family, friends, or rescue or ambulance personnel.
   1. ***History—AMPLE.***
      a. Allergies.
      b. Medications.
      c. Past medical history.
      d. Last meal.
      e. Events preceding injury or illness.
   2. ***Physical examination—ABCs.***
      a. Airway.
      b. Breathing.
      c. Circulation.

II. PHYSICIAN ORDERS

A. **Admission**—A helpful mnemonic is ADCA-VAN-DIMLS.
   1. ***Admit*** to ward, ICU or recovery room, surgery service, attending/resident.
   2. ***Diagnosis***—illness/disease.
   3. ***Condition*** (see also "Pre-Operative Preparation," section II.C).
      a. I = excellent.
      b. II = good.
      c. III = fair.
      d. IV = serious.
      e. V = critical.
   4. ***Allergies.***
   5. ***Vital signs*** and frequency; record inputs and outputs as indicated; specify neurologic or vascular checks. Include parameters to notify physician–BP $< 90/60$, $> 180/110$; P > 110;

P < 60; T > 101.5; urine output < 30 cc/h x 2 h; change in neurologic/vascular status; respiratory distress; respiratory rate > 30/min.

6. ***Activity*** or position; type of bed; elevation of head or foot of bed as needed; foot-board; measures for prevention of decubiti and thromboembolism (e.g., turn side-to-side q 2 h, OOB to chair tid, ambulate with assistance in the halls bid).
7. ***Nursing*** orders.
   a. Tubes–nasogastric, bladder catheter, chest tubes, drains.
   b. Dressings.
   c. Monitors.
   d. Respiratory care–supplemental O_2, ventilator settings, incentive spirometry.
   e. Compression boots or TED® hose.
8. ***Diet***—When in doubt, keep patient N.P.O. until decisions about patient disposition are finalized.
9. ***IV orders*** (e.g., D_5½ NS + 20 mEq KCl/liter @ 125 cc/h).
10. ***Medications***—Dose, route, frequency; sedatives, hypnotics, analgesics, laxatives, antiemetics, antipyretics, antibiotics, patient's regular medications, thromboembolism prophylaxis.
11. ***Laboratory tests.***
12. ***Special***—radiographs, special tests.

B. Pre-operative—Very important, since operations may be canceled if orders are inappropriately written.
1. NPO post midnight.
2. Hydration (D_5½ NS with 20 mEq KCL @ 100 cc/h).
3. Antibiotics/steroids on call to OR if needed.

C. Post-operative—Same as admission, but list procedure as part of diagnosis.

III. NOTES—*DATE AND TIME* ALL MEDICAL RECORD ENTRIES

A. Pre-operative notes (see also "Pre-operative Preparation").
1. Pre-operative diagnosis.
2. Procedure planned.
3. Surgeons.
4. Anesthesia anticipated.
5. Laboratory data.
   a. Minor operations–CBC and UA required.
   b. Major operations–CBC, renal profile, UA, PT, PTT, EKG if patient > 40 years old; CXR if patient has not had a normal CXR in past 6 months; type and screen or crossmatch if needed for specific procedure (verify crossmatch with the bloodbank); ABG, hepatic profile, bone profile, and other labs or specific radiographs as indicated by the patient's disease processes.
6. Identify–any specific risk factors related to cardiac, renal, pulmonary, hepatic, coagulation, and nutritional status.
7. Current medications or allergies; major medical illnesses.

8. Pre-operative Order checklist.
   a. Blood on hold (see "Pre-operative Preparation" for number of units).
   b. Antiseptic scrub.
   c. Incentive spirometry training.
   d. Thromboembolic prophylaxis.
   e. Prophylactic antibiotics.
   f. IV fluid overnight.
   g. Special medications (i.e., steroids, insulin, antihypertensives).
   h. NPO after midnight.
9. Document that potential risks and benefits of intended operation have been explained to the patient (and family or guardian), questions answered, and patient (or guardian) consents to the procedure.

B. Post-operative notes.

1. Mental status–neurologic exam, adequacy of pain control.
2. Vital signs, urine and drain outputs.
3. Physical exam–including inspection of surgical dressings, wounds, drains.
4. Laboratory data.
5. Assessment of condition.
6. Plan.

C. Progress notes—use *Problem Oriented Medical Records* by Lawrence Wood.

1. ***Daily notes***—Written to document status of current problems and identifying new problems. Identify post-operative day number, hospital day number, antibiotic or hyperalimentation day number, etc.
2. ***S.O.A.P.*** notes.
   a. Subjective data (patient's complaints, nurses' observations).
   b. Objective data (vital signs, physical findings, lab data).
   c. Assessment.
   d. Plans–diagnostic, therapeutic, patient education.
3. ***Flow sheets***—For complex data and time relationships, e.g., hyperalimentation data, diabetes control, hemodynamic parameters, etc.

IV. DICTATION—ALWAYS DICTATE IMMEDIATELY AFTER AN OPERATION

A. Operative report.

1. Identifying data–patient name, hospital number, dictator's name, date of dictation.
2. Service and Attending Surgeon.
3. Date of procedure.
4. Pre-operative diagnosis.
5. Post-operative diagnosis.
6. Procedure performed.
7. Surgeon, assistants.

8. Type of anesthesia used: Note the specific agents used.
9. Estimated blood loss.
10. Intra-operative fluid administered and blood products given.
11. Specimens–pathology, microbiology, etc.
12. Drains and tubes placed.
13. Complications.
14. Indications for surgery–brief history (reason for surgery).
15. Operative findings, including an itemized description of findings, both normal and abnormal, found at the time of surgery.
16. Details of operation–patient position, skin prep and draping, type and location of incision and technique, *specific details of procedure*, hemostatic technique, closure technique, dressings, disposition of patient, condition of patient, and sponge and needle counts as reported by nursing staff in attendance; send copies to surgeons and referring physicians.

NOTE: The above description is a formal, dictated note. A written note consisting of "3-15" above should be recorded in the chart immediately after all procedures.

B. Discharge summary.

1. Identifying data–patient name, chart number, service, attending surgeon, dictator's name.
2. Dates of admission and discharge.
3. Primary and secondary diagnoses.
4. Operation and procedures performed and dates.
5. Consultations.
6. Discharge medications.
7. Discharge diet.
8. Activity limitations.
9. Disposition and follow-up appointments.
10. Brief history on the reason that the patient was admitted.
11. Pertinent findings on physical exam, appropriate lab data, and brief narrative description of hospital course.
12. Copies to be sent to attending and referring physicians.

NOTE: It is useful if a simple written note consisting of "2-11" is included in the medical record. This is useful in follow-up visits if the dictated summary is not yet in the chart.

V. SUMMARY

A. Communication—The goal for all documentation is to provide a continuing commentary of the patient's care. This commentary is used by all the health care team members in providing the best care for the patient. Therefore, your notes must effectively communicate to health care workers your impression of the patient and your plans for the patient.

B. Standard documentation.

1. Admission history and physical.
2. Daily SOAP notes.
3. Procedure notes.
   a. Include any bedside procedures.
   b. Describe complications and findings.

4. Operative notes.
   a. Pre-operative note should include consent.
   b. Operative note is written and dictated. Check with your department/institution for any required format or elements. Dictate notes *immediately* after operation for optimal accuracy.
   c. Post-operative note is a documented examination of the patient after surgery.
5. Description of discussions with patients and their families, especially as it pertains to decisions regarding patient care.
6. Consult notes–indicate your thorough review of the patient's history, physical exam, and pertinent labs results and findings. Detail your impression and recommendations; include references to patient input and relevant discussion with other clinicians.
7. Discharge summary.

C. Litigation—Remember, in the event of litigation, nothing can be supported without written and legible documentation in the chart.

2

Medico-Legal Aspects

Michael D. Johns, J.D.

I. GENERAL LEGAL CONCEPTS

A. **Variance by state**—Most of the legal issues in medical care are governed by state law. Consequently, these standards vary, often significantly, from state to state.

B. **Questions of Fact *versus* Law**—Issues at trial are either questions of fact (for the jury to decide, where there is one) or questions of law (for the judge to decide). Most key issues in medical malpractice are factual and will be decided by a jury, which heightens the need for documentation and witnesses.

C. **Proof and documentation**—Details of patient care should be documented in detail, especially any conversations with the patient regarding care. Witnesses also are helpful.

D. **Legal action**—Lawsuits against physicians typically come in two forms: negligence and battery. A *negligence* theory looks to a standard of care and alleges a breach of that standard; whereas *battery* is merely the consequence of lack of adequate consent (negligence may be alleged here as well).

II. DUTY OF CARE

A physician has a duty to provide the type of care that would be given to similar patients under similar circumstances by a minimally qualified physician in good standing in the same field, given the facilities, resources, and options available. Inexperienced practitioners are not held to a lower standard of care.

A. **Elements**—In a court of law a plaintiff has the burden to prove four elements in a negligence malpractice case: standard of care, breach of that standard, injury to the patient, and causation between the breach and the injury.

B. **Good Samaritan exception**—Many states provide that the rendering of aid to patients outside the hospital setting, with no expectation of compensation, is insulated from liability for mere negligence; however, gross negligence as measured by reckless, willful, or wanton misconduct is still actionable.

C. Res Ipsa Loquitor—When a patient is injured in a setting where the patient cannot possibly provide proof of injury (e.g. while under anesthetic) and the injury would not likely have occurred without negligence, then courts will often shift the burden of proof to the physician to show that the injury was not due to negligence.

III. CONSENT

A. Generally—Prior to any examination or treatment, a physician must obtain informed consent from the patient for the particular procedure. Failure to obtain consent can lead to liability under a theory of battery (unconsented touching) or negligence (as to adequacy of the consent).

B. Types of Consent.

1. ***Written*** (most preferred)–Hospitals, in accordance with the AMA and legal authorities, provide standardized forms that physicians may modify for the particular situation. To complete written consent, physicians must discuss the treatment and then obtain the patient's signature on the form. Note that the physician must not delegate this duty.
2. ***Oral***–A patient may also agree orally to treatment. Differing recollections can lead to conflicting testimony at trial, however, making this method of consent significantly less desirable.
3. ***Implied***—Similar to oral consent, the conduct of a patient can indicate acquiescence to treatment. Again, evidentiary problems may exist as a jury decides the reasonable inferences that can be drawn from the patient's conduct. Avoid reliance on oral or implied consent.

C. Scope of Consent—Consent is generally limited to the specific procedures to which the patient originally gave written, oral, or implied consent.

1. ***Extending***—Caution should be used whenever treatment exceeds the scope of the consent.
   a. **General consent**–When the patient consents to treatment of a condition, rather than a specific procedure, the scope encompasses all measures reasonably necessary to remedy the condition.
   b. **Unexpected circumstances**–When an unexpected condition arises in performing the consented procedure or treatment and the patient is unable to grant consent (e.g. under anesthesia), then the physician must use medical judgment to decide on the appropriate action. If time permits, the physician should consult a family member or other legal representative.
2. ***Limiting.***
   a. **Procedure**–A patient may expressly limit consent to a particular procedure or expressly prohibit a particular procedure. Unless circumstances dramatically change to present

essentially an emergency, then the physician is bound by these limits. The physician should try to convince the patient to forgo such limitations when medical judgment suggests such procedures may become necessary.

b. **Physician**–A patient may also expressly limit consent to a particular physician. Again, this limitation is binding absent an emergency. In the academic or joint practice settings especially, the potential substitution of physicians is likely and must be included in consent.

D. Who may consent—The law presumes that persons 18 and over are competent to consent to treatment. For minors, the physician must look to the parents or legal guardians for consent. Substituted consent must also be sought for incompetent adults and may be required for those whose judgment is impaired by medication.

E. Adequacy: Informed Consent—The basis for the informed consent doctrine is rooted in personal autonomy–the patient should be free from non-consensual interference with his/her person. Thus, a physician has the duty to facilitate a reasonably informed decision by the patient as to treatment.

1. ***Measured by disclosure*** — A slight majority of the states have adopted the *professional disclosure* standard, which measures disclosure based upon the reasonable medical judgment of a practitioner who is similarly situated. A large minority of states, however, follow the *reasonable patient* standard, which asks whether the physician disclosed risks that a reasonable person would find material for making an informed decision. Disclosure must include but is not limited to the following:
   a. The nature, purpose, and material elements of the proposed treatment.
   b. The material risks of the treatment.
   c. The probability of both the risks and success.
   d. Treatment alternatives, including probability of risks and success.
   e. Side effects.
   f. Prognosis without any treatment.
   g. Any other items that a patient might find material to the decision. This discussion should be carefully and fully documented in the chart.
2. ***Exceptions: Consent or Disclosure not required*** — The law presumes that informed consent is required; a heavy burden of proof lies with the physician who proceeds without it.
   a. **Waiver**–A patient's request to waive disclosure on any or all of the items above must be treated with care and accepted only in writing.
   b. **Emergency**–When life-threatening injuries demand immediate treatment, the patient is unable to consent, and time does not allow any other person to be reached for substituted consent, then a physician may proceed without

consent. The physician should carefully document the nature of the emergency and any attempts to obtain alternative consent.

c. **Therapeutic privilege**—If disclosure would result in actual physical or emotional harm to the patient, jeopardize treatment, or result in an unreasonable election of nontreatment, then a doctor may use reasonable medical judgment to restrict disclosure. A heavy burden of proof lies on the physician in this situation.

IV. END-OF-LIFE/LIFE-SUSTAINING TREATMENT ISSUES

A. General interests—Both the law and the AMA support a presumption in favor of life while recognizing the competent patient's right to forgo life sustaining treatment. When the physician has doubts as to the appropriate course of action in end-of-life situations, the best course is to err in favor of life. In addition, in-house counsel and judicial intervention may be appropriate to resolve conflicts between the physician and the consenting party.

1. ***Personal autonomy***—Competent adults have a basic right to refuse treatment. In addition, the refusal, unless waived, should be an informed one (i.e., the patient must be told of the risks and prognosis for failing to accept treatment).
2. ***Doctors***—Have an ongoing interest in exercising the best medical judgment in treating patients. This interest tends to be strongly tied to doctors' reverence for the sanctity of life.
3. ***The State***—Preserves life and the quality thereof through appropriate legislation while recognizing individual interests of both patients and doctors.

B. Proxy decision-making in end-of-life or life-sustaining treatment situations.

1. ***Incompetent adults***—Physicians must obtain consent for incompetent adults from a proxy decision-maker. States vary as to whom the court or the physician may call upon to act as proxy. In addition, the substantive standard governing the proxy may vary according to the nature of the incompetence.
   a. **Substituted judgment**—The interest being served is the autonomy of the patient. Thus, the proxy decision-maker must apply the values and interests of the patient as opposed to his/her own. The person consenting says that the other, faced with this situation (typically terminal), would or would not have consented to the particular treatment at issue. The difficulty is that the patient has rarely thought of the exact situation.
   b. **Best interests**—When a patient has never been competent, "substituted judgment" is logically impossible, so the proxy is allowed to use his/her own judgment as to the "best interests" of the patient.
2. ***Minors***—Although children are deemed incompetent to make medical decisions, they are typically treated differently from

other incompetents. Of course, the physician must obtain consent from a proxy.

a. **Generally**—Parents or legal guardians are deemed to be the appropriate decision-maker for children. Physicians who fail to obtain consent for treatment of a minor will be liable.

b. **Limits**—The presumption in favor of life is applied more stringently with respect to children. Physicians should know any special rules of their institution pertaining to end-of-life/life-sustaining treatment cases in which minors are concerned.

C. Types of direction—Virtually all states have statutes that deal, in varying degrees, with living wills, durable powers of attorney, and family consent. The applicability may be exclusively for "terminal conditions" or may include conditions such as "irrevocable comas" and/or "persistent vegetative states". The laws also vary according to treatment (e.g., hydration and nutrition, ventilation). Physicians should consult the appropriate authority in their institutions for the governing rules.

1. ***Advanced directives.***

   a. **Living Wills**—This document specifies in detail the sort of treatment and discontinuance of treatment that a person desires in the event that he/she becomes incapacitated.

   b. **Durable Power of Attorney**—This document appoints a particular person(s) to act as decision-maker for a person in the event that he/she becomes incapacitated.

2. ***Family***—When the patient is unable to make an informed choice, then the family or other legal representative is often allowed to step in and determine whether the patient would want particular life-sustaining treatment. States vary in the procedural controls for these decisions, but a typical requirement might be that the family must show "clear and convincing" evidence that the patient would have agreed to suspend a particular life-sustaining treatment. Unanimous family decisions typically will be supported by a court when all other legal requirements are met.

3. ***DNR (Do Not Resuscitate)***—These situations are driven by institutional and other legal regulations. Again, the first step for a physician is to consult the appropriate authority in the institution in which he/she works.

   a. **Determination**—The physician must consult with the family or other legal representative. This discussion must be documented and witnessed by those involved. The following factors may be included in the decision:

      (1) Lack of significant benefit from further therapy.

      (2) Lack of productivity in prolonging life in cases of terminal illness or end-stage chronic disease.

      (3) An extension of the patient's physical or mental pain through prolonged ICU care.

   b. **Specificity**—The DNR should specify exactly what is to be done (e.g., "do not resuscitate in the event of cardiac or respiratory arrest", "no pressors, mechanical ventilatory support, or CPR in the event of cardiac or respiratory arrest," etc.). Hospitals typically have checklist forms of the usual directives.

c. **Level of care**—Maintain the standard level of nurse and physician care with particular attention to avoiding unnecessary patient discomfort. Additional treatment such as lab work, antibiotics, added nutritional support, and changes in ventilatory support typically are unnecessary.

D. Other distinctions.

1. ***Medically futile treatment***—Generally speaking, doctors are only required to provide medically reasonable treatment. When the family demands a "full court press", however, the physician is obligated to continue treatment in the absence of a judicial order to the contrary.
2. ***In life-sustaining treatment situations,*** many states still distinguish between active/passive, withholding/withdrawing, and ordinary/extraordinary treatments. Again, the physician must be aware of these distinctions and consult the appropriate authority in the institution where he/she works.

E. Patient Self-Determination Act of 1990—This requires that health care providers do four things:

1. Provide patients with written information about their rights under state law with respect to advance directives.
2. Provide patients with a written explanation of the provider's policies with respect to advance directives.
3. Indicate in the patient record the existence of any directives presented to the provider.
4. Train staff with respect to these issues.

3

Fluids and Electrolytes

WILLIAM J. O'BRIEN, M.D.

I. BASIC PHYSIOLOGY

A. Body fluid compartments.

1. Total body water (TBW).
   a. 50-70% of total body weight.
   b. Higher in males and in muscle tissue.
   c. Decreases with age. Highest in the newborn at 75-80%.
2. Intracellular fluid (ICF).
   a. 40% TBW, primarily in muscle.
3. Extracellular fluid (ECF).
   a. Interstitial water–15% TBW.
   b. Intravascular water–5% TBW.
      (1) Plasma volume–50 cc/kg body weight.
      (2) Blood volume–70 cc/kg body weight.

B. Fluid balance—management of fluid and electrolytes requires consideration of (1) normal daily requirements; (2) replacement of ongoing losses; and (3) correction of abnormalities. Trauma, surgery, and many disease states impose a much greater impact on fluid and electrolyte balance than simple starvation.

1. Basal requirements.
   a. Adult–35 cc/kg/day or 1500 cc/m^2/day.
   b. Pediatric.
      (1) 0-10 kg = 100 cc/kg.
      (2) 10-20 kg = 1000 cc + 50 cc/kg over 10 kg.
      (3) >20 kg = 1500 cc + 20 cc/kg over 20 kg.
2. Fluid turnover.
   a. Gastrointestinal tract (Table 1).
      (1) 6000-9000 cc/day.
      (2) 200-400 cc/day lost in stool.
   b. Renal 1000-1500 cc/day.
   c. Insensible losses.
      (1) 400 cc/m^2/day or 600-800 cc/day for adults (approximately 10 cc/kg/day).

TABLE 1
Composition of GI Secretions

Secretion	Volume (ml/24 h)	Na (mEq/L)	K (mEq/L)	Cl (mEq/L)	HCO_3 (mEq/L)
Salivary	1500	10	26	10	30
	(500-2000)	(2-10)	(20-30)	(8-18)	—
Stomach	1500	60	10	130	—
	(100-4000)	(9-116)	(0-32)	(8-154)	—
Duodenum	140	140	5	80	—
	(100-2000)	—	—	—	—
Ileum	3000	140	5	104	30
	(100-9000)	(80-150)	(2-8)	(43-137)	—
Colon	—	60	30	40	—
Pancreas	—	140	5	75	115
	(100-800)	(99-185)	(3-7)	(54-95)	—
Bile	—	145	5	100	35
	(50-800)	(99-164)	(3-12)	(89-180)	—

(2) 60% as water vapor (free water) from lungs; 40% as perspiration and water vapor from skin.

3. ***Increased requirement in patients with abnormal losses.***
   a. Fever–15% increase in insensible losses for each 1°C above 37°C.
   b. Tachypnea–50% increase for each doubling of respiratory rate.
   c. Evaporation–perspiration, ventilator, open abdominal wound.
   d. GI–diarrhea, fistula, tube drainage (see Table 1 for composition of losses).
   e. "Third space losses."
   f. Operative losses–may be 600-1000 cc/h in major abdominal operations.

C. Electrolyte composition.

1. Sodium.
   a. Major determinant of body tonicity, primary extracellular cation.
   b. Serum value is not indicative of total body sodium or volume status.
   c. Requirements: Adult–100-150 mEq/day, Child–3-5 mEq/kg/day.
2. Potassium.
   a. Important in glucose transport, intracellular protein deposition, and myoneural conduction.
   b. One of the two major intracellular cations, along with magnesium.

c. Serum levels do not reflect intracellular values; 1 mEq/L ECF = 200 mEq/L ICF. Affected by acid-base balance, nutritional state, sodium metabolism, renal function, and diuretic use.
d. Requirements: Adult–50-100 mEq/day, Child–2-3 mEq/kg/day.

3. Bicarbonate (section V)–major extracellular anion with chloride.
4. Chloride.
    a. Closely related to sodium metabolism.
    b. Requirements: Adult–90-120 mEq/day, Child–5-7 mEq/kg/day.
5. Calcium.
    a. Important in neuromuscular and enzyme physiology.
    b. Body stores 1-1.2 kg.
    c. Requirements:1-3 g/day (po), or 7-10 mmole/day (IV).
    d. Metabolism controlled by Vitamin D and parathyroid hormone.
    e. Physiologically active form in ionized state. Acidosis increases ionized form.
    f. Protein bound in serum. Correction for albumin level: Corrected Ca = (3.5 - patients albumin) x 0.8 + patient's Ca
6. Magnesium.
    a. Involved in myoneuronal conduction, enzyme phosphorylation, and protein anabolism.
    b. Distribution is similar to potassium, effects similar to calcium.
    c. Requirement: 20 mmole/day.
7. Phosphorus.
    a. Important mediator of cellular energy.
    b. Metabolism is related to calcium.
    c. Major intracellular anion, as is protein.
    d. Requirement: 30 mmole/day.

II. ASSESSMENT

A. History.

1. Medical conditions that predispose to fluid and electrolyte abnormalities (congestive heart failure, renal failure, cirrhosis, history of GI losses).
2. Usual and present weight.
3. Significant medications (steroids, diuretics, cardiac medications).

B. Physical exam.

1. Tissue turgor is decreased by contraction of interstitial fluid secondary to loss of sodium-containing fluids. May take 24-48 h.
2. Jugular venous distentionis indicator of volume status if cardiac disease is absent.

TABLE 2
Azotemia

Value	Prerenal	Renal
BUN	Increased	Increased
BUN/Creatinine	Normal	Increased
Urine Na	<10 mEq/L	>20 mEq/L
Urine Osmolality	>500	<350
FeNa	<1%	>1%
Response to Fluid	Increased Output	No Response

3. Orthostatic blood pressure changes are present with 10% loss of ECF.
4. Edema and lung crackles are due to increased body water and sodium.

C. Laboratory.

1. Serum electrolytes.
2. Hematocrit–slow reflection of changes in volume and tonicity.
3. Serum osmolality–"tonicity" of body fluids.
   a. Defined as ions per unit volume, primarily determined by sodium.
   b. Calculated by: Osmolality (mOsm/L) = 2(Na) + glucose/18 + BUN/2.8
4. Urine.
   a. Volume should be 0.5 to 1.0 cc/kg/h if there are adequate intravascular volume, renal function, and cardiac function.
   b. Specific gravity and osmolality vary inversely with volume status. Exceptions: diabetes insipidus, diuretic use, congestive heart failure.
   c. Urine indices can be obtained from "spot" urine and simultaneous serum samples. F_eNa (fractional excretion of Na) = (Urine Na x serum Cr/Serum Na x Urine Cr)100
   d. Hypovolemia and cardiogenic shock can both cause prerenal azotemia, and their urine indices will be identical.
5. Arterial blood gas–acid-base status.

III. VOLUME DISORDERS

A. Hypovolemia.

1. Clinical setting–trauma, prolonged gastrointestinal losses (vomiting, tube suction output, diarrhea), "third-spacing" (ascites, effusions, bowel obstruction, crush injuries, burns), increased insensible losses.
   a. Mild–4% loss total body water (TBW), 15% of blood volume.
   b. Moderate–6% TBW loss, 15-30% blood volume.

   c. Severe–8% TBW loss, 30-40% blood volume.
   d. Shock–> 8% TBW loss, > 40% blood volume.
2. Signs and symptoms.
   a. Mental status changes–sleepiness, apathy, coma.
   b. Cardiac–orthostatic hypotension, tachycardia, decreased pulse pressure, decreased CVP and PCWP.
   c. Tissue–decreased skin turgor, hypothermia, pale extremities, dry tongue, soft globe, depressed fontanelle in infants.
   d. Others–ileus, oliguria, weakness.
3. Laboratory.
   a. Increased BUN out of proportion to creatinine (> 20:1).
   b. Increased hematocrit, 3% rise for each liter deficit.
   c. Fractional excretion of sodium (F_eNa) < 1%; increased urine specific gravity and osmolality.
4. Treatment.
   a. Acute, life-threatening hypovolemia is usually secondary to trauma or major vascular catastrophe. Requires rapid infusion of isotonic fluid (crystalloid, plasma, and blood).
   b. Non-acute hypovolemia requires determination of volume deficit and associated electrolyte imbalances.
      (1) Hypotonic and isotonic deficits secondary to GI and "third space" losses are replaced with isotonic fluid; normal saline or lactated Ringer's solution.
      (2) Hypertonic deficits result from hyperosmolar nonketotic dehydration and jejunal feeding.
         a) Replace free water with D5W or D5W1/4 NS.
         b) Give D5W for excess free water losses: ventilator, high fever, tracheostomy, excessive perspiration.
   c. Administration of fluid.
      (1) Bolus therapy–250-1000 cc of fluid (depending on cardiac status and rate of losses), with frequent monitoring of heart rate, blood pressure, urine output. Use bolus therapy to achieve euvolemia.
      (2) Adjust rate and composition of fluids for maintenance, replacement of deficits, and ongoing losses to maintain euvolemia.

B. Hypervolemia.

1. Usually secondary to parenteral over-hydration, fluid-retaining states such as cardiac or renal failure, or mobilization of previously sequestered fluid.
2. Clinical findings.
   a. Weight gain over baseline. Fasting patient in ideal fluid balance should lose 0.25-0.5 kg body weight per day from catabolism.
   b. Pedal or sacral edema, pulmonary rales or wheezing, jugular venous distention, elevated CVP and PCWP.
   c. Pulmonary edema on chest radiograph.
3. Laboratory findings.
   a. Decreased hematocrit and albumin.

b. Serum sodium may be low, normal, or elevated; but total body sodium is usually increased.

4. Treatment.
   a. Water restriction to 1500 cc/day.
   b. Judicious use of diuretics.
   c. Sodium restriction to 0.5 g/day.
   d. Anasarca may respond to combined colloid (albumin) infusion followed by parenteral loop diuretics.

IV. COMPOSITIONAL DISORDERS

A. Hyponatremia—secondary to excess free water excess or salt deficit.

1. Forms.
   a. Hypotonic.
      (1) Hypovolemic is due to loss of isotonic fluids or replacement with inadequate volume of excessively hypotonic fluid.
      (2) Hypervolemic is due to fluid-retaining states: congestive heart failure, nephrosis, hepatic failure, malnutrition.
      (3) Isovolumic is due to iatrogenic free water overloading, SIADH, renal insufficiency, hypokalemia (sensitizes kidney to ADH).
   b. Isotonic ("pseudohyponatremia") occurs in presence of hypertriglyceridemia and hyperproteinemia.
   c. Hypertonic.
      (1) Due to non-sodium osmotic substances with intracellular water osmotic redistribution (glucose, mannitol).
      (2) For each 100 mg/dl of serum glucose > 100 mg/dl, serum sodium is decreased 3 mEq/L.
2. Signs and symptoms.
   a. Neurologic–muscle twitching, hyperactive deep tendon reflexes (DTR's), seizures, and hypertension secondary to increased ICP.
   b. Tissue–salivation, lacrimation, watery diarrhea.
   c. Usually asymptomatic if slow development to below 120 mEq/L. Symptoms may appear at 130 mEq/L in children, or in rapid onset of hyponatremia.
3. Treatment.
   a. Correct underlying disorder.
   b. Water restriction to < 1500 cc/day.
   c. Loop diuretics followed by hourly potassium and sodium replacement in hypervolemic forms.
   d. Hypertonic saline (3%, 5%) is reserved for symptomatic patients. Rate of infusion should increase sodium by 2-3 mEq/h, up to a serum Na of 125-130. Maximum rate of infusion 100 cc of 5% saline/h. Rapid correction may produce central demyelination.

B. Hypernatremia—free water deficit or water loss greater than salt loss. Always associated with hyperosmolar state.

1. Forms.
   a. Hypovolemic is due to loss of hypotonic fluids with inadequate volume replacement or hypertonic fluids. Each 3 mEq rise in serum Na reflects a 1 liter loss of free water.
   b. Isovolemic is actually subclinical hypovolemia. Frequent with diabetes insipidus.
   c. Hypervolemic is usually iatrogenic (large amounts of parenteral sodium bicarbonate, certain antibiotics). Also seen in disorders of adrenal axis; Cushing's syndrome, Conn's syndrome, congenital adrenal hyperplasia, steroid use.
2. Signs and symptoms.
   a. Neurologic–restlessness, seizures, coma, delirium, mania.
   b. Tissue–sticky mucous membranes, decreased salivation and lacrimation, increased temperature, and a red, swollen tongue.
   c. Other–thirst, weakness.
3. Treatment.
   a. Reversal of underlying disorder.
   b. Provision of free water: Water deficit = (0.6 x Kg body weight) (Serum Na/140-1). Hypotonic fluids, such as D5W, dextrose are metabolized in the liver to leave electrolyte free water.
   c. Replacement should be slow to avoid cerebral edema; half the calculated deficit is given over 8 h, with the remaining half over the next 16-24 h.

C. Hypokalemia.

1. Etiology.
   a. Redistributional losses from intracellular uptake of potassium; significant in acute alkalosis, insulin therapy, and anabolism.
   b. Depletion causes such as external losses from GI tract, renal losses (diuretics), steroid use, and renal tubular acidosis.
2. Signs and symptoms.
   a. Clinical–muscle weakness, fatigue, decreased deep tendon reflexes, paralytic ileus. Insulin resistance in diabetics or encephalopathy in cirrhotic patients may be seen.
   b. EKG findings include low voltage, flattened T waves, ST segment depression, and prominent U waves.
3. Treatment.
   a. Assure adequate renal function prior to repletion.
   b. Deficit is usually greater than the serum value indicates because of depleted body stores.
   c. Treat alkalosis, decrease sodium intake.
   d. Enteral replacement preferred–20-40 mEq doses.
   e. Parenteral replacement–7.5 mEq KCl in 50 cc D5W over 1 hour with peripheral IV; 20 mEq KCl/h with central line.

May increase amount of KCl in maintenance IVF's. Maximum KCl replacement 20mEq/h.

D. Hyperkalemia.

1. Etiology.
   a. Pseudohyperkalemia in leukocytosis, hemolysis, thrombocytosis.
   b. Redistributional–acidosis, hypoinsulinism, tissue necrosis (crush injury, burn, electrocution), reperfusion syndrome, digoxin poisoning.
   c. Elevated total body potassium in renal insufficiency, excessive intake, mineralocorticoid deficiency, diabetes mellitus, spironolactone use.
2. Signs and symptoms.
   a. Clinical–nausea/vomiting, intestinal colic, weakness, diarrhea.
   b. EKG changes include peaked T waves, decreased ST segments, widened QRS complex progressing to sine wave formation and ventricular fibrillation.
   c. Cardiac arrest occurs in diastole.
3. Treatment.
   a. Remove exogenous source–medications, IV fluids, diet.
   b. Emergent measures–if > 7.5 mEq/L or EKG changes present.
      (1) Calcium gluconate–1 g over 2 minutes IV.
      (2) Sodium bicarbonate–1 ampule, repeat in 15 minutes.
      (3) D50W–(1 ampule = 50 g) and regular insulin–10 units IVPB.
      (4) Emergent hemodialysis or peritoneal dialysis.
   c. Hydration and forced diuresis to promote renal excretion.
   d. Kayexalate®–20-50 g in 100-200 cc 20% sorbitol orally every 4 hours, 50 g in 200 cc water with 50 g sorbitol as retention enema, repeat every hour as needed.
   e. Kayexalate® and dialysis deplete total body potassium. Other measures only temporize by producing intracellular shifts of potassium.

E. Hypocalcemia.

1. Etiology.
   a. Frequently seen in hypoalbuminemic patients with normal ionized fraction.
   b. Usually asymptomatic until serum level < 8 mEq/dl.
   c. Ionized calcium may be subnormal with normal serum calcium in acute alkalotic states.
   d. If albumin is normal, check parathyroid hormone (PTH) level.
      (1) Low PTH–hypoparathyroidism, magnesium deficiency.
      (2) High PTH–pancreatitis, hyperphosphatemia, hypovitaminosis D, pseudohypoparathyroidism, massive ci-

trated blood transfusion, certain drugs (gentamicin), renal insufficiency, massive soft tissue infection.

2. Signs and symptoms.
   a. Numbness and tingling in extremities, circumoral paresthesia, muscle and abdominal cramps, tetany, increased DTRs, and seizures.
   b. Chvostek's sign–twitching of facial muscles after percussion over masseter muscle.
   c. Trousseau's sign–carpopedal spasm induced by inflation of blood pressure cuff above systolic pressure for 3 minutes.
   d. EKG findings–prolonged QT interval.
3. Treatment.
   a. Acute management (IV).
      (1) Calcium chloride 10 cc 10% solution = 6.5 mmole calcium (potential for tissue necrosis if infiltrated).
      (2) Calcium gluconate 10% solution = 2.2 mmole calcium.
   b. Chronic management (PO).
      (1) Calcium carbonate.
         a) Titralac®–1 cc = 1 g $CaCO_3$ = 400 mg Ca.
         b) OsCal®–1 tab = 1.25 g $CaCO_3$ = 500 mg Ca.
         c) Tums®–1 tab = 0.5 g $CaCO_3$ = 200 mg Ca.
      (2) Phosphate-binding antacids improve GI absorption of calcium.
      (3) Vitamin D (Calciferol®)–begin once serum phosphate is normal. Start at 50,000 units/day and increase up to 200,000 units/day as needed.

F. Hypercalcemia.

1. Etiology.
   a. Usually secondary to malignancy or hyperparathyroidism.
   b. Other causes–thiazide diuretics, milk-alkali syndrome, granulomatous disease, acute adrenal insufficiency, hyperthyroidism, prolonged immobilization in young patient, and Paget's disease of bone.
   c. Acute crisis with serum calcium > 12 mg/dl. Critical levels at 16-20 mg/dl. Requires immediate treatment.
2. Signs and symptoms–nausea, vomiting, anorexia, abdominal pains, constipation, polyuria, confusion, lethargy, and mental status changes. "Bones, stones, abdominal groans, and psychic overtones."
3. Treatment.
   a. Hydration with normal saline (dilution).
   b. Diuresis using loop diuretic, promotes renal excretion.
   c. Steroids–used in lymphomas, multiple myeloma, non-PTH secreting tumors metastatic to bone, vitamin D intoxication. May take several days to work.
   d. Mithramycin is used in malignant-induced hypercalcemia unresponsive to other treatments. Use 15-25 μg/kg IVP

over 4-6 h. Onset of action is 12 h, peak action at 36 h. Duration of action 3-7 days. Bone marrow suppression main side-effect.

e. Calcitonin used in malignancy-associated increased PTH. Skin test 1 unit SQ; usual dosage 4 units/kg SQ or IM every 12-24 h.

f. Hemodialysis.

g. Primary treatment of hypercalcemic crisis due to hyperparathyroidism is parathyroidectomy.

G. Hypomagnesemia.

1. Etiology–malnutrition of any type (alcoholism, prolonged fasting, TPN without adequate replacement, short gut syndrome, malabsorption, and fistulas), burns, pancreatitis, SIADH, vigorous diuresis, post-parathyroidectomy, and primary hyperaldosteronism.
2. Signs and symptoms–weakness, fasciculations, mental status changes, seizures, hyperreflexia, cardiac dysrhythmias.
3. Treatment.
   a. Parenteral–1-2 g $MgSO_4$ (8-16 mEq) IV as 10% solution over 15 minutes; continue with 1 g IM or IVPB every 4-6 h. Monitor replacement closely in oliguric patients.
   b. Oral–magnesium oxide 35-70 mg q/day.
   c. Follow replacement with decreasing patellar reflexes, serial serum measurements, and resolution of symptoms. ECG monitoring recommended for large doses.

H. Hypermagnesemia.

1. Causes–renal insufficiency, antacid overuse, adrenal insufficiency, hypothyroidism, excessive intake (i.e., treatment of eclampsia).
2. Signs and symptoms.
   a. Clinical–nausea, vomiting, weakness, mental status changes, hyperreflexia, hyperventilation.
   b. EKG findings include AV block and prolonged QT interval.
3. Treatment.
   a. Discontinue or remove external sources; large amounts found in antacids and cathartics.
   b. IV calcium gluconate for emergent symptoms.
   c. Dialysis in renal failure patients.

I. Hypophosphatemia.

1. Causes–hyperalimentation, nutritional recovery after starvation, diabetic ketoacidosis, malabsorption, phosphate binding antacids, alcoholism, acute tubular necrosis, prolonged alkalosis, hemodialysis, and starvation.
2. Signs and symptoms.
   a. Myocardial depression secondary to low ATP levels.
   b. Shift in oxyhemoglobin curve secondary to decreased 2,3-DPG levels.
   c. Clinical–anorexia, bone pain, weakness, rhabdomyolysis,

CNS changes, hemolysis, platelet and granulocyte dysfunction, and cardiac arrest.

3. Treatment.
   a. Parenteral if unable to take po or if severe hypophosphatemia (1 mg/dl).
      (1) Recent onset–0.08-0.20 mM/kg over 6 h.
      (2) Prolonged–0.16-0.24 mM/kg over 6 h.
   b. Enteral.
      (1) Neutraphos®–2 caps bid-tid (250 mg phosphorus/tab).
      (2) Phosphosoda®–5 cc bid-tid (129 mg phosphorous/cc).

J. Hyperphosphatemia.

1. Etiology–renal insufficiency, hypoparathyroidism, catabolism, vitamin D metabolites.
2. May produce metastatic calcification.
3. Treatment.
   a. Restrict external sources.
   b. Phosphate-binding antacid (Amphogel®, Alternagel®).

K. Zinc.

1. 1-2 g in body, with high concentrations in brain, pancreas, liver, kidney, prostate, testis.
2. Functions as enzyme activator and cofactor in enzymatic reactions.
3. Absorbed via ligand binding.
4. Deficiencies seen in malnutrition, malabsorption, trauma, inflammatory bowel disease, refeeding syndrome, cancer, and diarrhea.
5. Signs and symptoms.
   a. 4 Ds–diarrhea, dermatitis, depression, and dementia.
   b. Others–alopecia, night blindness, tremor, loss of taste.
6. Treatment with zinc sulfate 3-6 mg/day if patient having normal number of stools.

V. ACID-BASE DISORDERS

A. Physiology.

1. Most enzymatic reactions occur in narrow pH range.
2. Metabolism accounts for large proton load.
3. Three primary systems to buffer pH.
   a. Buffer systems.
      (1) Bicarbonate-carbonate system in RBCs is most important and rapid system: $HCl + NaHCO_3 \rightleftarrows NaCl + H_2CO_3 \rightleftarrows H_2O + CO_2$.
      (2) Others include intracellular proteins and phosphates, hemoglobin, and bone minerals.
      (3) Henderson-Hasselbach equation: $pH = pK + \log BHCO_3/H_2CO_3$.
   b. Respiratory system eliminates CO_2 ("volatile acid") generated during reduction of bicarbonate by metabolism. Pro-

vides rapid and inexhaustible source of acid elimination as long as ventilation is not compromised.

c. Renal system responsible for excretion of acid salts as well as reclamation of filtered bicarbonate and generation of *de novo* bicarbonate.

B. Disorders.

1. Metabolic acidosis.
   a. Etiology–due to overproduction or underexcretion of acids or depletion of buffer stores. Characterized by anion gap; normal = 8-12. Anion gap = Na − (Cl + HCO_3).
      (1) Increased anion gap–renal failure, ketoacidosis, lactic acidosis, various toxins (methanol, ethylene glycol, ethanol salicylates, paraldehyde).
      (2) Normal anion gap (hyperchloremic)–renal tubular acidosis, diarrhea, biliary or pancreatic fluid losses, Sulfamylon®, acetazolamide, ureteral diversions.
   b. Treatment.
      (1) Correct underlying disorder.
      (2) Mild to moderate acidosis requires no treatment unless complications ensue. Excessive use of sodium bicarbonate can lead to volume overload, hypernatremia, hyperosmolar state, and central alkalosis.
      (3) For pH < 7.25 or $HCO_3 < 15$, treatment may be required. Enzymes and catecholamines function poorly or not all below pH 7.2.
      (4) Base deficit = 0.4 x wt (kg) x (25 − measured HCO_3).
      (5) Correct 1/2 deficit, then recheck laboratory tests.
      (6) 1 ampule bicarbonate = 50 mEq $NaHCO_3$.
2. Metabolic alkalosis.
   a. Etiology.
      (1) Due to loss of acid or gain in base, aggravated by hypokalemia and volume contraction.
      (2) Chloride responsive (Urinary Cl < 10-20 mEq/L)–contraction alkalosis, diuretic induced, protracted vomiting or NG suction, exogenous bicarbonate loading, villous adenoma.
      (3) Chloride unresponsive (Urinary Cl > 10-20 mEq/L)–severe potassium depletion, mineralocorticoid excess.
   b. Diagnosis–elevated bicarbonate and pH, compensatory hypercapnia; frequently associated with hypokalemia.
   c. Treatment.
      (1) Correct underlying disorder.
      (2) Correct hypovolemia with chloride-containing solutions (0.9% NaCl).
      (3) Correct hypokalemia (assure adequate renal function first).
      (4) Provide acid solutions in refractory cases.
         a) Chloride deficit = wt (kg) x 0.4 x (100 − measured Cl).

TABLE 3

Replacement Therapy—Parenteral Fluids

Solution	Na (mEq/L)	K (mEq/L)	Cl (mEq/L)	Base (mEq/L)	mOsm/L	Dextrose (g/L)	Kcal/L
D5W	—	—	—	—	278	50	170
D10W	—	—	—	—	556	100	340
D50W	—	—	—	—	2780	500	1700
0.9% NaCl	154	—	154	—	286	—	—
0.45% NaCl	77	—	77	—	143	—	—
3% NaCl	513	—	513	—	1026	—	—
D5W 0.9% NaCl	154	—	154	—	564	50	170
D5W 0.45% NaCl	77	—	77	—	421	50	170
D5W 0.2% NaCl	39	—	39	—	350	50	170
LR	130	4	109	28	272	—	9
D5W LR	130	4	109	28	524	50	170

TABLE 4
Acid-Base Disorders

Disorder	Primary Change	Secondary Change	Effect
Metabolic Acidosis	↓ HCO_3	↓ pCO_2	Last 2 digits pH = pCO_2 HCO_3 + 15 = last 2 digits pH
Metabolic Alkalosis	↑ HCO_3	↑ pCO_2	HCO_3 + 15 = last 2 digits pH
Respiratory Acidosis			
Acute	↑ pCO_2	↑ HCO_3	Δ pH = .08 per 10 Δ in pCO_2
Chronic	↑ pCO_2	↑ ↑ HCO_3	Δ pH = .03 per 10 Δ in pCO_2
Respiratory Alkalosis			
Acute	↓ pCO_2	↓ HCO_3	Δ HCO_3 = .2 × Δ in pCO_2
Chronic	↓ pCO_2	↓ ↓ HCO_3	Δ HCO_3 = .3 × Δ in pCO_2

b) Calculate amount of 0.1 N HCl acid solution required to replace deficit.

(5) Acetazolamide (Diamox®) inhibits carbonic anhydrase, preventing renal reclamation and synthesis of bicarbonate. Dosage 500 mg q 6 h. Loses effect as serum bicarbonate decreases.

(6) For prolonged gastric suctioning, H_2 antagonists may decrease gastric acid production and minimize acid loss.

3. Respiratory acidosis.
   a. Etiology–results from acute or chronic hypercapnia secondary to inadequate ventilation.
   b. Diagnosis.
      (1) Characterized by increased pCO_2, decreased pH.
      (2) Acutely, HCO_3 may be normal; in chronic states there is a compensatory increase in HCO_3.
   c. Treatment.
      (1) Any measure designed to improve alveolar ventilation–aggressive pulmonary toilet, treatment of pneumonia, removal of obstruction (foreign body, secretions, misplaced endotracheal tube), bronchodilators, and avoidance of respiratory depressants.
      (2) Mechanical ventilation if conservative methods fail.
      (3) Maximize minute ventilation on ventilator–tidal volume of 12-15 cc/kg, then increase rate.
4. Respiratory alkalosis.
   a. Etiology.
      (1) Secondary to acute or chronic hyperventilation.
      (2) Caused by anxiety, metabolic encephalopathy, CNS infections, cerebrovascular accidents, early sepsis, pulmonary embolism, hypoxia, early asthma, pneumonia,

congestive heart failure, cirrhosis, or in severe head injury.

b. Diagnosis–characterized by hypocapnia and elevated pH.

c. Treatment.

(1) Treat underlying disorder.

(2) If symptomatic, use rebreather device; 5% CO_2 was used in past but is hazardous and is not recommended.

C. Evaluation of acid-base disorders (Table 4).

1. Obtain simultaneous blood gas and electrolyte panel.
2. Calculate anion gap.
3. Calculate expected compensation from chart and locate on acid-base nomogram.
4. If compensation is not within predicted values, suspect "mixed" disorder.
5. Correlate suspected diagnosis with clinical picture.

4

Shock

Patricia A. Abello, M.D.

Shock is equivalent *not* to hypotension, but rather to inadequate tissue perfusion, which leads first to reversible then irreversible cellular injury. "Syndrome precipitated by a systemic derangement of perfusion leading to widespread cellular hypoxia and vital organ dysfunction" (Fink). "Disordered response . . . to an inappropriate balance of substrate supply and demand at a cellular level" (Cerra).

I. PATHOPHYSIOLOGY OF SHOCK

- **A. Hypovolemic shock**—hemorrhagic vs. non-hemorrhagic (e.g., burn shock).
- **B. Septic shock.**
- **C. Neurogenic shock**—loss of autonomic vascular control.
- **D. Impaired cardiac function**—cardiac compressive shock *vs.* pump failure.
- **E. Anaphylactic shock.**

II. HEMODYNAMIC CONSIDERATIONS—CARDIOVASCULAR ABNORMALITIES

A. Frank-Starling relationship.

1. With the exception of septic shock, all forms of shock have low cardiac outputs: CO = HR x SV.
2. Stroke volume is determined by preload, myocardial contractility, and afterload (Frank-Starling curve).

B. Important principles.

1. Stroke volume, and thus cardiac output, increases as end-diastolic ventricular volume increases.
2. For a given end-diastolic volume, stroke volume increases with increase in myocardial contractility and decrease in afterload.
3. Shock can stem from abnormalities in either preload, afterload, or myocardial function.

C. Preload.

1. Preload reflects filling of the ventricle, and theoretically the LV-end diastolic volume.

2. In the absence of right ventricular dysfunction, central venous pressure can be used as an indirect measurement of central blood volume. In many elderly patients with cardiac disease or pulmonary dysfunction, the CVP will be an inaccurate assessment of left-sided filling volume.
3. Pulmonary artery (Swan-Ganz®) catheters measure pulmonary capillary wedge pressure (PCWP), an estimation of left ventricular end diastolic pressure (LVEDP). Optimal PCWP is 8-15 mm Hg (LVEDP by Swan-Ganz® measurement is inaccurate when mitral value disease is present.).

NOTE: LVEDP is* not *LV-end diastolic volume, which is the parameter directly correlating to stroke volume. Thus, changes in ventricular compliance, such as previous infarction or LV hypertrophy, may require higher filling pressures to effect the same LV-end diastolic volume. Newer pulmonary artery catheters can measure volume directly and may be more helpful.

D. Afterload.

1. Afterload of the ventricle is estimated by systemic vascular resistance (SVR), a calculated value.
2. A reduction in SVR can optimize cardiac output for a given preload and contractility. In cardiogenic shock with reduced myocardial function, a reduction in SVR can greatly improve cardiac output.
3. Hypovolemic patients may also demonstrate high SVRs. This reflects compensatory peripheral vasoconstriction to maintain adequate blood flow to vital organs. Afterload reduction is inappropriate until volume status has been corrected.
4. Common agents for afterload reduction.
   a. Nitroglycerin–increases venous capacitance.
   b. Nitroprusside–decreases arterial resistance.
5. In neurogenic shock, there is an inappropriate decrease in SVR due to loss of vasomotor tone. There is also a decrease in SVR in septic shock, with inappropriate vasodilation in the face of hypovolemia that is an inflammatory mediated event. In these instances, vasopressors are often used to improve vascular tone to help maintain adequate perfusion. Common agents include the following:
   a. Phenylephrine (Neosynephrine®)–α effect.
   b. Norepinephrine (Levophed®)–α and β_1 effects.
   c. Dopamine–see below.

E. Myocardial contractility.

1. Defined as the strength of myocardial contraction at a given preload and afterload. Compromised myocardial contractility is the primary pathology in cardiogenic shock. Treatment is directed toward increasing myocardial function with various inotropic agents.
2. Dopamine–increasing doses can lead to selective dopamine, α and β effects. Renal doses: 3-5 μg/kg/min; β–5-10 μg/kg/min; α–$\geq$ 10 μg/kg/min. At higher doses, dopamine is purely α.

3. Dobutamine–synthetic dopamine analog with β_1 and β_2 effects. Positive inotrope also acts as a mild to moderate vasodilator.
4. Amrinone–both inotropic and vasodilator effects. Load with 0.75 mg/kg, then 5-10 μg/kg/min infusion. Usually used with dopamine.
5. Epinephrine–α and β effects. Inotropic and chronotropic effects.
6. Norepinephrine–α and β effects. Used with Regitine® in cardiac patients to counteract peripheral vasoconstriction.

III. SHOCK STATES

A. Hypovolemic shock—Signs and symptoms depend upon degree of blood volume depletion, duration of shock, and the body's compensatory reactions to the shock itself.

Mild shock (< 20% blood volume)–adrenergic constriction of blood vessels in the skin with cool extremities; delayed capillary refill; patient may complain of thirst.

Moderate shock (20-40% blood volume)–low urinary output (< 0.5 cc/kg/h in adult). Oliguria reflects the effects of circulating aldosterone and vasopressin. Patient may be restless.

Severe shock (> 40% blood volume)–decreased urinary output, hypotension. May show myocardial ischemia on EKG. May be agitated, restless, or obtunded.

Exception: Inebriated or cirrhotic patients will maintain skin perfusion despite inadequate cardiac indices, making early shock difficult to assess. In addition, young patients, who have particularly effective compensatory responses, may be able to maintain a normal blood pressure and heart rate up to the point of cardiovascular collapse and arrest. It is important to recognize early signs of shock in these patients.

B. Traumatic shock.

1. Initially caused by both internal and external volume losses (i.e., loss of blood or plasma externaly from wound or burn surface, loss of blood or plasma into the damaged tissues). Worsened by plasma extravasation into tissues distal to injured areas.
2. Characterized by generalized systemic intravascular inflammatory response, which is generated by release of inflammatory mediators from damaged tissues, and free radicals from tissue reperfusion injury.
3. Mechanism of injury.
   a. Activation of the coagulation system, activating complement, kinins, and thromboxanes.
   b. Mobilization and activation of WBC and platelets with release of various inflammatory mediators, including TNF, IL-1, O_2 radicals, leukotrienes, kinins, serotonin, and histamine.

c. Generalized increase in systemic vascular permeability, with plasma extravasation into tissue and aggravation of preexisting hypovolemia.

4. Initial resuscitation.
   a. Remember ABCs. Establish airway, ensure adequate oxygenation and ventilation.
   b. Control of external hemorrhage.
   c. IV access and administration of crystalloid, preferrably lactated Ringer's solution. Lactate buffers hydrogen ion from ischemic tissues that is washed out with reperfusion.
   d. Supply blood products as needed.
   e. Operative control of hemorrhage if necessary.
5. Additional treatment.
   a. Debridement of ischemic or nonviable tissue.
   b. Immobilization of fractures to prevent further tissue damage.
   c. Pulmonary artery catheterization may be necessary for fluid management, especially in elderly patients.

C. Hypovolemic shock—non-hemorrhagic.

1. Similar as for hemorrhagic shock, except that blood is usually not necessary.
2. Examples include third space losses in bowel obstruction, GI losses from diarrhea, vomiting, biliary drainage, pancreatic fistula.
3. Replacements should be crystalloid with appropriate electrolyte composition of fluid lost. Good rule of thumb: $D_5$1/2NS + 10 mEq KCl/L for GI losses proximal to ligament of Treitz, lactated Ringer's solution for losses distal.

D. Septic shock.

1. Inappropriate host inflammatory response to initial infectious initiator.
2. Bacterial products from both gram-positive and gram-negative bacteria may initiate inflammatory, metabolic, endocrinologic, and immunologic pathways.
3. ***Gram-positive*** – massive fluid losses secondary to dissemination of potent exotoxin, often without bacteremia.
   a. Causative organisms–*Clostridium* sp., *Staphylococcus* sp., *Streptococcus* sp.
   b. Characterized by hypotension with normal urine output and unaltered mental status. Acidosis is infrequent.
   c. The prognosis is generally good with treatment.
   d. Treatment–appropriate antibiotics, surgical drainage or debridement if necessary, and intravenous fluids to correct volume deficit.
4. ***Gram-negative*** – initiated by endotoxins in cell walls of gram-negative bacteria.
   a. Causative organisms–GI flora, including coliforms and anaerobic bacilli such as *Klebsiella, Enterobacteriaceae, Serratia, Bacteroides.*

b. Common sources in order of decreasing frequency.
   (1) Urinary tract, pulmonary, alimentary tract, burns, and soft-tissue infections.
   (2) Always consider line sepsis.
c. Endotoxin, or lipopolysaccharide (LPS), in outer membrane of gram-negative bacteria can elicit marked host inflammatory response in absence of viable bacteria.
d. Host mediators implicated in pathogenesis of septic shock: Cytokines TNF-α and IL-1, reactive oxygen radicals, vasoactive peptides, complement activation, and platelet activating factor (PAF).
e. Hemodynamic changes and myocardial dysfunction.
   (1) Decreased SVR, increased or normal CO, decreased or normal PAO.
   (2) Increase in microvascular permeability leading to decreased intravascular volume, third space losses.
   (3) LVEF often depressed, but sepsis-induced tachycardia and LV dilatation maintain SV.
   (4) LV dysfunction coupled with RV dysfunction may be related to myocardial depressant factors.
   (5) Inappropriate vasodilation, pooling of blood in cutaneous venous bed.
   (6) Multiple organ dysfunction may ensue.
f. Treatment.
   (1) Early identification of source of infection and appropriate antibiotic treatment.
   (2) Foley catheter to monitor urine output.
   (3) Invasive hemodynamic monitoring.
   (4) Intravenous fluid resuscitation to achieve normal filling pressures.
   (5) Vasopressors, inotropes as needed.
   (6) Support of individual organ system.
g. New therapies directed at specific inflammatory mediators of sepsis.
   (1) Neutralizing microbiologic toxins–antibodies against core epitypes of LPS.
   (2) Modulating host mediators.
      a) Anti-TNF antibody.
      b) IL-1 receptor antagonists.
      c) PAF receptor antagonists.
      d) Anti-C5A antibodies.
      e) Antioxidant therapy.
   (3) Mixed results in animal and clinical trials, likely secondary to redundancy of inflammatory cascade.

5. ***Fungal.***
   a. Causative organisms–commonly *Candida* sp.
   b. Seen in neutropenic, immunosuppressed, multi-trauma, or burn patients.

c. Risk factors–hyperalimentation, invasive monitors, and broad-spectrum antibiotics.
d. When *Candida* reaches the intravascular compartment, widespread dissemination occurs.
   (1) Fungi lodge in the microcirculation, forming microabscesses.
   (2) Characterized by high fevers and rigors.
   (3) Blood cultures negative in 50% of patients.
   (4) Ophthalmologic evaluation may reveal evidence of ocular involvement in dissemination.
e. Treatment–Amphotericin B intravenously qd or qod as renal function permits, until target dose has been reached. Overall mortality rate approaches 50%.

E. Neurogenic shock.

1. Usually results from spinal cord injury, regional anesthetic agent, or autonomic blockade. Diagnosis based on history and neurologic exam.
2. Mechanism.
   a. Loss of vasomotor control.
   b. Expansion of venous capacitance bed with peripheral pooling of blood.
   c. Inadequate ventricular filling.
3. Manifested by the following:
   a. Warm, well-perfused skin.
   b. Low blood pressure.
   c. Urine output low or normal.
   d. Heart rate may be slow if adrenergic nerves to heart are blocked.
   e. Cardiac output normal, SVR low, PCWP low to normal.
4. Treatment.
   a. Correct ventricular filling pressure with IV fluids.
   b. Vasoconstrictors to restore venous tone. *Risks:* Vasculature to those parts of the body with an intact autonomic nervous system may constrict excessively, resulting in ischemia to vital organs or necrosis of fingers.
   c. Trendelenburg position if necessary.
   d. Maintain body temperature.

F. Cardiac compressive shock.

1. Distended neck veins in the injured patient should suggest cardiac compression and should be acted upon immediately. Absence of distended neck veins does not rule out cardiac compression in the hypovolemic patient. Distension may become evident only after adequate fluid resuscitation.
2. Common causes.
   a. Tension pneumothorax–shift of trachea to uninvolved side, decreased breath sounds, distended neck veins. This is not a radiographic diagnosis!
   b. Cardiac tamponade–hypotension, muffled heart sounds, distended neck veins (Beck's triad); low voltage on EKG;

enlarged cardiac silhouette on CXR with classic "water bottle" shape.
   (1) Pulsus paradoxus: drop in systolic blood pressure > 10 mm Hg with inspiration.
   (2) Kussmaul's sign: rise in CVP with inspiration (infrequently present).
  c. Positive pressure ventilation–patients receiving tidal volumes > 12 ml/kg or PEEP > 10 cm H_2O.
   (1) Compression of cavae, RA, and RV, limiting RV filling.
   (2) Compression of pulmonary microvasculature between inflated alveoli, to hinder RV emptying.
   (3) Compression of large pulmonary veins, LA and LV, to limit LV filling.
 3. Treatment–fluid administration and correction of underlying mechanism.
  a. Decompression of tension pneumothorax with 14 ga. angiocatheter in 2nd intercostal space, midclavicular line. Definitive treatment by chest tube placement in 5th intercostal space, anterior axillary line.
  b. Acute cardiac tamponade.
   (1) Stable hemodynamics.
    a) Pericardiocentesis–insert needle to left of xiphoid process, direct it upward and posteriorly. Fluid removal should return hemodynamics to normal.
    b) Pericardial window (Trinkle maneuver)–incise over xyphoid, exposing pericardium which is then incised.
   (2) Unstable–prompt operative thoracotomy or sternotomy. Cardiac compression caused by mechanical ventilation usually responds to volume expansion, adjustment of ventilator.

G. Cardiogenic shock—usually caused by cardiac disease. Penetrating trauma may result in direct damage to heart, valves, or coronary arteries, and blunt cardiac trauma may result in myocardial contusion, but these are rare causes for cardiogenic shock.
 1. Etiologies of cardiogenic shock.
  a. Arrhythmias.
  b. Myocardial failure.
  c. Valvular dysfunction.
  d. Increased PVR or SVR. Obstruction of pulmonary vasculature from pulmonary embolism as well as tension pneumothorax or high positive pressure ventilation (see above).
  e. Increased ventricular resistance (from scar tissue, hypertrophy, constrictive pericarditis, ischemia).
 2. Manifestations–cool skin, oliguria, cardiac output low, high SVR, elevated PCWP.
 3. Treatment.
  a. Identification and correction of hemodynamically significant arrhythmias.

b. Optimization of filling pressures.
c. Reduction of elevated vascular resistances–nitroglycerin, nitroprusside.
d. Inotropic support–dopamine, dobutamine.
e. Acute myocardial infarction–thrombolytic therapy, surgical treatment.

IV. MULTIPLE ORGAN DYSFUNCTION SYNDROME

A. Can result from prolonged or inadequately controlled shock. The most common cause of mortality in the surgical ICU.

B. Defined as "a syndrome of progressive but potentially reversible dysfunction involving two or more organs or organ systems that arises after resuscitation from an acute disruption of normal homeostasis."

C. Preventative measures.

1. Hemodynamic support–maintenance of adequate tissue oxygenation and substrate delivery.
2. Nutritional support–provision of adequate nutrition and reversal of catabolism.
3. Prevention of infection–maintenance of optimal antimicrobial defenses and prompt antimicrobial therapy at first sign of infection.

5

Blood Component Therapy

Scott M. Berry, M.D.

The judicious use of blood products is critical in the care of surgical patients. Because of the risk of metabolic, immunologic, and infectious complications, the clinician must be aware of the indications and contraindications of blood product use. The recommendations herein are derived from guidelines established by the American Association of Blood Banks, the American Red Cross, the FDA, the Center for Biologics Evaluation and Research, Hoxworth Blood Center, and the Council of Community Blood Centers.

I. ESTIMATION OF VOLUMES

A. **Total blood volume** (TBV) is approximately 7.5% of total body weight. It is slightly higher (8.0-8.5%) in males and newborns. TBV = 75 cc/kg total body weight.

B. **Red blood cell** (RBC) volume is TBV x hematocrit.

C. **Plasma volume** (PV) is TBV − RBC volume.

II. BLOOD COMPONENTS

Blood should be thought of in terms of its separate components (see Chart). Therapy should be directed at the specific deficit.

A. **Volume**—adequate intravascular volume maintains cardiac preload, cardiac output, and mean arterial perfusion pressure. Oxygen-carrying capacity is the responsibility of the RBC. Hypovolemia without significant red cell mass deficit is managed with *volume expanders.*

1. ***Crystalloid***—volume expander of choice in the acute setting. Isotonic fluids that will remain in the intravascular space are lactated Ringer's or normal saline solution. Potassium should not be added until adequate urine output is established.
2. ***Colloid solutions***—same hemodynamic effects as crystalloid in 1/3 the volume.

Summary Chart of Blood Components

Component	Major Indications	Action	Not Indicated For—	Special Precautions	Hazards	Rate of Infusion
Whole Blood	Symptomatic anemia with large volume deficit	Restoration of oxygen-carrying capacity, restoration of blood volume	Condition responsive to specific component	Must be ABO-identical; labile coagulation factors deteriorate within 24 hours after collection	Infectious diseases; septic/toxic, allergic, febrile reactions; circulatory overload	For massive loss, fast as patient can tolerate
Red Blood Cells	Symptomatic anemia	Restoration of oxygen-carrying capacity	Pharmacologically treatable anemia; coagulation deficiency	Must be ABO-compatible	Infectious diseases; septic/toxic, allergic, febrile reactions	As patient can tolerate, but less than 4 hours
Red Blood Cells, Leukocytes Removed	Symptomatic anemia, febrile reactions from leukocyte antibodies	Restoration of oxygen-carrying capacity	Pharmacologically treatable anemia; coagulation deficiency	Must be ABO-compatible	Infectious diseases; septic/toxic, allergic reactions (unless plasma also removed, e.g., by washing)	As patient can tolerate, but less than 4 hours

(Continued.)

Summary Chart of Blood Components (Cont.)

Component	Major Indications	Action	Not Indicated For—	Special Precautions	Hazards	Rate of Infusion
Red Blood Cells, Adenine-Saline Added	Symptomatic anemia with volume deficit	Restoration of oxygen-carrying capacity	Pharmaco-logically treatable anemia; coagulation deficiency	Must be ABO-compatible	Infectious diseases; septic/toxic, allergic, febrile reactions; circulatory overload	As patient can tolerate, but less than 4 hours
Fresh Frozen Plasma	Deficit of labile and stable plasma coagulation factors and TTP	Source of labile and non-labile plasma factors	Condition responsive to volume replacement	Should be ABO-compatible	Infectious diseases; allergic reactions, circulatory overload	Less than 4 hours
Liquid Plasma and Plasma	Deficit of stable coagulation factors	Source of non-labile factors	Deficit of labile coagulation facators or volume replacement	Should be ABO-compatible	Infectious diseases; allergic reactions	Less than 4 hours

Cryo-precipitated AHF	Hemophilia A, von Willebrand's disease, hypofibrinogenemia, Factor XIII deficiency	Provides Factor VIII, fibrinogen, VWF, Factor XIII	Conditions not deficient in contained factors	Frequent repeat doses may be necessary	Infectious diseases; allergic reactions	Less than 4 hours
Platelets: Pheresis	Bleeding from thrombocytopenia or platelet function abnormality	Improves hemostasis	Plasma coagulation deficits and some conditions with rapid platelet destruction (e.g., ITP)	Should not use some micro-aggregate filters (check manufacturer's instructions)	Infectious diseases; septic/toxic, allergic, febrile reactions	Less than 4 hours
Granulocytes	Neutropenia with infection	Provides granulocytes	Infection responsive to antibiotics	Must be ABO-compatible; do not use depth-type micro-aggregate filters	Infectious diseases; allergic, febrile reactions	One Pheresis unit over 2-4 hr period; closely observe for reactions

From American Red Cross, Council of Community Blood Centers, and American Association of Blood Banks: Circular of Information for the Use of Human Blood and Blood Components, Washington, DC, American Red Cross, Publication #1751, Feb. 15, 1991, pp. 14–15. Used by permission.

a. Albumin–patients with hypovolemia and hypoalbuminemia. Its intravascular half-life is short. Only proven benefit is earlier return of bowel motility in post-operative patients with hypoalbuminemia.
b. Purified protein fraction (Plasmanate®)–83% albumin, 17% globulin.
c. Hetastarch (Hespan®)–artificial colloid of 6% hetastarch in saline. Effectiveness decreases over 24 h. Will exacerbate bleeding disorders and congestive heart failure.

B. Red blood cells—given when inadequate oxygen-carrying capacity exists.

1. If intravascular volume is adequate (see section A), a hemoglobin of 8 will provide adequate oxygen-carrying capacity for most patients. In elderly patients and those with cardiovascular disease, a hemoglobin of 10 may be more desirable. Do not use RBCs when anemia can be corrected with specific medications (iron, B12, folate, erythropoeitin).
2. In the trauma setting, priorities are immobilization and direct pressure to control hemorrhage, volume repletion with crystalloid, then restoration of oxygen-carrying capacity with RBCs.
   a. If hemostasis and volume replacement with 2 L of crystalloid stabilize the patient, transfusion can await specific indications.
   b. If 2 L of crystalloid fail to produce hemodynamic stability, this suggests greater than 30% blood volume loss, and transfusion should begin immediately with O-negative universal donor blood; if the patient is sufficiently stable, use type-specific (ABO, Rh compatible) blood.
   c. Each unit of PRBCs has a volume of approximately 300 cc, a hematocrit of 35-80, and should raise the patient's hematocrit by 3 points.
3. ***Complications.***
   a. Hemolytic transfusion reaction–1:50-100 occurs when donor RBCs and recipient plasma are incompatible. Characterized by chills, fever, back pain, chest pain, dyspnea, abnormal bleeding, headache, and shock. In anesthetized patients hypotension and bleeding may be the only signs. Hemoglobinemia, hemoglobinuria, hyperbilirubinemia, and renal failure may all ensue. The transfusion should be stopped with institution of volume expansion and diuresis. A delayed form may also occur 4-14 days after transfusion. Continued anemia despite transfusions, fever, hemoglobinuria, and hyperbilirubinemia suggest delayed hemolytic transfusion reaction.
   b. Infectious complications.
      (1) Viral hepatitis–1:3300 for hepatitis C and 1:200,000 for hepatitis B.
      (2) HIV–1:40,000 to 1:300,000.

(3) CMV, EBV, HTLV-I, HTLV-II viruses–1:50,000-1,000,000.
(4) Others–*Babesia, Bartonella, Borrelia, Brucella,* Colorado tick fever, plasmodia, and some trypanosomes.

c. Bacterial contamination–gram-negative bacilli can lead to endotoxic shock.
d. Alloimmunization to red cell, white cell, platelet, or protein antigens can occur. It does not cause immediate problems but sensitizes the recipient to future transfusions.
e. Graft versus host disease (GVHD)–may occur in immunocompromised recipients as a result of infused lymphocytes. Irradiation of the blood product reduces this risk.
f. Febrile reactions–occur in 1-2% of recipients and are usually caused by antibodies that agglutinate with leukocytes.
g. Allergic reactions with urticaria, wheezing, and angioedema occur in about 1% of patients. Premedication with antihistamines pre-transfusion will lessen this complication.
h. Anaphylactoid reaction with bronchospasm, dyspnea, and pulmonary edema can occur. Treatment–epinephrine and steroids.
i. Circulatory overload–can occur in patients with congestive heart failure. Each unit of PRBCs contains 20 mEq of sodium. Blood should be given over 3-4 h in this situation, and IV furosemide should be given between units.
j. Hemosiderosis–occurs with prolonged transfusion requirements. Desferrioxamine may be helpful.
k. Depletion of coagulation proteins and platelets–can occur if more than 1 blood volume is transfused in less than 24 h. Therapy is with specific components as directed by clinical and laboratory evaluation, but in general repletion with FFP and cryoprecipitate should be considered once 4-6 units of PRBCs are given.
l. **Metabolic complications**–can occur when large volumes of banked blood products are transfused.

(1) Hypothermia–most common, may lead to cardiac arrhythmias. Warming the blood to 37°C will decrease this risk.
(2) Citrate toxicity due to complexing of ionized calcium can occur in liver failure patients who are unable to metabolize citrate to pyruvate and HCO_3. Treatment–IV calcium.
(3) Acidosis–can occur with liver failure patients because of citric acid buildup.
(4) Alkalosis–more common as the citrate is metabolized to pyruvate and HCO_3 in patients with normal liver function.
(5) Potassium abnormalities–either hypokalemia secondary to the alkalosis of citrate metabolism or hyperkalemia due to PRBC lysis from transfusion of old units of blood.

C. Autologous blood—intra-operative salvage and pre-operative donation should be considered when feasible to reduce the risk of disease transmission and immune reactions.

1. Reinfusion of blood from body cavities not contaminated by bacteria or malignant cells. Must be used within 4 h and is devoid of clotting factors.
2. Intra-operative hemodilution–when 1-3 units of blood are removed at the beginning of a procedure with immediate volume replacement. The whole blood is then infused post-operatively. Platelets and coagulation factors remain intact.
3. Pre-operative donation 4-6 weeks prior to a planned procedure–this blood may or may not be screened for infectious agents. If positive testing occurs (hepatitis, HIV, etc.), the units may still be suitable for use.

D. Coagulation factors (Figure 1)–blood vessels, platelets, and soluble protein coagulation factors are all critically important in hemostasis. Failure of any of these three can lead to life-threatening hemorrhage.

1. The most common cause of post-operative bleeding is poor surgical hemostasis, followed by thrombocytopenia, thrombocytopathia, acquired coagulation defects, and congenital coagulation defects.
2. A medical history is the single best screening test available for detecting bleeding problems.
   a. Family history of coagulopathy (hemophilia A or B, von Willebrand's disease).
   b. Abnormal bleeding during minor trauma, teeth extractions, or menses.
   c. Medications–aspirin, warfarin, bile salt binders, dipyridamole, NSAIDs, cephalosporins.
   d. Concurrent illnesses–liver disease, biliary obstruction, renal disorders, blood dyscrasias, or colon cancer with obstruction.
   e. Medical/surgical history of malabsorption, ileal resection, or prosthetic valves.
3. Laboratory tests.
   a. Platelet count.
   b. Bleeding time–evaluates platelet function and blood vessel integrity.
   c. Prothrombin time (PT)–evaluates production of the vitamin K-dependent clotting factors and therefore is used to monitor Coumadin® therapy and the extrinsic pathway.
   d. Activated partial thromboplastin time (PTT)–evalutes the intrinsic pathway and heparin therapy.
   e. Thrombin time–measures polymerization of fibrinogen. Prolonged with heparin, disseminated intravascular coagulation, dysfibrinogenemia, and primary fibrinolysis.
   f. Fibrinogen level–decreased in disseminated intravascular coagulation (DIC) and primary fibrinolysis.

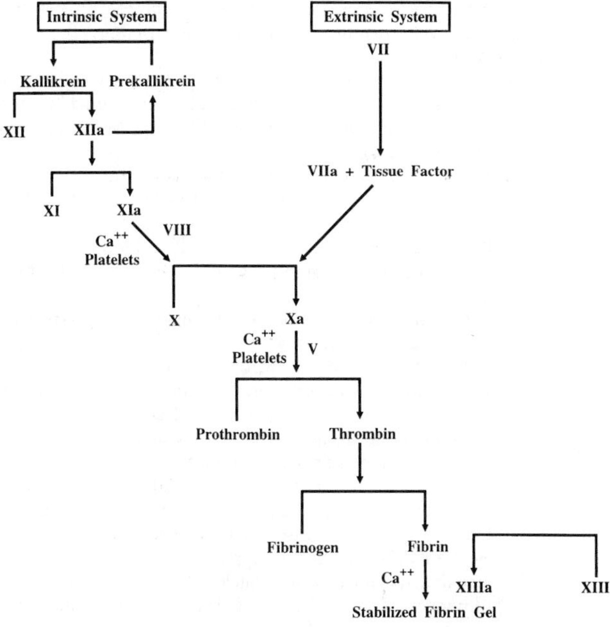

FIG. 1 Coagulation Cascade

g. Fibrin split products–measure fibrinolysis and are increased in DIC and primary fibrinolysis.

4. Congenital coagulopathy states–absence of each of the factors has been reported, only some of which are of clinical significance.
   a. Hemophilia A (classic hemophilia)–prolonged PTT x linked recessive deficiency of factor VIII. The most common congenital bleeding disorder. Surgery and trauma require 75-100% factor VIII activity for 7-10 days. The calculation is:

   $$\frac{\text{Desired VIII \% activity x plasma volume}}{80}$$

   This will determine the number of bags of cryoprecipitate required to achieve desired activity. This amount should be given every 8 h to maintain hemostasis.
   b. Hemophilia B ("Christmas disease")–prolonged PTT x linked recessive deficiency of Factor IX. Treated like hemophilia A.
   c. Von Willebrand's disease–prolonged PTT, prolonged bleed-

ing time. Autosomal dominant deficiency of factor VIII:vWF. Treat like hemophilia A or with dDAVP.

5. Acquired coagulopathy states.
   a. Vitamin K deficiency–due to inadequate intake, malabsorption, biliary obstruction, TPN, antibiotics, coumadin therapy. Treat with vitamin K 10 mg SQ/IV q AM x 3. FFP will correct the coagulopathy rapidly.
   b. Hypothermia–especially in the trauma patient.
   c. Liver failure–due to decreased clotting factors except VIII. Treat with FFP.
   d. Heparin acts with ATIII to prolong PTT. Protamine 1 mg/100 U heparin will rapidly reverse heparin effects. Half-life is 4 hours.
   e. Renal failure–leads to uremic bleeding secondary to platelet dysfunction. Treatment is dialysis and dDAVP.
   f. DIC–secondary to release of thromboplastic substances with simultaneous clotting and bleeding. Caused by trauma, sepsis, malignancy, burns, obstetrical accidents (amniotic fluid embolus, abruptio placentae, retained fetus), envenomation, anaphylaxis. Large amounts of FDP (fibrin degradation products) worsen the coagulopathy by inhibiting fibrin polymerization. Characterized by diffuse bleeding, prolonged PT, PTT, decreased platelets, decreased fibrinogen, elevated FDP. Treatment supportive with transfusions directed by specific defecits: platelets, FFP, cryoprecipitate for fibrinogen, vitamin K, and treatment of the underlying disease.
   g. Primary fibrinolysis–occurs acutely with heat stroke, hypoxia, and hypotension, or chronically with neoplasms or cirrhosis. Consists of a hemorrhagic state characterized by a shortened euglobulin lysis time, decreased fibrinogen, and elevated FDP without thrombocytopenia. May treat with Amicar®.
6. Components.
   a. Fresh frozen plasma–contains 200 units of Factors VIII, V, and all other coagulation factors. No cross-match. For bleeding due to elevated PT/PTT.
   b. Cryoprecipitate–contains 80 units of Factor VIII, 150 mg of fibrinogen in 15 cc volume. Indicated for hemophilia A, low fibrinogen states, and von Willebrand's disease.

E. Platelets—active in normal hemostasis. Masses of platelets occlude breaks in small blood vessels and are a source of phospholipid, which is required for coagulation of blood. No cross-match is required for their use.

1. Indicated in patients actively bleeding due to thrombocytopenia or thrombocytopathia.
2. Indicated to raise platelet count to 100,000 in pre-operative patients.

3. Indicated to keep platelet counts above 20,000 in thrombocytopenic patients.
4. Do not use platelets in patients with thrombotic thrombocytopenia purpura (TTP) or idiopathic thrombocytopenia purpura (ITP) unless life-threatening hemorrhage is occurring, as the infused platelets will be rapidly degraded.
5. One unit of platelets will raise the platelet count by 10,000.
   a. Platelets usually are pooled in a package that contains 8-10 units.
   b. Each 8-10 pack contains the equivalent of stable clotting factors (all except V, VIII) in 2 units of FFP.
   c. Platelet infusion will need to be repeated q\1-3 days due to degradation.
   d. Rarely contaminated by bacteria, but are the most likely of blood components to be contaminated.
   e. In sensitized individuals, pheresis of platelets from a HLA-matched individual may replace pooled platelets.

F. Granulocytes—Used as supportive therapy in neutropenic patients (< 500 neutrophils/μL of blood) with a documented bacterial infection.

1. Usually prepared by pheresis of a single donor's blood.
2. Rarely increases the patient's granulocyte count.
3. If bone marrow recovery is not anticipated, granulocyte infusion is unlikely to alter the patient's course.
4. Granulocyte colony stimulating factor has supplanted most uses of granulocyte infusions.
   a. Recombinant DNA technology, infectious transmissions are non-existent.
   b. Stimulates the patient's own marrow to produce native granulocytes, so sensitization and graft *vs.* host disease are not seen.

6

Nutrition

Scott M. Berry, M.D.

Forty to 60% of hospitalized patients are malnourished to some degree. This may be due to (a) inadequate intake, (b) impaired absorption, (c) increased requirements.

I. NUTRITIONAL ASSESSMENT

A. Subjective global assessment.

1. A clinical impression performed on the basis of history (attention to recent reduction in oral intake, recent unintentional weight loss of > 7-10 lbs, underlying disease, and functional status).
2. The presence of low serum albumin (< 3.0 g/dl). No single laboratory test is more accurate than subjective global assessment of nutritional status on admission.
3. Physical examination–wasting of muscle mass (temporalis muscle) and fat, presence of edema or ascites, glossitis, skin lesions (vitamin deficiencies).
4. Weight change or unintentional weight loss is important.
   a. Weight loss of ≥ 10% of ideal body weight (IBW) suggests mild to moderate malnutrition.
   b. Weight loss of ≥ 20% suggests severe malnutrition.
   c. Weight loss of ≥ 30% is premorbid.

B. Biochemical indicators of malnutrition.

1. Visceral proteins.
   a. **Albumin** adequate indicator of malnutrition in absence of other causes of hypoalbuminemia (hepatic insufficiency, protein-losing nephropathy or enteropathy). Synthesis decreases with malnutrition.
      (1) Long half-life (21 days) and extravascular space distribution make it unreliable as a short-term index of nutrition.
      (2) Albumin > 3.5 g/dl suggests adequate nutritional status; < 3.0 g/dl suggests malnutrition.
2. Rapid-turnover proteins–shorter half-life; early indicator of

nutritional depletion; falling levels suggest ongoing malnutrition.

a. **Transferrin:** half-life of 8 days; a sensitive indicator of malnutrition, although anemia may stimulate transferrin synthesis. Level < 220 mg/dl suggests malnutrition.
b. **Thyroxin-binding prealbumin (TBPA)**: half-life of 2 days.
c. **Retinol-binding protein (RBP)**: half-life of 12 h.

3. ***Nitrogen balance.***
   a. Calculate from intake and excretion of nitrogen.
      (1) Total nitrogen loss (g/day) = 24-h urinary urea nitrogen (UUN) (g/day) + 4 g/day fecal and non-urinary nitrogen loss.
   b. Requires accurate 24-h urine collection and accurate assessment of grams of nitrogen given daily, in conjunction with the appropriate amount of carbohydrate for proper nitrogen utilization (calories:nitrogen).

C. Immunologic function—malnutrition is associated with decreased cellular and humoral immunity.

1. Delayed cutaneous hypersensitivity–reflects cellular immunity. Anergy to antigens suggests malnutrition. Anergy may also occur with cancer, severe infection, renal or hepatic failure, post chemo- or radiation therapy.
2. Total lymphocyte count–calculated as WBC x % lymphocytes. Count < 1500 cells/mm^3 suggests severe malnutrition (must rule out other causes such as hematologic disorder or AIDS).
3. Complement levels, measurements of neutrophil function, and opsonic index may be useful measurements of response to infection, but are not widely available for clinical use.

II. NUTRITIONAL REQUIREMENTS IN STRESS

A. Basic needs.

1. In basal state, 25-30 kcal/kg/day, 30% as fat.
2. Protein needs are 0.8-1 g protein/kg/day.
3. In stressed, burned, or multiple-trauma patient, needs may increase up to 50 kcal/kg/day and 2.0 g protein/kg/day.

B. Determination of caloric needs on individual basis.

1. 35 kcal/kg/d rough estimate.
2. Calculate basal energy expenditure (BEE) using the *Harris-Benedict equation*:

$$\text{BEE (Men)} = 66.47 + 13.75\ W + 5.0\ H - 6.76\ A$$

$$\text{BEE (Women)} = 655.1 + 9.56\ W + 1.85\ H - 4.68\ A$$

$$\text{BEE (Infants)} = 22.10 + 31.05\ W + 1.16\ H$$

W = weight in kg; H = height in cm; A = age.

3. Calculate increase in energy needs imposed by *illness or injury* (i.e., BEE x activity factor x injury factor) using *Calvin-Long injury factor*:

Minor operation: 1.2 (20%)
Skeletal trauma: 1.35 (35%)
Major sepsis: 1.60 (60%)
Severe thermal injury: 2.10 (100-120%)

4. Calculate increase in energy needs imposed:
   Confined to bed: 1.2
   Out of bed: 1.3
5. Indirect calorimetry–measurements of the patient's oxygen consumption and carbon dioxide production.
   a. Determines resting energy expenditure by measuring respiratory gas exchange (i.e., O_2 consumption, CO_2 production).
   b. Gives index of fuel utilization – respiratory quotient (RQ) = VCO_2/VO_2.
      RQ:carbohydrate = 1.0; mixed substrate = 0.80; lipid = 0.70; lipogenesis $>$ 1.0 (also induced spuriously by hyperventilation); ketogenesis $<$ 0.70. RQ of 0.8-1.0 is desirable; $<$ 0.70 suggests "underfeeding" and $>$ 1.0 "over-feeding".

III. INDICATIONS FOR NUTRITIONAL SUPPORT

A. Factors.

1. Age–in a previously healthy adult, adequately hydrated and mildly catabolic.
   a. Up to age 60 will tolerate up to 10 days of starvation.
   b. 60-70 years will tolerate up to 7 days of starvation.
   c. $>$ 70 years will tolerate 5 days of starvation.
2. Previous state of health–including prior nutritional status. Patients with chronic medical problems (i.e., diabetes mellitus; COPD; renal, cardiac, or hepatic insufficiency) are probably at more nutritional risk than those patients described in section A.1 above.
3. Current condition–metabolic demands per Section II.

B. Pre-operative nutritional supplementation—requires consideration of the above and anticipated duration of dietary deprivation. If evidence of moderate to severe malnutrition exists, 7-10 days of pre-operative nutritional support may be beneficial.

C. Post-operative nutritional supplementation—in the malnourished patient, post-operative nutrition is necessary until adequate oral intake is resumed. For the healthy patient, follow guidelines (see "Factors" above).

1. If the GI tract is functional, enteral nutrition is preferable. Placement of a nasoenteric feeding tube for short-term feeding is recommended.
2. If prolonged support is anticipated, a feeding gastrostomy or jejunostomy should be considered (see below).

IV. ENTERAL NUTRITION

A. Indications.

1. Prolonged period without caloric intake.
2. Functional GI tract.

3. Inadequate oral intake.
4. Avoid gut mucosal atrophy.
5. In major burns and trauma may decrease hypermetabolism.

B. Short-term supplementation—for nasogastric or nasointestinal feeds, use small-bore (7-9 Fr) soft tubes to improve patient comfort.

1. ***Nasogastric (NG).***
   a. Adequate gastric emptying required.
   b. Alert patient with intact gag reflex is necessary.
   c. Maintain gastric residuals ≤ 50% of total infusion over last 4 h.
2. ***Nasointestinal—***patients with higher risk of aspiration (i.e., neurologic impairment, poor gastric motility).

C. Long-term supplementation (> 6 weeks).

1. ***Gastrostomy—***placed operatively or percutaneously.
   a. Adequate gastric emptying required.
   b. Evidence of reflux or impaired gag reflex is contraindication.
   c. Intermittent bolus feeds, or continuous infusion.
2. ***Jejunostomy—***placed operatively.
   a. Anticipate long-term enteral supplementation in patient for whom gastrostomy is contraindicated.
   b. Requires continuous infusion.

D. Products.

1. ***Oral supplements.***
   a. Indications–supplementation for inadequate caloric intake.
   b. Must be palatable (flavoring increases osmolarity and cost).
   c. Examples–Ensure®, Ensure Plus®, Sustacal®, Carnation Instant Breakfast®.
2. ***Tube feedings.***
   a. Blenderized food.
   b. Blenderized (pureed) diet–Complete B®.
      (1) Primarily used with gastrostomies.
   c. Polymeric–Isocal®, Osmolite®, Jevity®, Ultracal®.
      (1) Complete diet, with intact protein; generally lactose-free.
      (2) Iso-osmolar, fairly well tolerated.
      (3) 1 kcal/cc.
   d. High-caloric density–Magnacal®.
      (1) Complete diet, with intact protein; generally lactose-free.
      (2) Hyperosmolar–May provoke diarrhea.
      (3) Used for patients with increased caloric needs and decreased volume tolerance.
      (4) 2 kcal/cc.
   e. Monomeric–Vivonex TEN®, Criticare HN®.
      (1) Amino acids with or without peptides as protein source.
      (2) Requires no digestion.

(3) Essentially complete small-bowel absorption (low residue).
(4) Hyperosmolar.

f. Disease-specific formulas–most are of unproven benefit.
   (1) Renal failure–Amin-Aid®, Nepro®, Suplena®.
      a) Elemental diet, essential L-amino acids, reduced nitrogen.
      b) Hyperosmolar, 2 kcal/cc.
      c) Best when administered by tube (not very palatable).
   (2) Acute or chronic hepatic failure–HepaticAid II®.
      a) Enriched with branched chain amino acids.
      b) Low in aromatic and sulfur-containing amino acids.
      c) May be used as tube feeding or to supplement a protein-restricted oral diet.
   (3) Immunomodulatory–Impact®, Alitraq®.
      a) Enriched with immunostimulatory amino acids, lipids, and nucleic acids.
      b) May benefit critically ill patients by reducing infectious complications.

E. Administration.

1. Generally, all types of tube feedings should be iso-osmolar (i.e., 300 mosm) for initial administration. Hypertonic feeds require dilution.
2. Gastric feeding–due to the greater diluting capacity of the stomach and the protective mechanism of the pylorus, concentration is advanced first, then rate is advanced. Bolus feeds may be used.
3. Intestinal feedings–increase *rate first*, then concentration. Continuous infusion.
4. Elevate the head of the bed 30 degrees and check gastric residuals every 4 h ($<$ 50% of total administered over the past 4 h is a high residual).
5. Metoclopramide (Reglan®) 10 mg IV or PO q 6 h may aid gastric emptying.
6. Most feeds can be started at 40 cc/h and advanced by 20 cc/h increments at 12-h intervals as tolerated.
7. If the infusion is stopped for any prolonged period, the tube must be flushed with water in order to prevent clogging.
8. If there is any doubt, the position of the tube should be confirmed radiographically.

F. Major complications of enteral feeding.

1. Aspiration pneumonia–may be minimized by jejunal feeding and by precautions indicated under "Administration" above.
2. Feeding intolerance–evidenced by vomiting, abdominal distention, cramping, diarrhea. Treat by decreasing infusion rate or diluting feedings.
3. Diarrhea–defined as $>$ 5 stools per day.
   a. Minimized by a continuous, appropriate administration schedule, assuming intact GI function and no pancreatic insufficiency; rule out antibiotic-associated colitis.

b. May be a symptom of too rapid advancement of hyperosmolar tube feedings.
c. Minimized by clean technique in formula preparation and administration (avoid bacterial overgrowth in formulation). Time limits on formula life and duration of administration should be observed.
d. Treatment–depending upon severity, either decrease administration rate or add an antidiarrheal agent when infectious cause is ruled out.
   (1) Kaolin Pectin safe to use even in patients with infectious diarrhea.
   (2) Diphenoxylate (Lomotil®) elixir–2.5-5 mg\GT q 6 h prn.
   (3) Loperamide (Imodium®) elixir–2-4 mg\q 6 h prn.
   (4) Psyllium seed (Metamucil®)–1 package in 6 oz water bid (bulking agent).

4. Metabolic–in general, the metabolic complications are the same as for parenteral nutrition. Hyperglycemia should be treated with frequent, short-acting insulin, or a peripheral drip. If new onset, should rule out sepsis.
5. Hyperosmotic non-ketotic coma–caused by too many calories without enough free water to excrete the obligatory renal osmotic load.

V. PARENTERAL NUTRITION

A. Indications.

1. Prolonged period without caloric intake.
2. Enteral feeding contraindicated or not tolerated.
3. Presence of malnutrition.

B. Role in primary therapy.

1. Efficacy demonstrated in the following situations:
   a. Gastrointestinal fistulas–allows for total bowel "rest" while providing adequate nutrition. Rate of spontaneous closure is increased, but doesn't affect overall mortality.
   b. Short bowel syndrome–to maintain nutritional status until remaining bowel can undergo hypertrophy. May be required for long-term survival.
   c. Acute tubular necrosis–mortality rate is decreased, with earlier recovery from renal failure. Hypercatabolism of renal failure is met by TPN.
   d. Acute-on-chronic hepatic insufficiency–normalization of amino acid profiles results in improved recovery from hepatic encephalopathy and possibly in decreased mortality.
2. Efficacy not completely established:
   a. Inflammatory bowel disease–Crohn's disease limited to small bowel responds best. Course of ulcerative colitis not affected, but allows for bowel rest and improved postoperative course when given prior to ileoanal pull-through operations.
   b. Anorexia nervosa.

TABLE 1
TPN Solutions: Composition

Solution	Amino Acid	Glucose	Calories
Standard	4.25%-42.5 g/L	D15-150 g/L	510 Kcal/L
	5.00%-50.0 g/L	D25-250 g/L	850 Kcal/L
Renal	1.70%-17.0 g/L	D47-470 g/L	1598 Kcal/L
Hepatic	3.50%-35.0 g/L	D35-350 g/L	1190 Kcal/L
Peripheral	3.00%-30.0 g/L	D10-100 g/L	340 Kcal/L

C. Supportive therapy.

1. Efficacy established:
   a. Radiation enteritis.
   b. Acute GI toxicity due to chemotherapeutic agents.
   c. Hyperemesis gravidarum.
2. Efficacy not yet established:
   a. Pre-operative nutritional support for malnourished patients. Studies have shown improvement in metabolic endpoints, but no statistically significant improvement in mortality or complication rate.
   b. Cardiac cachexia.
   c. Pancreatitis.
   d. Respiratory insufficiency with need for prolonged ventilatory support.
   e. Prolonged ileus (> 5 days).
   f. Nitrogen-losing wounds.

D. Indications currently under investigation:

1. Cancer–generally, nutritional support indicated in patients undergoing antineoplastic therapy (e.g., surgery, radiation, chemotherapy) during times of ileus, GI mucosal damage, etc; goal of nutritional support is for weight *maintenance*, not gain.
2. Sepsis–some evidence exists concerning use of 45% branched chain amino acid (BCAA) solution to improve hepatic protein synthesis as well as improve septic encephalopathy.

E. Basic composition of formulations (Tables 1 & 2).

1. Carbohydrate–dextrose used exclusively in U.S. Concentrations range from 15% to 47%.
2. Amino acids–either balanced or disease-specific (renal, hepatic, stress formulations).
3. Lipid emulsions.
   a. Available as 10% or 20% solutions (1 kcal/cc or 2 kcal/cc, respectively).
   b. Infusion of 100 ml of 10% solution per week is adequate to prevent essential fatty acid deficiency (EFAD).
   c. Important to check baseline measurements of serum triglycerides to avoid exacerbation of pre-existing hypertriglyceridemia.

TABLE 2
Additional Components to TPN Solution

Trace Elements (add to 1st bottle each day):			
Zn—3.0 mg			
Cu—1.2 mg		Stress formula	
Cr—12 μg	Se—60 mg	Hepatic formula	
Mn—0.3 mg			
Vitamins (add to 1st bottle each day):			
MVI—12 (1 amp. 10 cc)			
Vitamin K (add to 2nd bottle every Monday):			
5 mg (for patients not requiring anticoagulants)			
Electrolytes and Insulin:		Usual	Range
Na^+ (mEq/L)		20-80	0-150
K^+ (mEq/L)		13-40	0-80
Cl^- (mEq/L)		10-80	0-150
Ca^{++} (mEq/L)		4.7	0-10
Mg^{++} (mEq/L)		8	0-15
P (mM)		14	0-21
Acetate (mEq/L)		45-81	45-220
Human regular insulin (units/L)		0-25	0-60

d. Lipid emulsion substituted for carbohydrate calories in certain situations (decrease overall volume given, carbohydrate overfeeding, TPN hepatotoxicity).
e. Safe to provide 20-60% of total calories as lipid.

4. Minor components.
   a. Vitamins–including 5 mg Vitamin K weekly.
   b. Trace elements–Zn, Cu, Cr, Mn, Se.
   c. Insulin and electrolytes as ordered.
   For solutions with dextrose concentrations of 25% and above lipids can be given twice weekly; all others should get daily lipids.
   Electrolytes may be adjusted as appropriate. Some patients with ongoing electrolyte losses may require up to 140 mEq/L NaCl and 80 mEq/L K^+.

F. Central formulas—administered into vena cava.

1. ***Standard central formula***—Most patients requiring parenteral nutrition can use a formula containing 15-25% dextrose.
2. ***Renal formulation.***
   a. Nephramine® (essential L-amino acids only).
   b. Indicated in patients with acute renal failure who are not being dialysed.
   c. Electrolyte composition offsets abnormalities in acute renal failure (ARF). Useful in preventing rise in potassium and BUN, and may delay dialysis.
   d. Higher [glucose] D47, limits volume.
   e. Once converted to chronic dialysis, parenteral nutrition should be changed to standard.

3. ***Hepatic formulation.***
   a. Indicated for patients with grade 2 (impending stupor) or greater (3–stupor, 4–coma, unresponsive to pain) hepatic encephalopathy.
   b. Hepatic formulation is enriched with 35% branched chain amino acids (BCAA), alanine, arginine, and reduced amounts of aromatic and sulfur-containing amino acids.

G. Peripheral parenteral nutrition.
1. Contains 3% amino acids in 10% dextrose.
2. To provide adequate calorie:nitrogen ratio, the equivalent of 500 ml of 10% lipid emulsion should be administered with each liter of peripheral formulation to a maximum of 100 g fat/day. Must follow lipid profile to avoid hyperlipidemia.
3. Indicated in patients in whom central venous catheterization is contraindicated (*Candida* sepsis, blood dyscrasias, thrombosis).
4. Difficulties include increased cost and difficulties with long-term venous access due to phlebitis from administration of hypertonic solution.
5. Peripheral parenteral nutrition may be indicated for 3-5 days of nutritional support in patients who may not be able to take an adequate oral intake, and are felt to be at increased risk for complications of malnutrition.
6. Only major advantage is elimination of risks associated with central venous catheterization.

H. Administration.
1. The institution of central formulation should always be via a new central line.
2. The tip of the catheter should reside within the innominate vein, or preferably the SVC, due to increased blood flow and mixing (*not* right atrium or subclavian vein to avoid perforation or thrombosis, respectively); this should be documented in the patient's chart.
3. Long-term catheters (Hickman(TM), Portacath(TM)) may be placed in SVC to avoid catheter clotting.
4. Insertion of this catheter is *never* an emergency; patient should be stable, well hydrated, and without serious coagulopathy.

I. Subclavian catheter insertion—(see "Vascular Access").

J. Infusion.
1. Rate.
   a. All formulations begin at 40-50 ml/h with exception of renal formulation, which generally begins at 30 ml/h due to higher glucose content, and peripheral formulation, which begins at target rate.
   b. Rate increased in increments of 20-25 ml/h per 8-24 h (if blood sugar well controlled) until caloric needs are matched.
   c. With renal formula advance in increments of 10 ml/h each day.

2. With exception of lipid emulsion, single-lumen catheters should not be used for any other infusion of maintenance fluid, medication, blood products, or CVP readings.

K. Monitoring.

1. Vital signs q 6 h for initial 24-48 h.
2. Urine S & A's q 6-8 h for initial 24-48 h, then every 8-24 h. Finger-stick glucose determinations are more accurate if the patient is glucose intolerant.
3. Intake and Outputs (I's & O's) recorded q 8 h.
4. Weigh patient every other day.
5. Twice-weekly blood work–electrolytes, glucose, liver enzymes, calcium, phosphorus, PT, PTT, CBC, short-turnover proteins, if available.

L. Complications.

1. ***Technical*** (placement).
   a. Pneumothorax–should occur < 3% of all insertions in elective, well-prepared patients.
   b. See Vascular Access chapter.
2. ***Late technical***— thrombosis of subclavian vein or SVC.
   a. Clinically silent in up to 35% of patients.
   b. If clinically apparent, treat as follows:
      (1) Local heat.
      (2) Remove catheter.
      (3) Heparinization until symptoms resolve.
      (4) Long-term anticoagulation is usually unneccessary, but should be considered for continued symptoms.
   c. Prophylactic heparin is of little benefit in prevention of thrombosis.
3. ***Septic complications*** (Figure 1).
   a. Catheter sepsis–clinical sepsis in a patient receiving parenteral nutrition for which no anatomic septic focus is identified, and which resolves following removal of the catheter.
   b. Major source of catheter sepsis is bacteria from the skin around the insertion site of the catheter and, thus, catheter sepsis is best prevented by *meticulous* adherence to dressing change and catheter access protocols.
4. ***Metabolic complications.***
   a. Disorders of glucose metabolism.
      (1) Hyperglycemia (blood sugar > 200 mg/dl).
         a) From either parenteral or tube feeding, may lead to hyperosmolar, hyperglycemic, non-ketotic dehydration with shock/death resulting if untreated.
         b) If blood sugar is > 200 mg/dl, the rate of infusion of the formulation should not be increased; SQ regular insulin should be administered acutely, and the amount of insulin in each liter of solution should be increased appropriately. Causes of sepsis should be ruled out.

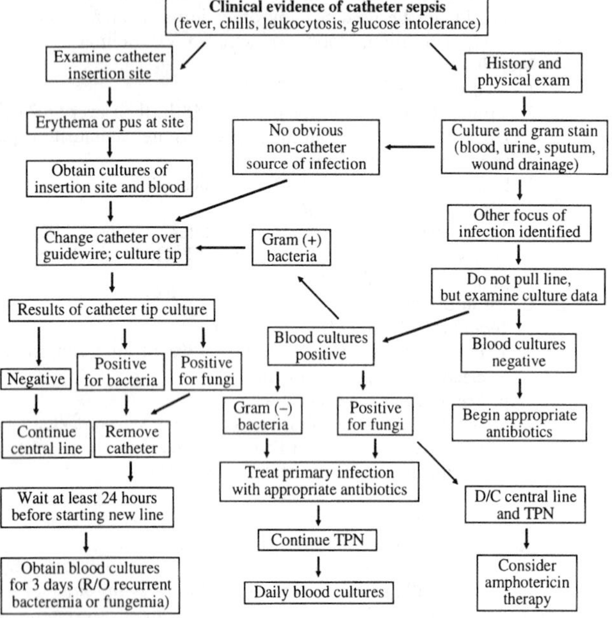

FIG. 1 Algorithm for Management of Suspected TPN Catheter Sepsis

c) If urine glucose 3+ or greater, obtain STAT blood glucose.

(2) Hypoglycemia–rare complication.

a) If TPN suddenly discontinued for any reason, IV administration of any 5% dextrose solution is sufficient to prevent hypoglycemia.

b) Rarely occurs with endogenous insulin response to very high rates of infusion. Treat by slowing infusion.

b. Liver dysfunction.

(1) Excess carbohydrate stored in liver as fat.

(2) Reversible, self-limited in adults.

c. Deficiency states.

(1) Requirements for electrolytes, vitamins, and trace elements vary according to age, previous nutritional state, disease, and external losses.

(2) As patients become anabolic, there is an increased re-

quirement for intracellular ions (potassium, magnesium phosphate).

(3) Deficiencies of trace elements and vitamins are generally avoided by the administration (daily) of recommended amounts.

7

Pre-Operative Preparation

Susan E. MacLennan, M.D.

Preparation of a patient for surgery begins with establishing a diagnosis and determining the course of surgical management. This requires thoughtful consideration of both the risks and benefits of a contemplated operation. Much of pre-operative care involves optimizing the patient's physiologic status and taking steps to prevent peri- and post-operative complications.

I. NEED FOR OPERATION

A. Determine relative risks and benefits of surgery.

Requires consideration of the following:

1. Natural history of disease if left untreated.
2. Benefit of surgical therapy *vs.* medical therapy.
3. Urgency of operation–may limit the time available for pre-operative preparation.
4. Patient's physiologic reserve and overall ability to undergo anesthesia and operation.
5. Potential complications of the procedure.

II. ASSESSING OPERATIVE RISK

The patient's age, pre-operative physiologic status, and the urgency and magnitude of the planned operation are major determinants of operative morbidity and mortality.

A. Age.

1. Elderly patients often have either limited reserve or impaired function of the major organ systems: cardiovascular, pulmonary, renal, hepatic, and immunologic.
2. True even for "healthy" septuagenarian–"There is nothing like an operation or an injury to bring a patient up to chronological age" (W.R. Howe).

B. Urgency of operation—in one study, emergent nature of surgery doubled risk of operative mortality in low- and moderate-risk patients.

C. Organ system dysfunction—impairment of more than one organ system, disease severity, and adequacy of control profoundly influences risk of operative mortality. American Society of Anesthesiologists classification of physical status (Dripps-ASA Scale):

1. ASA I–healthy individual with no systemic disease, undergoing elective surgery; patient not at extremes of age.
2. ASA II–individual with one-system, well-controlled disease. Disease does not affect daily activities. Other anesthetic risk factors, including mild obesity, alcoholism, and smoking, are incorporated at this level.
3. ASA III–individual with multiple system disease or well-controlled major system disease. Disease status limits daily activity.
4. ASA IV–individual with severe, incapacitating disease. Normally, disease state is poorly controlled or end-stage. Danger of death due to organ failure is always present.
5. ASA V–patient in imminent danger of death. Operation is last-resort attempt at preserving life. Patient with little chance for survival. Always an emergency procedure.
6. Each class above may be subclassified with an "E", denoting an emergency procedure.

Relation of Physical Status to Anesthetic Mortality

Physical status	Patients	Deaths	Ratio
I	16,192	0	0/16,000
II	12,154	7	1/1740
III	4,070	11	1/370
IV	720	17	1/40
V	87	4	1/20

Adapted from Dripps RD, Lamont A, and Eckenhoff JE: *JAMA* 178(3):216, 1961, American Medical Association, with permission.

D. The following conditions identify those patients at risk for increased peri-operative and post-operative morbidity and mortality:

1. Cardiovascular (see Goldman criteria below)–coronary artery disease, congestive heart failure, presence of arrhythmias, peripheral vascular disease, or severe hypertension.
2. Respiratory (see "Respiratory Care")–smoking history > 20 pack-years, morbid obesity, pre-existing pulmonary disease (pO_2 < 60 mmHg, pCO_2 > 50 mmHG; FEV_1/FVC < 70%), thoracic or upper abdominal surgery, or pulmonary hypertension.
3. Renal–renal insufficiency (BUN > 50 mg/dl; creatinine > 3.0 mg/d); highest risk in acute renal failure.

TABLE 1
Goldman Classification

Class (number)	Point Total	No or Minor Complication	Major Complication	Cardiac Death
I (1127)	0-5	1118 (99%)	7 (0.6%)	2 (0.2%)
II (769)	6-12	735 (96%)	25 (3%)	9 (1%)
III (204)	13-25	175 (86%)	23 (11%)	6 (3%)
IV (41)	≥26	20 (49%)	5 (12%)	16 (39%)

Adapted from Goldman L, et al: *N Engl J Med* 297:845, 1977. Reprinted by permission of *New England Journal of Medicine.*

TABLE 2
Computation of Cardiac Risk Index

History	Age > 70	5
	Myocardial infarction within 6 months	10
Physical	S_3 gallop or JVD	11
	Important valvular aortic stenosis	3
Electrocardiogram	Rhythm other than sinus or PACs on	7
	More than 5 PVCs per min at any time prior to	7
Poor general medical status	$PO_2 < 60$ or $PCO_2 > 50$	
	$K^+ < 3.0$ or $HCO_3^- < 20$ mEq/L	
	BUN > 50 or creatinine > 3 mg/dl	3
	Abnormal SGOT	
	Chronic liver disease	
	Bedridden due to non-cardiac cause	
Operation	Intraperitoneal, intrathoracic, aortic surgery	3
	Emergency surgery	4

4. Hepatic–cirrhosis, hepatitis (see "Cirrhosis").
5. Endocrine–diabetes mellitus, steroid therapy (adrenal insufficiency), hyper- or hypothyroidism.
6. Hematologic–anemia, leukopenia, thrombocytopenia, coagulopathy.

E. Goldman cardiac risk in non-cardiac surgery.

1. Computation of the cardiac risk index (Table 2).
2. Risks of cardiac complications in unselected patients over age 40 years who underwent major non-cardiac surgery.
3. General concepts.
   a. Class III and IV patients warrant routine pre-operative cardiology consultation.
   b. Class IV–life-saving procedures only.
   c. 28 of the 53 points are potentially correctable pre-operatively.

d. Index correctly classified 81% of the cardiac outcomes.
e. Criticisms–cardiac risks only and based on mixed patient population (e.g., vascular patients have higher morbidity and mortality).

III. INTERVENTION TO REDUCE OPERATIVE RISK

A. Emergent operations—procedure should not be delayed for most situations. Exception: Volume-depleted patients (e.g., those with intestinal obstruction, peritonitis, perforated viscus, etc.) should undergo fluid and electrolyte repletion prior to operation.

B. Cardiovascular.

1. Coronary artery disease (CAD)–A history of angina or previous myocardial infarction increases the risk for new myocardial infarction or sudden death. Risk of myocardial infarction following a recent infarction:

	Steen (1978)	Rao (1983)
0-3 months	27%	5.8%
4-6 months	11%	2.3%
>6 months	5%	1%

   a. Suspected CAD should be evaluated by EKG, exercise thallium scan or dipyridamole thallium scan, and MUGA or echocardiogram. Coronary angiography may be indicated.
   b. Coronary artery bypass grafting has been shown to decrease risk of post-operative myocardial infarction.
   c. Patients with severe disease should undergo major operations with peri-operative pulmonary artery monitoring to assess cardiac output and filling pressures (see "Cardiopulmonary Monitoring").
2. Congestive heart failure (CHF)–risk factors for post-operative CHF are CAD, elderly patients, and major operations.
   a. Pre-existing CHF should be optimally controlled (e.g., diuretics, digoxin).
   b. Pre-operative pulmonary artery monitoring recommended to guide manipulation of hemodynamic performance (i.e., fluids, inotropes, vasodilators) and guide peri-operative fluid management.
3. Arrhythmias–optimal medical control required prior to operation (see "Cardiopulmonary Monitoring"). High-grade block and bradyarrhythmias may require pre-operative temporary or permanent pacing.
4. Hypertension (HTN)–no increased risk for non-labile mild HTN and diastolic blood pressure (DBP) < 110 mm Hg.
   a. Anti-hypertensive agent should be continued to time of surgery, except monoamine oxidase inhibitors (should discontinue 2 weeks before surgery).
   b. New onset HTN, severe HTN with DBP > 110 mm Hg, SBP > 250 mm Hg, or suspicion of unusual causes of HTN should lead to further work-up and treatment.

c. Should check for evidence of end-organ deterioration (e.g., renal insufficiency, CHF).

C. **Respiratory.**
1. Have patient discontinue smoking as long before surgery as possible. May take up to 8 weeks to decrease risk of pulmonary complications.
2. Arterial blood gas and pulmonary function tests are needed for suspected or documented pulmonary disease or for patients undergoing thoracic surgery.
3. Initiate or continue use of bronchodilators (e.g., inhalants, theophylline) for patients with bronchospastic disease (COPD or asthma).
4. Utilize chest physiotherapy as indicated; initiate incentive spirometry and cough, deep-breathing exercises pre-operatively.
5. Pneumonia, bronchitis–delay elective surgery; treat with pulmonary toilet and antibiotics.
6. Pulmonary artery monitoring–consider use peri-operatively for fluid management.

D. **Renal.**
1. Reduce azotemia–peritoneal or hemodialysis.
2. Correct electrolyte abnormalities.
3. Optimize volume status–ultrafiltration, diuretics; consider use of pulmonary artery monitoring.

E. **Hepatic** (see "Cirrhosis").

F. **Endocrine** (see "Management of the Diabetic Patient" and section VII below).

G. **Hematologic** (see "Blood Component Therapy").

H. **Nutrition** (see "Nutrition").

IV. GENERAL PRE-OPERATIVE PREPARATION

A. **Overall assessment of patient, history, physical examination, and operative risk** (see section II above).

B. **Documentation of indications for procedure, informed consent** (see "Medical Record" and "Medico-Legal Aspects").

C. **Routine pre-operative laboratory evaluation—**although several studies have documented that certain pre-operative labs are not cost-effective, these are the standard pre-operative studies performed at our institution.
1. Labs–CBC, urinalysis, electrolytes, BUN, creatinine, PT, PTT.
2. Room-air arterial blood gas (ABG) if predisposed to respiratory insufficiency ($>$ 20 pack-year smoker, can't blow out match, short of breath on 1-2 flights of steps, etc.), or if anticipate prolonged post-operative ventilatory support.
3. Radiographs–PA and lateral chest radiographs unless previously normal within the past six months or $<$ 35 years old; radiographs of specific areas of interest in relation to the upcoming procedure.
4. EKG if patient $>$ 35 years old or if otherwise indicated by past cardiac history.

D. Blood Orders—type and screen or type and cross for number of units appropriate to procedure.

E. Skin Preparation.

1. Hair removal is best performed the day of surgery with an electric clipper. Shaving the night prior to surgery is associated with an increased risk of infection
2. Pre-operative (the night before) scrub or shower of the operative site with a germicidal soap (Hibiclens®, pHisoHex®, etc.).

F. Pre-operative Antibiotics.

1. When used, should have an established blood level at the time of initial skin incision. Administer prophylactic antibiotics 30 minutes prior to incision.
2. Indications for prophylactic antibiotics.
   a. Clean/contaminated procedures–GI/GU tract, gynecologic, respiratory tract.
   b. Contaminated procedures (i.e., trauma).
   c. Insertion of synthetic material (e.g., vascular grafts, artificial valves, prosthetic joints).
   d. High-risk patients.
   e. Patient with prosthetic heart valves or history of valvular heart disease (see VI: Bacterial Endocarditis Prophylaxis).

G. Respiratory Care.

1. Pre-operative incentive spirometry on the evening prior to surgery when indicated (upper abdominal operations, thoracic operations, predisposed to respiratory insufficiency).
2. Bronchodilators for moderate to severe COPD.

H. Decompression of GI tract—NPO after midnight.

I. Intravenous fluids—maintenance rate overnight.

J. Access and Monitoring Lines.

1. At least one 18-ga. IV needed for initiation of anesthesia.
2. Arterial catheters and central or pulmonary artery catheters when indicated (see "Cardiopulmonary Monitoring").

K. Thromboembolic prophylaxis—when indicated (see "Thromboembolic Prophylaxis and Management of DVT").

L. Void—on call to the operating room.

M. Pre-operative sedation—as ordered by anesthesiologist (see "Anesthesia").

N. Special Considerations.

1. Maintenance medications (i.e., antihypertensives, cardiac medications, anticonvulsants, etc.) may be given the morning of surgery with a sip of water before routine operations.
2. Pre-operative diabetic management (see "Management of the Diabetic Patient").
3. SBE prophylaxis (see VI below).
4. Peri-operative steroid coverage (see VII below).

O. Stomas—marking of site by stomal therapist in elective situations.

P. Pre-operative note (see "Medical Records").

V. BOWEL PREP

The purpose of a bowel preparation is to remove all solid and most liquid from the bowel and to reduce the bacterial population in anticipation of procedures or complications of procedures that may contaminate the wound and the peritoneal cavity.

A. Non-colonic surgery.

1. Stomach decompression prior to induction of anesthesia by remaining NPO after midnight before surgery or by NG suction.
2. Bowel preparation required if any of the upper or lower GI tract is to be opened.
   a. Surgery may involve colon (e.g., extensive surgery for gynecologic malignancy or abdominal masses that impinge upon the colon or when there is a potential for mechanical or ischemic bowel damage [aneurysmectomy]).
   b. Achlorhydria, gastric carcinoma, prolonged H_2 blocker usage, and obstructive peptic ulcer disease will allow bacterial growth in the stomach. Consider using an oral antibiotic prep (i.e., neomycin) for gastric surgery in these patients (see below).

B. Colonic surgery—mechanical or whole gut lavage prep with or without oral antibiotic prep. Many variations exist.

1. Mechanical prep.
   a. Day 1–clear liquid diet, laxative of choice (castor oil 60 cc, Milk of Magnesia® (MOM) 30 cc, magnesium citrate 250 cc), tap water or soap-suds enema until clear.
   b. Day 2–clear liquid diet, IV fluids, laxative of choice.
   c. Day 3–operation.
   or:
   d. Day 1–clear liquid diet, IV fluids, Fleet® phosphosoda 1-2 oz. with water (repeat x 1), Dulcolax® suppository in the evening.
   e. Day 2–operation.
2. Whole gut lavage–GoLYTELY® (a polyethylene glycol base, electrolyte balanced solution).
   a. Day 1–GoLYTELY® 4 L po or per NG tube over 5 h.
   b. Metaclopramide 10 mg po to reduce bloating and nausea.
   c. Clear liquid diet after above.
   d. Day 2–operation.
3. Oral antibiotic prep–mechanical prep or whole gut lavage should be completed prior to the administration of the oral antibiotic prep.
   a. Nichols-Condon prep–on day prior to surgery , neomycin 1 g and erythromycin base 1 g po at 1 p.m., 2 p.m., 11 p.m. for case scheduled at 8 a.m.
   b. Metronidazole (500 mg) po may be substituted for erythromycin base in the Nichols-Condon prep (less nausea than with erythromycin base).
4. Peri-operative IV antibiotics may be used in conjunction with or in place of the oral antibiotic prep.

a. These antibiotics should be administered immediately pre-operatively (see above) and intra-operatively for prolonged operations. Any further doses post-operatively have not been shown to be effective in the prevention of wound infection; however, most surgeons administer at least 1 dose of antibiotic post-operatively, and it is common to continue the antibiotic for 24 h post-operatively.

b. Choice of antibiotic–need broad coverage of enteric organisms (gram-negative bacteria, anaerobes) (e.g., gentamicin and clindamycin, cefazolin and metronidazole, or cefotetan).

VI. BACTERIAL ENDOCARDITIS PROPHYLAXIS

A. Indications—patients with the following are particularly vulnerable to bacteriologic seeding during very transient bacteremia.

1. Prosthetic valve.
2. Congenital valve disease.
3. Rheumatic valve disease.
4. History of endocarditis.
5. Idiopathic hypertrophic subaortic stenosis.
6. Mitral valve prolapse with murmur (Barlow's syndrome).

B. Antibiotic Recommendations.

Prevention of Bacterial Endocarditis (Dental, Upper Respiratory, Genitourinary, and Gastrointestinal Procedures)

Drug	Adult Doses	Pediatric Doses
Oral—Amoxicillin	3 g 1 h before and 1.5 g 6 hours after procedure	50 mg/kg 1 h before and 25 mg/kg 6 h after procedure
Oral—Erythromycin (PCN Allergy)	1 g 2 h before and 500 mg 6 h after procedure	20 mg/kg 2 h before and 10 mg/kg 6 h after procedure
IV/IM—Ampicillin and IV/IM—Gentamicin	2 g 30 min before procedure 1.5 mg/kg 30 min before procedure	50 mg/kg 30 min before procedure 2 mg/kg 30 min before procedure
*IV Vancomycin (PCN Allergy)	1 g 1 h before procedure	20 mg/kg 1 h before procedure

* Add gentamicin to IV vancomycin for gastrointestinal and genitourinary procedures.

Notes:

1. For patients with valvular heart disease, prosthetic heart valves, most forms of congenital heart disease (but not uncomplicated secundum atrial septal defect), idiopathic hypertrophic subaortic stenosis, and mitral valve prolapse with regurgitation.
2. Data are limited on the risk of endocarditis with a particular procedure. For a review of the risk of bacteremia with various procedures, see Everett ED and

Hirschmann JV, *Medicine* 56:61, 1977, and Shorvon PJ, et al, *Gut* 24:1078, 1983. For useful guidelines on which procedures justify prophylaxis, see Shulman ST, et al, *Circulation* 70:1123A, 1984.

3. Oral regimens are more convenient and safer. Parenteral regimens are more likely to be effective; they are recommended especially for patients with prosthetic valves, those who have had endocarditis previously, or those taking continuous oral penicillin for rheumatic fever prophylaxis.
4. A single dose of the parenteral drugs is probably adequate, since bacteremias after most dental and diagnostic procedures are of short duration. One or two follow-up doses may be given at 8-12 h intervals in selected patients, such as hospitalized patients judged to be at higher risk.

From *The Medical Letter*, Vol. 31, #807, p. 112, 1989 with permission.

VII. STEROIDS

A. Indications.

1. Any patient currently on steroids, or those who have taken them within 1 year.
2. Pre-operative for adrenalectomy.
3. Known history of adrenal insufficiency.
4. History of adrenal or pituitary surgery, or surgery for renal cell carcinoma.

B. Endogenous Cortisol Output.

1. Normal unstressed adult–8-25 mg/day.
2. Adult undergoing major surgery–75-100 mg/day.

C. Guide to Steroid Coverage.

1. Correct electrolytes, blood pressure, and hydration if necessary.
2. Hydrocortisone phosphate or hemisuccinate, 100 mg IVPB on call to OR.
3. Hydrocortisone phosphate or hemisuccinate, 100 mg IVPB in recovery room and every 6 h for the first 24 h.
4. If progress is satisfactory, reduce dosage to 50 mg every 6 h for 24 h, then taper to maintenance dosage over 3 to 5 days. Resume previous fluorocortisol or oral steroid dose when patient is taking oral medications.
5. Maintain or increase hydrocortisone dosage to 200-400 mg per 24 h if fever, hypo-tension, or other complications occur.
6. If patient has potassium wasting, may switch to methylprednisolone (Solumedrol®).

NOTE: High-dose (300-600 mg/day) regimens are potentially deleterious secondary to impaired wound healing, increased catabolism, electrolyte abnormalities, and increased infectious complications.

8

Anesthesia

David J. Shelley, M.D.
Francis Nazareno, M.D.

While most patients are seen pre-operatively by an anesthetist or anesthesiologist, the surgeon should be familiar with anesthesia and its influence on surgical patients. Many ancillary local techniques are commonly used by the surgeon. Communication between the surgeon and the anesthesiologist is paramount to the successful peri-operative treatment of the patient.

I. PRE-OPERATIVE ASSESSMENT AND PREPARATION

A. History and physical.

B. Airway.

1. Assessment: Anatomic characteristics associated with difficult exposure of the glottic opening–short muscular neck, receding mandible, inability to visualize uvula, limited C-spine mobility, obesity, large tongue.

C. American Society of Anesthesiologists (ASA) classification (see "Pre-operative Preparation" section II. C).

D. Indications for delaying or postponing elective surgery.

1. Uncontrolled medical disease (cardiac, respiratory, hepatic, renal, endocrine).
2. Upper respiratory infection.
3. Recent food ingestion (commonly wait 6 h after ingestion).
4. No informed consent.

E. Suggested guidelines for pre-operative fasting.

1. No solids the day of surgery.
2. Clear liquids up to 6 h prior to surgery.
3. Oral medications up to 1 h before surgery with sips.

F. Pre-operative medication—goals.

1. Anxiety relief.
2. Sedation.

3. Analgesia.
4. Amnesia.
5. Control oral and bronchial secretions.
6. Increase gastric pH and decrease gastric secretions.
7. Anti-emetic effects.

II. TECHNIQUES OF ANESTHESIA

A. General anesthesia.

1. Mask.
2. Laryngeal mask airway.
3. Endotracheal intubation.
4. Inhalation *vs.* total intravenous anesthesia.
5. "Balanced anesthesia"–refers to combining multiple drugs to produce surgical anesthesia.

B. Regional anesthesia.

1. Spinal.
2. Epidural.
3. Combined spinal/epidural.
4. Caudal.
5. Peripheral nerve blocks; local/field blocks with or without sedation.
6. Monitored Anesthesia Care (MAC).

C. Stages of anesthesia.

1. Amnesia/analgesia.
2. Delirium/excitement.
3. Surgical anesthesia.
4. Overdosage/apnea.

III. INTRAVENOUS ANESTHESIA

May be used as induction agents, supplemental anesthesia agents, or as the sole anesthetic agent.

A. Ultrashort-acting barbiturates.

1. ***Thiopental*** [Pentothal®]–dose: 3-5 mg/kg over 30-45 sec.
   a. Onset–immediate; duration–awakening may occur in 5-10 min due to redistribution.
   b. Side-effects–myocardial depression, respiratory depression, peripheral vaso-dilatation; use with caution in patients with coronary artery disease and shock. Induces histamine release. Decreases cerebral blood flow and intracranial pressure.
2. ***Methohexital*** [Brevital®]–dose: 1 mg/kg.
   a. Onset–immediate, used for induction and intubation, respiratory depression may be prolonged.
   b. Side-effects–myocardial depression, significant hypotension.
   c. *Contraindicated* in patients with porphyrias.

B. Etomidate—dose: 0.1-0.4 mg/kg

1. Onset–30-60 sec. Induction and intubation.
2. Side-effects–hypo/hypertension, adrenocortical suppression.

C. Ketamine [Ketalar®]–dose: 2.5-5 mg/kg IM, 0.5-1 mg/kg IV.

1. Dissociative anesthetic with good analgesia. Maintains hypoxic pulmonary vasoconstrictive reflexes. Does not relieve visceral sensation. Useful in burn, pediatric, and thoracic surgery.
2. Side-effects–tachycardia, hypertension, increased cardiac output and myocardial oxygen demand. Respiratory depression. Emergence hallucinations can be avoided by pretreatment with a benzodiazepine.

D. Propofol [Diprivan®]–dose: 2.0-2.5 mg/kg, titrate 40 mg q 10 sec IVP; 0.1-0.2 mg/kg/min constant infusion IV.

1. Intravenous hypnotic with immediate onset.
2. Awakening may occur within 8 min because of both drug redistribution out of the CNS and metabolism.
3. Metabolism.
   a. Conjugation in the liver to inactive metabolites, which are excreted by the kidney.
   b. Extrahepatic metabolism is suspected.
   c. Pharmacokinetics not changed by chronic hepatic or renal failure.
4. Lacks analgesic and amnestic properties.

E. Narcotics useful for both analgesia and anesthesia.

1. ***Fentanyl*** [Sublimaze®]–dose: 0.04 mg/kg IV.
   a. Short-acting agent, 75 times more potent than morphine. Minimal myocardial effects make fentanyl useful in cardiac surgery.
   b. Side-effects–respiratory depression, muscle rigidity, hypotension, bradycardia, occasional truncal rigidity ("wooden chest").
   c. Reversible with *naloxone* [Narcan®] 0.04 mg IVP. *Caution:* short half-life of naloxone can result in return of opioid effect; analgesic effects will also be reversed.
   d. Analgesic dose–0.05-0.1 mg (1-2 cc); consider decreased dose in the elderly or debilitated.
2. ***Morphine sulfate*** – dose: 2.5-15 mg IV.
   a. Side-effects–hypotension, bradycardia, biliary tract spasm.
3. ***Meperidine*** [Demerol®]–dose: 0.5-2mg/Kg IV/IM/PO.
4. ***Naloxone*** [Narcan®]–Reversal of narcotic depression, dose: 0.1-2 mg.
   a. Titrate to response, may repeat at 2-3 min intervals; max 10 mg.

F. Benzodiazepines—good amnesia; based upon dose and route of administration, can produce a level of consciousness from sedation to unconsciousness.

1. ***Diazepam*** [Valium®]–dose: 10 mg IM 1-2 h pre-operative; or 5-10 mg slow IVP (do not exceed 2.5 mg/min) for sedation.
   a. Useful as pre-operative medication, or sedation for endo-

scopic or minor surgical procedures. Use cautiously in elderly or cachectic patients.

b. Side-effects–respiratory depression, disorientation, unpredictable IM absorption.

2. ***Midazolam*** [Versed®]–dose: 0.07-0.08 mg/kg deep IM 1-2 h pre-operative; or 0.07-0.1 mg/kg IV for sedation.
   a. Short duration of action. Useful as pre-operative medication or for minor surgical procedures. Water soluble, predictable IM absorption.
   b. Use cautiously in the elderly (reduce dose 50%).
3. ***Lorazepam*** [Ativan®] dose: 0.05 mg/kg deep IM up to 4 mg, 2 h pre-operative. Recommended in liver disease. More predictable IM absorption than diazepam.
   a. Contraindicated in patients with egg allergy.
   b. Adverse reactions.
      (1) Pain at injection site.
      (2) Hypotension.
      (3) Apnea.

G. Neuroleptanalgesia.

1. Combination of tranquilizer and narcotic analgesic.
2. ***Droperidol*** + ***fentanyl*** [Innovar®] (50:1)–preanesthetic used in conjunction with general anesthetic.
3. Amnesia, analgesia, and somnolence without complete unconsciousness.

IV. MUSCLE RELAXANTS

Achieve skeletal muscle relaxation without deep levels of anesthesia. Depolarizing agents mimic the action of acetylcholine, whereas non-depolarizing agents compete for cholinergic receptors on the post-synaptic membrane. The choice of an agent depends upon the desired duration of effect and the potential side-effects, particularly cardiovascular. The degree of neuromuscular blockade is assessed by electrical stimulation of peripheral motor nerves.

A. Depolarizing agents.

1. ***Succinylcholine*** [Anectine®]–dose: 1 mg/kg.
   a. Onset of action: 1 min; duration: 5-15 min.
   b. Most commonly used agent.
   c. Side-effects–may cause hyperkalemia in cases of severe muscle damage (i.e., burns, crush injury). Can cause bradycardia and hypotension, and post-operative muscle pain (secondary to fasciculations). Reported cases of malignant hyperthermia.
   d. *Contraindicated* in patients with eye injury due to increased intraocular pressure.

B. Non-depolarizing agents.

1. ***Pancuronium*** [Pavulon®]–dose: 0.04-0.1 mg/kg.
   a. Onset of action: 1-3 min; duration: 40-65 min.
   b. Renal and hepatic elimination.

c. Side-effects–interacts with halothane to increase ventricular irritability. May cause *tachycardia* and *hypertension* due to vagolytic effect.

2. ***Atracurium*** [Tracrium®]–dose: 0.3-0.5 mg/kg.
   a. Onset of action: 2-3 min; duration: 20-40 min.
   b. Hoffmann elimination; can use in hepatic or renal failure.
   c. Side-effects–less histamine release than d-tubocurarine and pancuronium.
3. ***Vecuronium*** [Norcuron®]–dose: 0.1 mg/kg.
   a. Onset of action: 2-3 min; duration: 20-40 min.
   b. Hepatic elimination.
   c. Very little histamine release, less cardiovascular effects than other neuromuscular blocking agents.
4. ***Rocuronium*** [Zemuron®]–dose: 0.6-1.2 mg/kg IV.
   a. Onset of action:1 min (only rapid onset non-depolarizing agent); duration 20-35 min.

C. Reversal of neuromuscular blockade—non-depolarizing agents can be antagonized by anticholinesterase drugs. Atropine (0.6-1.2 mg) or glycopyrrolate (Robinul®) should be added to block muscarinic side-effects (salivation, bronchospasm, and bradycardia).

1. ***Edrophonium*** [Tensilon®]–dose: 0.75-1.0 mg/kg IV.
   a. Onset of action: 3-5 min.
   b. Always use with atropine.
2. ***Neostigmine*** [Prostigmine®]–dose: 0.4-1.0 mg/kg IV.
   a. Onset of action: 7-10 min.
   b. Always use with glycopyrrolate (Robinul®) 0.01 mg/kg.
3. ***Pyridostigmine*** [Mestinon®]–dose: 0.1 mg/kg IV.
   a. Onset of action 12-15 min.
   b. Must add either atropine or glycopyrrolate.

V. INHALATIONAL ANESTHESIA

A. Induction—achieved via short-acting barbiturate or inhalation of O_2-anesthetic mixture.

1. ***MAC (Minimum Alveolar Concentration)*** is the minimum alveolar concentration that prevents movement in 50% of patients in response to a skin incision.
2. Rapidity of induction of inhalation anesthesia depends upon inspired concentration, volume of pulmonary ventilation, solubility of the agent in blood, and cardiac output clearing the agent from the alveoli.

B. Nitrous oxide (MAC = 104% with oxygen).

1. Commonly used; nonflammable and odorless (good patient acceptability). Rapid recovery with low potency; potentiates other inhalational anesthetics and narcotics, allowing reduction in dosage of other agents. Results in increased peripheral resistance and cardiac depression.

2. Complications:
    a. Diffusion anoxia–O_2 administration post-operatively to prevent hypoxia.
    b. Expansion of air-filled cavities (e.g., bowel [dangerous in bowel obstruction] and pneumothorax).

C. Halothane [Fluothane®] (MAC = 0.77%).

1. Potent, rapid onset of action. Bronchial smooth muscle relaxant (excellent for asthmatics).
2. Complications:
    a. Myocardial depression, profound hypotension.
    b. Sensitizes myocardium to catecholamines with increased risk of *ventricular arrhythmias.*
    c. Potent vasodilator increases cerebral perfusion and intracranial pressure (harmful with CNS space occupying lesions).
    d. Halothane hepatitis (cumulative with repeat exposures)–marked elevation of LFTs 2 to 5 days post-operative and preceded by fever and eosinophilia. More common in females.

D. Enflurane [Ethrane®] (MAC = 1.68%).

1. Rapid induction, quick recovery, profound muscle relaxation.
2. Complications:
    a. Similar cardiovascular effects as halothane, but less likely to produce arrhythmias.
    b. Potential to elicit grand mal seizures at high MAC with hyperventilation.

E. Isoflurane [Forane®] (MAC = 1.2%).

1. Potent muscle relaxant, with minimal hepatic, CNS, or renal impairment. Less cardio-vascular depression than with enflurane or halothane.
2. Complications–increased incidence of coughing and *laryngospasm.*

F. Desflurane (MAC = 6-7%).

1. New inhalation agent with very rapid induction and rapid recovery (similar to that of N_2O).
2. Low toxic potential.
3. Hemodynamic effects similar to isoflurane.
4. Potent muscle relaxant.

VI. MALIGNANT HYPERTHERMIA

A. 1:50,000 adults, 1:15,000 children—highest incidence in young, athletic males with a mortality rate of 10%. A genetic predisposition exists. **Halothane** and **succinylcholine** are most often involved, but may occur with all anesthetic agents except N_2O. May occur during induction, anesthesia, or post-operatively. The syndrome is characterized by a hypermetabolic state.

B. Clinical signs.

1. Masseter rigidity following succinylcholine administration.
2. Unexplained tachycardia and tachypnea.
3. Arrhythmias.
4. Cyanosis.
5. Metabolic and/or respiratory acidosis.
6. Fever is a *late* sign (may reach 107°F).

C. Treatment.

1. Discontinue anesthetic agent and change all tubing.
2. Hyperventilate with 100% O_2.
3. ***Dantrolene sodium*** (2-10 mg/kg)–treatment of choice, can also be used prophylactically with suspected family history.
4. $NaHCO_3$–for severe metabolic and respiratory acidosis.
5. Hyperkalemia–treat with $NaHCO_3$, insulin (0.15 mg/kg), 20% dextrose.
6. Iced cooling of IV fluids and patient.
7. Procainamide 1 g IV–effective in arresting "runaway" metabolism.

D. Late complications.

1. Consumptive coagulopathy.
2. Acute renal failure.
3. Hypothermia.
4. Pulmonary edema.
5. Skeletal muscle swelling.
6. Neurologic sequelae.
7. Suspected family members should undergo evaluation.

VII. LOCAL ANESTHETICS

A. Analgesia/anesthesia without risks of general anesthesia. Used in spinal, regional, and local anesthesia.

B. Limit total anesthetic dose to prevent seizures.

1. Add vasoconstrictor to slow vascular absorption.
2. Avoid inadvertent vascular injection by pre-injection aspiration.
3. Impending toxicity muscle twitching, restlessness, sleepiness.
4. Treatment of toxicity–Trendelenburg position, O_2, IV Valium® (5-10 mg), Thiopental® (50-100 mg).

C. Never inject solutions containing epinephrine into digits, ear, tip of nose, or penis—may cause local ischemic necrosis.

D. Commonly used local anesthetics:

1. Procaine [Novocaine®, Planocaine®]–dose: 14 mg/kg; duration: 0.5 h.
2. Lidocaine [Xylocaine®, Xylotox®]–dose: 7 mg/kg; duration: 1-2 h.
3. Mepivacaine [Carbocaine®, Polocaine®]–dose: 7 mg/kg; duration: 1-2 h.

4. Tetracaine [Pontocaine®, Pantocaine®]–dose: 1.5 mg/kg; duration: 2-3 h.
5. Bupivacaine [Marcaine®]–dose: 3 mg/kg; duration: 5-7 h.

E. **Systemic toxicity effects—**numbness of tongue, visual disturbances, unconsciousness, seizures, coma, respiratory arrest, CNS depression.

VIII. SPINAL ANESTHESIA

A. **Injection of local anesthetic into subarachnoid space.**
   1. Order of blockade–preganglionic sympathetic fibers, somatic sensory fibers, somatic motor fibers.
   2. Denervation can extend about 2 spinal segments above the anesthetic areas.

B. **Level of anesthesia** is controlled by specific gravity of injected mixture (hyperbaric solution, e.g., D10W) and adjusting Trendelenburg position.

C. **Best for procedures below the umbilicus.**
   1. T4 dermatome–nipple.
   2. T6 dermatome–xiphoid.
   3. T10 dermatome–umbilicus.
   4. L1 dermatome–pubic crest.

D. **Complications.**
   1. Diminished sympathetic tone, vasodilatation, hypotension, and decreased cardiac output.
   2. ***Spinal headache*** – produced by leakage of CSF from puncture site occurring about 36-48 h post spinal puncture.
      a. Most frequent after use of large-bore spinal needles in young adults. Uncommon when finer needles used.
      b. May last for weeks.
      c. Treatment–bedrest, hydration, prone position, IV hydration, "epidural blood patch" (patient's blood injected into epidural space).
   3. Intercostal paralysis if agent extends into thoracic area.
   4. Spinal block of cardiac nerves (T2-4) can produce hypotension and bradycardia.
   5. Total spinal (above C3) block of all intercostal and phrenic nerves, requires ventilatory and hemodynamic support.
   6. Urinary retention.

E. **Advantages of spinal and epidural anesthesia.**
   1. Blunts "stress response" to surgery.
   2. Reduces intra-operative blood loss and thromboembolic complications.
   3. Provides means of post–operative pain control.
   4. Maintains upper airway reflexes, protecting against aspiration.

F. **Contraindications—**coagulopathy, infection at site, current neurological dysfunction, uncorrected hypovolemia.

IX. EPIDURAL ANESTHESIA

A. Epidural space.

1. Bordered by the dura mater internally and the spinal canal periosteum.
2. Contains fat and blood vessels.

B. Anesthetic injection blocks sympathetic/parasympathetic ganglia and motor/sensory impulses. These opioid receptors in spinal cord allow opioid epidural administration for acute/chronic pain states.

C. Less dependent on position of patient than spinal anesthesia.

D. Larger amounts of local anesthetic required (*vs.* spinal).

E. More demanding technically.

F. Surgical advantages (see VIII E).

1. Blockade of all nerve functions without requirements for endotracheal intubation.
2. In combination with light general anesthesia, lessens postoperative complications.

G. Complications.

1. Profound hypotension if block above T5.
2. Infection of indwelling catheter (especially immunocompromised patients).
3. Respiratory depression (especially epidural opioid administration). May last much longer than equivalent IV dose.
4. Urinary retention.
5. CNS toxicity.

X. COMBINED SPINAL/EPIDURAL

Takes advantage of the beneficial aspects of both; i.e., a rapid, reliable block with spinal and the ability to supplement the block and provide post-op pain relief with an epidural.

XI. CAUDAL ANESTHESIA

A. Injection—at S5 through sacrococcygeal membrane.

B. No spinal headache.

C. Continuous anesthesia for long procedures—useful for rectal surgery.

D. Similar degree of hypotension as with spinal anesthetic; lessened amount of motor paralysis.

XII. REGIONAL NERVE BLOCKS

A. Cervical block (anterior divisions of C1-C4).

1. Indications–carotid endarterectomy, lymph node biopsies.
2. Provides anesthesia in anterior/posterior cervical triangles between jaw and clavicles with relaxation of strap musculature.
3. Lateral approach injection at midpoint of posterior border of SCM to anesthetize superficial cervical plexus. Fan out with 10-20 cc 1% lidocaine.

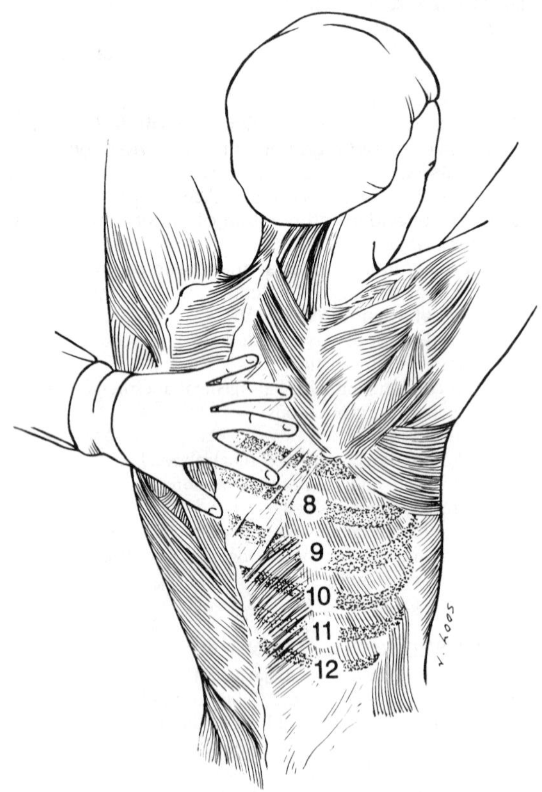

FIG. 1

4. 2nd, 3rd, and 4th nerves individually blocked at anterior tubercles of transverse processes using 5 cc 1% lidocaine at 4th process just above midpoint of posterior border of SCM where external jugular crosses the muscle.
5. *Note:* Cervical block also blocks phrenic nerve. Bilateral block will produce phrenic paralysis and hypoventilation.

B. Intercostal block (12 thoracic nerves) [Figures 1 & 2].

1. Intercostal nerve courses from intervertebral foramen to rib angle along subcostal groove: nerve-inferior, artery-middle, vein-superior.

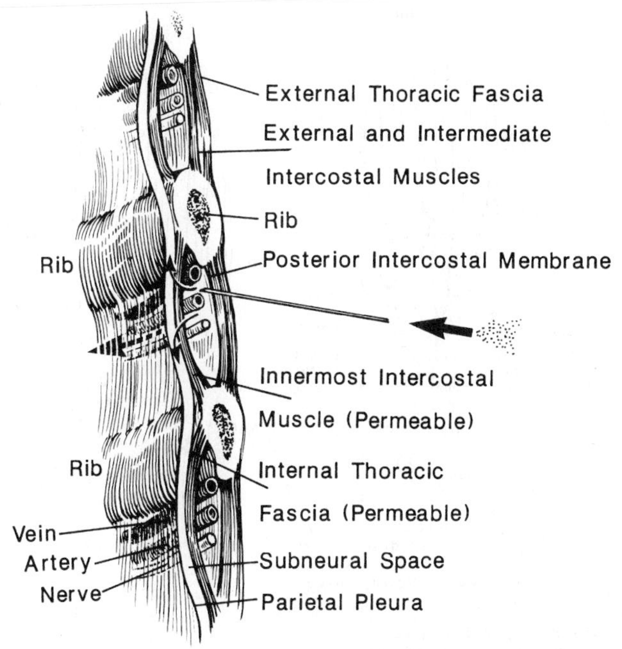

FIG. 2

2. May also provide anesthesia of abdominal wall (T5-T11 must be blocked).
3. Technique.
   a. Prone position for bilateral block; lateral position for unilateral block.
   b. Insert needle over selected rib at 5 cm from posterior midline until needle point touches rib. Walk down rib (2-3 cm); aspirate (no air or blood); inject 3-4 cc 1% lidocaine.
   c. For successful intercostal space block, 3 intercostal nerves (one on each side) must be anesthetized.

C. Wrist and hand blocks [Figures 3-6].

1. Hand procedures may be performed through blockage of the median, ulnar, and radial nerves, or with wrist bracelet infiltration. Minor procedures in digits can be accomplished using a digital block.

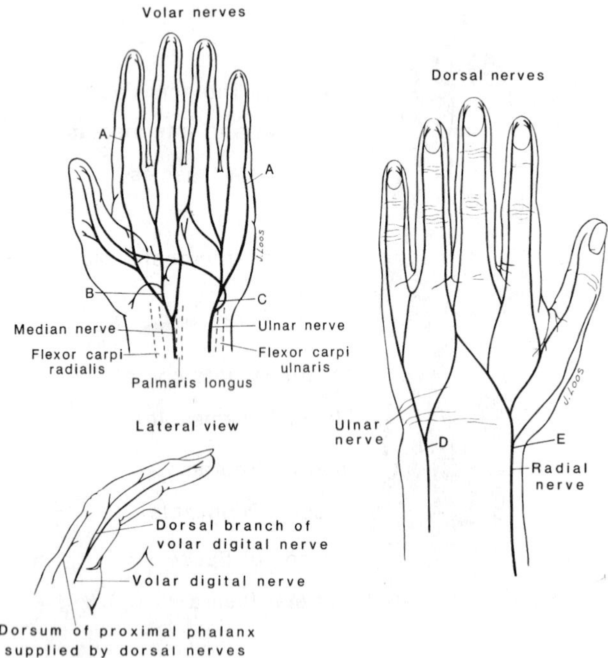

FIG. 3 Anatomy of sensory nerve blocks and sites for injection: **A,** volar digital nerve; **B,** median nerve, **C,** ulnar nerve; **D,** dorsal branch of ulnar nerve; **E,** dorsal branch of radial nerve.

2. General considerations.
   a. Always complete the sensory exam prior to injection.
   b. Do *not* use epinephrine or inject into an infected area.
   c. Always aspirate first to avoid intra-arterial injection.
3. ***Median nerve***—located between tendons of palmaris longus (PL) and flexor carpi radialis (FCR) with wrist flexed. Enter 2 cm proximal to the distal crease and just radial to the PL tendon or 1 cm medial to the FCR tendon. Penetrate to a length of 1 cm and inject 5 cc 1% lidocaine (Figures 3 & 4).
4. ***Ulnar nerve***—medial to ulnar artery and lateral to flexor carpi ulnaris (FCU). Enter to the ulnar side of the FCU and just proximal to the pisiform bone, aiming about 1.5 cm below tendon. Aspirate, then inject 5 cc 1% lidocaine (Figures 3 & 4).

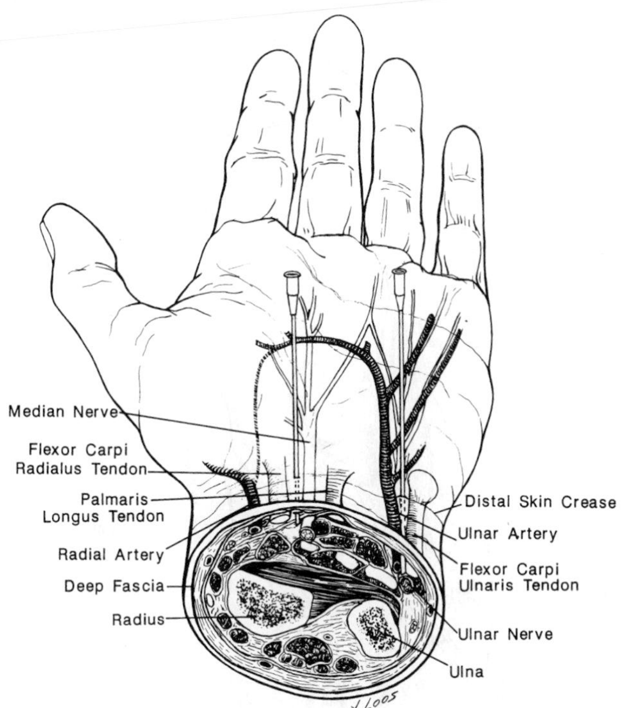

FIG. 4

5. ***Radial nerve***—superficial branch of radial nerve located in anatomical snuff box; inject 5 cc 1% lidocaine in snuff box (Figures 3-5).
6. ***Wrist bracelet***—achieved by individual block of median, ulnar, and radial nerves and subcutaneous infiltration of wrist circumferentially.
7. ***Digital block***—inject 1-2 cc 1% lidocaine into web space just dorsal to palmar (plantar) and dorsal skin junction. Then redirect needle dorsally and inject additional 1 cc to include dorsal branch. Avoid circumferential injections in the digits (Figures 3 & 6).

D. Femoral nerve block.

1. Level below inguinal ligament.
2. NAV (**n**erve-**a**rtery-**v**ein)–lateral to medial.
3. Lateral to artery with 5-10 cc 1% lidocaine.

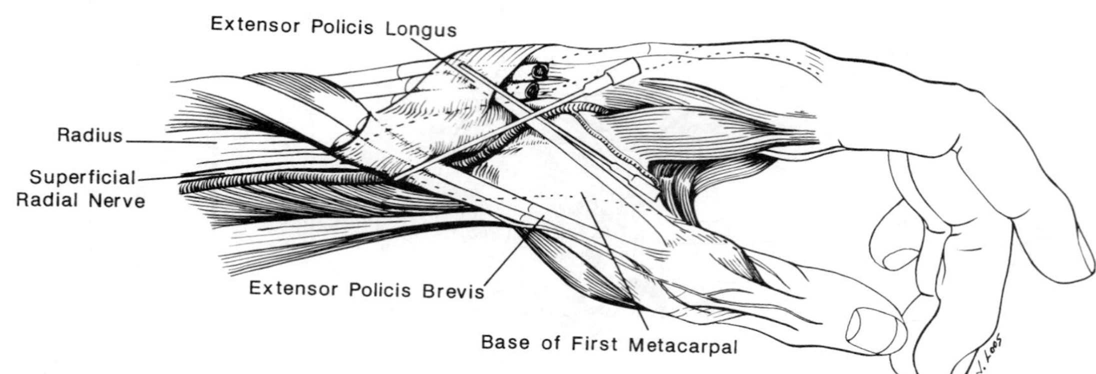
Extensor Policis Longus
Radius
Superficial
Radial Nerve
Extensor Policis Brevis
Base of First Metacarpal

FIG. 5

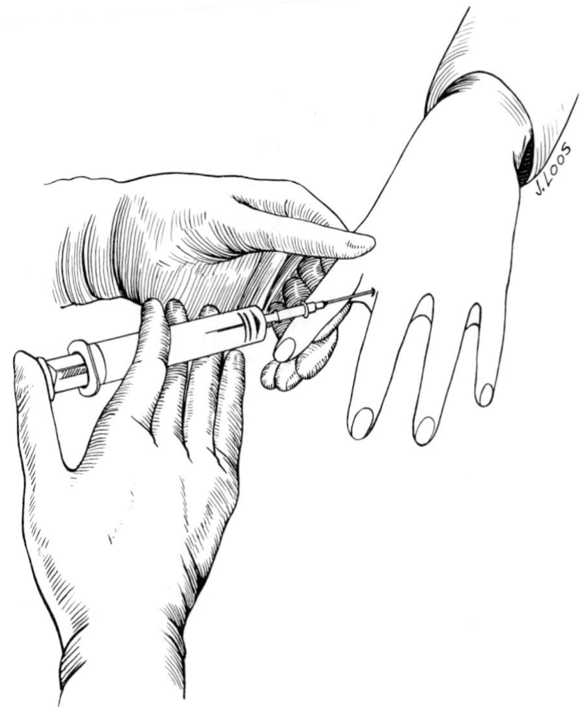

FIG. 6

4. Most combine lateral femoral cutaneous nerve block (L2, L3)–beneath inguinal ligament, just medial to anterior superior iliac spine (fanwise) with 5-10 cc 1% lidocaine.

E. Ankle nerve block.

1. Must block anterior/posterior tibial nerves.
2. Knee flexed with sole of foot on table.
3. Anterior tibial nerve located between tendons of tibialis anticus and extensor hallucis longus, with liberal infiltration of 1% lidocaine.
4. Posterior tibial nerve located medial to calcaneous tendon, lidocaine as above.
5. Add superficial "bracelet" cutaneous block and posterolateral compartment block (deep infiltration) for sural nerve block.

F. Bier block (intravenous regional anesthesia).

1. Excellent for forearm, hand, or foot procedures.

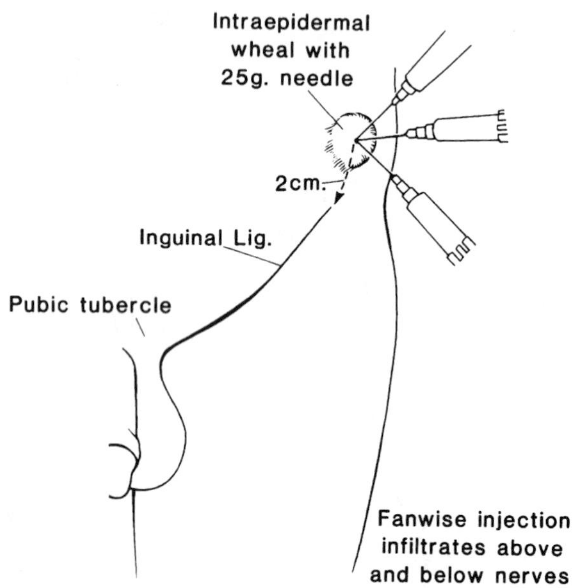
Intraepidermal
wheal with
25g. needle
2cm.
Inguinal Lig.
Pubic tubercle
Fanwise injection
infiltrates above
and below nerves

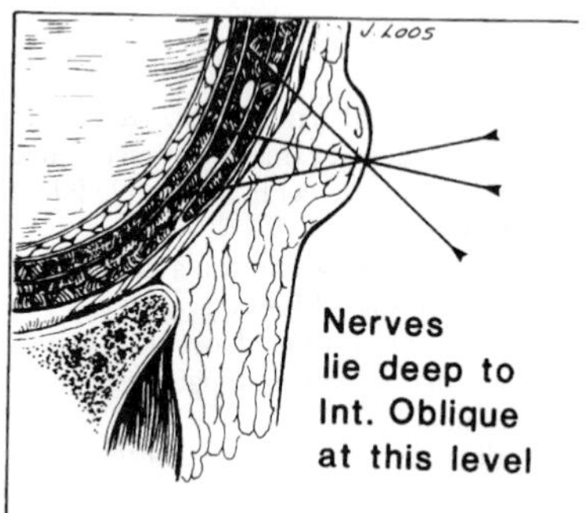
J. Loos
Nerves
lie deep to
Int. Oblique
at this level

FIG. 7

2. Usually limited to 1 hour.
3. Double pneumatic tourniquet applied above elbow (calf).
4. Initially inflate above venous pressure to distend vein, venipuncture with 22-ga. IV.
5. Release tourniquet, exsanguinate extremity with elevation, and wrap with elastic bandage, inflate distal tourniquet then proximal tourniquet, then release distal tourniquet (> 100 mm Hg above arterial).
6. 0.5% lidocaine injection–IV 3 mg/kg.
7. With onset of tourniquet pain (at 45 min), inflate distal tourniquet and release proximal tourniquet for slow release of lidocaine into systemic circulation.

XIII. LOCAL ANESTHESIA FOR INGUINAL/FEMORAL HERNIA REPAIR (7 STEPS)

A. **Intraepidermal wheal**—2-3 cm above and slightly lateral to anterior superior iliac spine (Figure 7). At least 5 cc of anesthetic injected superiorly, horizontally, and inferiorly (fanwise) deep to the external oblique muscle to anesthetize the ilioinguinal and iliohypogastric nerves, which lie deep to the external and internal oblique muscles (Figure 7).

B. **Inject anesthetic**—subcutaneously and intradermally in a medial direction toward the umbilicus (anesthetize the 11th thoracic nerve), inferiorly toward the anterior superior iliac spine and obliquely in the direction of the proposed line of incision (Figure 8).

C. **Multiple injections of small amounts**—placed just under the external oblique fascia (Figure 9).

D. **Injections about the base of the spermatic cord** (Figure 10).

E. **3-5 cc of anesthetic**—injected into the pubic tubercle and in the area in proximity to Cooper's ligament (Figure 11).

F. **Injections of the peritoneal sac**—under direct vision (Figure 12).

XIV. ACUTE POST–OPERATIVE PAIN MANAGEMENT

A. **Patient-controlled analgesia (PCA).**

1. Allows patient to self-administer narcotics with a programmable infusion pump.
2. Attempts to provide optimal pain relief and safety by avoiding peak and trough levels out of the therapeutic range caused by delays in administration, improper dosage, and pharmacokinetic and pharmacodynamic variability.
3. Pumps are programmable to be able to deliver intermittent boluses on demand, a continuous infusion, or a continuous background infusion with intermittent bolus doses.
4. The dose, dose interval, and infusion rate are determined by the physician.

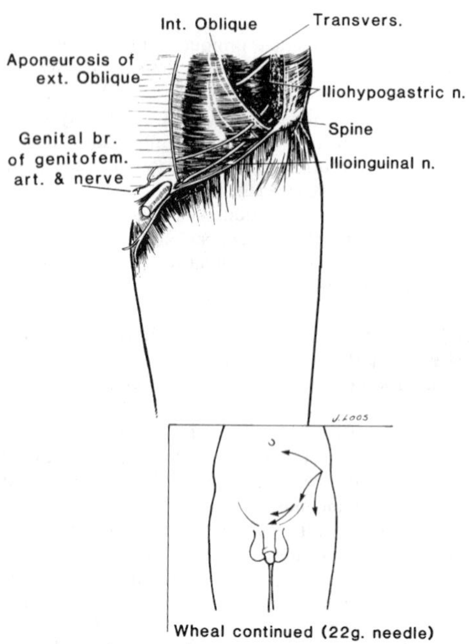

FIG. 8

Points of injection *

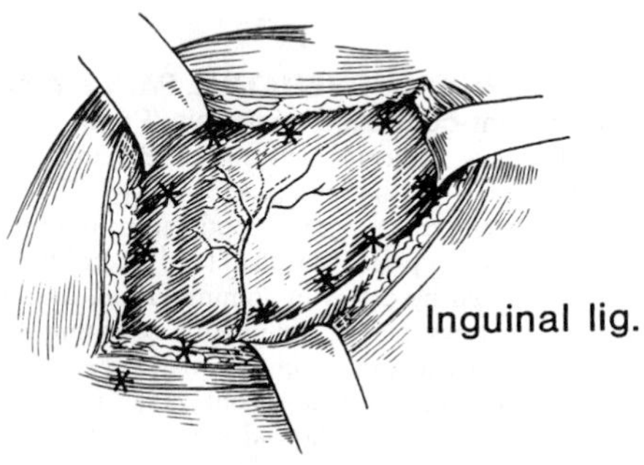

FIG. 9

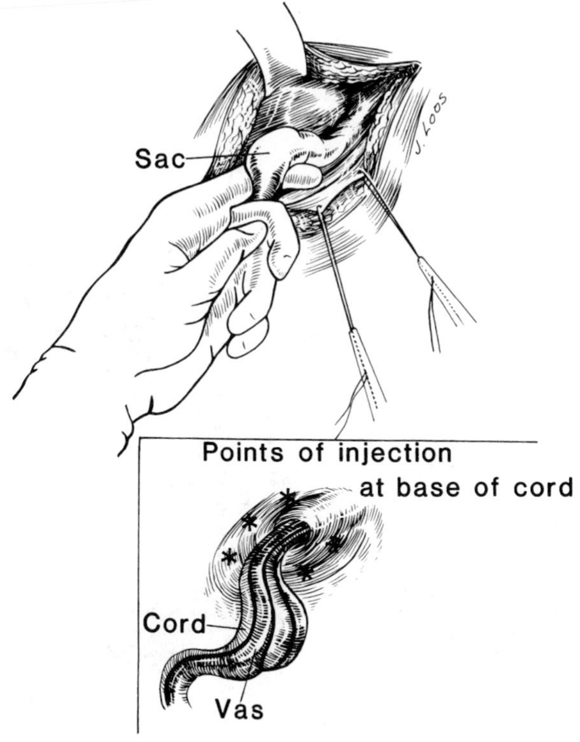

FIG. 10

5. Morphine and meperidine are used often for intermittent dosing because of an intermediate duration of action. Typical morphine bolus doses are 0.5-2.0 mg with a 5-20 min lockout interval.
6. A *loading dose* is administered post-operatively in the recovery room prior to starting PCA therapy. When fully awake, the patient is given the control button. Dose and interval can be adjusted as needed to achieve adequate analgesia.
7. Bolus doses and/or infusion rates can be increased at night to provide more sedation and rest.
8. Potential complications are respiratory depression, tolerance, physical dependence, nausea, vomiting, and pruritus.

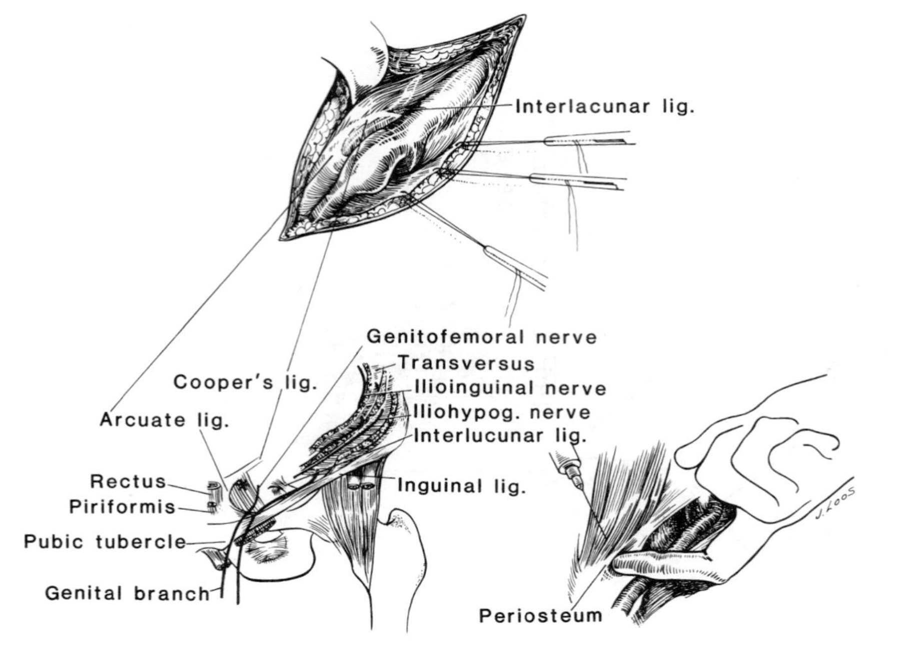
Interlacunar lig.
Genitofemoral nerve
Transversus
Cooper's lig.
Ilioinguinal nerve
Iliohypog. nerve
Arcuate lig.
Interlucunar lig.
Rectus
Inguinal lig.
Piriformis
Pubic tubercle
Genital branch
Periosteum
J. Loos

FIG. 11

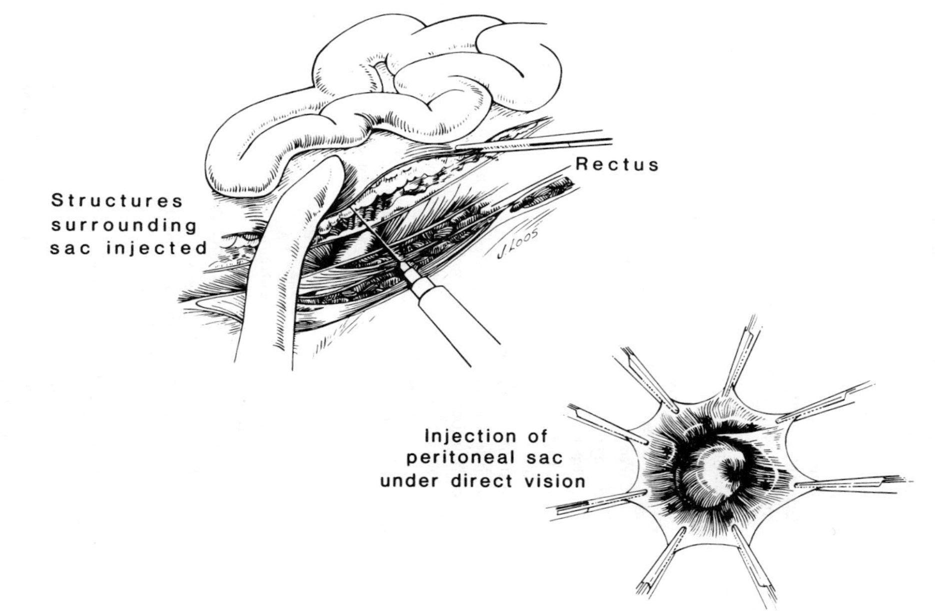
Rectus
Structures surrounding sac injected
J. Loos
Injection of peritoneal sac under direct vision

FIG. 12

B. Intrathecal analgesia.
1. Provides short-term analgesia (24 h).
2. Morphine is drug of choice. Dosage is 0.5 mg or less.
3. Local anesthetics are not used because of a shorter duration of action and dose-dependent side-effects of hypotension and motor block.
4. Limited to single-dose administration by risk of spinal headache and nerve damage from multiple punctures.
5. Side-effects are respiratory depression, nausea, and vomiting.

C. Epidural analgesia—attempts to provide pain relief without high systemic levels and side-effects of analgesics. Narcotics or local anesthetics can be used.
1. Advantages.
    a. Prevents muscle spasm and splinting, avoiding pulmonary complications.
    b. Less sedation allows earlier ambulation.
    c. Possible earlier return of GI function post-operatively.
    d. Excellent for patients with chest trauma, including rib fractures, pulmonary contusion, and flail chest.
2. Catheter tip placed at vertebral level corresponding to targeted dermatome.
3. Narcotic analgesics.
    a. Effect is most likely by direct action on spinal cord.
    b. Number of nerve roots involved affected by lipid solubility, infusion rate (continuous infusion), and volume of dose (intermittent dosing).
    c. Narcotics with poor lipid solubility (morphine) have greater nerve root spread, slower onset of action, and longer duration of action.
    d. Side-effects–respiratory depression, pruritus, nausea, vomiting, urinary retention.
    e. COPD is a relative contraindication.
4. Local anesthetics.
    a. Blocks conduction and operation of nerve impulses of spinal nerves and spinal cord.
    b. Number of nerve roots involved affected by infusion rate, volume of intermittent dose.
    c. Bupivacaine used most frequently because of rapid onset of action, good analgesia, long duration, and absence of motor block.
    d. Side-effects are hypotension, motor block, systemic toxicity, and urinary retention. Epidural blocks above T5 can cause bradycardia and cardiac failure.
    e. Contraindications are severe heart disease, shock, and hypovolemia.
5. Dosing.
    a. Intermittent dosing causes peak systemic levels above those required for analgesia, causing more side-effects.

b. Continuous infusion prevents peaks and troughs of intermittent dosing. Side-effects occur slowly over time.
c. Combining infusions of local anesthetics and narcotics lowers the total dose of each, reducing the chance of side-effects.
d. Continuous infusion of local anesthetics should be weaned off slowly over 2-4 h as increased fluid mobilization secondary to vasoconstriction can precipitate pulmonary edema.

9

Cardiopulmonary Monitoring

Stephen B. Archer, M.D.

I. MONITORING

Basic principle is periodic objective assessment of patient's clinical condition. Ideal monitors are nonvinvasive, reliable, and accurately convey physiologic information in "real-time". Often, in critically ill patients, noninvasive monitors are either unreliable and/or inaccurate, and invasive techniques are required.

A. "Vital signs"–evaluation of pulse, blood pressure (BP), temperature, respiratory rate. In its simplest form, these parameters are measured using a watch, thermometer, and sphygmomanometer. Although such assessments made at 4-h or 8-h intervals are adequate for the "stable" patient, the seriously ill patient requires closer evaluation on a more frequent schedule. Continuous assessment is the ideal situation.

B. Monitoring techniques—invasive *vs.* non-invasive.

1. *Non-invasive.*
   a. Continuous ECG monitoring–heart rate, rhythm.
   b. Apnea monitoring–respiratory drive.
   c. Pulse oximetry–arterial O_2 saturation.
   d. Capnography–end-tidal CO_2.
   e. Ultrasonic BP monitor (Dynamap®)–blood pressure.
   f. Doppler ultrasonography–presence or abscense of nonpalpable pulse.
2. *Invasive.*
   a. Arterial catheterization–BP, arterial waveform, and continuous arterial blood gas analysis.
   b. Central venous catheterization–central venous pressure (CVP).
   c. Pulmonary artery catheterization–CVP, pulmonary artery systolic (PAS) and diastolic (PAD) pressures, pulmonary capillary wedge pressure (PCWP), cardiac output.

3. In practice, often a combination of non-invasive and invasive techniques are applied. Invasive monitoring (placement of intravascular catheters) provides more direct measurement and provides data from which other measurements can be calculated.

C. Indications for Invasive Monitoring.

1. Complex surgical procedures associated with large volume shifts.
2. Circulatory instability.
3. Fluid management problems.
4. Deteriorating cardiac function.
5. Deteriorating pulmonary function.
6. Inappropriate response to volume challenge.
7. Unexplained hypoxemia.
8. Severe head injury.
9. Surgical procedures in patients with baseline poor cardiac, respiratory, or renal function.

II. PULMONARY MONITORING

A. Apnea monitoring—sensitive to chest wall motion. Monitors respiratory rate. Alarms usually set for bradypnea or apnea.

B. Pulse oximetry—non-invasive; transcutaneous measurement of arterial oxygen saturation by light absorption technique. Probe is attached to body areas where capillary bed are accessible (i.e., fingernail bed, earlobes, toes). Does not function under conditions of hypoperfusion (such as in hypothermia) or inadequate pulsatile flow or in situations in which light pulse cannot reach capillaries such as with stained fingernails.

C. Capnography—direct measurement of end-tidal CO_2.

D. Arterial blood gas—direct measure of a patient's ability to exchange O_2 and CO_2 and support oxidative metabolism. Reflects oxygenation, ventilation, and acid-base disturbances.

III. HEMODYNAMIC MONITORING TECHNIQUES

A. Indirect monitoring of BP—sphygmomanometer (notoriouslyinaccurate in hypotensive conditions; wide inter-observer variation), ultrasonic BP monitor. Work well in euvolemic patients. Doppler devices give no measure of diastolic pressure.

B. Arterial catheterization—provides direct measure of arterial pressure as well as arterial access for blood sampling. In conjunction with continuous EKG monitor, affords indirect evaluation of electromechanical function of the heart.

1. Arterial pressure–the displayed pressure tracing is a synthesis of harmonics of the ejection pressure of the ventricular stroke volume into the elastic arterial tree. Diastolic run-off pressures represent the relationship between systemic vascular resistance, arterial pressure, and intravascular blood volume. An undamped arterial pressure tracing will show a distinct dicrotic notch separating the systolic and diastolic pressures.

a. In hypovolemia with decreased stroke volume, a smaller pressure wave will be generated.
b. If myocardial contraction is diminished, there will be prolongation of the upslope of the arterial pressure tracing.

2. Access for arterial blood samples.
   a. Sequential analysis of blood gas tensions and acid/base status in the arterial blood are necessary in any acute illness involving cardiovascular or respiratory dysfunction. Continuous arterial blood gas analysis via an arterial line is available; however, it is not widely used.
   b. Access to other blood samples necessary to chart the progression of multisystemic illness.
   c. Arterial blood cultures.
      (1) Fungal organisms may be more reliably cultured from arterial blood.
      (2) Risk of catheter-induced sepsis is a danger with any invasive monitoring–sequential arterial cultures are necessary whenever these catheters are maintained for a long time. Arterial catheter colonization occurs much less frequently than with venous catheters.
3. Pitfalls.
   a. Kinked catheters or inappropriately zeroed transducers may give misleading information.
   b. Arterial BP is not the "*sine qua non*" of shock and should not be used as the sole criterion of effectiveness of therapy.
   c. BP measurement alone is inadequate to assess the relationship between systemic resistance and cardiac output. If there is a question about low cardiac output or the level of peripheral resistance, then cardiac output should be determined.
4. Method of insertion (see "Vascular Access Techniques").

C. **Central venous pressure (CVP) monitoring—**permits assessment of the ability of the right ventricle to accommodate the volume being returned to it.
   1. Accurate method of estimating right ventricular filling pressure (relevant in interpreting right ventricular function).
   2. CVP is a function of 4 independent forces.
      a. Volume and flow of blood in the central veins.
      b. Compliance and contractility of the right side of the heart during filling of the heart.
      c. Venomotor tone of central veins.
      d. Intrathoracic pressure.
   3. ***Clinical uses of CVP catheter.***
      a. Infusion of TPN, vasoactive substances, hypertonic solutions, or chemically irritating medications for prolonged period of time.
      b. Monitoring right atrial pressures.
      c. Aspiration of venous samples for chemical analysis (cannot be used as a substitute for true mixed venous blood).

d. Head injury–increasing right atrial pressure will result in increased intracranial blood volume and may increase intracranial pressure (ICP).
e. Sensitive in reflecting increased transmyocardial pressure in pericardial tamponade.

4. Pitfalls of using CVP in critically ill patient.
   a. Water manometer system cannot reliably represent right ventricular filling pressure–transducer-monitor system is necessary. Transducer systems also need to be accurately zeroed: position of transducer is critical.
   b. Misinterpretation of CVP data when extrapolating information relative to left ventricular performance in critically ill patients.
      (1) In normal situations, right ventricular filling pressure *may* correlate with left ventricular filling pressures.
      (2) In specific pathophysiologic states (e.g., ARDS, cor pulmonale, pulmonary fibrosis, pulmonary hypertension, myocardial contusion, septic shock), when invasive monitoring is used, right and left atrial pressures may differ significantly. CVP cannot be substituted for assessment of left ventricular filling pressures in these situations. Thus, in a critically ill patient, placement of a pulmonary artery catheter is more appropriate.
5. Method of insertion–see "Vascular Access Techniques".

D. Balloon-tipped pulmonary artery catheter (Swan-Ganz® catheter).

1. Advantages over CVP measurements.
   a. Allows independent assessment of right and left ventricular function, which may be dissimilar during critical illness.
   b. Permits measurement of pulmonary arterial diastolic and wedge pressures that approximates left atrial filling pressure (preload).
   c. Continuous monitoring of pulmonary artery systolic and mean pressures reflects changes in pulmonary vascular resistance (PVR) secondary to hypoxemia, pulmonary edema, pulmonary emboli, and pulmonary insufficiency. It helps distinguish cardiogenic pulmonary edema from noncardiogenic.
   d. Allows sampling of global mixed venous blood.
      (1) Global mixed venous blood saturations provide an index of tissue perfusion and oxygenation. Increasing SV_2 correlates with increasing cardiac output and tissue perfusion or decreased oxygen extraction (in sepsis or liver failure). Decreasing SVO_2 signifies decreasing cardiac output or tissue perfusion with increased oxygen extraction. (SVO_2 *cannot,* however, reflect the changes in regional perfusion that are often present in critically ill patients.)

TABLE 1

Determinants of Cardiac Output

Determinant	Definition	Effect on Cardiac Output	Measurement	Treatment
Pre-load	Length of myocardial fibers at end-disastole, which is the result of vertricular filing pressure	Direct, up to physiologic limit	End-diastolic volume and pressure of the ventricles Pulmonary diastolic pressure Pulmonary capillary wedge pressure Direct left atrial pressure measurements CVP (right atrial)	Volume expansion Pericardiocentesis Reduction of PEEP
Contractility	The inotropic state of the myocardium; length/tension/velocity relationship of the myocardium independent of initial length and after-load	Direct	Ventricular function curves Ejection fraction Vmax Vcf PEP/LVET *dP/dt* iP	Dopamine Norepinephrine Epinephrine Isoproterenol Dobutamine Digitalis Glucagon GKI
Afterload	Systolic ventricular wall stress, which is produced by the force against which the myocardial fibers must contract	Inverse, as long as coronary flow is maintained	Aortic pressure for left ventricle Pulmonary artery pressure for right ventricle	Diuretics Phentolamine Sodium nitroprusside Nitroglycerine Intra-aortic balloon pumping External counter-pulsation
Pulse Rate	The numbers of cardiac systoles per minute	Direct >60 and <180 per minute	ECG Count pulse	Bradycardia: Atropine Pacemaker Tachycardia: Digitalis Lidocaine Electroversion

From Hardy JD: Textbook of Surgery, Philadelphia, 1983, J.B. Lippincott, p. 54, with permission.

(2) Allows calculation of arteriovenous oxygen content difference (A-VDO$_2$) and physiologic shunt (Qsp/Qt), which is helpful in the management of respiratory failure (see Appendix).

e. Permits accurate, reproducible measurement of cardiac output by thermodilution technique.

f. Permits monitoring of right ventricular filling pressure through the CVP access port.

g. Evaluation of myocardial function–preload, contractility, and afterload (Table 1).

(1) Myocardial perfusion pressure can be estimated from the difference between systemic diastolic pressure and pulmonary capillary wedge pressure (PWCP).

(2) Heart rate and systolic pressure can be combined to provide a "time tension index."

(3) Systemic vascular resistance (SVR) as an estimation of aortic impedence (afterload) can be calculated.

(4) Effect of therapeutic interventions can be quantitated in terms of physiologic cost.

h. Specialized pulmonary artery catheter permits atrial, ventricular, or sequential A-V pacing simultaneously.

2. Clinical indications for PA catheter–myocardial infarction, acute respiratory failure, sepsis, peritonitis, multiple trauma, noncardiogenic pulmonary edema, near-drowning, overdoses, pulmonary edema in pregnancy, fat emboli, and elderly or critically ill patients undergoing non-cardiac surgical procedures (see "Pre-operative Preparation").

3. Pitfalls.

a. Pulmonary capillary wedge pressure (PCWP) is at best an estimation of LV filling pressures. The gold standard for measuring preload is LV end-diastolic volume, which is not practical clinically. PWCP is an extrapolation of left atrial pressure, which in turn is an estimate of LV end-diastolic pressure. Thus, in cardiac disease states with changes in myocardial compliance or valvular function, PCWP may be an inaccurate estimation of preload.

b. Catheter artifact (whip) and high PEEP's may produce inaccrate measurements.

c. Catheters may be difficult to "float" in patients with cardiomegaly or low cardiac output. Placing patient upright and with the left side down may alleviate this problem

d. Arrhythmias during insertion include ventricular irritability (PVC's and V-tach) and right bundle branch block. Catheter placement in a patient with previous left bundle branch block may produce complete heart block. If pulmonary artery monitoring is essential, preparation for emergency pacing should be made.

4. Method of insertion (see "Vascular Access Techniques").

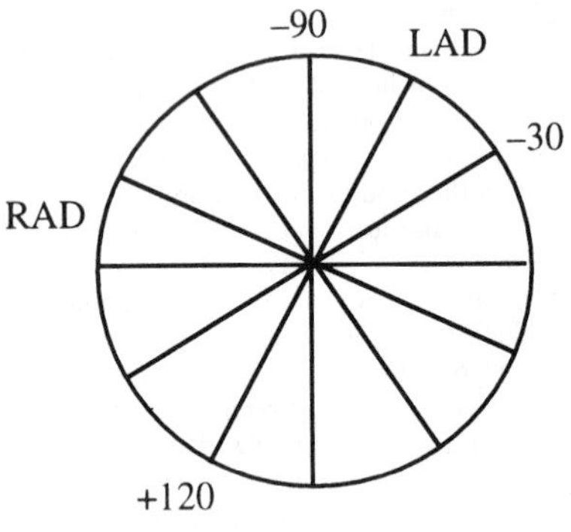

FIG. 1

IV. CARDIAC MONITORING

Surgeons should be versed in basic ECG interpretation and dysrhythmia recognition.

A. Rate—at a standard paper speed of 25 mm/sec, each 5-mm block is 0.2 sec in duration. Bradycardia is < 60 BPM (beats per min), whereas tachycardia is > 100 BPM.

B. Rhythm—cardiac rhythm is described as *regular* or *irregular*.

C. Axis (Figure 1)–an estimate of the cardiac axis can be obtained from line leads I and AVF:

1. Normal axis is between +120° and −30°. The QRS complex will be positive (above the isoelectric line) in I and AVF (+I, +AVF).
2. LAD (left axis deviation) is −30° to −90°; QRS is positive in lead I and negative (below isoelectric line) in AVF (+I, −AVF).
3. RAD (right axis deviation) is +120° to −90°; QRS is negative in I, and above or below isoelectric line in AVF (−I, +/-AVF).
4. Alternatively, the mean cardiac axis will be perpendicular to a frontal QRS complex with a net amplitude of ZERO.

D. Waves, intervals, and segments—by analyzing the"PQRST" complex in systematic fashion, EKG interpretation is simplified, and pathology can be readily identified.

1. ***P waves.***
   a. Reflect electrical activity of the atria. Abnormalities include "P pulmonale" or tall P wave (> 2.5 mm) in lead II, III, AVF. This reflects RA pathology in conditions such as pulmonary hypertension, COPD, pulmonary embolus, and tricuspid stenosis or insufficiency.
   b. "P mitrale" is wide P waves (> .10 sec) in lead II, or a notched P wave in lead VI. Left atrial pathology, secondary to mitral stenosis or regurgitation, may cause P mitrale.

2. ***P-R interval***—normally 0.12 to 0.20 sec, but may be as long as 0.14 sec in young individuals. A-V block is reflected in the P-R interval.
   a. First degree–delayed A-V conduction, with prolonged P-R.
   b. Second degree.
      (1) "Type I" (Wenckebach)–P-R interval is progressively prolonged until a QRS complex is dropped.
      (2) "Type II"–P-R intervals are constant, but QRS complexes are unexpectedly dropped.
   c. Third degree–atrial and ventricular activity are independent. Conduction is interrupted. Also termed "complete" heart block.
3. QRS complex–reflects ventricular activity. Normal QRS width is up to .09 sec.
   a. **LVH**–increased leftward forces result in large R waves in leads I, AVL, V_5 and V_6 ("large" = > 20 mm high in limb leads and > 30 mm in precordial leads). Inverted T waves and depressed ST segments accompany this finding, which is called a "strain" pattern.
   b. **RVH**–increased rightward forces lead to large S waves in I, AVL, V_5 and V_6, as well as tall R waves in V_1 and/or V_2. Again, an "RV strain" pattern is manifested as inverted T waves and depressed ST segments in leads with dominant R waves.
   c. **LBBB**–a mid-conduction delay causes prolonged ventricular depolarization in left bundle branch block; the QRS interval will be > 0.12 sec. Note that ventricular hypertrophy criteria are invalid if LBBB is present (see above). The following are seen in LBBB:
      (1) Broad R waves in I, AVL, V_5 and V_6.
      (2) Broad S waves in V_1 and/or V_2.
      (3) Absent septal Q waves in I, AVL, V_5 and V_6.
   d. **RBBB**–a terminal delay in ventricular conduction results in characteristic changes. Again, the QRS is > 0.12 sec in duration, and has:
      (1) Broad R waves in V_1.
      (2) Broad S waves in I, AVL, V_5 and V_6.
   e. Incomplete block defined as QRS between 0.10-0.12 sec in duration.
4. ***ST segment changes***—may be the only changes seen in infarction or ischemia.
   a. ST depression seen in subendocardial infarction, myocardial ischemia, and in patients on digitalis.
   b. ST elevation seen in transmural infarction, LV aneurysm, and pericarditis.
5. ***T waves***—this indicator of depolarization changes the morphology in several clinical settings.
   a. Ventricular hypertrophy (see above).
   b. Transient ischemia.

c. Late transmural infarction.
d. High/low serum potassium.

V. DYSRHYTHMIAS: RECOGNITION AND MANAGEMENT

A. Bradycardia (rate < 60 beats/min).

1. *Sinus bradycardia.*
   a. Decreased rate from within the sinus node (disease; increased parasympathetic tone; drugs: digitalis or β-blockers).
   b. Rhythm–regular.
   c. **Therapy**–immediate treatment required only when accompanied by hypotension, angina, dyspnea, altered mental status, myocardial ischemia, or ventricular ectopy.
2. ***Second-degree A-V block, Möbitz Type I (Wenckebach)*** occurs at level of A-V node and is often due to increased parasympathetic tone or drug effect (digitalis, propranolol). Usually transient. Characterized by progressive prolongation of the PR interval, which is indicative of decreasing conduction velocity through the A-V node before an impulse is completely blocked. Usually only a single impulse is blocked; then the cycle is repeated. The atrial rhythm is usually regular. There is no risk of progression to complete heart block.
3. ***Second-degree A-V block, Möbitz Type II*** occurs below level of A-V node either at the bundle of His (uncommon) or bundle branch level. Associated with an organic lesion in the conduction pathway. Poor prognosis; the development of complete heart block should be anticipated. The P-R interval does not lengthen prior to a dropped beat. Atrial rhythm is usually regular. Placement of a transvenous pacemaker is usually required.

B. Sinus tachycardia.

1. Increased rate within sinus node from demands for higher cardiac output (exercise, fever, anxiety).
2. Rate ≥ 100.
3. P wave–upright in I, II, AVF.
4. ***Therapy***— usually none, other than to treat underlying cause. In older patients with cardiac disease, beta blockers or calcium channel blockers may be needed acutely to prevent the increase in myocardial oxygen demand that occurs at high heart rates.

C. Paroxysmal supraventricular tachycardia (PSVT)/ paroxysmal atrial tachycardia (PAT).

1. Sudden onset of tachycardia originating in atria, lasting minutes to hours.
2. Rate–atrial rate 160-200.
3. Rhythm–regular.
4. P waves–may not be present (i.e., buried in previous T wave).
5. P-R–normal or prolonged.
6. QRS–normal with rapid rate.

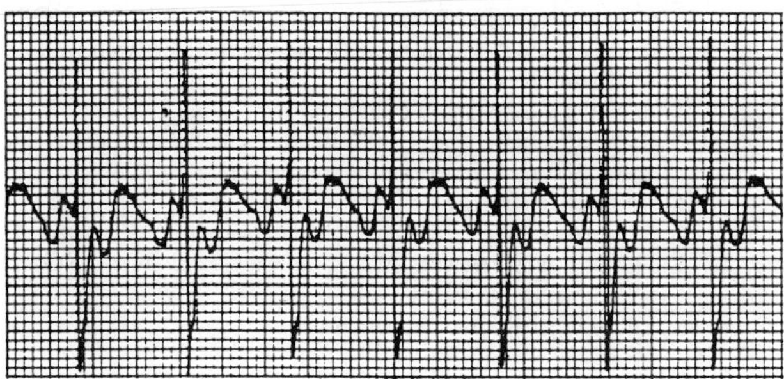

FIG. 2 **Atrial Flutter** (From Textbook of Advanced Cardiac Life Support, 1994, copyright American Heart Association, p. 3-12.)

7. RBBB or less often LBBB with PAT/SVT may appear like ventricular tachycardia, but can be discerned by presence of P waves and BBB.
8. ***Therapy.***
   a. For symptomatic (unstable) patients, use low-voltage DC cardioversion.
   b. For stable patients, initially try vagal maneuvers. If unsuccessful, intravenous diltiazem, verapamil, or adenosine (Adenocard®) is indicated.
   c. If conversion occurs but PSVT recurs, repeated electrical cardioversion is *not* indicated. Sedation should be used as time permits.
   d. Other therapies may include α-receptor stimulation (phenylephrine 30-60 mg/500 ml D_5W to raise systolic BP 30-40 mm Hg in patients who are not significantly hypertensive) or edrophonium 1 mg IV; if no response, use up to 10 mg and watch for bronchospasm.

D. Premature atrial contraction (PAC).

1. Originates in atria, not in sinus node. May be caused by stimulants (caffeine, tobacco, ETOH), drugs, hypoxia, digitalis intoxication.
2. Rate–variable.
3. Rhythm–irregular.
4. P wave–abnormal, premature; may be buried in preceding T.
5. P-R–normal or prolonged (PAC with first-degree A-V block).
6. QRS–normal or wide if aberrancy (usually RBBB). QRS absent with complete block.
7. ***Therapy***—discontinue stimulating factor (drug), correct hypoxia.

E. Atrial flutter (Figure 2).

Atrial rate is 250/min and rhythm is regular. Every other F (flutter) wave is conducted to ventricles (2:1 block), resulting in regular ventricular rhythm at rate of 125/min.

1. F-wave", "sawtooth", or "picket-fence" waves between QRS complexes with varying conduction ratios, best seen in leads II, III, and AVF. Seen in organic heart disease (mitral or tricuspid valve) or coronary disease.
2. Rate–atrial rate about 300/min (220-350); ventricular rate about 150/min, but varies with ratio (2:1, 3:1, etc.).
3. Rhythm–atrial regular.
4. P waves–absent.
5. Flutter waves between QRS complexes. *Hint:* Turn EKG upside down to see waves.
6. QRS–normal, may be aberrant.
7. ***Therapy.***
   a. If clinically symptomatic (hemodynamically), low-voltage DC countershock.
   b. Drugs to increase degree of A-V block (digitalis, propranolol).
   c. Overdrive pacemaker–atrial pacing at a rate faster than the intrinsic atrial rate may result in the conversion of atrial flutter to NSR or to atrial fibrillation.
   d. Watch for development of atrial fibrillation with digitalis or pacing.

F. Atrial fibrillation [Figure 3].

1. Originates from multiple areas within atria, with only a small area of depolarization. Multiple causes, including valvular heart disease, pulmonary embolus, digitalis intoxication, pulmonary disease, electrolyte abnormalities, and idiopathic causes.
2. Rate–atrial rate 400-700 (may not be clearly seen); ventricular rate 60-180 (variable).
3. Rhythm–irregularly irregular.
4. P waves–absent.
5. QRS–normal.
6. ***Therapy.***
   a. Digoxin to prolong A-V conduction.
   b. Synchronized DC cardioversion if clinically significant (pulmonary edema, low BP). Precautions include holding digoxin 24-48 h if possible, normalizing potassium and renal function, and stopping if ventricular arrhythmias occur.
   c. Quinidine, procainamide.
   d. Propranolol.

G. Premature ventricular complex (PVC) [Figure 4].

1. Early depolarization arising within a ventricle from one or more sites. Ventricles depolarize sequentially, followed by a compensatory pause (usually twice the regular sinus interval).
2. Rate–variable.
3. Rhythm–variable, irregular.
4. P wave–usually obscured in previous S or T wave, or may be present.
5. QRS–prolonged, bizarre $\geq$ 0.12 sec. Complexes may have different appearances with different ectopic sites.

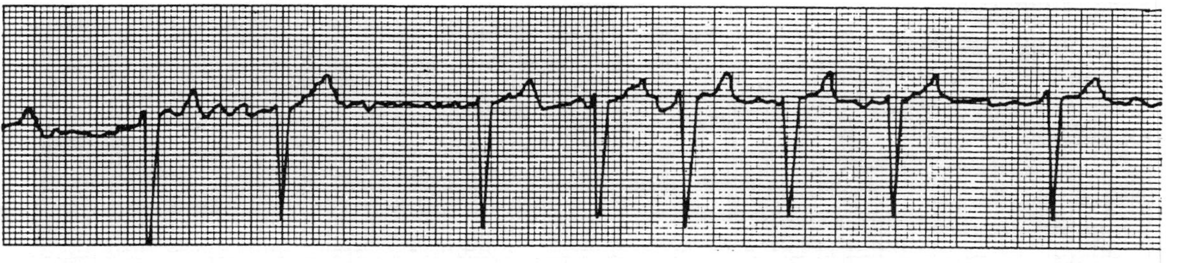

FIG. 3 **Atrial Fibrillation** (From Textbook of Advanced Cardiac Life Support, 1994, copyright American Heart Association, p. 3-11.)

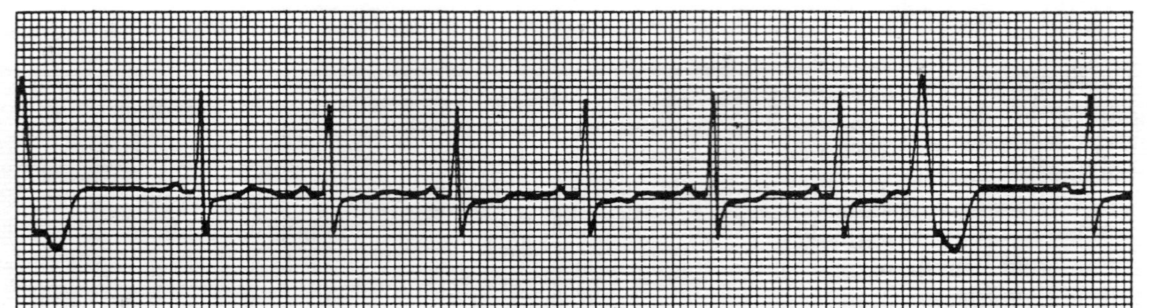

FIG. 4 Premature Ventricular Complex (From Textbook of Advanced Cardiac Life Support, 1994, copyright American Heart Association, p. 3-8.)

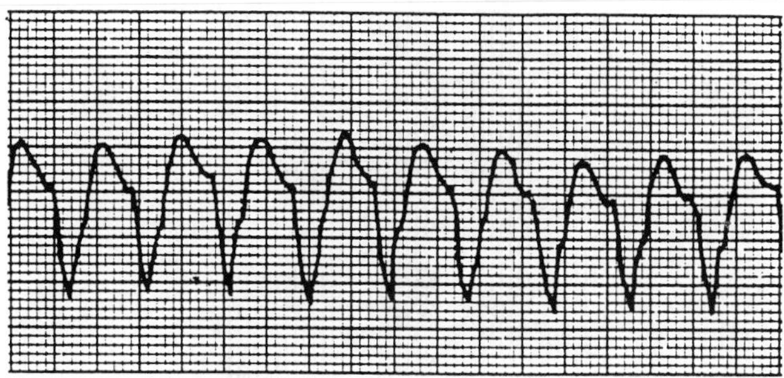

FIG. 5 Ventricular Tachycardia (From Textbook of Advanced Cardiac Life Support, 1994, copyright American Heart Association, p. 3-6.)

6. ST segments–slope away from QRS (inverted).
7. T waves–inverted.
8. Variations.
   a. Bigeminy–alternating normal beats and PVCs.
   b. Trigeminy–every third beat is a PVC.
   c. R-on-T–PVC falls on previous T wave; is especially dangerous because it may precipitate ventricular tachycardia or ventricular fibrillation.
9. ***Therapy.***
   a. Acute treatment for frequent or multifocal PVCs is usually a lidocaine drip, titrated to maintain suppression.
   b. Procainamide is recommended if lidocaine is unsuccessful. Bretylium is then used if ectopy continues or progresses to ventricular tachycardia.

H. Ventricular tachycardia (VT) [Figure 5].

1. Three or more PVCs together; may or may not cause clinical symptoms.
2. Rate–$\geq$ 100; usually $\leq$ 220.
3. Rhythm–variable, usually regular.
4. P waves–may or may not be present.
5. QRS–wide; usually no Q in $V_{5,6}$.
6. Fusion beats–early sinus-like, later like PVC. These occur prior to and at the end of a run of ventricular tachycardia; thus, are characteristic.
7. ***Therapy.***
   a. Stable patient–lidocaine, followed by cardioversion if not successful.
   b. Unstable patient–epinepherine, followed by cardioversion.
8. Unstable–symptoms (e.g., chest pain, dyspnea), hypotension (systolic BP < 90 mm Hg), CHF, ischemia, or infarction.

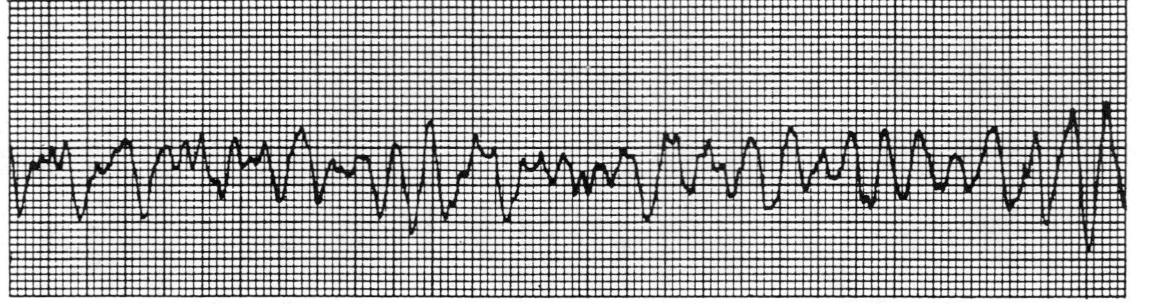

FIG. 6 Ventricular Fibrillation (Coarse) (From Textbook of Advanced Cardiac Life Support, 1994, copyright American Heart Association, p. 3-5.)

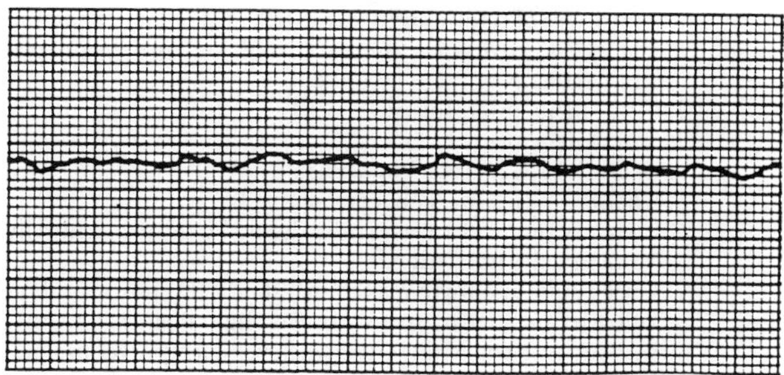

FIG. 7 Ventricular Fibrillation (Fine) (From Textbook of Advanced Cardiac Life Support, 1994, copyright American Heart Association, p. 3-5.)

9. If patient becomes unstable at any time, move to "unstable" arm of algorithm (see Appendix).
10. Sedation should be considered for all patients, including those defined as unstable, except those who are hemodynamically unstable (e.g., hypotensive, in pulmonary edema, or unconscious).
11. If hemodynamically stable, a precordial thump may be employed prior to cardioversion.
12. Once VT has resolved, begin IV infusion of the antiarrhythmic agent that has aided resolution of the VT. If hemodynamically unstable, use lidocaine if cardioversion alone is unsuccessful, followed by bretylium. In all other patients, the recommended order of therapy is lidocaine, procainamide, and then bretylium.

I. Torsade de pointes.

1. A form of ventricular tachycardia characterized by gradual alteration in the amplitude and direction of the electrical activity.
2. Treated differently than other types of VT.
   a. Electrical pacing is treatment of choice.
   b. Bretylium, magnesium sulfate + isoproterenol and lidocaine have been reported as effective.
   c. Quinidine-like drugs are *contraindicated*.
3. Polymorphic VT (PVT) can masquerade as *torsade de pointes*—pay close attention to the length of the QT interval of complexes preceding the tachycardia.
   a. When QT interval is long, pacing is indicated.
   b. If QT interval is normal, the arrhythmia is more likely to be PVT and may therefore respond to antiarrhythmic drugs.

J. Ventricular fibrillation (Figures 6 & 7).

1. Multiple areas of ectopic ventricular activity, but no effective contraction of the heart; hence, no cardiac output. It is a com-

mon cause of cardiac arrest due to ischemia or infarction. Amplitude of activity determines "coarse" *vs.* "fine" ventricular fibrillation.
2. Rate–rapid, disorganized.
3. Rhythm–none.
4. P, QRS, ST, T waves all undefinable.
5. ***Therapy*** — cardioversion, epinephrine.
6. Pulseless ventricular tachycardia should be treated identically to ventricular fibrillation.
7. Check pulse and rhythm after each shock. If ventricular fibrillation recurs after transiently converting (rather than persists without ever converting), use whatever energy level has previously been successful for defibrillation.
8. The value of sodium bicarbonate is questionable during cardiac arrest, and it is *not* recommended for the routine cardiac arrest sequence. Consideration of its use in a dose of 1 mEq/kg is appropriate at the point noted in the algorithm. One-half of the original dose may be repeated q 10 min if it is used.

K. Ventricular asystole (agonal rhythm).
1. No effective electrical activity, resulting in no cardiac contraction.
2. P waves, QRS, ST, T waves may appear in ever-increasing intervals until no impulses or only isolated impulses are seen.
3. Asystole should be confirmed in two leads.

L. Pulseless electical activity (PEA)—formerly known as electrical-mechanical dissociation (EMD)—electrical activity (usually QRS-type activity) depicted on EKG, but no pulse. Consider possible causes:
1. Hypovolemia–volume infusion.
2. Hypoxia–ventilation.
3. Cardiac tamponade–pericardiocentesis.
4. Tension pneumothorax–needle decompression followed by thoracostomy tube.
5. Hypothermia–warming.
6. Massive pulmonary embolism–surgery, thrombolytics.
7. Drug overdoses such as tricyclics, digitalis.
8. Hyperkalemia.
9. Acidosis–sodium bicarbonate.
10. Massive myocardial infarction.

APPENDIX A: FORMULAS UTILIZED IN CARDIOPULMONARY CRITICAL CARE

1. **Mean arterial pressure (MAP):**
   MAP = DP + 1/3 (SP-DP) [normal = 80-90 Torr]
2. **Stroke volume (SV):**
   SV = CO/HR [normal = 50-60 ml]
3. **Cardiac index (CI):**
   CI = CO/BSA [normal = 3.5-4 ICU population]

4. **Stroke index (SI):**
SI = SV/BSA [normal = 35-40 ICU population]
5. **Right ventricular stroke work (RVSW):**
RVSW = SV x (MPA-CVP) x .0136 [normal = 10-15 g/meters]
6. **Left ventricular stroke work (LVSW):**
LVSW = SV x (MAP-PAO) x .0136 [normal = 60-80 g/meters]
Ratio = LVSW/PAO
7. **Systemic vascular resistance (SVR)** (also referred to in the literature as total peripheral resistance):
$SVR = \frac{(MAP\text{-}CVP) \times 80}{CO}$ [normal = 800-1200 dynes/sec/cm^{-5}]
8. **Pulmonary vascular resistance (PVR):**
$PVR = \frac{(MPA\text{-}PAO) \times 80}{CO}$ [normal = 100-200 dynes/sec/cm^{-5}]
9. **Myocardial oxygen consumption** (correlate–a fair calculated measure of how much O_2 the heart is requiring):
$MVO_2C = \frac{SP \times HR}{100}$ [higher values = greater consumption]
10. **Alveolar PO_2:**
$P_AO_2 = (P_B\text{-}P_{H2O})\ FiO_2 - P_ECO_2/R$
P_B = Barometric pressure (760 mm Hg at sea level).
P_{H2O} (at body temp.) = 47 mm Hg.
$P_ECO_2 \approx P_ACO2$.
R = 0.8 (assumed).
Thus: $P_AO_2 = (760\text{-}47)\ FiO_2 - PaCO_2/0.8$
11. **Capillary O_2 content:**
$Cc'_{O2} = (P_AO_2) \times .0031) + Hb \times 1.39 \times 1$
(assumes 100% Hb sat.) [normal = 18.3 ml/100 ml]
12. **Mixed venous O_2 content:**
$Cv_{O2} = Pv_{O2} \times .0031 + (Hb \times 1.39 \times \text{Ven. Sat.})$ [normal = 13 ml/100 ml]
13. **Arterial O_2 content:**
$Ca_{O2} = Pa_{O2} \times .0031 + (Hb \times 1.39 \times \text{Art. Sat.})$ [normal = 18 ml/100 ml]
14. **O_2 delivery:**
O_2 Del = C_A x CO x 10 [normal = 1000 ml/min]
15. **A-V O_2 difference ($A\text{-}V_{DO2}$):**
$A\text{-}V_{DO2}$ = Ca – Cv [normal = 3.5-4.5 ml/100 ml]
16. **O_2 consumption:**
O_2 Cons = (Ca – Cv) x CO x 10 [normal = 250 ml/min]
17. **O_2 utilization:**
% Util = Ca – Cv/Ca [normal = 0.2-0.25]
18. **Shunt (intrapulmonary):**
$Qsp/Qt = \frac{Cc'O_2 - CaO_2}{Cc'O_2 - CvO_2}$ [normal < 0.10]
19. **Body surface area (BSA):**
Use DuBois' BSA chart (see Reference Data)

APPENDIX B: ARRHYTHMIA TREATMENT ALGORITHMS

(From *JAMA* 259:2946-2949, 1986, with permission.)

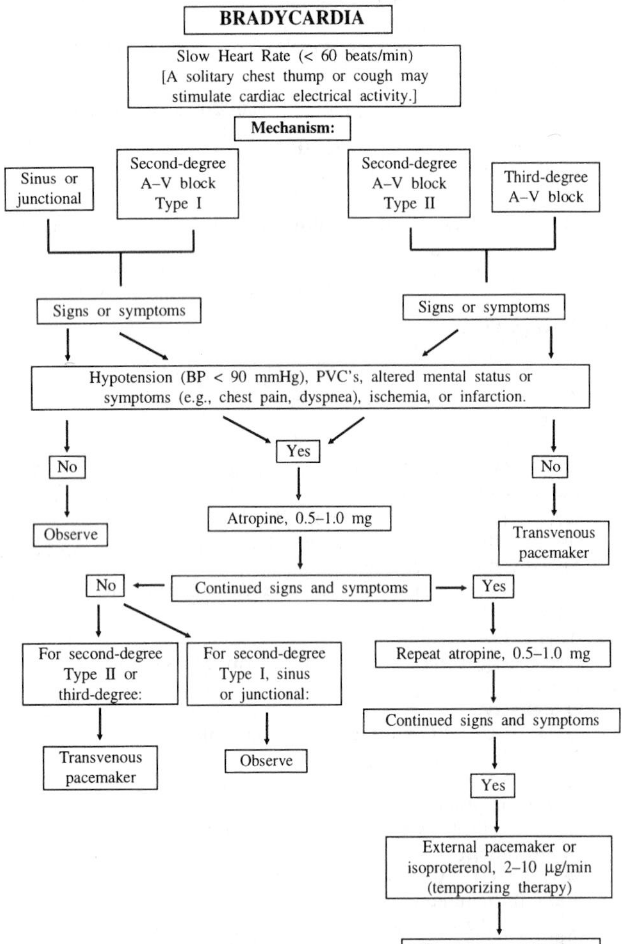

PREMATURE VENTRICULAR CONTRACTION

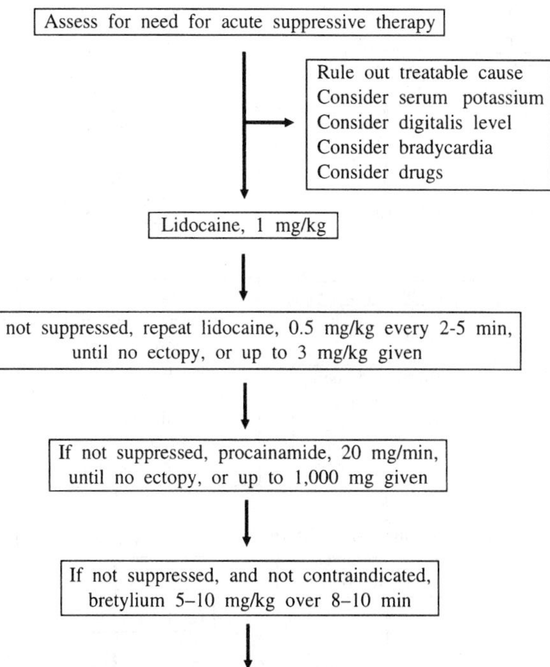

Once ectopy resolved, maintain as follows:

- After lidocaine, 1 mg/kg . . . lidocaine drip, 2 mg/min
- After lidocaine, 1–2 mg/kg . . . lidocaine drip, 3 mg/min
- After lidocaine, 2–3 mg/kg . . . lidocaine drip, 4 mg/min
- After procainamide . . . procainamide drip, 1–4 mg/min (check blood level)
- After bretylium . . . bretylium drip, 2 mg/min

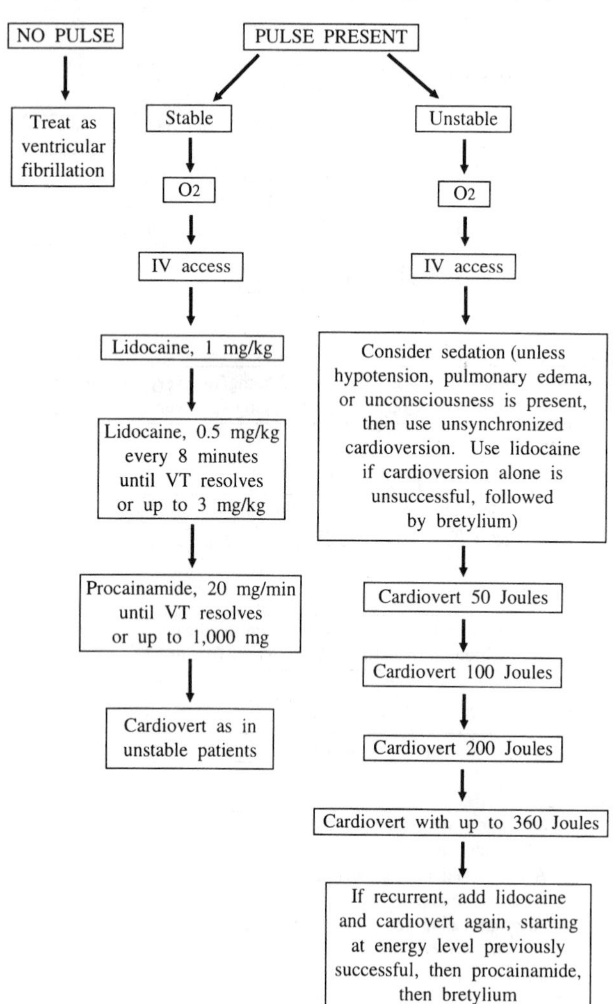
SUSTAINED VENTRICULAR TACHYCARDIA
NO PULSE
Treat as ventricular fibrillation
PULSE PRESENT
Stable
O2
IV access
Lidocaine, 1 mg/kg
Lidocaine, 0.5 mg/kg every 8 minutes until VT resolves or up to 3 mg/kg
Procainamide, 20 mg/min until VT resolves or up to 1,000 mg
Cardiovert as in unstable patients
Unstable
O2
IV access
Consider sedation (unless hypotension, pulmonary edema, or unconsciousness is present, then use unsynchronized cardioversion. Use lidocaine if cardioversion alone is unsuccessful, followed by bretylium)
Cardiovert 50 Joules
Cardiovert 100 Joules
Cardiovert 200 Joules
Cardiovert with up to 360 Joules
If recurrent, add lidocaine and cardiovert again, starting at energy level previously successful, then procainamide, then bretylium

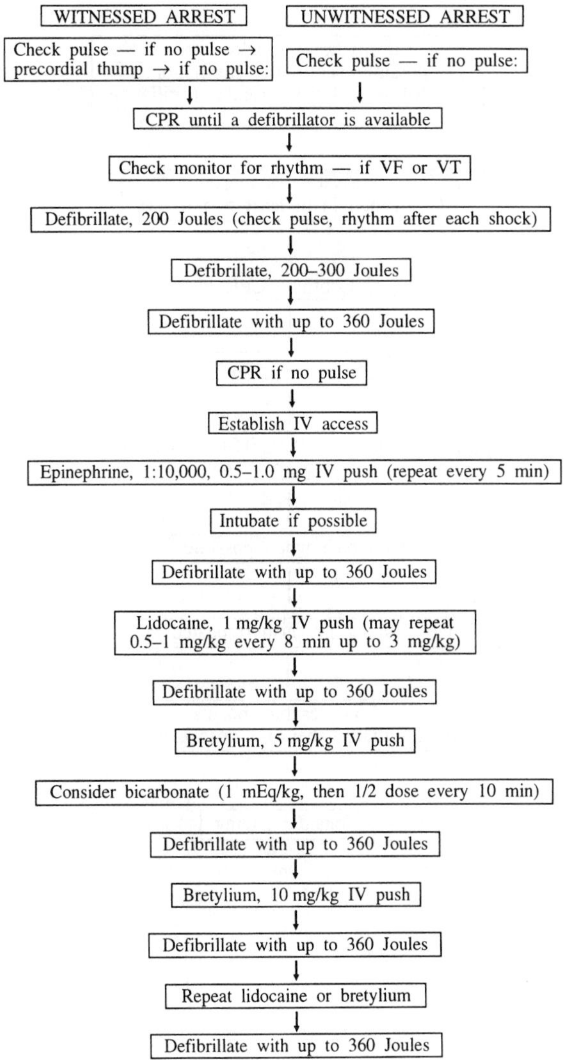
VENTRICULAR FIBRILLATION
WITNESSED ARREST
UNWITNESSED ARREST
Check pulse — if no pulse → precordial thump → if no pulse:
Check pulse — if no pulse:
CPR until a defibrillator is available
Check monitor for rhythm — if VF or VT
Defibrillate, 200 Joules (check pulse, rhythm after each shock)
Defibrillate, 200–300 Joules
Defibrillate with up to 360 Joules
CPR if no pulse
Establish IV access
Epinephrine, 1:10,000, 0.5–1.0 mg IV push (repeat every 5 min)
Intubate if possible
Defibrillate with up to 360 Joules
Lidocaine, 1 mg/kg IV push (may repeat 0.5–1 mg/kg every 8 min up to 3 mg/kg)
Defibrillate with up to 360 Joules
Bretylium, 5 mg/kg IV push
Consider bicarbonate (1 mEq/kg, then 1/2 dose every 10 min)
Defibrillate with up to 360 Joules
Bretylium, 10 mg/kg IV push
Defibrillate with up to 360 Joules
Repeat lidocaine or bretylium
Defibrillate with up to 360 Joules

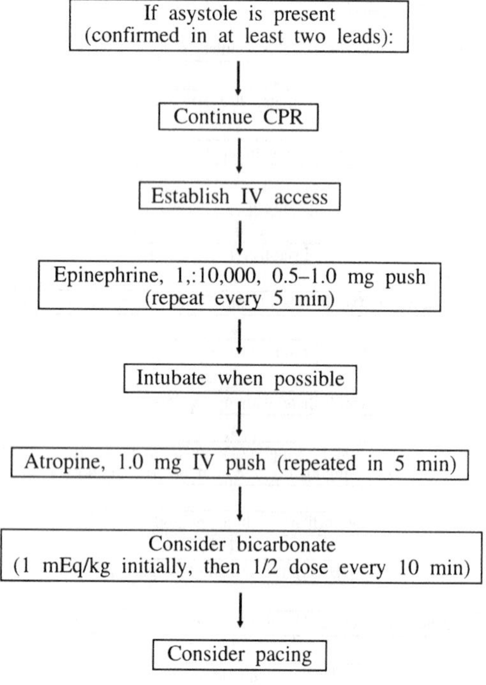
VENTRICULAR ASYSTOLE
If rhythm is unclear and possibly ventricular fibrillation, defibrillate as for ventricular fibrillation.
If asystole is present (confirmed in at least two leads):
Continue CPR
Establish IV access
Epinephrine, 1,:10,000, 0.5–1.0 mg push (repeat every 5 min)
Intubate when possible
Atropine, 1.0 mg IV push (repeated in 5 min)
Consider bicarbonate (1 mEq/kg initially, then 1/2 dose every 10 min)
Consider pacing

ELECTROMECHANICAL DISSOCIATION

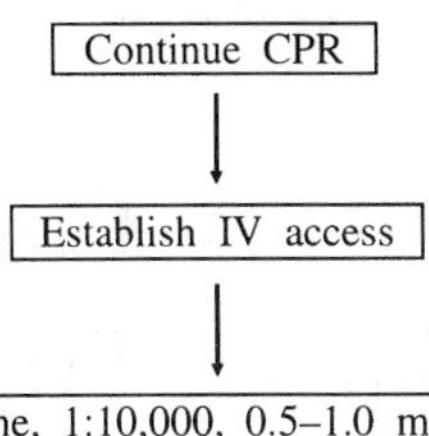

↓

Epinephrine, 1:10,000, 0.5–1.0 mg IV push (should be repeated every 5 min)

↓

Intubate when possible (If intubation can be accomplished simultaneously with other techniques, then the earlier the better; however, epinephrine is more important initially if the patient can be ventilated without intubation.)

↓

Consider bicarbonate (The value of sodium bicarbonate is questionable during cardiac arrest and is not recommended for the routine cardiac arrest sequence. Consideration of its use in a dose of 1 mEq/kg is appropriate at this point. One-half of the original dose may be repeated every 10 min if it is used.)

↓

Consider hypovolemia, cardiac tamponade, tension pneumothorax, hypoxemia, acidosis, pulmonary embolism

10

Respiratory Care and Ventilatory Support

David A. Rodeberg, M.D.

I. PRE-OPERATIVE EVALUATION

A. History.

1. Exercise intolerance, dyspnea at rest or exertion–unable to climb two flights of stairs.
2. Cigarette smoking–risk proportional to pack-years.
3. Cough–sputum production.
4. Age > 60 years.
5. Previous diagnosis of chronic obstructive pulmonary disease (COPD), asthma, fibrosis, silicosis, heart failure.

B. Physical examination.

1. Wheezing.
2. Rales.
3. Rhonchi.
4. Obesity.
5. Clubbing/cyanosis.
6. Tobacco stains.

C. Operative risk factors.

1. Anesthesia > 3.5 h.
2. Upper abdominal or thoracic incisions.
3. Use of nasogastric tube peri-operatively.

D. Pre-operative laboratory evaluation.

1. Chest radiograph.
   a. Any patient with pulmonary abnormality detected on history and physical, undergoing thoracotomy, or > 40 years old.
   b. Observe for bullae, hyperexpanded lungs (flat diaphragms), CHF (perivascular cuffing, Kerley b lines, edema), pneumonia, opacifications, atelectasis.
2. Pulmonary Function Test (PFT)–any patient with risk factors

detected by history and physical exam, or undergoing thoracotomy.

a. If lung volume and flow are normal range, risk is minimal.
b. Values < 70% or > 120% of predicted normal indicate problems.
c. Need to be performed with and without bronchodilators.
d. Important values.
   (1) TV–tidal volume–normal quiet breathing ≈ 0.5 L.
   (2) FRC–functional residual capacity–volume of lung after quiet expiration ≈ 3 L.
   (3) VC–vital capacity–volume from maximal inspiration to maximal expiration ≈ 4 L.
   (4) FVC–forced vital capacity.
   (5) FEV1.0–forced expiratory volume in 1 sec.
   (6) MVV–maximal voluntary ventilation over 1 min.
   (7) D_LO_2–diffusing capacity of the lung for oxygen.
e. Types of lung pathology.
   (1) Restrictive–reduction of lung volumes due to decreased compliance. Causes:
      a) Extrinsic–skeletal deformity, space-occupying lesions in chest cavity, obesity, extensive pleural scar, previous thoracotomy.
      b) Intrinsic–deposition of material in alveoli or interstitium that decreases pulmonary compliance (e.g., interstitial fibrosis, interstitial edema, silicosis, or granulomatous disease).
      c) Muscular weakness (e.g., myasthenia gravis, polio).
   (2) Obstructive–reduction of airflow due to airway narrowing. Causes:
      a) Asthma–intermittent reversible obstruction.
      b) Bronchitis–obstruction secondary to thickening of bronchial walls.
      c) Emphysema–airway collapse on expiration secondary to destruction of alveolar walls.
      d) Mixed–COPD connotes a mixed disorder that may include all three of the above components.
   (3) Diffusion defects–inability of gas to diffuse from alveoli to capillary. Causes:
      a) Loss of alveolar membranes (emphysema).
      b) Thickening of membranes (fibrosis, granuloma, edema, silicosis, etc.)
      c) Decrease in ventilation or perfusion.
      d) Removal of a portion of lung.
f. MVV is greatest indicator of pulmonary reserve, and a value < 50% of predicted normal is best correlate of post-operative pulmonary complications.

3. ABG–baseline for post-operative comparison, decision for post-operative ventilatory measure, and collaboration of type/severity lung pathology.

a. pH: < 7.35 or > 7.45–acute process.
7.35-7.45–normal or chronic process.
b. P_aCO_2: > 45 mm Hg–hypoventilation.
< 35 mm Hg–hyperventilation.
c. P_aO_2: < 70 mm Hg–hypoxic.
> 70 mm Hg–not hypoxic.
d. Ventilation/perfusion (V/Q) mismatch–many causes:
(1) V > Q–ventilation of nonperfused tissue (dead space) (i.e., pulmonary embolus).
(2) V < Q–perfusion of nonventilated tissue (shunt)–cannot be improved by increasing inspired O_2 content (F_iO_2) (i.e., atelectasis).

4. V/Q scan–should be performed on patients with compromised pulmonary function who are undergoing lung resection.

	Non-Hypoxic	Hypoxic	
Hyperventilation	Pain—anxiety	Pulmonary embolus Pneumonia ARDS Pulmonary edema Bronchospasm Aspiration Mucous plug	Acute
	Decreased compliance (Fibrosis)	COPD—non CO_2 retainer ARDS	Chronic
Hypoventilation	Always associated with some degree of hypoxia	Narcotics CNS disorder Increased ICP	Acute
		COPD—CO_2 retainer	Chronic

II. PREVENTION

A. Pre-operative.

1. Exercise and training respiratory muscle–incentive spirometry and deep breathing.
2. Quit smoking–requires 8 weeks for risk of complications to reverse; less time may be more detrimental than continued smoking.
3. Loss of excess weight.
4. Bronchodilators if bronchospasm is a problem or if bronchodilators improve PFT results.
5. Treat bronchitis with antibiotics.
6. Inotropic support if congestive heart failure is present.

B. Operative.

1. Use transverse incision if possible.
2. Consider gastrostomy instead of NG tube.

3. Spinal or local anesthesia. If problems are severe, may need to control airway, so use a light general anesthesia combined with epidural.
4. Large (15-20 ml/kg) tidal volumes.
5. Keep IV fluids to a minimum.

C. Post-operative.

1. Deep breathing–negative pressure generated by deep inspiration prevents atelectasis. Frequent ≈ 10-15 min.
2. Clear mucus and sputum–suctioning, mist inhalation, mucolytic agents.
3. Coughing–beneficial in chronic bronchitis, but if lungs are well ventilated, not always needed; only removes debris from ventilated alveoli, not atelectatic areas; very painful.
4. Frequent change of position, early ambulation.
5. Avoid IV or IM narcotics because they suppress respiratory drive–use regional or epidural analgesia for pain control, and consider IM ketoralac (Toradol®).
6. Intermittent positive pressure breathing (IPPB) or continuous positive pressure breathing (CPAP) if the patient is unable to take large breaths.
7. May require prolonged intubation until patient is fully alert, cardiac and vascular fluid status optimized, and patient able to maintain adequate gas exchange spontaneously.
8. Supplemental oxygen should be used if needed but should be used for as short a time as possible and at the lowest concentration needed. *Remember*–in CO_2 retainers the hypoxic drive keeps the patient spontaneously breathing. If you remove this with supplemental O_2, the patient may develop CO_2 narcosis and become apneic.
9. Monitor patient with pulse oximetry.
10. Avoid overfeeding–high carbohydrate meals or excess enteral or parenteral nutrition may cause CO_2 production, which can cause P_aCO_2 accumulation if patient is not able to provide adequate ventilation.

III. PULMONARY INSUFFICIENCY

A. Etiology.

1. After operation, shallow breathing with incomplete alveolar inflation (atelectasis) ⇒ decreased compliance ⇒ increased work of breathing and hypoxemia (due to V/Q mismatch).
2. This is superimposed on the patient's pre-existing pulmonary status.
3. Excessive tracheobronchial debris, aspiration, and fluid overload compound the problem.
4. Pulmonary edema due to increased hydrostatic pressure (fluid overload), decreased intravascular oncotic pressure (malnutrition, large crystalloid fluid replacement), and increased capillary permeability (due to toxic substances of ischemia or infection).

B. Complications.

1. Atelectasis.
2. Pneumonia.
3. Cardiogenic pulmonary edema.
4. Bronchospasm.
5. Aspiration.
6. ARDS.
7. Pulmonary embolism.
8. Mucous plugging.

C. Diagnosis.

1. Syndrome of dyspnea, tachypnea, tachycardia, fever, confusion, cyanosis, suprasternal and intercostal retractions, paradoxical respiration.
2. ABG, chest radiograph.
3. Bronchoscopy.
4. V/Q scan if diagnosis of pulmonary embolus is questioned.

D. Treatment—at all times ask "Does this patient need to be monitored in ICU and/or mechanically ventilated?"

1. Atelectasis.
   a. Incentive spirometry and deep breathing.
   b. Supplemental O_2 and airway humidification.
   c. Pulmonary toilet–nasotracheal suction.
   d. Pain control.
   e. Bronchoscopy for lobar collapse.
2. Pneumonia.
   a. Supplemental O_2.
   b. Appropriate antibiotic.
   c. Pulmonary toilet, percussion, and postural drainage.
   d. May require bronchoscopy.
3. Edema.
   a. Supplemental O_2.
   b. Diuresis.
   c. Negative fluid balance.
   d. Inotropic support (dopamine, dobutamine) as needed.
   e. Pulmonary artery catheterization.
4. Bronchospasm.
   a. Supplemental O_2.
   b. Bronchodilator (albuterol, alupent).
5. Aspiration.
   a. Supplemental O_2.
   b. Bronchodilator.
   c. Bronchoscopy–remove visible debris.
   d. Effects lessened if gastric fluid pH neutral (ranitidine)–controversial. Neutral gastric pH leads to colonization of stomach; some studies suggest that this exacerbates effects of aspiration.
6. Pulmonary embolism.
   a. Supplemental O_2.
   b. V/Q scan–if positive ⇒ treat, if equivocal and clinical suspicion high ⇒ angiogram.

c. Continuous heparin infusion.
d. Vena caval filter if not candidate for anticoagulation.

7. Mucous plugging.
   a. Supplemental O_2.
   b. Humidification, mucolytic and bronchodilator therapy (if indicated).
   c. Nasotracheal suction.
   d. Bronchoscopy.
8. ARDS.
   a. Supplemental O_2.
   b. Pulmonary artery catheterization.
   c. Optimize cardiac and fluid status.
   d. Mechanical ventilation as needed.

IV. MECHANICAL VENTILATION

A. Modes.

1. CMV–Controlled Mechanical Ventilation.
   a. Ventilator delivers only preset tidal volume and respiratory rate.
   b. Patient unable to breathe spontaneously.
   c. Minute ventilation determined solely by preset tidal volume and respiratory rate.
   d. Usually used intra-operatively or with apneic (paralyzed or CNS injured) patients.
   e. Requires heavy sedation or chemical paralysis.
2. ACMV–Assist Controlled Mechanical Ventilation.
   a. Ventilator delivers preset tidal volume when patient initiates a breath. If spontaneous rate is less than the machine backup rate, the ventilator will initiate a breath.
   b. Minute ventilation determined by preset tidal volume, respiratory rate, and patient respiratory rate.
   c. Used in patients with normal brain stem and respiratory center function.
3. IMV–Intermittent Mandatory Ventilation.
   a. Ventilator delivers preset tidal volume and respiratory rate and provides gas for patient spontaneous respiration.
   b. Patient able to breathe spontaneously.
   c. Minute ventilation is combination of preset tidal volume and rate and patient-generated ventilation independent of ventilator.
   d. SIMV–synchronized intermittent mandatory ventilation–tidal volume is delivered as assist control mode breath.
   e. IMV is preferred to ACMV because it allows a lower mean intrathoracic pressure and the patient is allowed to breathe spontaneously, thus preventing disuse muscle atrophy and facilitating weaning. This is a controversial topic among medical and surgical intensivists.
4. PS–Pressure Support.
   a. Ventilator delivers gas at preset pressure only when initiated by patient.

b. Minute ventilation determined by patient's respiratory rate and tidal volume.
c. Decreases the inspiratory effort to generate the tidal volume.
d. Helpful in prolonged or difficult weaning.

B. Ventilator types.

1. Time-cycled ventilator.
   a. Timed delivery of gas flow; tidal volume = flow rate x inspiratory time.
   b. Delivers relatively constant tidal volume to ventilator circuit.
   c. Allows precise control and variability in waveform of delivered gas.
2. Volume-cycled ventilator.
   a. Inspiratory gas flow terminated after pre-selected volume delivered into circuit–regardless of pressure generated.
   b. Pressure in circuit determined by tidal volume and lung compliance. Patient-delivered tidal volume varies with changes in pressure (compliance).
3. Pressure-cycled ventilator.
   a. Gas flow continued until preset pressure developed.
   b. Tidal volume = flow rate x time until pressure is reached.
   c. Variable volume if circuit pressure varies (changes in compliance).
   d. Lower peak airway pressures than volume cycled–usually requires longer inspiratory times.
4. High-frequency ventilators.
   a. Types.
      (1) High-frequency positive pressure ventilation.
      (2) Jet ventilation.
      (3) Flow interruption.
      (4) Oscillation.
      (5) Percussive ventilation.
   b. Physiologic effects.
      (1) Lower mean airway pressure. *Note:* The site of pressure measurement is important to avoid unintentional PEEP.
      (2) Cardiac output–no clear benefit.
      (3) Lung volume–increased.
      (4) Mucociliary clearance–increased.
   c. Clinical indications.
      (1) Closed head injury–maintains lower intracranial pressure.
      (2) Large pulmonary air leaks/flail chest with contusions–presents as over-PEEPing undamaged lung.
      (3) Refractory respiratory failure.

C. Criteria for initiation of ventilatory support.

1. Inadequate ventilation.
   a. Apnea.

b. Deteriorating alveolar ventilation.
   (1) Increasing P_aCO_2 (>50 mm Hg).
   (2) Decreasing pH (<7.25).
c. Result from increased airway resistance, neuro- or muscular impairment, or decreased respiratory drive.

2. Inadequate oxygenation.
   a. Decreasing P_aO_2.
      (1) P_aO_2 <70 mm Hg on 50% O_2 mask.
      (2) P_aO_2 <55 mm Hg on room air.
   b. Result of venous admixture (shunt) due to ventilation/perfusion (V/Q) mismatch (edema, pneumonia, atelectasis).
3. Tracheal intubation.
   a. Impaired airway patency.
   b. Inadequate airway protection.
   c. Inadequate pulmonary toilet.
4. Common clinical entities requiring ventilatory support.
   a. Severe pulmonary edema.
   b. Suspected or impending ARDS (sepsis, shock, prolonged hypotension, massive transfusion, severe pancreatitis, head trauma, multiple trauma).
   c. Massive resuscitation in the face of multiple trauma.
   d. Severe chest trauma (flail chest, pulmonary contusion).
   e. COPD/bronchospasm.
   f. Decreased mental status (lack respiratory drive, airway protection).
   g. Aspiration of gastric contents.
   h. Pneumonia.
   i. Inhalation injury (chemical or smoke).

D. Operation of the conventional mechanical ventilator.

1. Control variables.
   a. F_iO_2–fraction of inspired gas that is O_2.
      (1) Ideally maintained to < 50% to avoid O_2 toxicity.
      (2) Maintain hemoglobin saturation > 90%.
   b. V_T–tidal volume.
      (1) Initially 10-15 cc/kg body weight; volumes > 20 cc/kg should be avoided (cause high airway pressures and barotrauma).
      (2) Actual V_T delivered may be different from preset volume due to pulmonary compliance. Always measure exhaled volume.
   c. Ventilatory rate.
      (1) Initial rate 10 breaths/min.
      (2) Rates greater than 20/min should be avoided.
      (3) Ventilatory efficiency decreases as respiratory rate increases (the percentage of minute ventilation that is alveolar ventilation decreases).
   d. PEEP–Positive End Expiratory Pressure.
      (1) Positive airway pressure is maintained at the end of expiration.

(2) Usually begun at 5 cm H_2O and increased in increments of 2-3 cm.
a) Continue to increase PEEP until pulmonary shunt < 15-20% or the P_aO_2/F_iO_2 ratio exceeds 250.
b) Alternatively, adjust PEEP until attaining adequate oxygenation (high saturation > 90%) at non-toxic levels of F_iO_2 (<50%).
(3) Re-expands collapsed alveoli, prevents alveolar collapse by maintaining functional residual capacity (FRC) above the critical closing volume (i.e., volume at which alveolar collapse begins).
(4) Decreases V/Q (ventilation/perfusion) mismatching that results from perfusion of collapsed alveoli (decreases intrapulmonary shunt).
(5) Improves pulmonary compliance and therefore reduces the work of breathing.

e. PIP–Peak Inspiratory Pressure.
(1) Maximum airway pressure.
(2) Usually 20-30 cm H_2O.
(3) Should be kept < 45 cm H_2O to minimize barotrauma.
(4) Influenced by $V_{T,}$ compliance, inspiratory flow rate, inspiratory wave pattern.

f. I/E–Inspiratory/Expiratory times–regulates respiratory rate.
(1) Usually 0.5-3 ratio.
(2) Increased inspiratory time causes improved oxygenation.

g. Inspiratory sighs and holds are generally not needed.

2. Monitoring of ventilated patient.
a. Peripheral O_2 saturation–continuous monitor.
(1) Less reliable below 80% saturation.
(2) Should be correlated with ABG result.
b. End tidal CO_2–continuous monitor. Should be correlated with ABG result.
c. Arterial line–for frequent ABGs.
d. Pulmonary artery catheter.
(1) Indications–PEEP > 15 cm H_2O, cardiac disease, intracranial injury, questionable fluid status.
(2) Mixed venous blood gas.

E. Use of conventional mechanical ventilation.

1. Ventilation–correlates with P_aCO_2. Controlled by $V_{T,}$ respiratory rate, expiratory time. Worsening ventilation (increasing P_aCO_2) corrected by:
a. Increasing RR.
b. Increasing $V_{T.}$
c. Decreasing CO_2 production (reducing muscular activity, improving hypermetabolic state, minimizing exogenous carbohydrate nutritional load).

2. Oxygenation–correlates with P_aO_2.
   a. Controlled by F_iO_2, PEEP, inspiratory time. Worsening ventilation (decreasing P_aO_2) corrected by:
      (1) Increasing PEEP.
      (2) Increasing F_iO_2.
      (3) Increasing inspiratory time.
   b. Oxygen delivery to tissues is determined by cardiac output, Hgb, and O_2 saturation. By increasing those values, O_2 delivery is maximized. Little accomplished by increasing O_2 saturation > 90%.
3. Complications.
   a. Decreased cardiac output secondary to decreased venous return.
      (1) Due to increased intrathoracic pressure (increased PEEP, PIP, mean airway pressure).
      (2) Treat by decreasing PEEP, V_T, PIP, and fluid bolus to increase CVP (must be cautious of edema and CHF).
   b. Pulmonary barotrauma (pneumothorax, pneumomediastinum, subcutaneous emphysema, interstitial emphysema).
      (1) Due to elevated PIP (> 45), PEEP (> 15), F_iO_2 (> 50%).
      (2) Prevent by minimizing above values.
      (3) Treat symptomatically.
   c. Ventilation/perfusion (V/Q) mismatch. V > Q–ventilation of non-perfused tissue (dead space), V < Q–perfusion of non-ventilated tissue (shunt); cannot be improved by increasing F_iO_2.
      (1) Treat by increasing PEEP and V_T.
      (2) Beware of pathologically high airway pressures.

F. Weaning from ventilatory support.

1. Initiated only after the primary process responsible for pulmonary insufficiency has been reversed.
2. Priorities of weaning.
   a. Decrease F_iO_2 to < 50% (below toxic level).
   b. Decrease mechanical rate.
      (1) Reduces mean intrathoracic pressure and frequency of exposure to peak inspiratory pressure (PIP).
      (2) Minimizes barotrauma.
      (3) Improves V/Q matching.
   c. Decrease PEEP.
      (1) Increments of 2-3 cm per step.
      (2) Check PO_2 and/or shunt, and if satisfactory, reduce PEEP again.
      (3) Allow approximately 6 h between successive drops in PEEP.
      (4) Decrease PEEP to a base of 5 cm H_2O (approximates end expiratory pressure in extubated patients as a result of epiglottic closure; so-called "physiologic PEEP").

G. Criteria for extubation.

1. Traditional extubation criteria.
   a. Ventilation (mechanical) factors.
      (1) Vital capacity > 15 cc/kg.
      (2) Negative inspiratory force < -20 cm H_2O.
      (3) Respiratory rate < 30.
      (4) Spontaneous tidal volume ≥ 5 cc/kg.
      (5) 48% false-negative prediction of outcome.
   b. Oxygenation factors–P_aO_2 > 300 mm Hg on F_iO_2 of 100%.
2. "Blow by" T-piece trial should be *avoided.*
   a. Fails to provide physiologic levels of PEEP.
   b. Promotes alveolar collapse.
3. Gas exchange criteria–trial of room air CPAP.
   a. IMV rate of zero, F_iO_2 of 21% and CPAP of 5 cm H_2O.
   b. After 1/2 hour, extubate if:
      (1) P_aO_2 > 55 mmHG.
      (2) Ventilatory rate < 30 breaths/min.
      (3) pH > 7.35.
      (4) P_aCO_2 < 45 mmHG.
      (5) 95% predictive of the patient tolerating extubation.
      (6) Modify criteria for patients with underlying pulmonary disease (e.g., hypoxemia (chronic), CO_2 retention).

11

Wound Healing, Care, and Complications

Michael A. Helmrath, M.D.

Healing and tissue repair form the foundation of surgical practice. Although healing generally proceeds without complication, impaired healing and wound infection are leading causes of morbidity in surgical patients.

I. THE PHYSIOLOGY OF WOUND HEALING

A. Fibroplasia—creation of a scar.

1. ***Inflammatory phase (0-4 days)***—the initial response to injury. Tissue damage initiates the inflammatory response, which includes activation of coagulation, complement, prostaglandins, and cytokines. Erythrocyte adhesion can be seen histologically as rouleaux formation. Platelets are deposited and platelet plugs are formed. Fibrin incorporates these elements into a fibrous coagulum that bridges the defect. Migration of cells into the wound begins with **polymorphonuclear leukocytes (PMNs)** a few hours after injury and usually peak in number at 28-48 h. Although not essential for wound healing, they are responsible for the killing and phagocytosis of bacteria. **Macrophages,** derived from circulating monocytes, enter the wound and peak in number approximately 72 h postinjury. Besides their phagocytic role in clearing the wound of debris, macrophages orchestrate the complex cellular interrelationships necessary in normal healing.
2. ***Proliferative phase (2-22 days)***—marked by the beginning of collagen deposition, which increases steadily before it plateaus. Fibroblasts migrate into the wound and proliferate, becoming the predominant cell type by the fifth day. They begin the deposition of the extracellular matrix, including collagen. At this point the wound begins to gain strength. After 5 weeks the number of fibroblasts decreases.

3. ***Maturation phase (21 days to 2 years)***—characterized by increasing strength without an increase in collagen content. The predominant phase after 3 weeks, it continues for the life of the wound. A dynamic equilibrium exists between collagen breakdown and synthesis. Strength is gained with increasing cross-links and alignment of collagen fibers along lines of tension.

B. Epithelialization—involves migration of epithelial cells from the wound edge across the wound. Migration begins within 12 h and an intact monolayer may be formed between well-approximated tissues within 24 h.

C. Contraction—the decrease in size of the wound due to contraction of the myofibroblast or fibroblast. This markedly decreases the time required to heal a large or gaping wound.

D. Wound strength—the wound gains very little strength during the first several days of the inflammatory phase. As the wound enters the proliferative phase, the strength of the wound will parallel the rapid rise in collagen content for about 3 weeks. At this time the collagen content and the rate of increasing wound strength plateau. This time point would theoretically be ideal for the removal of all sutures were it not for the adverse cosmetic results. Even at 3 weeks the wound only has 40% of the strength of undivided tissues and far less strength than strong suture material. At 6 to 8 weeks a wound will achieve 70% of its strength. Wound remodeling will increase wound strength for at least two years, although ultimate strength will never reach that of unwounded tissue.

II. GROWTH FACTORS IN WOUND HEALING

A. Growth factors are polypeptides or glycoproteins that are synthesized by one cell for local communication with other cells. In the healing wound they appear to be responsible for the orderly procession of cells into a wound, the proliferation of cells, and the production of extracellular proteins.

B. Epidermal Growth Factor (EGF)—a mitogen for all epithelial cells and fibroblast in the cornea, lung, breast, GI tract, and keratinocytes in skin. EGF increases hyaluronic acid in the extracellular matrix and inhibits gastric secretions.

C. Transforming Growth Factor Alpha (TGF-α)—related to and having effects similar to EGF. TGF-α stimulates epithelial growth and migration as well as angiogenesis. Derived from activated macrophages and many tissues.

D. Transforming Growth Factor Beta (TGF-β)—strongly chemotactic for monocytes and fibroblasts. It increases collagen and fibronectin production by fibroblasts and inhibits their breakdown to increase the extracellular matrix. TGF-β is thought to be very important as a down-regulator of mitogenesis and as such may be involved in neoplasia by inhibiting NK cell activity and

T/B cell proliferation. Derived from platelets, PMNs, T-lymphocytes, and macrophages.

E. Platelet-Derived Growth Factor (PDGF)—the active dimer is found in high concentrations in platelets, macrophages and other cells. It is chemotactic for fibroblasts, smooth muscle cells, monocytes, and neutrophils. PDGF is mitogenic for fibroblasts, neutrophils, mononuclear, and smooth muscle cells. May be important in pathologic proliferative disorders such as malignancies, atherosclerosis, cirrhosis, pulmonary fibrosis, and rheumatoid arthritis.

F. Fibroblast Growth Factor (FGF)—exists in several forms, including acidic and basic; all forms bind strongly to heparin. FGF is chemotactic and mitogenic for endothelial cells and fibroblasts. Its major role may be in angiogenesis.

G. Careful orchestration of growth factors is responsible for normal healing at a near maximal rate. Alterations in the production and responsiveness to these potent compounds likely contributes to a large number of proliferative disorders, such as excessive scarring and neoplasms, as well as impaired wound healing.

III. TYPES OF WOUND HEALING

A. Primary intention—healing of reapproximated tissues.

B. Secondary intention (spontaneous healing)—healing occurs by the processes of granulation, contraction, and epithelialization.

C. Delayed primary healing—the wound is closed after a time. Contaminated wounds may be closed after 2 to 5 days of dressing changes to improve the cosmetic outcome, decrease the time of closure, and decrease the risk of infection.

IV. MANAGEMENT OF SOFT TISSUE WOUNDS

A. Traumatic wound care.

1. Address more urgent problems first. Bleeding is initially controlled with direct pressure.
2. Obtain radiographs for suspected foreign bodies or fracture.
3. Clean the skin around the wound with antiseptic. Use chlorhexidine or hexachlorophene on the face. These agents are damaging to exposed tissues and should be kept out of the wound. Cut the hair as needed, but never shave eyebrows because they occasionally fail to grow back.
4. Before closure, a careful neurovascular exam and local wound exploration should be undertaken to identify injury to nerves, vessels, tendons, joints, or other structures in anatomic proximity.
5. Anesthetize with local agents if there is no history of allergy (see "Anesthesia"–local anesthetics). Epinephrine is useful to control skin bleeding, particularly on the face, but avoid areas where distal ischemia may occur (e.g., fingers, toes, nose, ear, and penis).

6. Saline irrigation will remove clot and gross contaminates. No amount of irrigation will sterilize the wound. Perform careful debridement of all devitalized tissue.
7. Bleeding vessels should be clamped and tied under direct vision.

B. Wound closure.

1. Wounds with minimal contamination, controlled bleeding, adequate debridement, and no foreign body or debris may be closed primarily.
   a. Close wounds with minimum tension; use subcutaneous sutures to obliterate dead space in deep wounds.
   b. Observe periodically for drainage or infection.
2. Contraindications for primary closure.
   a. Inflamed or infected wounds.
   b. Dirty, neglected, or wounds older than 8 h, except when on the face.
   c. Wounds with gross bacterial contamination.
   d. Wounds that cannot be debrided adequately.
   e. Human or animal bites, except for selected bites to the face.
3. Wounds that are left open should be cleaned, debrided, and packed with gauze.
4. Antibiotics are indicated for cellulitic or infected wounds, immunocompromised or diabetic patients, and all bites.
5. Delayed primary closure may be performed after several days of dressing changes, when the wound is free of devitalized tissue and active infection.

C. Dressings.

1. For clean surgical wounds, dressings should be left in place for 48-72 h to allow time for epithelialization to occur. Dressings should be removed earlier if saturated by blood or serum or if there is suspicion of infection. The ideal dressing is sterilely applied, splints the skin around the incision, absorbs excess drainage, and is semi-permeable.
2. For contaminated wounds, after thorough cleansing and debridement, the wound should be packed open to promote hemostasis and drainage. Wet-to-dry dressings should be changed every 6 to 8 h to further debride the wound.
   a. Normal saline is isotonic and non-toxic.
   b. Dakin's solution, 2% boric acid, 0.25% acetic acid, and povodine-iodine may inhibit granulation tissue. In heavily contaminated, heavily colonized, or infected wounds, however, their antiseptic benefits often justify their use.

D. Tetanus and Rabies prophylaxis.

1. Tetanus is caused by the toxin of *Clostridium tetani.*
2. Tetanus-prone wounds are old (> 6 h), deep (> 1 cm), and contaminated, especially those involving rusty metal, feces, or soil. Missile, crush, stellate, or avulsion wounds with devitalized tissue are also at risk.
3. Adequate immunization for adults requires at least three injec-

tions of toxoid, with a booster every 10 years. In children younger than 7 years old, immunization requires four injections of DPT. A fifth dose may be given at 4-6 years of age. Thereafter, adult type (Td) is recommended for routine or wound boosters.

4. Specific measures for patients with wounds.
   a. Previously immunized individuals.
      (1) If the patient is fully immunized and the last dose of toxoid was given within 10 years, for non-tetanus-prone wounds no booster of toxoid is indicated. For tetanus-prone wounds and if more than 5 years have elapsed since the last dose, 0.5 ml of adsorbed toxoid should be given IM.
      (2) When the patient has had 2 or more prior injections of toxoid and received the last dose more than 10 years previously, 0.5 ml of adsorbed toxoid should be given for both tetanus- and non-tetanus-prone wounds. Passive immunization is not required.
   b. Individuals *NOT* adequately immunized (or unknown).
      (1) For non-tetanus-prone wounds, 0.5 ml of adsorbed toxoid should be given.
      (2) For tetanus-prone wounds, 0.5 ml of adsorbed toxoid and 250 Units (or more) of human tetanus immune globulin should be given using different needles, syringes, and sites of injection. Administration of antibiotics should be considered, although their effectiveness in prophylaxis is unproven.
5. ***Rabies*** is a routinely fatal disease caused by the rabies virus, a single-stranded RNA virus of the rhabdovirus group. Fewer than 5 cases usually are reported in the U.S. each year.
   a. Prophylaxis is indicated for bites by carnivorous wild animals (esp. skunks, raccoons, foxes, coyotes, and bats). Prophalaxis is not indicated for bites by domestic animals (unless thought to be rabid) or rodents such as mice, rats, or squirrels.
   b. Previously unimmunized persons should receive five 1 ml doses of human diploid cell vaccine (HDCV) by IM injection on days 0, 3, 7, 14, and 28. Rabies immune globulin (RIG) 20 IU/kg (preferable) or equine anti-rabies serum (ARS) 40 IU/kg should be given prior to day 8, with half the dose infiltrated in the area of the wound and the remainder given IM. RIG or ARS is not indicated after day 8.

V. WOUND COMPLICATIONS

A. Factors affecting wound healing.

1. Age—not an important independent factor. Although age does play some role in healing, age-related failures are most likely due to associated chronic disease.
2. Anemia—associated hypovolemia and hypoperfusion.

3. Blood supply–adequate wound perfusion is important for healing.
4. Chemotherapy–particularly detrimental to early stages of healing and should be delayed for at least 1 week after surgery.
5. Diabetes–peripheral vascular disease, neuropathy, and poor leukocyte function all contribute to poor wound healing in diabetics.
6. Foreign body–may cause chronic inflammation or infection.
7. Immunosuppression–cyclosporin has no significant effect.
8. Malnutrition–deficiencies in basic cellular building blocks and energy have profound effects on healing.
9. Obesity–problems are due to underlying illness such as diabetes, and relative malnutrition. Poorly vascularized fatty tissue is prone to infection.
10. Radiation–dose-related, both acute and chronic effects are seen. Waiting 1 week will significantly decrease the incidence of wound complication.
11. Sepsis–infection can impair healing.
12. Steroids–impair every phase of wound healing. The inflammatory phase is decreased and the production of cytokines, kinins, and other active factors is impaired.
13. Tension–leads to hypoperfusion and hypoxia as well as direct mechanical disruption.
14. Trauma–devitalized tissue and inadequate debridement pose a mechanical barrier to healing as well as a culture media for infection.
15. Uremia–healing is improved by careful dialysis and nutritional support.

B. Management of wound complications.

1. ***Wound infection***—50% of all post-operative complications are wound related. Most of these are infections.
   a. Increased incidence with prolonged pre-operative stay, breaks in surgical technique, long operation, abdominal procedures, and anything that adversely affects wound healing.
   b. Usually noted 3-7 days post-operative with fever. The wound will be red, warm, tender, and often fluctuant. There may be drainage.
   c. Wound infections within 24-48 h are often caused by *Clostridia* or Group A *Streptococci.*
   d. Common pathogens are *Staphylococci* and *Streptococci.* If a hollow viscus has been entered, consider gram-negative bacteria.
   e. **Necrotizing fasciitis**–aggressive surgical debridement is essential in the treatment of this polymicrobial infection of the subcutaneous tissue and fascia.
   f. Treatment of wound infections includes opening the wound and debriding as necessary. Cultures should be

taken, and dressing changes are begun. The fascia should be visually and manually inspected for integrity. Antibiotics are indicated for significant cellulitis or systemic sepsis.

2. Wound collections–**seromas and hematomas.**
   a. Use closed-suction drains when flaps are created. These are removed when drainage decreases. Seromas after drain removal may be sterilely aspirated. Drains may increase the incidence of infection but are effective in preventing seromas.
   b. Expanding hematomas must be evacuated and ongoing bleeding controlled. Small non-expanding hematomas may be left alone but should be watched for infection. Evacuated hematomas may be resutured if clean and without infection.
3. Vascular compromise–ischemic necrosis. This is caused by compromised arterial inflow or venous outflow or by local tension, which may strangulate tissues. Necrotic tissue should be debrided.
4. ***Wound dehiscence.***
   a. **Superficial**–separation of skin edges. May be reclosed if not infected. Otherwise treat as an open contaminated wound.
   b. **Fascial**–separation of fascia with potential for evisceration. Associated with a 15% mortality.
      (1) No one type of incision or type of closure is most prone to dehiscence. The most common causes are local ischemia, increased intra-abdominal pressure, underlying or concomitant illness, and technical problems. Typical occurrence at POD 5-8 is heralded by sudden drainage of pink, serosanguinous, "salmon-colored", peritoneal fluid.
      (2) If **evisceration** occurs, cover the wound with sterile saline-soaked towels and arrange immediate operative repair. Minor fascial separation without evisceration may be treated expectantly with later repair of the resultant hernia.
   c. Retention sutures are used to prevent evisceration in the event of fascial dehiscence and have no influence on whether dehiscence will occur. They are usually placed in high-risk patients and should be removed around POD 21.

VI. PRINCIPLES OF DRAIN MANAGEMENT

A. Drains—rarely indicated in non-infected wounds unless flaps are created or fluid collections are anticipated. Closed suction drains have the lowest incidence of infection and are removed as drainage decreases.

B. Intra-abdominal drains—use closed suction drains. Penrose drains work best with the help of gravity, but provide a two-way route for bacteria.

1. Infection–drains are placed in abscess cavity or dependent areas for drainage and to produce a tract. They are usually left in place for at least 7-10 days and then slowly advanced out.
2. Peritonitis–drains are not effective in draining the whole peritoneal cavity and should not be used for generalized infection.

C. Infected wounds—infected wounds are generally best opened and treated with local wound care.

12

Surgical Infections

Robert C. Bass, M.D.

I. DEFINITIONS

A. Infection—invasion of tissue by pathogens. A surgical infection is an infection that either is the result of, or requires, surgical intervention.

B. Virulence—the tissue-invading potency of a pathogen.

C. Bacteremia—the presence of bacteria in the circulation, with or without systemic toxicity.

D. Septicemia—the presence of bacteria and their toxins in the circulation with characteristics of systemic toxicity.

E. Toxemia—intoxication of the circulation, with or without the presence of the producing organism. Toxemia may result from infection by a toxin-producing bacteria (*Clostridia* in gas gangrene) or ingestion of pre-formed toxin without infection (botulinum or staphylococcal enterotoxin).

F. Abscess—localized collection of pus and devitalized tissue surrounded by inflamed tissue. Treatment requires drainage because antibiotics cannot penetrate abscess cavity owing to poor local blood supply.

G. Phlegmon—mass of inflammatory tissue.

II. DIAGNOSIS

A. General—history and physical, followed by directed laboratory and radiologic tests.

B. Signs and symptoms—the body's response to infection. Five cardinal signs: *dolor* (pain), *rubor* (redness), *calor* (heat), *tumor* (swelling), and *functio laesa* (loss of function). In addition:

1. Local–fluctuance, crepitance, drainage.
2. Systemic–fever, rigors, tachycardia, tachypnea.

C. Laboratory.

1. WBC count–with differential.
   a. Increased in presence of infection.

b. Differential shows "left shift"–presence of bands and immature WBCs in the blood.
c. Neutropenia may be seen in overwhelming sepsis.
2. Erythrocyte sedimentation rate–nonspecific indicator of inflammation.

D. Culture techniques.
1. Aspiration of fluid collection–send for **gram stain** and aerobic and anaerobic culture.
2. Aspiration of *edge* of cellulitic area (instillation of 1-2 cc sterile nonbacteriostatic saline may increase yield).
3. Wound or fluid swab.
4. Tissue biopsy.
5. Blood cultures–2 sets each time from a peripheral vein and/or indwelling catheters at time of fever or timed intervals.

E. Imaging techniques.
1. Radiograph (x-ray)–may visualize air-fluid levels or gas in tissue.
2. CT scan–most useful when intra-abdominal or intrathoracic pathology is suspected. Accurate localization of abscess and can be used to guide percutaneous drainage.
3. Ultrasound–good for defining nature of fluid collections and localizing intra-abdominal abscess. Also helpful in guiding percutaneous drainage.
4. Tagged (radiolabelled) WBC scan–patient's WBCs labelled with indium, and reinfused. Cells pool at site(s) of inflammation. Very nonspecific and poor localization.
5. Gallium scan–gallium taken up by WBCs. Radiolabelling scans are most useful in identifying and localizing occult abscesses. Both require 12-72 h for completion.

III. PRINCIPLES OF THERAPY

A. Incision and drainage of purulent material.
B. Debridement of necrotic or devitalized tissue.
C. Removal of colonized foreign bodies.
D. Open wound management—pack wound open, dressing changes.
E. Antibiotics.
1. Empiric choice based on likely pathogens.
2. Adjust antibiotics according to sensitivities.
3. Adequate dosage.
4. Adequate blood supply to infected tissue.
5. No improvement in 24-48 h suggests treatment failure; reconsider antibiotic regimen.

IV. SOFT TISSUE INFECTION

A. Focal infections.
1. Cutaneous abscesses.
a. Furuncle ("boil")–abscess in a sweat gland or hair follicle.
b. Carbuncle–multilocular suppurative extension of a fu-

runcle into adjacent subcutaneous tissue. Usually caused by *Staphylococci.*

c. Impetigo–intraepithelial abscesses, usually caused by *Staphylococci* or *Streptococci*; contagious.

2. Pyoderma gangrenosum–rare.
   a. Painful, raised pustular lesion with necrotic center, which progresses to spreading ulceration.
   b. 60-80% are associated with underlying condition: inflammatory bowel disease, polyarthritis, leukemia.
   c. Treat by local wound care, antimicrobials. Treatment of underlying condition is essential.
3. Meleney's progressive synergistic gangrene.
   a. Appears after injury or operation on purulent pleural or peritoneal infection, usually after 2 weeks or longer.
   b. Characterized by necrotic center, bluish undermined edges, and surrounding erythema.
   c. Synergistic infection with *S. aureus* and microaerophilic *Streptococcus.*
   d. Treat by wide excision, open wound care, and high-dose penicillin or vancomycin.

B. Diffuse non-necrotizing infections.

1. Cellulitis.
   a. Nonsuppurative inflammation of subcutaneous tissues.
   b. Presents with redness, swelling, pain; often fever and chills.
   c. *Streptococci* and *Staphylococci* are the most common organisms. Gram-negative bacilli may be present, especially in diabetic patients.
   d. Failure to improve after 72 h of antibiotics suggests abscess formation or necrotizing process (see C below), requiring incision and drainage.
2. Lymphangitis.
   a. Inflammation of lymphatic channels manifested by erythematous streaks.
   b. Often accompanies cellulitis, usually associated with streptococcal infections.
   c. Regional lymphadenopathy usually seen.
   d. Appropriate antibiotic therapy is usually sufficient treatment.
3. Erysipelas.
   a. Acute spreading streptococcal cellulitis and lymphangitis. Lesions are raised with defined margins.
   b. Usually responds well to antibiotic therapy.

C. Diffuse necrotizing infections.

1. Nonclostridial.
   a. A spectrum of life-threatening necrotizing infections, including necrotizing fasciitis, Fournier's gangrene (necrotizing fasciitis of the perineum), gram-negative synergistic necrotizing cellulitis that manifests as extensive necrosis

of subcutaneous tissue, and superficial fascia with widespread undermining of surrounding tissues and severe systemic toxicity. More common in diabetics.

b. Causal organisms are anaerobic *Streptococci, Staphylococcus,* and *Bacteroides.*

c. Characterized by erythematous skin, edema beyond erythema, crepitance, hemodynamic derangements due to systemic sepsis.

d. Diagnosis–confirmed by serosanguinous exudate, necrotic fascia with extensive undermining. Gram stain demonstrates gram-positive organisms, WBCs.

e. Treatment–emergent aggressive wide debridement and broad-spectrum antibiotics. Hyperbaric oxygen may be helpful but is used as secondary treatment. May require daily operative debridement to prevent ongoing infection.

2. Clostridial myonecrosis (gas gangrene).
   a. Rapidly progressive invasion of muscle by anaerobic *Clostridium.*
   b. Treatment–emergent wide debridement or amputation, and antibiotics (IV high-dose penicillin). Delay of treatment may be fatal. Hyperbaric oxygen may be helpful, but again as secondary treatment.

V. OTHER INFECTIONS

A. Intra-abdominal abscess.

1. Localized collection of pus walled off from the rest of the peritoneal cavity by inflammatory adhesions and viscera.
2. Usually polymicrobial, with aerobic and anaerobic organisms.
3. Clinical manifestations–fever (initially spiking, eventually sustained) anorexia, paralytic ileus, leukocytosis, abdominal tenderness. Symptoms may be masked by antibiotics. Subphrenic or retroperitoneal abscesses may not be associated with abdominal pain.
4. Diagnosis–usually by ultrasound or CT scan with confirmatory aspiration for gram stain and culture.
5. Treatment–drainage essential. May be percutaneous, transrectal, transvaginal, or open surgical. Antibiotic therapy should cover aerobic and anaerobic organisms.

B. Antibiotic-associated (pseudomembranous) colitis.

1. Usually caused by an overgrowth of *Clostridium difficile.* Most frequently following use of clindamycin, ampicillin, or cephalosporins, but may be associated with any antibiotic.
2. Presents with watery, nonbloody diarrhea. Fever, leukocytosis, and abdominal pain and distention may be present.
3. Diagnosis–isolation of organism or its toxin from the stool. Sigmoidoscopy reveals yellow-white, exudative pseudomembranes.

4. Treatment–discontinue offending antibiotic. Oral vancomycin has been the treatment of choice; oral metronidazole is currently used initially due to good efficacy and lower cost. Cholestyramine is sometimes used to bind toxin but is of questionable efficacy.

C. Wound infections.

1. Clinically defined as discharge of any purulent material regardless of whether bacteria are identified.
2. Conditions associated with increased wound infection rates–extremes of age, malnutrition, decreased blood flow to wound, cirrhosis, steroids, immunosuppression, leukopenia, foreign body, devitalized tissue, fluid collections, cancer, irradiated tissue, diabetes mellitus.
3. Expected wound infection rates depend on type of operation.
   a. Clean (skin, vascular): 1.5-5%.
   b. Clean-contaminated (GI, GU, GYN, respiratory tract surgery): ~ 7% if prophylactic antibiotics used.
   c. Contaminated (penetrating trauma, bowel spillage): 10-15%.
   d. Dirty/infected (gross pus, gangrene, bowel perforation): 15-40%.
4. Superficial wound infections–75% of wound infections.
   a. Involve skin and subcutaneous tissues, superficial to fascia and muscle.
   b. Signs/symptoms–fever, erythema, drainage with or without bacteria, wound erythema with seroma, fluctuance, tenderness, nonhealing.
   c. Management–open wound.
      (1) Complicated wounds (extreme obesity, uncooperative patient, wound failure, fistula) should be explored in OR.
      (2) Prep widely, and make a generous opening where signs and symptoms are greatest.
      (3) Obtain cultures–swab and if possible a capped syringe for aerobic and anaerobic cultures.
      (4) Probe wound with finger, insure patency of fascia.
      (5) Begin wet to dry saline dressing changes 3x/day. Showers may be helpful to clean wound.
      (6) Systemic antibiotics indicated if patient is immunocompromised or if prosthetic devices, signs of systemic toxicity, or significant cellulitis are present.
      (7) Wound may be closed secondarily when infection has cleared and healthy granulation tissue is present.
5. Deep wound infections.
   a. Involves muscles, fascia, and/or structures deep to them.
   b. Signs and symptoms are those of superficial wound infections, fascial dehiscence, drainage between fascial sutures, evisceration, ileus.

c. Management.
   (1) Explore in operating room.
   (2) For fascial dehiscence–explore abdominal wound to rule out fistula or abscess, debride necrotic fascia, and close. Consider retention sutures, as they can prevent evisceration if there is subsequent dehiscence. Retention sutures may not prevent dehiscence, however. Leave skin and subcutaneous tissue open.
   (3) Antibiotics.

6. Prevention.
   a. Pre-operative antimicrobial shower.
   b. Remove hair immediately before operation by clipping.
   c. Prophylactic antibiotics (when indicated, see VII D below) 30 min before incision, maintain therapeutic levels throughout case.
   d. Vigilance for breaks in aseptic technique.
   e. Appropriate skin preparation and sterile draping.
   f. Meticulous surgical technique.
      (1) Monofilament sutures.
      (2) Minimize sutures and ligatures (foreign bodies).
      (3) Do not strangulate tissues.
      (4) Meticulous skin closure.
   g. Avoidance of post-operative hypoxia.
   h. Surveillance of wounds for early signs of infection.

VI. POST-OPERATIVE FEVER

Fever is a common post-operative finding. The presence of fever does not necessarily imply the presence of infection (nor does absence of fever rule out presence of infection). The timing of a fever may help to identify the source. In general, when working up post-operative fevers, the 5 Ws should be considered–**w**ound, **w**ind (pulmonary), **w**alk (DVT or pulmonary embolus), **w**ater (urine), and **w**onder drugs (drug fever, diagnosis of exclusion).

A. Fever at 0-48 h—usually due to atelectasis; treat with incentive spirometry, cough and deep breathing, ambulation, and/or pulmonary toilet.

1. Important exceptions.
   a. Soft-tissue infection with *Clostridia* or group A *Streptococcus*. Rapidly spreading wound erythema, lymphangitis, gram-positive cocci or rods in wound. Treatment is immediate opening of wound, and antibiotics. All wounds should be examined in patients with early post-operative fever, as these infections spread rapidly and have high mortality rates if treatment is delayed.
   b. Leakage of bowel anastomosis–tachycardia, hypotension, decreased urine output, diffuse abdominal tenderness.
   c. Aspiration pneumonia–rales, rhonchi that do not clear with pulmonary toilet, infiltrate on chest radiographs.

B. By post-operative day 3, infections become an increasingly likely source of fever.

1. Urinary tract infection–especially common in instrumented patients. Diagnose by both urinalysis and culture.
2. Wound infection–usually not seen until post-operative day 3-5 (See above for treatment).
3. I.V. site–infection rate increases after a line has been in 3 days.
   a. Local catheter-related infection.
      (1) Manifestations include redness, streaking, tenderness, purulence, lymphangitis.
      (2) Removal of catheter is usually adequate. Culture tip.
   b. Catheter-related sepsis.
      (1) Manifestations–signs of local catheter infection and isolation of same organism from blood and catheter, signs of systemic toxicity, and no other source of septicemia.
      (2) Treat by removal of catheter. If temperature and WBC return to normal within 24 h, no antibiotics are needed.
   c. Septic thrombophlebitis.
      (1) Should be suspected when signs of sepsis, positive blood cultures, and local inflammation persist after removal of offending catheter.
      (2) Surgical removal of affected vein is required.
4. Intra-abdominal abscess–usually not seen until post-operative days 5-10 (see above).
5. DVT–usually post-operative days 7-10, but can occur anytime. Diagnose with noninvasive lower extremity scan.
6. Cholecystitis.
   a. Acalculous–seen in critically ill patients, associated with NPO status and parenteral nutrition.
   b. Calculous–occurs post-operatively in patients with known cholelithiasis.
   c. Diagnosis by ultrasound with/without HIDA scan.
7. Other causes–pulmonary embolus, sinusitis (especially in patients with endotracheal or nasogastric tubes), salivary/parotid glands (check amylase), prostate, perirectal abscess, drug fevers, inflammation in ears or throat, factitious fever.
8. New and unrelated diseases should be considered–appendicitis, neoplasm, etc.

VII. PRINCIPLES OF ANTIBIOTIC THERAPY

A. Types of antibiotics.

1. Bacteriostatic–prevent growth and multiplication of bacteria, but does not kill them. Rely on defense mechanisms of the host to clear infection.
2. Bactericidal–kills bacteria. Must be employed in immunocompromised patients.

B. Selection of antibiotics.

1. Empiric choices–based on likely infecting organism, often related to endogenous flora of involved organ.
2. Specific choices–based on culture results and sensitivities.
3. Other factors.
    a. Assure adequate contact between drug and the infecting agent.
        (1) Adequate dosage.
        (2) Adequate tissue perfusion.
        (3) Drug will reach site or organism (i.e., biliary excretion, CNS penetration).
    b. Minimize potential side effects.
    c. Maximize host defenses.

C. Complications of antibiotic therapy.

1. Direct toxicity–drug fever, rashes, anaphylaxis, neurologic problems (seizures, neuropathy), GI symptoms, renal dysfunction, blood/bone marrow dyscrasias, visual and auditory losses.
2. Emergence of resistant strains.
3. Superinfection with microorganisms resistant to current regimen (gram-negative bacteria, *Candida*).

D. Antibiotic prophylaxis.

1. Directed at preventing wound infections, prophylaxis is effective when properly employed, but is not a substitute for good surgical technique.
2. Indications.
    a. Traumatic wounds with contamination, delay of treatment, injury to a hollow viscus.
    b. Clean-contaminated and contaminated operations.
    c. Resection/anastomosis of colon or intestine.
    d. Prosthetic devices are or will be present.
    e. Valvular heart disease.
    f. Immunocompromised patient.
    g. Shock.
    h. Ischemic tissue present.
    i. Open fractures, penetrating joint injuries.
3. Unless there is gross intra-operative contamination, discontinue antibiotics 24-48 h after surgery.
4. Intestinal asepsis–involves systemic and intraluminal antibiotics and mechanical cleansing (see "Pre-operative Preparation").

VIII. ANTIMICROBIAL AGENTS

Antibiotics should be targeted toward an organism, not a disease.

A. Penicillins—bactericidal, β-lactam ring blocks bacterial cell wall synthesis.

1. Streptococcal penicillins–penicillin G, drug of choice for *Streptococcus pyogenes* and *Clostridia*. *Bacteroides* usually resistant.

2. Staphylococcal penicillins–β-lactamase resistant. Methicillin, also nafcillin, oxacillin, dicloxacillin. Active only against gram-positive organisms such as *S. aureus* and *S. epidermidis*.
3. Enterococcal penicillins–ampicillin, also amoxicillin.
4. Anti-pseudomonal penicillins–piperacillin, carbenicillin, and ticarcillin. Used in conjunction with an aminoglycoside as an antipseudomonal regimen.
5. Gram-negative penicillins–mezlocillin and piperacillin: active against most Enterobacteriaceae and some anaerobes.
6. Penicillin/β-lactamase inhibitor combinations–ampicillin-sulbactam, amoxicillin-clavulanate and ticarcillin-clavulanate. Covers gram-positives, most *Bacteroides*, and gram-negative aerobes. Does not cover methicillin-resistant *S. aureus* (MRSA).

B. Cephalosporins—bactericidal, mechanism of action similar to penicillins. There is a 5-10% allergic cross-reactivity with the penicillins in patients with a history of anaphylactic reactions to penicillin.

1. Staphylococcal cephalosporins–cefazolin, also cefamandole, cefuroxime, ceforanide, and cefoperazone. Cephalexin, cephradine, and cefaclor are acid-stable and can be given PO. Active against *Staphylococcus, Streptococcus*, and some aerobic coliforms. Primarily used for surgical prophylaxis and treatment of skin infections.
2. Anaerobe cephalosporins–cefoxitin, cefotetan, cefmetazole, moxalactam. Enhanced activity against aerobic gram-negatives and anaerobes including most *B. fragilis*.
3. Anti-pseudomonal cephalosporins–ceftazidime.
4. Coliform cephalosporins–cefotaxime, also ceftizoxime, ceftriaxone and cefmenoxime. Effective against most coliforms, as well as *S. aureus* and streptococci. Enterococci, *Pseudomonas* and *B. fragilis* are resistant.

C. Monobactams—monocyclic β-lactams, bactericidal–aztreonam–only active against gram-negative aerobes, including *Pseudomonas*.

D. Carbapenems—bactericidal–imipenem-cilastatin.

1. Cilistatin prevents breakdown of the antibiotic.
2. Very broad spectrum. Diphtheroids, *P. maltophilia* and *Proteus mirabilis* are resistant. Useful for intra-abdominal infections.

E. Aminoglycosides—bactericidal, interfere with protein synthesis–gentamicin, also tobramycin, amikacin, kanamycin.

1. Effective against all gram-negative aerobic coliforms. Also effective against staphylococci and streptococci. Enterococci and anaerobes are resistant. Primarily used with a β-lactam as an antipseudomonal regimen.
2. Adverse effects include ototoxicity and nephrotoxicity. Nephrotoxicity is increased by concurrent use of loop diuretics, NSAIDs, cyclosporin or cisplatin, preexisting renal in-

sufficiency; usually reversible with cessation of aminoglycoside. Ototoxicity is usually *not* reversible.
3. Kinetics may be unpredictable, dosage must be adjusted to serum levels to insure efficacy and prevent toxicity (gentamicin desired levels: peak 4-10 mg/L, trough 1-2 mg/L).

F. **Sulfonamides**—sulfamethoxazole-trimethoprim–covers gram-negative aerobic coliforms including *Proteus*, *Morganella* and *Shigella*. Useful for urinary tract infection and is drug of choice for *Pneumocystis carinii* and *Nocardia*.

G. **Fluoroquinolones**—ciprofloxacin, also norfloxacin–bactericidal. Broad spectrum of activity, including gram-negative aerobes and *Chlamydia, Mycoplasma, Salmonella,* and *Shigella*. Useful as PO broad-spectrum agent and for refractory urinary tract infection.

H. **Tetracyclines**—tetracycline, doxycycline–bacteriostatic, inhibit protein synthesis.
1. Variable broad-spectrum coverage against many gram-positives and gram-negatives, and effective against *Rickettsiae*, mycoplasma, and spirochete. Frequently used with ceftriaxone in the empiric treatment of gonococcal/chlamydial sexually-transmitted diseases.
2. Should not be used in children or lactating mothers due to dental discoloration.

I. **Other agents.**
1. ***Vancomycin***—bactericidal.
   a. Potent antistaphylococcal agent, no gram-negative activity. Drug of choice for methicillin-resistant *S. aureus* (MRSA) and useful orally for *C. difficile* pseudomembranous colitis refractory to metronidazole.
   b. May cause ototoxicity and phlebitis at IV site. Need to monitor serum levels.
2. ***Erythromycin***—bacteriostatic, bacteriocidal in high doses.
   a. Broad gram-positive and gram-negative coverage. Drug of choice for *Legionella* and *Mycoplasma*. Erythromycin base is used for pre-operative oral bowel prep (Nichols-Condon prep).
   b. Resistance common with long-term treatment, causes GI upset when given orally.
   c. Also used as a motilin agonist.
3. ***Metronidazole.***
   a. Bactericidal for anaerobes and effective against amoebae and trichmonads. Initial drug of choice orally for pseudomembranous colitis.
   b. Disulfuram-like (Antabuse®) activity with alcohol intake, also stocking-glove peripheral neuropathy and convulsions with long-term use.
4. ***Clindamycin.***
   a. Active against gram-positive cocci except enterococci; anaerobes except *C. difficile*. Primarily used for anaerobic

coverage in intra-abdominal infections and aspiration pneumonia.

b. Overgrowth of enteric *C. difficile* leading to pseudomembranous enterocolitis is major adverse effect.

J. Anti-fungal agents.

1. ***Amphotericin B.***
   a. The only fungicidal drug available. Effective against all species of fungus.
   b. Begin therapy with 1 mg test dose; if well tolerated increase dose by 5-10 mg/day up to maximum of 15-30 mg/kg total dose. Pretreatment with acetaminophen and diphenhydramine and perhaps hydrocortisone is recommended.
   c. Major toxicity is renal. Dosing interval may have to be extended to every other day or every third day to avoid renal insufficiency.
2. ***Fluconazole.***
   a. Active against most pathogenic fungi of surgical importance.
   b. Can be administered PO or IV.
   c. Less toxicity than associated with amphotericin.
3. ***Flucytosine.***
   a. For serious *Candida* and *Cryptococcus* infections.
   b. May act synergistically with amphotericin.
4. ***Nystatin/clotrimazole***—nonabsorbed oral agent used prophylactically in immunosuppressed patients or those on broad-spectrum antibiotics to prevent GI overgrowth of *Candida.*

IX. ACQUIRED IMMUNE DEFICIENCY SYNDROME (AIDS)

A. General.

1. With the prevalence of human immunodeficiency virus (HIV)-infected patients increasing, surgeons will be more frequently asked to treat surgical problems in AIDS patients and HIV-seropositive patients.
2. HIV is a retrovirus that attaches to the CD4 receptor on T4 lymphocytes. The virus is internalized and incorporated into cellular DNA. Replication of the virus leads to cell destruction and infection of other cells.
3. Patient usually converts to seropositivity 6-8 weeks after infection with the virus.
4. When damage to the T4 helper cell population becomes severe enough, a generalized state of immunocompromise develops.
5. Serotesting.
   a. ELISA–good screening test.
   b. Western blot–definitive confirmatory test.

B. Epidemiology.

1. Homosexual males 10-70% HIV positive, average 25%.
2. IV drug abusers–5-60%.
3. Hemophiliacs–A: 70%, B: 35%.
4. Sexual partners of 1-3 above, 5%.
5. Study in Baltimore revealed 3% of critically ill patients and 16% of young trauma patients were HIV positive.

C. Clinical stages—Center for Disease Control (CDC) classification system.

1. Category A–asymptomatic carrier (largest group), generalized lymphadenopathy, acute retroviral infection (mononucleosis-like illness).
2. Category B–AIDS-related complex (ARC)–endocarditis, oral candidiasis, herpes zoster, idiopathic thrombocytopenic purpura (ITP), tuberculosis. Diseases must be attributed to HIV infection.
3. Category C–AIDS–disseminated candidiasis, coccidioidomycosis, cytomegalovirus (CMV), Kaposi's sarcoma, lymphoma, *Pneumocystis carinii* pneumonia, atypical mycobacterium.

D. Risk to health care workers.

1. Studies of needle sticks with contaminated needles demonstrate a seroconversion rate of 0.3-0.5% per stick.
2. Risk to surgeons may be underestimated. Three factors determine surgeon's risk:
   a. Number of contaminated needle sticks.
   b. Percent of HIV-positive patients in a surgeon's patient population.
   c. Number of years at risk.
3. Precautions.
   a. Wear gloves when at risk for body fluid exposure.
   b. Use protective clothing, mask, and goggles during procedures where material may be aerosolized or body fluid exposure is likely.
   c. Wash hands after body fluid contact.
   d. Treat all sharps as infective, do not recap needles.
   e. *Clean up sharps after procedures to prevent injury to others.*
   f. Clean spills with ammonia, bleach, or other sterilant.
   g. Double-bag and label infective fluids.
4. Post-exposure prophylaxis–immediate administration of AZT after injury with a contaminated sharp may prevent infection. Confirmatory studies pending.

E. Risk to patients.

1. Transfusion.
   a. Whole blood, PRBC, platelets, plasma, cryoprecipitate, and leukocytes can carry HIV.
   b. With antibody testing, the risk of transfusion-related transmission is now 1 in 36,000 to 1 in 100,000 per unit transfused.

2. Transplantation—potential donor tissues must be tested.
3. Surgeon to patient—a theoretical risk. No documented cases.

F. Surgical considerations.

1. Role of surgeons involves diagnostic biopsies, supportive care, and managing complications of infectious and malignant processes.
2. Surgical problems in HIV patients.
   a. Central venous access for chemotherapy.
   b. Acute cholecystitis, cholangitis secondary to cryptosporidiosis and CMV infection.
   c. Splenectomy for marked splenomegaly or thrombocytopenia.
   d. GI perforations and obstructions from infectious agents and malignancies.
   e. Spontaneous pneumothorax due to *Pneumocystis* pneumonia.
3. Patient's risk of post-operative complications is related to their underlying condition.
   a. Patients with CD4 counts of 500 or greater are not at increased risk of opportunistic infections.
   b. Asymptomatic HIV patients are not at increased risk of wound-healing complications.
   c. Emergent procedures in AIDS patients are associated with a high morbidity and mortality.

13

Management of the Diabetic Patient

M. Ryan Moon, M.D.

Diabetes mellitus is the most common metabolic disease that surgeons encounter. Not only do these patients suffer from acute problems such as increased susceptibility to infections, poor wound healing, diabetic ketoacidosis, and nonketotic hyperosmolar coma, but they present with the chronic problems of retinopathy, neuropathy, nephropathy, and advanced atherosclerosis, which may complicate their peri-operative management.

I. GENERAL PRINCIPLES

A. Diagnosis—fasting plasma glucose > 140 mg/dl on two separate occasions, or patients with abnormal glucose tolerance test. Patients can develop glucose intolerance in response to stress (trauma, surgery, infection, pregnancy).

B. Classification.

1. ***Type I****—Insulin Dependent Diabetes Mellitus (IDDM)*–20% of all diabetics; childhood or adolescent onset; prone to hyperglycemia and ketoacidosis.
2. ***Type II****—Non-Insulin Dependent Diabetes Mellitus (NIDDM)*–onset usually after 30 years of age; usually obese; prone to nonketotic hyperosmolar coma (ketoacidosis is rare); patients usually require exogenous insulin during stress or peri-operative period.
3. ***Secondary diabetes.***
   a. Pancreatic insufficiency–chronic pancreatitis, hemochromatosis, post-pancreatic resection.
   b. Hormonal excess–Cushing's disease, adrenal cortical tumors.
   c. Medications–steroids, thiazide diuretics.

C. Pre-operative evaluation—for presence and severity of diabetic complications.

1. Cardiovascular.
   a. Atherosclerosis; history of angina, myocardial infarction,

congestive heart failure, hypertension, claudication, and stroke or transient ischemic attacks.

   b. Examine for evidence of congestive heart failure (CHF) and bruits, and to document distal pulses.
   c. Lab work–baseline EKG; MUGA scan or echocardiogram, and dipyridamole-thallium scan for major procedures in patients with symptoms of angina, CHF, or previous myocardial infarction. Remember, diabetic patients may also have "silent" or asymptomatic myocardial ischemia.
2. Nephropathy.
   a. Evidence of proteinuria or elevated creatine.
   b. Sensitive to nephrotoxic effects of IV contrast; hydrate before study and follow renal function afterwards. Mannitol may be given IV after study to expedite contrast excretion.
3. Neuropathy–autonomic and somatic nerves.
   a. Peripheral–examine for lower extremity neuropathy (e.g., Charcot joint).
   b. Gastrointestinal–gastroparesis with resulting gastric dilitation may require metoclopramide, cisapride, erythromycin, and/or nasogastric decompression during stress/surgery.
   c. Hemodynamic–postural hypotension.
4. Infections.
   a. Leukocyte dysfunction (decreased chemotaxis and phagocytic activity) when blood glucose > 250 mg/dl.
   b. Evidence of urinary tract infection (most common), pneumonia, bronchitis, skin infections, diabetic foot ulcers.
   c. At risk for development of candidiasis–should be prophylaxed with nystatin 10 cc s/s q 8 h and antifungal vaginal suppository while on antibiotics.
5. Metabolic.
   a. Duration of diabetes, need for oral hypoglycemics, insulin dosage and schedule.
   b. History of episodes of hypoglycemia, diabetic ketoacidosis, and hyperglycemic coma.

II. PERI-OPERATIVE MANAGEMENT

In general, hospitalized diabetic patients are maintained at a slightly higher blood glucose than at home, since the consequences of prolonged hypoglycemia are much more severe than those of mild hyperglycemia.

A. Pre-operative.

1. Patients on oral hypoglycemic agent–discontinue 1 day preoperative.
2. Schedule early morning operation if possible.
3. Start IV containing dextrose (i.e., D51/2 normal saline) the night prior to surgery at 50-75 cc/h (the minimum carbohydrate requirement is 100 g/day).
4. Give 1/2 of usual dose and type (i.e., NPH, Lente, Regular) of insulin subcutaneously (SQ) the morning of surgery.

5. Continuous IV infusion of regular insulin may be preferred for peri-operative control of the brittle diabetic.

B. Post-operative.

1. Continue intravenous dextrose.
2. Follow glucose q 4-6 h with finger-stick blood sugar (FSBS) (must be correlated initially with serum glucose). Urine S & A (sugar and acetate) are not reliable for dosing insulin. Use insulin sliding scale (see section IV) to maintain serum glucose between 100-250 mg/dl. Absorption may be erratic with SQ administration in patients with poor peripheral perfusion (i.e., hypotensive, hypothermic).
3. Adjust insulin dose with resumption of oral diet or enteral feeding. Convert to intermediate (NPH) regimen by giving 80% of the previous 24-h insulin requirements as 2/3 NPH and 1/3 Regular. Continue to monitor FSBS.
4. Resume oral hypoglycemic agent when feasible.

III. MANAGEMENT OF COMPLICATIONS

A. Hypoglycemia (< 60 mg/dl)–occurs most commonly in brittle diabetics. Must be suspected in obtunded patients receiving insulin.

1. Treat with oral carbohydrates (milk or orange juice). If patient is obtunded, give one ampule of D50 (Dextrose 50%) IVP and repeat as needed; failure to respond at this point should lead one to question diagnosis; start D5W via peripheral IV and continue to monitor FSBS.
2. Adjust insulin sliding scale or infusion.

B. Nonketotic hyperosmolar hyperglycemia—condition of extreme hyperglycemia (> 600 mg/dl), hyperosmolality with mental status changes. Usually precipitated by stress, trauma, surgery, sepsis, or TPN.

1. Findings–include CNS changes from lethargy to coma and/or seizures, hypotension, tachycardia (extreme dehydration secondary to osmotic diuresis), and nausea/vomiting (ileus).
2. ***Therapy.***
   a. ICU setting, may require invasive monitoring. Place NG tube and Foley catheter.
   b. Begin hydration with normal saline solution to correct extreme dehydration. Cannot use urine output as indicator of fluid resuscitation because of osmotic diuresis.
   c. Serial electrolyte, glucose, and arterial blood gas determinations.
   d. Give 10 U insulin IV and begin insulin drip at 5-10 U/h. Should not decrease serum glucose more than 100 mg/dl/h to avoid cerebral edema.
   e. Once serum glucose is < 300 mg/dl, add 5% dextrose to IVFs.
   f. Replace potassium, magnesium, and phosphate levels as needed.
   g. Investigate precipitating cause (i.e., infection).

C. Diabetic ketoacidosis—similar to nonketotic hyperglycemia except patient is severely acidotic secondary to ketone production.

1. Findings–include CNS changes, tachycardia, hypotension secondary to dehydration, dysrhythmias secondary to hypokalemia, Kussmaul respirations (rapid deep breathing), and abdominal pain. Serum potassium may be high initially secondary to acidosis, but will fall with hydration and correction of acidosis.
2. ***Therapy***—see treatment of nonketotic hyperosmolar hyperglycemia. May need to correct acidosis with $NaHCO_3$ IV if pH < 7.20. Continue insulin therapy until ketonemia resolved.

IV. INSULIN SLIDING SCALE

This varies among patients, but this is good starting point.

A. Recommendations for SQ:

< 60	one amp D50 IVP and call house officer
61-200	0 U
201-250	5 U Regular SQ
251-300	10 U Regular SQ
301-350	15 U Regular SQ
351-400	20 U Regular SQ
> 400	25 U Regular SQ and call house officer

(for sugars > 400, blood glucose should be re-checked 2 h after dose is given)

B. Recommendations for IV:

1. ICU only.
2. Q 2 h blood sugar measurements.
3. Start IV insulin infusions at 5 U/h, increase by 2-3 U/h for sugars greater than 150, for sugars greater than 250, bolus 10 U IV then increase by 2-3 U/h as needed.

V. TYPES OF INSULIN

A. Human insulin (Humulin®) should be used as the standard class of insulin (as opposed to bovine or porcine). Recombinant DNA source. Useful in the diabetic with antibodies to animal-derived insulin.

B. Insulin characteristics (see "Formulary"):

Action	Type	Onset	Peak	Duration
Short	Regular	0.5-1 h	2-4 h	6 h
	Semilente	0.5-1 h	4-8 h	12-16 h
Intermediate	NPH	1-2 h	8-12 h	18-24 h
	Lente	1-2 h	8-12 h	18-24 h
Long	Protamine Zinc	4-8 h	12-24 h	36 h
	Ultralente	4-8 h	12-24 h	36 h

14

Thromboembolic Prophylaxis and Management of Deep Venous Thrombosis

Tory A. Meyer, M.D.

I. INTRODUCTION

A. Epidemiology—deep venous thrombosis (DVT) is a common problem in surgical patients of all types. Estimates of DVT after surgical procedures in patients without prophylaxis:

1. General surgery (intra-abdominal)–22-33%.
2. Orthopedic procedures–45-66%.
3. Prostatectomy–50%.
4. Trauma–20%.
5. Postpartum–3%.

B. Etiology—3 factors that contribute to the development of venous thrombosis and are known as **Virchow's Triad**:

1. Venous stasis.
2. Endothelial injury.
3. Hypercoagulability.

C. Risk factors for the development of DVT.

1. Age > 60.
2. Malignancy (especially prostate cancer, pancreatic cancer, and carcinomatosis).
3. Prior history of DVT, pulmonary embolism, or varicose veins.
4. Prolonged immobilization or bed rest.
5. Cardiac disease, especially congestive heart failure.
6. Obesity.
7. Major surgery, especially pelvic surgery.
8. Trauma.

9. Hypercoagulability, either congenital or acquired.
10. Pregnancy.
11. Oral contraceptives.

D. Clinical presentation is nonspecific and may include signs and symptoms of extremity swelling, tenderness, calf pain on ankle dorsi-flexion (Homan's sign), or fever. Clinical diagnosis is inaccurate.

1. Less than 50% of patients with the above signs and symptoms will have a DVT.
2. Signs and symptoms are present in only about 50% of patients documented to have DVT by venography.
3. ***Diagnosis*** — best made by venography, Doppler ultrasonography, or impedance plethysmography. Radiolabelled iodine fibrinogen studies are poor in diagnosing proximal vein thrombosis.
4. If the diagnosis of DVT is established in a patient without any risk factors, an occult malignancy should be suspected and sought.

E. Sequelae.

1. ***Pulmonary embolism*** is potentially the most lethal result of DVT. One in every 200 patients undergoing a major operation dies from massive pulmonary embolus. It accounts for 50,000 deaths/year. Ten percent of the deaths occur within 60 minutes of the first symptom, underscoring the importance of prophylaxis versus treatment.
   a. Calf vein thrombosis rarely gives rise to pulmonary embolism, unless there is propagation into the femoral vein.
   b. Pulmonary embolism can originate from the iliofemoral, pelvic, ovarian, axillary, subclavian, and internal jugular veins, as well as the IVC and cavernous sinuses of the skull.
   c. Clinical manifestations are inconsistent and nonspecific, but may include dyspnea, chest pain, hemoptysis, tachycardia, recent fever, rales, accentuated P_2 heart sound, elevated venous pressures, and EKG changes such as arrhythmias, enlarged P waves, ST depression, and T-wave inversions (particularly in III, AVF, V1, V3, and V4).
   d. Diagnosis established conclusively by pulmonary arteriography. High probability ventilation/perfusion scans coupled with a high clinical suspicion to PE may obviate the need for arteriography; low probability scans effectively exclude PE.
2. ***Post-thrombotic syndrome*** — occurs in 50% of patients with acute DVT and reflects chronic venous insufficiency. Brawny, non-pitting edema, and ulcer formation eventually occur.
3. Extreme cases of DVT may cause phlegmasia cerulea dolens—a loss of sensory and motor function secondary to compromised arterial supply to the limb from severe leg swelling.

F. Thrombosis of other deep veins.

1. **Axillary and subclavian vein thrombosis** are occurring with

increasing frequency in surgical patients as a result of more widespread use of indwelling catheters for TPN, chemotherapy, and central cardiovascular monitoring.

2. "Effort thrombosis"–occurs in the dominant arm of an otherwise healthy individual after straining, and represents axillary or subclavian thrombosis due to thoracic outlet compression.
3. SVC obstruction is usually related to tumor invasion; however, it may also be due to primary thrombosis, chronic fibrosing mediastinitis, or granulomatous disease.
4. IVC thrombosis in adults is generally a consequence of extension of thrombi from pelvic or thigh veins.

II. METHODS OF PROPHYLAXIS

A. Mechanical.

1. ***Leg elevation***—has been historically advised but lacks substantive support.
2. ***Graduated compression stockings***—must be well fitted and even then have a modest if appreciable effect.
3. ***Early ambulation***—simple and effective.
4. ***Pneumatic compression boots***—intermittently inflate and deflate, causing compression of the limb, usually the calves.
   a. Mechanism of action is both by propulsion of blood flow proximally and by activation of fibrinolytic system. Boots have been shown to be effective even when placed on the arms.
   b. Effective at reducing DVT as much as 50-75% in general surgery patients and 66% in neurosurgery patients.
   c. Pneumatic compression boots confer no increased risk of bleeding and are therefore especially important in neurosurgical and ophthalmological patients.

B. Pharmacologic agents.

1. ***Aspirin*** acts by irreversibly inactivating platelet cyclooxygenase and has been shown to be effective only in hip surgery patients. Not a currently recommended method of prophylaxis.
2. ***Dextran solution*** (40 and 70) is a branched polysaccharide solution that causes decreased platelet adhesiveness, aggregation, and release reaction in addition to RBC and Factor VIII, and plasma volume effects.
   a. Disadvantages.
      (1) Increased rate of bleeding.
      (2) Pulmonary edema due to volume overload in patients with cardiac compromise.
      (3) Allergic reactions in 1% of patients.
   b. Recommended dose is 15-20 cc/h continuous IV infusion peri-operatively.
3. ***Warfarin*** (Coumadin®).
   a. Shown to decrease incidence of DVT by 66% and pulmonary embolism by 80% in hip surgery patients.

b. Disadvantages.
   (1) Severe hemorrhage in 2-7% of patients.
   (2) Must be started 2-3 days pre-operatively.
   (3) Requires careful monitoring of prothrombin time (PT).

4. **Heparin** (unfractionated) accentuates antithrombin III inhibition of Factor X and thrombin and may also potentiate disintegration of thrombi that form while it is being administered.
   a. "Low-dose" regimen of 5,000 units SQ 2 h pre-operatively, then every 12 h post-operative until the patient is fully ambulatory has been shown to decrease the incidence of DVT by 2/3, and pulmonary embolism by 1/2 in general, urologic, and orthopedic patients.
   b. For morbidly obese patients, a "micro-heparin" drip at 1 unit/kg/h is believed to be more effective.
   c. Disadvantages.
      (1) Risk of bleeding–4-6%.
      (2) Rarely associated with thrombocytopenia at this dose.
      (3) Contraindicated in patients with active peptic ulcer disease, uncontrolled hypertension, evidence of bleeding disorders, current acetylsalicylic acid (ASA) use.
5. ***Heparin and dihydroergotamine (DHE) combinations*** (Embolex®).
   a. DHE at these low dosages causes preferential vasoconstriction of capacitance vessels and increased venous return.
   b. Shown to be at least as effective as heparin alone and particularly effective in orthopedic procedures.
   c. Contraindicated in patients with hypotension, ischemic heart disease, and peripheral arterial occlusive disease.
6. ***Low molecular weight heparin (LMWH)*** (Enoxaparin®, Fragmin®) are heparin fragments made by depolymerizing a heparin ester. Standard (i.e., unfractionated) heparin is actually a mixture of compounds of varying molecular weight and anticoagulant activity. Characteristics of LMWHs.
   a. LMWHs have equivalent inhibition of Factor X, but have less inhibition of thrombin and platelet aggregation.
   b. A smaller increase is seen in the PTT. These effects are thought to explain the finding in some orthopedic patient studies that show LMWH is more effective than standard heparin in DVT prophylaxis, but is not associated with a higher risk of hemorrhagic complications.
   c. Studies to date in general surgery patients have been inconclusive in demonstrating a reduction in DVT and/or a decrease in bleeding complications.
   d. They have a longer half-life and may therefore be dosed once daily.
   e. LMWH is much more expensive than standard heparin .
7. ***Fibrinogen-depleting compounds*** (Ancrod ®) are a new class of anticoagulants that have been found to be safe anecdotally; however, no prospective, controlled trials have been performed.

C. Prophylactic IVC filter placement (Greenfield filter) may be performed in patients at extremely high risk who have contraindications to other forms of prophylaxis and/or cannot be anticoagulated. It is effective only in preventing pulmonary embolism, not DVT. (See section IV. D.)

III. AN APPROACH TO PROPHYLAXIS

A. Determine the patient's risk.

1. Low risk–age < 40, ambulatory or minor surgery.
2. Moderate risk–age > 40, abdominal, pelvic, or thoracic surgery.
3. High risk–age > 40, prior DVT or pulmonary embolism, malignancy, hip and other orthopedic surgery, immobility, hypercoagulable states.

B. Prophylaxis of choice.

1. Encourage all patients to ambulate as soon as possible.
2. Low-risk patients probably do not need prophylaxis.
3. Moderate-risk patients should have either pneumatic compression boots or low-dose heparin prophylaxis. LMWH may play a role in this group in the future.
4. High-risk patients should probably have a combination of therapies consisting of pneumatic compression boots plus low dose heparin or dextran. Full anticoagulation with Coumadin® or IVC filter placement can be considered in these patients. There are no data to support or refute combination *vs.* single therapy.
5. Prophylaxis should be started prior to the institution of anesthesia.
6. Ophthalmology and neurosurgery patients with intracranial or spinal lesions are not considered candidates for prophylaxis with anticoagulants because even minor bleeding may have disastrous consequences.
7. High-risk patients should be watched closely for clinical signs and symptoms of DVT in addition to undergoing frequent (every 3-4 days) objective testing. Duplex scanning is the least invasive of these methods and has a high (88%) sensitivity in the lower extremity.

IV. TREATMENT OF DVT AND PULMONARY EMBOLUS

A. Prevent death from pulmonary embolus.

1. Intubate and give mechanical ventilatory support if necessary.
2. Aggressive respiratory care and monitoring often obtainable only in intensive care setting.
3. Consider anticoagulation versus thrombolytic therapy.

B. Anticoagulation is done for treatment of both pulmonary embolism and DVT. It prevents further propagation of the thrombus and also minimizes the late complication of post-thrombotic syndrome in the leg.

1. Heparin bolus with 100-150 units/kg IV followed by a con-

stant infusion (starting at 1000 units/h) and titrated to maintain the PTT at 50-70 sec. The PTT should be checked at least daily and 4-6 h after every new bolus or rate change. Heparin is usually continued for 7-10 days while the patient's Coumadin® dose is manipulated into the therapeutic range.

2. Coumadin® is generally started 3-5 days after initiating heparin and is continued for 3-6 months. The PT should be maintained at 1.5 times normal (17-20 seconds), or an INR of 2.0-2.5.
3. Contraindications include recent neurosurgical or ophthalmic surgery or hemorrhage, serious active bleeding, or malignant hypertension. Relative contraindications include severe hypertension, recent major surgery, recent major trauma, recent stroke, active GI bleed, bacterial endocarditis, severe hepatic or renal failure.

C. **Thrombolytic therapy** (using streptokinase, urokinase, or tPA).
   1. Promotes rapid clot lysis and may preserve venous valve function.
   2. Useful in patients who have massive pulmonary embolism or who are hypertensive or severely hypoxic due to the mechanical effect of clot producing occlusion of a significant portion of the pulmonary circulation.

D. **Venal caval interruption** (as with a Greenfield filter) prevents further embolism of thrombi > 3 mm. Indications:
   1. Recurrent thromboembolism despite adequate anticoagulation.
   2. Pulmonary embolism in a patient with contraindications to anticoagulation.
   3. Chronic recurrent pulmonary embolism with ensuing pulmonary hypertension.
   4. Complications with anticoagulation.

E. **Venous thrombectomy**—not indicated for routine iliofemoral DVT; however, it may be necessary in cases of venous gangrene or in the event of septic thrombosis.

F. **Pulmonary embolectomy.**
   1. Open embolectomy, usually through a median sternotomy with cardiopulmonary bypass, carries a greater than 50% mortality as well as high morbidity.
   2. Transvenous embolectomy using a suction-cap tipped catheter passed via jugular or femoral vein has been described. Especially useful in massive pulmonary embolism in which there is a contraindication for fibrinolytic therapy.

PART II

Specialized Protocols in Surgery

15

Trauma

Scott W. Gibson, M.D.

Trauma is the leading cause of death in the first four decades of life in the United States and the third leading cause of death in all age groups. Penetrating trauma, particularly from handguns, is becoming more common in nearly all areas of the country, especially in urban areas. The total cost annually of trauma care in this country, including medical care, rehabilitation, and lost wages, exceeds $100 billion. Death from trauma has a trimodal distribution:

1. Seconds to minutes of injury–due to injury to brain, high spinal cord, heart, aorta, and other large vessels. These patients can rarely be salvaged.
2. Minutes to few hours of injury (the "golden hour")–these are due to subdural and epidural hematomas, hemopneumothorax, ruptured spleens, liver lacerations, femur fractures or multiple injuries with significant blood loss. Rapid assessment and resuscitation during this period can reduce trauma deaths, and it is toward this period that Advanced Trauma Life Support (ATLS) techniques are aimed.
3. Several days to weeks of injury–these are due to sepsis and organ failure.

The following chapter is based in part on the American College of Surgeons Committee on Trauma ATLS course, with additional information and some modifications as practiced at the University of Cincinnati Medical Center.

I. TRAUMA SCORING SYSTEMS

A. Physiologic scores—document body's response to injury.

1. ***Trauma score*** – based on the Glasgow Coma Score and hemodynamic assessments (systolic BP, respiratory rate and effort, capillary return). Range from 1 = worst to 16 = best (Table 1).
2. Acute Physiology and Chronic Health Evaluation System (APACHE II)–evaluation designed for the intensive care setting, not specifically for trauma patients. Based on 12 physio-

TABLE 1

Trauma Score	Value	Points	Score
A. **Respiratory Rate:**	20-24	4	
Number of respirations in 15 sec, multiply by four	25-35	3	
	> 35	2	
	< 10	1	
	0	0	A. ______
B. **Respiratory Effort:**	Normal	1	
Shallow — markedly decreased chest movement or air exchange	Shallow or retractive	0	
Retractive — use of accessory muscle or intercostal retraction			B. ______
C. **Systolic Blood Pressure:**	> 90	4	
Systolic cuff pressure — either arm auscultate or palpate	70-90	3	
	50-69	2	
No carotid pulse	< 50	1	
	0	0	C. ______
D. **Capillary Refill:**			
Normal — forehead, lip mucosa, or nail bed color refill in 2 sec.	Normal	2	
Delayed — more than 2 sec of capillary refill	Delayed	1	
None — no capillary refill	None	0	D. ______

E. **Glasgow Coma Scale (GCS)**

1. **Eye opening:**

Spontaneous	______ 4
To Voice	______ 3
To Pain	______ 2
None	______ 1

2. **Verbal response:**

Oriented	______ 5
Confused	______ 4
Inappropriate words	______ 3
Incomprehensible words	______ 2
None	______ 1

3. **Motor response:**

Obeys commands	______ 6
Purposeful movement (pain)	______ 5
Withdraw (pain)	______ 4
Flexion (pain)	______ 3
Extension (pain)	______ 2
None	______ 1

Total GCS Points (1+2+3) ______

Total GCS Points	Score
14-15	5
11-13	4
8-10	3
5-7	2
3-4	1

E. ______

Trauma Score
(Total A+B+C+D+E) ______

From Champion HR, Sallo WJ, Carnazzo AJ, et al.: *Crit Care Med* 9:672-676, 1981, with permission.

logic measurements, may not be properly predictive of outcome in trauma patients.

B. Anatomical scores—based on patient's anatomical injuries.

1. ***Abbreviated injury scale (AIS)***—list of hundreds of injuries, each scored from 1 (minor) to 6 (usually fatal). Complex, usually done with computer software.
2. ***Injury severity score (ISS)***—useful clinical score. Based on AIS, scores range from 1 (minimal injury) to 75 (usually fatal).

II. INITIAL MANAGEMENT

A. Overview.

1. ***Primary survey: ABCs***—life-threatening conditions are identified and simultaneous management begun.
   a. **A**–Airway maintenance with C-spine control.
   b. **B**–Breathing.
   c. **C**–Circulation with hemorrhage control.
   d. **D**–Disability: neurologic status.
   e. **E**–Exposure: completely undress the patient.
2. ***Resuscitation***—shock management is initiated, oxygenation is reassessed, and hemorrhage control is re-evaluated. Tissue aerobic metabolism is assured by perfusion of all tissue with well-oxygenated red blood cells. Volume replacement with crystalloid and blood (if needed) is begun. A Foley and nasogastric tube are placed if not contraindicated.
3. ***Secondary survey***—only begins after primary survey is completed and resuscitation has begun. This is a head-to-toe evaluation of the patient. It uses the look, listen, and feel techniques in a systematic total body/system evaluation. A complete neurologic exam is performed in the secondary survey. Chest, C-spine, and pelvic radiographs are obtained. Special assessment procedures (peritoneal lavage, other radiographs, blood/urine tests) are performed.
4. ***Definitive care***—the patient's less life-threatening injuries are managed. In-depth management, fracture stabilization and splinting, any necessary operative intervention, and stabilization in preparation for transfer are undertaken.

B. Primary survey.

1. ***Airway.***
   a. **General concepts**–the upper airway is assessed to ascertain patency. Maneuvers to establish a patent airway must be made with the knowledge of the possibility of a C-spine injury. C-spine injury should be assumed in all patients, especially those with injuries above the clavicle.
   b. **Airway obstruction–awareness.**
      (1) Head, neck, and facial trauma–typical injury mechanism is the unbelted passenger or driver thrown into the windshield or dashboard.
      (2) Altered level of consciousness–**TIPPS** on the vowels (**AEIOU**):

T—trauma	**A**—alcohol
I—infection	**E**—epilepsy
P—psych	**I**—insulin
P—poison	**O**—opiates
S—shock	**U**—urea/metabolic

c. **Airway obstruction—recognition.** The most important question to ask a trauma patient is "How are you?" No response implies an altered level of consciousness. Positive, appropriate verbal response indicates a patent airway, intact ventilation, and adequate brain perfusion.
   (1) Look—agitation (hypoxia), obtundation (hypercarbia), facial trauma.
   (2) Listen—snoring and gurgling sounds imply partial pharynx occlusion; hoarseness implies laryngeal obstruction/trauma.
   (3) Feel—air movement.

d. **Airway obstruction—management.**
   (1) Objectives—maintain an intact airway, protect the airway in jeopardy, and provide an airway when none is available. These principles must be applied with the assumption that a C-spine injury is present.
   (2) Chin lift and jaw thrust.
   (3) Suction—remove blood and secretions.
   (4) Oropharyngeal airway.
   (5) Nasopharyngeal airway—may also be used to facilitate placement of a nasogastric tube when a cribriform plate fracture is suspected.
   (6) Esophageal obturator airway (EOA)—use is controversial. Do not remove in the unconscious patient until an endotracheal airway is placed.
   (7) Pre-intubation ventilation—mandatory for the hypoxic or apneic patient, use bag-valve face-mask.
   (8) Endotracheal intubation—orally or nasally; neck extension must be avoided. Nasal route is preferred for the non-apneic patient with a non-cleared C-spine, but apneic patients should be orally intubated with manual cervical immobilization. Confirm endotracheal tube placement by auscultation and chest radiograph. Intubation is relatively contraindicated in the presence of severe maxillofacial injuries (one attempt with the patient prepped and locally anesthetized for surgical cricothyroidotomy may be acceptable in selected patients).

e. **Surgical airways.**
   (1) Indications—inability to intubate the trachea (glottic edema, oropharyngeal hemorrhage), contraindication to intubation (severe maxillofacial injuries, larynx fracture).
   (2) Needle cricothyroidotomy—preferred for children un-

der age 12. Place a 12-or 14-ga. plastic cannula into the trachea, connect to wall O_2 at 15 L/min (40-50 PSI) with Y-connector or side hole cut in tubing, and use intermittent ventilation by placing thumb over opening in system (1 second on, 4 seconds off). Effective for only 30-45 min due to poor CO_2 elimination.

(3) Surgical cricothyroidotomy–contraindicated in children under age 12. Surgically prep and locally anesthetize the area, stabilize thyroid cartilage, and make transverse skin incision over lower half of cricothyroid membrane, incise cricothyroid membrane. After scalpel handle or tracheal spreader is used to open airway, insert endotracheal tube or tracheostomy (5-7 mm) and secure.

2. ***Breathing.***
   a. General–expose patient's chest to assess ventilation adequately. Ventilate with a bag-valve device until the patient is stable.
   b. Traumatic conditions that compromise ventilation.
      (1) Tension pneumothorax.
      (2) Open pneumothorax.
      (3) Flail chest with pulmonary contusion.
3. ***Circulation.***
   a. Cardiac output–obtain rapid assessment from:
      (1) Pulse–assess quality, rate, regularity; site of palpable pulse is related to systolic BP (radial > 80, femoral > 80, carotid > 60).
      (2) Skin color.
      (3) Capillary refill–test on hypothenar eminence, thumb, or toenail bed; color should return within two seconds.
   b. **Bleeding.**
      (1) Identify exsanguinating hemorrhage and control it–direct pressure on wound.
      (2) Pneumatic splints and MAST suit are often helpful.
      (3) Major intra-thoracic and intra-abdominal bleeding require rapid operative repair, usually after brief resuscitative period.
4. ***Disability***—brief neurologic evaluation.
   a. **AVPU**–determine level of consciousness.
      (1) **A**–Alert.
      (2) **V**–responds to Vocal stimuli.
      (3) **P**–responds to Painful stimuli.
      (4) **U**–Unresponsive.
   b. Pupillary size and reaction.
   c. More detailed evaluation is done during secondary survey.
5. ***Expose***—completely undress the patient.

C. Resuscitation—after primary survey is completed and especially after an adequate airway has been established, the resuscitation phase begins.

1. ***Oxygen.***
   a. Nasal cannula or face-mask delivery for conscious patients with adequate airways.
   b. Ventilatory support for intubated patients.
   c. Monitor arterial blood gases and/or pulse oximetry O_2 saturation (unreliable in shock).
2. ***Fluid resuscitation***—hypovolemia and shock in trauma are almost always due to blood loss. Access to the circulation for crystalloid or blood resuscitation is mandatory (Table 2).
   a. Crystalloid resuscitation.
      (1) Initial fluid bolus is 1-2 L of isotonic electrolyte solution, preferably lactated Ringer's solution (20 cc/kg in pediatric patients).
      (2) Response (↑ BP, ↓ pulse, ↑ pulse pressure, ↑ CNS state, ↑ skin circulation, ↑ urinary output) to initial fluid bolus determines degree of shock and dictates decision regarding blood replacement.
         a) Rapid response–patient responds and remains stable as fluids are slowed, indicates class I (or less) hemorrhage without ongoing losses, no further fluid bolus or blood required.
         b) Transient response–initial response but subsequent deterioration, indicates class II-III hemorrhage and ongoing losses, continued fluid administration and initiation of blood transfusion are indicated.
         c) Minimal or no response–indicates class IV hemorrhage with or without ongoing losses, rapid blood administration and surgical intervention are needed, also consider error in diagnosis (tension pneumothorax, peri-cardial tamponade, cardiogenic shock).
   b. **Blood replacement.**
      (1) Type O blood–for class IV exsanguinating hemorrhage, Rh negative preferable for females.
      (2) Type-specific, saline crossmatched–for class II-III hemorrhage, usually ready in 10 min.
      (3) Crossmatched–usually ready in 30-60 min, have available in all patients and use when needed and ready.
      (4) Platelets and fresh frozen plasma should be given for multiple transfusion-induced coagulopathy. In general, after 4-6 units of blood have been given, coagulation factors should be ordered.
      (5) Calcium (2 ml of 10% $CaCl_2$ solution)–only needed while blood is being transfused at > 100 ml/min.
   c. **Military anti-shock trousers (MAST).**
      (1) Mechanism of action is translocation of blood from lower extremities, increased peripheral vascular resistance, increased myocardial afterload; it can raise BP but is not a substitute for and should not delay volume replacement.

TABLE 2
Estimated Fluid and Blood Requirements

	Class I	Class II	Class III	Class IV
Blood Loss (ml)	up to 750	750-1500	1500-2000	≥ 2000
Blood Loss (%BV)	up to 15%	15-30%	30-40%	≥ 40%
Pulse Rate	< 100	> 100	> 120	≥ 140
Blood Pressure	Normal	Normal	Decreased	Decreased
Pulse Pressure (mm Hg)	Normal or increased	Decreased	Decreased	Decreased
Capillary Blanch Test	Normal	Positive	Positive	Positive
Respiratory Rate (BPM)	14-20	20-30	30-40	> 35
Urine Output (ml/h)	≥ 30	20-30	5-15	Negligible
CNS-Mental Status	Slightly anxious	Mildly anxious	Anxious and confused	Confused-lethargic
Fluid Replacement (3:1 Rule)	Crystalloid	Crystalloid	Crystalloid + blood	Crystalloid + blood

(2) Indications.
  a) Pelvic fractures–splinting and hemorrhage control.
  b) Soft tissue hemorrhage–tamponade.
  c) Leg fractures–stabilization.
  d) Stabilize circulation for transport.
  e) Maintaining upper torso perfusion when IVs or volume replacement are inadequate.

(3) Contraindications (first 2 are absolute).
  a) Pulmonary edema.
  b) Circulatory instability due to myocardial dysfunction.
  c) Head injuries.
  d) Intrathoracic bleeding.
  e) Diaphragmatic rupture.

(4) Use.
  a) Remove MAST only after shock state is reversed; deflate gradually with abdominal compartment first, then each leg sequentially; if blood pressure falls ≥ 5 mm Hg, reinflate and increase volume resuscitation.
  b) Leave in place once deflated; may take to operating room if patient is unstable.

d. **Intravenous lines.**

(1) Location (order of preference).
  a) Antecubital.
  b) Peripheral upper extremity veins.
  c) Saphenous.
  d) Femoral.
  e) Jugular.
  f) Subclavian.
  g) Central lines–rarely used for resuscitation. Use only in extreme situations or when CVP monitoring is needed (suspected pericardial tamponade). Place on same side of pneumothorax or subcutaneous emphysema if present.

(2) Type (order of preference).
  a) Percutaneous 14- or 16-ga. angiocath.
  b) Large bore, single lumen catheter (8 Fr Traumacath®, sterile IV tubing, 8 Fr pediatric feeding tube).
  c) Cutdown (antecubital, saphenous, cephalic)–8 Fr pediatric feeding tube, sterile IV tubing, 8 Fr Traumacath®.

(3) Number of lines.
  a) 2 lines for stable patients (systolic BP > 100).
  b) 3 lines for marginally stable patients (systolic BP 80-100).
  c) 4-6 lines for unstable patients (systolic BP < 70-80).
  d) Lines on both sides of the diaphragm when injuries are suspected on both sides of the diaphragm.

3. ***Laboratory studies.***
   a. As soon as the first large-bore IV line is established and before infusion of IV fluid, 30-60 cc of blood is withdrawn and sent for STAT blood studies.
      (1) Type & cross for 6 units or more, depending upon the injury.
      (2) Complete blood count and platelet count.
      (3) PT, PTT.
      (4) Electrolytes, including calcium, creatinine, BUN, glucose, and measured osmolality.
      (5) Ethanol level.
      (6) Sickle cell prep as needed.
      (7) Pregnancy test as needed.
   b. Arterial blood gas.
   c. Urinalysis (also dipstick urine).
   d. Osmolality measured (serum and urine).
   e. Urine toxicology screen and serum toxicology screen as indicated.
   f. Liver, bone, and cardiac enzyme profiles as indicated.
   g. Serum amylase.
4. ECG monitoring.
5. ***Foley catheterization*** — monitor urinary output and decompress bladder in preparation for peritoneal lavage.
   a. Immediate insertion *contraindicated* in suspected urethral injury, usually associated with pelvic fracture.
      (1) Blood at the meatus.
      (2) Scrotal or perineal hematoma.
      (3) High-riding prostate (or non-palpable prostate)–rectal exam must be performed prior to Foley insertion.
   b. Prior to Foley insertion in suspected urethral injury, obtain radiographs.
      (1) Retrograde urethrogram–use 20 ml of half-strength contrast; inject gently into meatus, obtain AP and oblique radiographs views, look for disruption or extravasation.
      (2) Cystogram–after Foley placed, fill bladder with 50 cc of contrast; if no extravasation, fill bladder to 250-300 cc by gravity, clamp Foley, and obtain AP and oblique radiographs. Always obtain post-evacuation film.
6. ***Nasogastric tube placement.***
   a. Indications–to relieve and prevent gastric dilatation, remove gastric contents and prevent aspiration (especially prior to intubation), obtain gastric sample for analysis, rule out GI bleeding, decompress stomach prior to peritoneal lavage.
   b. Contraindications (pass NG tube via mouth)–suspected cribiform plate fractures (head trauma with non-clotting [CSF containing] blood coming from ears, nose, or mouth) to avoid intracranial placement, maxillofacial trauma.

D. Secondary survey—involves complete examination of patient in a systematic fashion.

1. ***History and mechanism of injury.***
   a. Pertinent past medical history (**AMPLE**):
      (1) **A**–Allergies.
      (2) **M**–Medications.
      (3) **P**–Past illness.
      (4) **L**–Last meal.
      (5) **E**–Events preceding injury.
   b. Nature of injury.
      (1) Motor vehicle accident (MVA).
         a) Type of collision.
         b) Speed of accident.
         c) Use of seat belts.
         d) Condition of windshield–head trauma.
         e) Condition of steering wheel–blunt chest trauma.
         f) Location of patient in car at time of impact.
         g) Need for extrication, length of time involved.
      (2) Stab wound.
         a) Type of weapon.
         b) Length of knife.
         c) Sex of attacker: Male–upward thrust. Female–downward thrust.
      (3) Gunshot wound.
         a) Caliber of gun.
         b) Distance from patient that gun was fired.
         c) Patient's position when shot.
         d) Number of shots fired.
   c. Condition at scene and on transport.
      (1) Blood pressure.
      (2) Pulse.
      (3) Respiration/airway.
      (4) Level of consciousness.
2. Examination–the secondary survey involves a head-to-toe examination of the patient. The detailed examinations of particular body areas are discussed later in this chapter.
3. ***Radiologic studies.***
   a. Initial mandatory films.
      (1) Lateral C-spine.
      (2) AP chest radiograph (usually supine until spine cleared).
      (3) AP pelvis.
   b. Secondary films.
      (1) CT scan of head, spine, chest, or abdomen as appropriate (see "Neurosurgical Emergencies" and "Specific Injuries")
      (2) C-spine series–additional lateral films if not all vertebra seen (C1-T1), AP, odontoid view.
      (3) T-spine series–AP and lateral.

TABLE 3
Tetanus Prophylaxis for the Wounded Patient

History of Tetanus Immunization (doses)	Clean, Minor Wounds		Tetanus-Prone Wounds	
	TD[1]	TIG	TD[1]	TIG[2]
Uncertain	Yes	No	Yes	Yes
0-1	Yes	No	Yes	Yes
2	Yes	No	Yes	No[3]
3 or more	No[4]	No	No[5]	No

KEY:
[1]TD = 0.5 ml absorbed toxoid. For children younger than 7 years old, DPT (DT if pertussis vaccine is contraindicated) is preferred to tetanus toxoid alone.
[2]TIG = 250 units tetanus immune globulin, human. When TIG and TD are given concurrently, separate syringes and separate sites should be used.
[3]Yes, if wound is more than 24 h old.
[4]Yes, if more than 10 years since last dose.
[5]Yes, if more than 5 years since last dose (more frequent boosters are not needed and can accentuate side-effects).

(4) L-spine series–AP and lateral.
(5) Specific bony films to evaluate suspected areas of injury–facial, skull, extremities.
(6) Upright chest radiograph–obtained after spine is cleared in blunt trauma, to fully evaluate mediastinum.

4. Diagnostic peritoneal lavage (DPL) (see "Specific Injuries," "Trauma Appendix," and "Diagnostic Peritoneal Lavage."
5. Antibiotics.
   a. Intraperitoneal injuries.
   b. Open orthopedic injuries.
6. Tetanus prophylaxis (Table 3).
7. Temperature–hypothermia is detrimental in trauma patients, and every effort should be made to keep the patient warm; use warm blankets, IV fluids, and peritoneal lavage fluid.

E. Definitive care.

III. SPECIFIC INJURIES

A. Abdominal.

1. *Types of injuries.*
   a. Penetrating.
      (1) The limits of the abdomen are the nipples superiorly, the perineum and gluteal folds inferiorly, and the posterior axillary lines laterally.
      (2) Gunshot wounds of the abdomen carry a 95% probability of significant visceral injury.
      (3) Stab wounds of the abdomen–only two-thirds pene-

trate the peritoneal cavity; of these, only half cause significant visceral injury that requires surgical repair.

b. Blunt.
   (1) Injury is produced by compression of the abdominal contents against the vertebral column or rib cage, by direct transfer of energy to an organ or by rapid deceleration with resulting tears of the structures.
   (2) Spleen and liver are most commonly injured organs.
   (3) CT scan, DPL, and ultrasound are key diagnostic aids in identifying patients who require exploration.

2. ***Physical examination.***
   a. *Look*–examine anterior and posterior walls of abdomen, flanks, lower chest, buttocks, and perineum. Look for contusions, abrasions, lacerations, and penetrating wounds.
   b. *Listen*–absence of bowel sounds may indicate ileus or early peritoneal irritation (blood, bacteria, GI secretions). Ileus is also associated with extra-abdominal injuries (thoracic/lumbar spine fractures, burns).
   c. *Feel*–palpate anterior abdominal wall, intra-abdominal contents, and posterior abdomen. Feel for early signs of peritoneal irritation:
      (1) Muscle guarding.
      (2) Percussion tenderness.
3. ***Areas of the abdomen for evaluation.***
   a. Intrathoracic abdomen–portion of abdomen protected by bony thorax (costal margins up to nipples); contains spleen, stomach, liver and diaphragm. Injured by blows to lower thorax and abdomen (sometimes associated with seat belts). Diagnostic modalities include chest radiographs, gastrografin swallow, DPL, CT scanning. Penetrating wounds of thorax below nipples may injure subdiaphragmatic organs; therefore, evaluate with DPL or abdominal exploration.
   b. True abdomen–contains small and large bowel, bladder, uterus, fallopian tubes, and ovaries. More readily accessible to examination. Injuries diagnosed by increasing abdominal pain, decreasing bowel sounds, positive DPL, CT scan, ultrasound, free air on upright chest radiograph or left lateral decubitus abdominal radiograph, blood on rectal exam, peritoneal penetration, evisceration.
   c. Retroperitoneal abdomen–difficult to evaluate and diagnose injuries in this area; there is a high rate of false-negative DPLs. A high index of suspicion is essential to avoid missing injuries here. Involved organs include kidneys, ureters, duodenum, pancreas, and retroperitoneal vascular structures (IVC, aorta, iliac vessels). Diagnostic modalities include IVP, abdominal radiographs (paraduodenal air), gastrografin swallow, CT scan, ultrasound, elevated serum or DPL fluid amylase.
   d. Rectal examination–look at perineum, feel sphincter tone,

feel rectal wall integrity, feel prostate position and mobility, look for gross and occult blood.

e. Vaginal examination–pelvic exam required in all female trauma patients. Look and feel for lacerations. Injuries are often associated with pelvic fractures.

4. ***Diagnoses of abdominal injuries.***
   a. Diagnostic Peritoneal Lavage (see "Diagnostic Peritoneal Lavage")
      (1) Indications.
         a) History of blunt abdominal trauma.
            1) Depressed sensorium or altered pain response leading to possible false-negative physical examination (ethanol intoxication, head injury, drug abuse, spinal cord injury).
            2) Manifestations of hemodynamic instability.
            3) Equivocal abdominal findings (nearly half of patients with hemo-peritoneum will not have positive abdominal findings).
            4) Positive abdominal exam findings.
            5) Unavailability of patient for continued monitoring.
            6) Low rib fractures, particularly on left side.
         b) Stab wound–hemodynamically stable patient without signs of peritoneal irritation.
         c) Gunshot wound–rarely indicated. May be useful in stable patient with low-caliber injury and question of penetration of the peritoneal cavity.
      (2) Contraindications.
         a) Absolute–clinically apparent need for laparotomy.
         b) Relative–multiple previous abdominal incisions, gravid uterus, inability to decompress bladder or stomach, pelvic fracture with pelvic hematoma, coagulopathy.
      (3) Advantages.
         a) Accuracy greater than 90%.
         b) Early diagnosis of serious injury.
         c) Easy to perform
         d) Possible cost savings when compared to other tests.
      (4) Disadvantages.
         a) Lack of organ specificity.
         b) Poor ability to detect retroperitoneal and diaphragm injury.
         c) Bleeding sufficient to create positive result frequently stops by time of laparotomy.
         d) Risk of iatrogenic injury.
   b. Abdominal CT scan.
      (1) Indications.
         a) Hemodynamically stable patient who otherwise meets criteria for DPL.
         b) Inability to perform DPL.

c) Contraindications to DPL.
d) Significant hematuria.
e) Pelvic fracture.
f) Delayed presentation after blunt abdominal injury.
g) Follow-up of a patient undergoing non-operative management of an identified injury.

(2) Contraindications.
a) Clinically apparent need for laparotomy.
b) Unavailability of the scanner for a long period.
c) Uncooperative patient.
d) Allergy to contrast dye.

(3) Advantages.
a) Ability to detect injury and characterize type or location.
b) Noninvasive.
c) Detects retroperitoneal and diaphragm injury.
d) Useful tool for identification and follow-up of non-operative solid organ injury.

(4) Disadvantages.
a) Limited to hemodynamically stable, cooperative patients.
b) Early pancreatic and hollow viscus injury can be missed.
c) Length of time required to perform.
d) Use of contrast dye.
e) Risk oral contrast aspiration.
f) Possible increased cost over other tests.

c. Abdominal ultrasound (a procedure that can be performed easily at the bedside in trauma patients; it is currently gaining acceptance in the United States).

(1) Indications–any patient that meets criteria for DPL or CT scan.

(2) Advantages.
a) Rapid and easy assessment of abdomen with potential for identification of abnormal fluid collections, estimation of fluid quantity, location of fluid in the peritoneal cavity, visualization of solid organ injury, evaluation of the retroperitoneum.
b) Noninvasive.
c) Equipment is portable.
d) Usually less expensive than other tests.
e) Ability to repeat test often if needed.

(3) Disadvantages.
a) Less sensitive than DPL and less specific than CT scan.
b) Difficulty identifying hollow viscus and pancreas injury.
c) Technical difficulties including user inexperience, inter-observer interpretation differences, obese pa-

tients, subcutaneous air, bowel gas that obscures areas of the abdomen.

d. Diagnostic laparoscopy ("minilaparoscopy" that can be performed at the bedside or in the operating room under local anesthesia using a 4-mm laparoscope through a 5-mm trochar).
   (1) Indications–stable patient that meets criteria for DPL or CT scan.
   (2) Contraindications.
      a) Clinically apparent diaphragmatic injury.
      b) Closed head injury (pneumoperitoneum can lead to increased intracranial pressure).
   (3) Advantages.
      a) Ability to assess the abdominal cavity for visible injury.
      b) Ability to select patients for conservative management of some injuries.
   (4) Disadvantages.
      a) Certain areas within the abdomen cannot be seen with laparoscopy including most retroperitoneal structures, the posterior surface of the liver, colon, and diaphragm, and the extraperitoneal urinary bladder.
      b) Possibility of gas embolism with exposed vessels.
      c) Cost if performed in the operating room exceeds that of other tests.
      d) Limited by availability of facilities and equipment, also experience of performing surgeon and technical staff.

5. ***Specific injuries.***
   a. Spleen–injuries usually result from blunt trauma. Management may consist of hemostatic control, splenorrhaphy, partial splenectomy, or splenectomy. Recent operative trend is toward splenic salvage procedures. In hemodynamically stable patients with lower grade injury, strict extended bedrest with serial hematocrit levels is gaining acceptance (see Table 4 for injury classification).
   b. Liver–usually injured from blunt trauma; injuries include capsular tears, simple lacerations, stellate lacerations, stellate lacerations with crush injury, and retrohepatic venous injuries (see Table 5 for injury classification). Management consists of simple repair with/without drainage, direct suture of bleeding vessels, debridement of devitalized tissue, lobectomy, or temporary packing. Lesser-grade injuries in hemodynamically stable patients are often managed nonoperatively with bedrest and serial hematocrit level. Adjuncts of management include the Pringle maneuver (clamping of porta hepatis–up to 60 min), placement of atrial-caval shunt, or hepatic artery ligation.

TABLE 4
Splenic Injury Scale

Grade*		Injury Description
I.	Hematoma	Subcapsular, nonexpanding, < 10% surface area
	Laceration	Capsular tear, nonbleeding, < 1 cm parenchymal depth
II.	Hematoma	Subcapsular, nonexpanding, 10-50% surface area; intraparenchymal, nonexpanding, <2 cm in diameter
	Laceration	Capsular tear, active bleeding, 1-3 cm parenchymal depth, does not involve a trabecular vessel
III.	Hematoma	Subcapsular, > 50% surface area or expanding; ruptured subcapsular hematoma with active bleeding; intraparenchymal hematoma, < 2 cm or expanding
	Laceration	> 3 cm parenchymal depth or involving trabecular vessels
IV.	Hematoma	Ruptured intraparenchymal hematoma with active bleeding
	Laceration	Laceration involving segmental or hilar vessel producing major devascularization (> 25% of spleen)
V.	Laceration	Completely shattered spleen
	Vascular	Hilar vascular injury which devascularizes spleen

*Advance one grade for multiple injuries to the same organ. Based on most accurate assessment of autopsy, laparotomy, or radiologic study.

c. Small bowel–injuries require primary repair or resection and anastomosis.
d. Colon–most injuries can be managed by primary repair or resection and anastomosis. Colostomy usually only required for left-sided injuries with gross fecal contamination, significant associated injuries, presence of shock, or delay in treatment.
e. Pancreas.
   (1) No ductal involvement–adequate drainage with or without suture repair.
   (2) Ductal involvement–distal pancreatectomy for injuries of body or tail, some advocate Roux-en-Y drainage or ductal repair; injuries in head may be drained alone with resultant fistula.
f. Duodenum.
   (1) Duodenal hematoma–may be managed expectantly if exploration is not performed for other reasons; if found

TABLE 5
Liver Injury Scale

Grade		Injury Description
I.	Hematoma	Subcapsular, nonexpanding, < 10% surface area
	Laceration	Capsular tear, nonbleeding, with < 1 cm deep parenchymal disruption
II.	Hematoma	Subcapsular, nonexpanding, hematoma 10-50%; intraparenchymal, nonexpanding, < 2 cm in diameter
	Laceration	< 3 cm parenchymal depth, < 10 cm in length
III.	Hematoma	Subcapsular, > 50% surface area or expanding; ruptured subcapsular hematoma with active bleeding; intraparenchymal hematoma > 2 cm
	Laceration	> 3 cm parenchymal depth
IV.	Hematoma	Ruptured central hematoma
	Laceration	Parenchymal destruction involving 25-75% of hepatic lobe
V.	Laceration	Parenchymal destruction > 75% of heptic lobe
	Vascular	Juxtahepatic venous injuries (retrohepatic cava / major hepatic veins)
VI.	Vascular	Hepatic avulsion

upon exploration, mobilize duodenum, evacuate hematoma, achieve hemostasis, rule out mucosal perforation.

(2) Duodenal injuries—most managed by primary closure with or without duodenostomy tube; more severe injuries require resection, serosal patching, and pyloric exclusion or duodenal diverticulization.

g. Diaphragm—traumatic rupture may be associated with blunt or penetrating trauma.

6. ***Indications for exploratory celiotomy.***
   a. Peritoneal signs.
   b. Diagnostic peritoneal lavage.
      (1) Gross blood > 5 cc.
      (2) RBC count > 100,000/mm^3 (blunt), > 10,000/mm^3 (penetrating).
      (3) WBC count > 500/mm^3.
      (4) Fecal contamination.
      (5) Amylase > serum amylase.
      (6) Lavage fluid of chest tube or bladder catheter.
   c. Diaphragmatic rupture shown by chest radiograph.
   d. Intraperitoneal bladder injury.

B. Chest.

1. Life-threatening injuries—identified in the primary survey.
   a. Tension pneumothorax.
      (1) Pathophysiology—one-way valve air leak from lung or

chest wall allows air to be forced into thoracic cavity (pleural space) without means of escape ⇒ collapse of affected lung ⇒ displacement of mediastinum and trachea to opposite side ⇒ kinking of SVC/IVC and impaired venous return to heart, compression of contralateral lung ⇒ hypotension, hypoxia.

(2) Causes–mechanical ventilation with PEEP and air leak, ruptured emphysematous bullae, blunt chest trauma with unsealed parenchymal lung injury, penetrating thoracic injury.

(3) Diagnosis–tracheal deviation, respiratory distress, unilateral absence of breath sounds, distended neck veins, cyanosis (late), hypertympanic on ipsilateral chest. It is a clinical, not radiographic, diagnosis. Do *not* wait for chest radiograph to diagnose and treat.

(4) Management–initially by inserting large-bore needle (14- or 16-ga. angiocath) into chest via 2nd intercostal space in midclavicular line (diagnosis confirmed by rush of air) to relieve tension; insertion of chest tube then follows.

b. Open pneumothorax.

(1) Pathophysiology–large chest defects often remain open, causing a "sucking chest wound" ⇒ intrathoracic pressure equilibrates with atmospheric pressure; if chest wall opening is greater than two-thirds the diameter of the trachea ⇒ air passes preferentially through the chest defect with each inspiratory effort (it is path of least resistance) ⇒ impairment of effective ventilation ⇒ hypoxia.

(2) Causes–penetrating injury to the thorax that results in a large defect.

(3) Diagnosis–presence of sucking chest wound, hypoxia, hypoventilation.

(4) Management–prompt closure of defect with sterile occlusive dressing taped on 3 sides (provides a flutter valve effect that prevents further air from entering), place chest tube in area remote from wound, surgical closure of defect is usually required.

c. Massive hemothorax.

(1) Pathophysiology–blood loss of 1500 ml into the chest cavity ⇒ compression/collapse of ipsilateral lung ⇒ hypoxia.

(2) Causes–usually due to penetrating thoracic injury that disrupts systemic or pulmonary vessels, can also result from blunt chest trauma. Also consider a ruptured hemidiaphragm with intra-abdominal injury.

(3) Diagnosis–hypoxia, hypoventilation, ipsilateral chest is dull to percussion, absent/decreased breath sounds, hypotension, equivocal neck veins. CXR demonstrates large effusion.

(4) Management–restoration of volume deficit (crystalloid and blood, often type-specific) and evacuation/decompression of chest cavity (36 or 40 Fr chest tube). Most will require operative intervention; emergency thoracotomy rarely needed in the Emergency Room.

d. Flail chest.

(1) Pathophysiology–occurs when a segment of chest wall does not have bony continuity with the rest of the thoracic cage, usually secondary to multiple rib fractures ⇒ paradoxical motion of the chest wall (flail segment sinks in during inspiration). Hypoxia results from underlying pulmonary contusion and associated bony pain, which hinders respiratory effort.

(2) Causes–severe blunt thoracic trauma, usually MVA.

(3) Diagnosis–usually apparent on visual examination of the patient's chest and inspiratory pattern, but may not be initially seen due to splinting. Flail segment and rib fractures may be palpated, rib fractures and pulmonary contusion may be seen on chest radiographs, and respiratory failure with hypoxia in severe cases.

(4) Management–initially involves adequate ventilation, O_2 therapy, and avoidance of overhydration. Stabilization of the chest wall defect is not important, and definitive treatment is re-expansion of lung and maintaining adequate oxygenation. Intubation and mechanical ventilation are needed in severe cases (CPAP mask use may preclude intubation). Adequate pain control (best achieved with thoracic epidural) is essential to allow for good ventilatory effort and respiratory care.

e. Cardiac tamponade.

(1) Pathophysiology–the pericardial sac is a fixed fibrous structure, and only a small amount of blood is required in an acute setting to severely restrict cardiac activity. Pericardial blood ⇒ impaired venous filling ⇒ signs of venous hypertension and systemic hypotension due to poor cardiac output.

(2) Causes–vast majority are penetrating injuries, rarely due to blunt trauma.

(3) Diagnosis–the diagnosis should be suspected in any patient who presents with penetrating injury (knife, bullet) to the anterior chest between the nipples or transmediastinal missile path. Beck's classic triad of distended neck veins, hypotension, and muffled heart sounds is uncommon. Other signs/symptoms include pulses paradoxus and mental anxiety or agitation. Diagnosis is confirmed by pericardiocentesis or sub-xyphoid pericardial window performed in the operating room. If available, ultrasound can demonstrate pericardial fluid.

(4) Management–immediate removal of pericardial blood

via pericardiocentesis may be life-saving, use of a plastic catheter that can be left in place allows repeated aspiration if necessary. Positive pericardiocentesis mandates emergent median-sternotomy and inspection and repair of the heart. False-negatives and false-positives do occur. Subxyphoid pericardial window is suitable for patients with a good possibility of tamponade and who are hemodynamically stable enough to make it to the operating room. Many authors prefer this approach in all patients in place of pericardiocentesis.

2. Potentially lethal injuries identified in the secondary survey.
   a. Pulmonary contusion with or without flail chest.
      (1) General–common, potentially lethal due to gradual development of respiratory failure similar to ARDS.
      (2) Clinically–presents in setting of appropriate blunt chest trauma, usually MVA related. Often with associated rib fractures. Chest radiograph may show localized infiltrate, but chest radiographic findings often lag behind or do not correlate with clinical course. Hypoxia is good indicator.
      (3) Management–analgesics (intermittent or continuous parenteral morphine, patient-controlled analgesia, thoracic epidural) and good pulmonary toilet are essential. Patients should be monitored in ICU setting for 24-48 h. Selective management without intubation is suitable for many patients. CPAP mask is another measure that may preclude intubation.
      (4) Factors predisposing toward intubation/mechanical ventilation:
         a) Severe contusion with hypoxia.
         b) Pre-existing chronic pulmonary disease.
         c) Impaired level of consciousness.
         d) Abdominal injury resulting in ileus, or exploratory laparotomy.
         e) Skeletal injuries requiring immobilization.
         f) Renal failure.
         g) Poor cough effort, atelectasis, lobar collapse.
   b. Thoracic aortic tear/rupture.
      (1) General–most common cause of sudden death after an MVA or fall (major deceleration injury); 90% of these are fatal either at scene or prior to arriving in the Emergency Room; of the 10% who make it to a hospital, half will die each day if left untreated/unrecognized. Tear usually occurs just beyond take-off of left subclavian artery, at the insertion of the ligamentum arteriosum.
      (2) Diagnosis–a high index of suspicion, along with appropriate radiologic findings, should prompt arteriography (arch and great vessels) to confirm the diagnosis. About 10% of aortograms will be positive if appropriate liberal

indications are used. Work-up should not take precedence over immediate life-threatening injuries such as hemoperitoneum or intracranial hematoma.

(3) Chest radiographic findings associated with aortic tear.
   a) Widened mediastinum–> 8 cm, preferably on an upright PA film.
   b) Fractures of the first and second ribs.
   c) Obliteration of aortic knob.
   d) Deviation of the trachea to the right.
   e) Presence of a pleural cap.
   f) Elevation and rightward shift of the right mainstem bronchus.
   g) Depression of the left mainstem bronchus.
   h) Obliteration of space between pulmonary artery and aorta.
   i) Deviation of the esophagus (NG tube) to the right.

(4) Management–immediate surgical repair, either direct repair or resection with grafting.

c. Tracheobronchial tree injuries.

(1) Tracheal injuries–due to blunt or penetrating injury.
   a) Fracture of larynx–triad of hoarseness, subcutaneous emphysema, and palpable fracture crepitus.
   b) Fiberoptic laryngoscopy may aid in diagnosis.
   c) Definitive surgical repair required.

(2) Bronchial injury.
   a) Clinically–unusual but potentially fatal injury, usually results from blunt trauma. Usually occurs about 1 inch from carina. May present with hemoptysis, subcutaneous emphysema, or tension pneumothorax. Pneumothorax with persistent large air leak is typical. Diagnosis is confirmed with bronchoscopy.
   b) Management–usually requires direct repair via a thoracotomy.

d. Esophageal injury.

(1) General–usually caused by penetrating injury, rarely blunt trauma.

(2) Clinically–presents similar to Boerhaave's syndrome, left pneumothorax or hemothorax without a rib fracture, history of severe blow to lower sternum or epigastrium, pain or shock out of proportion to injury, particulate matter in chest tube drainage, chest tube that bubbles continuously and equally during inspiration and expiration, and mediastinal air or empyema (usually on left side). Diagnosis confirmed by gastrograffin swallow or esophagoscopy. Esophageal injury due to penetrating trauma usually occurs in the neck.

(3) Management–treatment of choice is wide drainage of the pleural space and mediastinum and direct repair of the injury via thoracotomy. Esophageal diversion in the neck and gastrostomy is sometimes required.

e. Traumatic diaphragmatic hernia.
   (1) Clinically–more common on left side (liver protects right hemidiaphragm). Blunt trauma usually produces large diaphragmatic tears with acute herniation (stomach, small bowel). Penetrating trauma produces small perforations that often take years to develop into hernias. In a small percentage of cases, defects are found bilaterally. High index of suspicion is key to making the diagnosis, as is careful exploration of diaphragm at time of exploratory laparotomy.
   (2) Diagnosis–suggested by abnormal chest radiograph (elevated hemidiaphragm, loculated hydropneumothorax, NG tube in left lower chest) in appropriate clinical setting. Gastrografin upper GI series and CT scan are sometimes helpful. Rarely discovered when peritoneal lavage fluid fills chest.
   (3) Management–operative repair indicated. Best approached via abdomen in acute setting because of high incidence of associated intra-abdominal injuries. Approach via chest in delayed setting owing to presence of intrathoracic adhesions that require lysis.

f. Myocardial contusion.
   (1) Clinically–results from blunt chest trauma, usually unrestrained driver in head-on collision that results in bent or crushed steering wheel column. Often associated with chest wall contusion or fractures of the sternum and/or ribs.
   (2) Diagnosis–an abnormal ECG (PACs, PVCs, atrial fibrillation, bundle branch block, ST segment changes) may be present. Major contusions are associated with hemodynamic instability and unexplained hypotension. Diagnosis can be confirmed with serial cardiac enzyme determinations, echocardiography, or MUGA scanning. There is little or no role of work-up in patient who has normal ECG, no arrhythmias, and is hemodynamically stable.
   (3) Management–because of risk of dysrhythmias patients should be continuously monitored in ICU or monitored bed setting for 24 h. Patients with documented contusions and hemodynamic compromise who require surgery with general anesthetic for treatment of associated injuries should undergo invasive hemodynamic monitoring (A-line, pulmonary artery catheter) peri-operatively.

3. ***Serious chest injuries.***
   a. Subcutaneous emphysema.
      (1) May result from airway injury, lung injury, or rarely, blast injury.
      (2) A physical finding that often necessitates chest tube placement.

b. Pneumothorax.
   (1) Pathophysiology–results from entry of air (either from lung or atmosphere) into pleural space. May result from penetrating or blunt chest trauma. Most commonly caused by lung laceration associated with rib fractures from blunt trauma.
   (2) Diagnosis–usually seen on chest radiographs. Typical signs (hyper-resonance, decreased breath sounds) are often difficult to detect in noisy emergency room unless tension pneumothorax is present.
   (3) Management–placement of chest tube in 4th or 5th inter-costal space, anterior to mid-axillary line. Initially place tube to suction and confirm placement and lung re-expansion with repeat chest radiograph. Patients at risk for pneumothorax (rib fractures, significant blunt chest injury) should have chest tubes placed prophylactically prior to undergoing a general anesthetic for management of associated injuries.

c. Hemothorax.
   (1) Pathophysiology–due to lung laceration or laceration of an intercostal vessel or internal mammary artery, seen in penetrating or blunt trauma.
   (2) Diagnosis–effusion seen on chest radiograph, diminished breath sounds.
   (3) Management–any hemothorax sufficient to appear on chest radiograph requires placement of large-caliber chest tube. This provides immediate drainage to prevent a clotted hemothorax or fibrothorax with associated restrictive pulmonary function. Chest tube also provides a monitoring method to assess the severity of injury . . . initial drainage of $>$ 1000 cc blood or hourly output of $\geq$ 200 cc are indications for exploratory thoracotomy. Most hemothoraces, however, require chest tube placement only.

d. Rib fractures.
   (1) Pathophysiology–pain on motion results in splinting of thorax $\Rightarrow$ impaired ventilation, poor clearance of secretions $\Rightarrow$ atelectasis, pneumonia. Because of greater flexibility of chest in youth, rib fractures in young patients imply greater thoracic impact.
   (2) Clinically–upper ribs (1-3) are well protected, and their fracture implies major impact, often with associated head, neck, spinal cord, lung, or great vessel injury. Middle ribs (5-9) are the most commonly injured, often associated with pneumothorax, hydrothorax, pulmonary contusion, or flail chest.
   (3) Diagnosis–localized pain, tenderness on palpation, crepitus, palpable or visible deformity. Chest radiograph is important to exclude other intrathoracic injuries.

(4) Management–adequate analgesia and pulmonary toilet, intercostal blocks or epidural analgesia are helpful. Splinting or taping is of no value.

4. ***Emergency Department thoracotomy.***
   a. General–survival of trauma patients arriving in the Emergency Room in full cardiac arrest is not enhanced by thoracotomy.
   b. Indications.
      (1) Patients in full arrest with penetrating chest or high epigastric wounds.
      (2) Patients (blunt or penetrating) who arrest (witnessed) during initial evaluation and resuscitation.
   c. Technique.
      (1) Anterolateral thoracotomy, 4th-5th intercostal space (infra-mammary), left side (some recommend side of wound), incision may be extended across midline if needed.
      (2) Incise pericardium with scissors along longitudinal axis of heart anterior to phrenic nerve to evacuate hemopericardium.
      (3) If hemopericardium present, visualize and control cardiac wounds (finger, hand, Foley catheter).
      (4) Look for ruptured thoracic aorta (subadventitial hematoma).
      (5) Cross-clamp descending thoracic aorta.
      (6) Begin cardiac massage.
      (7) Transport to operating room for definitive care.

C. Genitourinary (see "Urologic Problems in Surgical Practice").

D. Head (see "Neurosurgical Emergencies").

E. Spinal cord (see "Neurosurgical Emergencies").

F. Extremity trauma (see also "Orthopedic Emergencies").

1. General considerations.
   a. Extremity trauma is rarely life-threatening; however, if not properly managed, permanent disability may occur.
   b. Except for direct control of bleeding, which includes maintaining traction on extremities with obvious or suspected fractures, the extremities receive little specific attention during the primary survey.
2. Extremity assessment–occurs during secondary survey.
   a. History–mechanism of injury, environment, predisposing factors, findings at the accident scene, pre-hospital care, status of tetanus prophylaxis.
   b. Physical examination.
      (1) *Look*–deformities, angulation, shortening, swelling, discoloration, bruising, muscle spasm, wounds, color and perfusion of the extremity.
      (2) *Feel*–tenderness, crepitation, pulse (Doppler signal), capillary filling, sensation, warmth.
      (3) *Movement*–active motion, passive motion (not of an obvious fracture).

c. Fracture assessment–fractures are either closed or open (associated with break in skin).
   (1) Life-threatening extremity injuries.
      a) Massive, open fractures with ragged, dirty wounds.
      b) Bilateral femoral shaft fractures–open or closed.
      c) Vascular injuries, with or without fractures, proximal to the knee or elbow.
      d) Crush injuries of the abdomen and pelvis, major pelvic fractures.
      e) Traumatic amputations of the arm or leg.
   (2) Limb-threatening injuries.
      a) Fracture-dislocation of the ankle with or without vascular compromise.
      b) Tibial fractures with vascular impairment.
      c) Dislocation of the knee or hip.
      d) Wrist and forearm fractures with circulatory interruption.
      e) Fractures or dislocations of the elbow.
      f) Crush injury.
      g) Amputations, complete or incomplete.
      h) Open fractures.
   (3) Associated fractures or dislocations–certain injuries, because of a common mechanism, are often associated with a second injury that is not immediately apparent; i.e., knee contusions may be a clue to patellar or supracondylar fractures of the femur in patients with posterior dislocations of the hip.
   (4) Occult fractures–beware of fractures in the multiple-injured patient with life-threatening injuries.

d. Blood loss assessment.
   (1) Closed injury–closed femur fractures can result in 2-3 units of blood loss, closed pelvic fractures can cause hypovolemic shock.
   (2) Open injury–blood loss from open fractures is usually far greater than estimated.

e. Dislocation and fracture-dislocation assessment. Radiographs are required for differentiation. Dislocations produce neurovascular stress that can be limb-threatening. Dislocations should be reduced as soon as possible.

f. Neurovascular assessment.
   (1) Vascular injuries–can result in bleeding or thrombosis with impairment of distal circulation and ischemia. Often suggested by brisk bleeding from wound, although complete arterial tears bleed less than partial tears. A large hematoma or injuries to adjacent neural structures are also suggestive. Examination of distal pulses is crucial, although the presence of a pulse does not rule out vascular injury. Proximity wounds must be evaluated, and all pulse abnormalities must be evaluated with angiography in symptomatic patients or with ultrasound

duplex scanning in asymptomatic patients. An arterial pressure index (ratio of blood pressure distal to extremity injury compared to uninjured extremity) of 0.9 or greater indicates a non-operative lesion with 95% accuracy. Current trend is to observe patients with clinically occult vascular injuries.

(2) Nerve injuries–may be complete disruption or contusion/stretch injury.

g. Vascular impairment (extremity ischemia).
   (1) Signs of vascular injury.
      a) Bleeding.
      b) Expanding hematoma.
      c) Bruit.
      d) Abnormal pulses.
      e) Impaired distal circulation.
   (2) Arterial intimal tears often are not immediately recognized, although they can rapidly lead to thrombosis.
   (3) Checklist for suspected vascular injury.
      a) Check immobilization device.
      b) Assess fracture alignment.
      c) Re-assess distal perfusion, Doppler signals.
      d) Consider compartment syndrome.
      e) Arteriogram vs. ultrasound duplex.
   (4) Goal of management is to identify vascular injuries prior to the development of ischemia (six P's–pain, paresthesias, paralysis, pallor, pulselessness, poikilothermia).

h. Compartment syndrome–can occur in lower leg or arm because neurovascular bundle is enveloped within the fascial planes. Associated with compartmental hemorrhage and edema, often with fractures and crush injuries.

i. Amputation–preserve amputated parts for possible reimplantation or use of skin/soft tissue for grafts to treat other injuries.

G. Penetrating neck injury.

1. ***Assessment by Zones*** (Figure 1).
   a. **Zone I** (base of neck)–from the suprasternal notch or cricoid cartilage and inferiorly, includes great vessels, difficult exposure and control.
   b. **Zone II** (neck)–between zones I and III, easy exposure and control.
   c. **Zone III** (base of skull)–from the angle of the mandible and superiorly, difficult exposure and control.
2. Management.
   a. Surgical exploration indicated for the following signs/symptoms.
      (1) Penetration of platysma (Zone II)–never probe defect.
      (2) Subcutaneous or retropharyngeal air on examination or plain films.
      (3) Hoarseness or stridor.

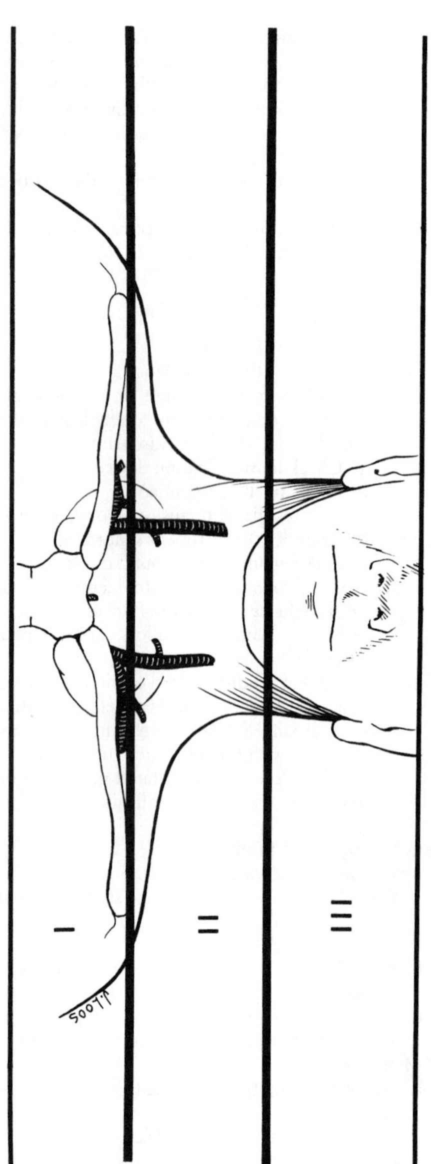

FIG. 1

(4) Active external or oropharyngeal hemorrhage.
(5) Absent carotid pulse.
(6) Bruit or thrill suggesting intimal flap or arteriovenous fistula.
(7) Neurologic deficit.

b. Zone I injuries–selective management.
c. Zone II injuries–mandatory exploration.
d. Zone III injuries–selective management.
e. Diagnostic modalities for selective management.
   (1) Arteriography–arch, great vessels, carotids, and vertebrals.
   (2) Carotid Duplex scanning.
   (3) Laryngoscopy, bronchoscopy–flexible and rigid.
   (4) Esophagoscopy, contrast esophagography.

H. Maxillofacial trauma.

1. ***Initial evaluation*** — beware of causes of sudden death or permanent disability.
   a. Cervical spine fractures–present in 2-4% of cases when facial fractures are present.
   b. Laryngeal fractures.
      (1) Symptoms.
         a) Laryngeal pain.
         b) Dysphonia or aphonia.
         c) Hemoptysis.
         d) Stridor.
         e) Dysphagia.
      (2) Physical findings.
         a) Distortion of normal external landmarks.
         b) Cervical ecchymosis.
         c) Subcutaneous emphysema.
         d) Air or salivary leakage from lacerations.
      (3) Treatment.
         a) Do not attempt endotracheal intubation.
         b) Early tracheostomy under optimum conditions at 3rd or 4th tracheal ring.
         c) Open reduction with internal fixation (ORIF).
2. ***History.***
   a. Important to note both pre-injury and post-injury visual acuity and occlusion.
   b. Also note special pre-injury problems (i.e., hearing deficits, nasal airway obstruction, or missing teeth).
3. ***Physical examination.***
   a. Note and diagram any lacerations or abrasions–photographs are best; determine whether tissue loss is present.
   b. Eye exam.
      (1) Visual acuity.
      (2) Extraocular muscle function.
      (3) Fundoscopic examination.
      (4) Eyelids and conjunctiva.

(5) Fluorescein exam if corneal abrasion is suspected.
(6) "Raccoon eyes" indicates basilar skull fracture until proven otherwise.
(7) Ophthalmology consult for suspected globe injury.

c. Ear exam.
(1) Look for distortion of normal landmarks on the external ear indicating hematoma.
(2) Otoscopic exam for foreign body, hemotympanum.
(3) Hemotympanum or CSF otorrhea–imply basilar skull fracture.

d. Nose exam.
(1) Palpation for fracture–radiographs play little or no role in establishing or excluding the diagnosis of nasal fracture.
(2) Check for septal hematoma.
(3) CSF rhinorrhea–basilar skull fracture.

e. Mouth exam.
(1) Check occlusion.
(2) Look for loose or missing teeth–if teeth missing, check posterior pharynx or chest radiograph for aspiration.
(3) Intra-oral laceration or ecchymosis.

f. Facial skeleton–bimanual exam of all facial bones to assess tenderness and/or motion.

4. Radiologic evaluation.
a. C-spine series.
b. Reverse Waters view for suspected zygomatic/maxillary complex fracture–may be done in the Emergency Room.
c. Panorex for patients with malocclusion or suspected mandibular fracture–patient needs to be able to sit up and be cooperative.
d. CT scan–patient should be stable hemodynamically and cooperative.
(1) Axial–good detail of zygomatic arches.
(2) Coronal/sagittal cuts–give excellent orbital detail; need clear C-spine.
(3) 3-D reconstructions not generally necessary.

5. Management.
a. Soft tissue.
(1) Anesthesia.
a) Local anesthesia with 1:200,000 epinephrine is helpful to control hemorrhage and prolong anesthetic effect.
b) Nerve blocks diminish volume required and minimize distortion (see "Anesthesia").
c) Mark normal landmarks before infiltration (i.e., lip vermilion).
(2) Cleansing–large-volume high-pressure irrigation, mild detergent soap.
(3) Sharp debridement.

a) All foreign material.
b) Any unequivocally dead tissue.
c) Preserve all viable tissue–narrowly based flaps on the face will survive because of excellent blood supply.
d) Black powder tattoos should go to the operating room for debridement under general anesthesia as soon as possible.
e) Drain any significant hematoma.

(4) Reapproximation of normal landmarks.
(5) Any residual soft tissue defect can be managed acutely by moist saline dressings and referral to plastic surgeon.
(6) For eyelid avulsion, keep the eye well lubricated with bland ophthalmic ointment and patch coverage; immediate ophthalmologic referral.
(7) Special cases.

a) Suspected laceration of Stensen's (parotid) duct.
 1) Location (Figure 2).
 2) Cannulation of duct for suspected injury.
 3) Treatment–repair soft tissue over stent with drain.

b) Lacrimal duct laceration.
 1) Location–laceration through lid margin medial to punta or through medial canthus.
 2) Treatment–ophthalmologic referral for cannulation of duct and repair of laceration over stent.

c) Facial nerve injury.
 1) Note functional defect and location of lesion.
 2) Those lateral to canthus should be repaired with the microscope.

b. Facial fracture management–operative considerations.

(1) Restore facial height and projection.
(2) Re-establish pre-traumatic occlusion.
(3) Wide exposure–through laceration or incisions: intraoral, lower lid, coronal incision.
(4) Thorough debridement.
(5) Meticulous reduction and fixation.
(6) Specific approach based on anatomic diagnosis.
(7) Treatment of complex cases.

a) Restore mandibular relation to cranial base.
b) Restore occlusion.
c) Reconstruct midface.

c. Facial fracture management based on diagnosis.

(1) Upper third–supraorbital ridge, orbital roof, frontal sinus, naso-orbitoethmoid.

a) Exam–pain, tenderness, edema, ecchymosis, palpable fracture; look for associated injuries.
b) Treatment.
 1) Posterior table intact, anterior table depressed.

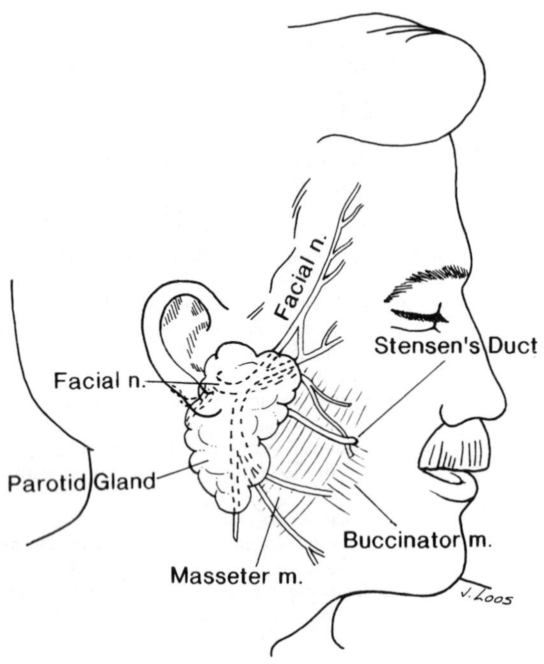

FIG. 2

(a) Duct open–ORIF of anterior table.
(b) Duct injured–obliterate sinus or fix duct, then ORIF.

2) Posterior table not intact.
   (a) Neurosurgery evaluation.
   (b) Nondisplaced.
   (c) Displaced–cranialization vs. obliteration.
3) Complications–meningitis, CSF leaks, sinusitis, residual deformity.

(2) Middle third–maxilla, zygoma, orbit, nose.
   a) Nasal bones.
      1) Symptoms–epistaxis, pain, nasal congestion.
      2) Exam–tenderness, edema, ecchymosis, displacement, instability, crepitance.
      3) Treatment–drain septal hematoma if present.
         (a) Closed reduction and splint.
         (b) May require revision.

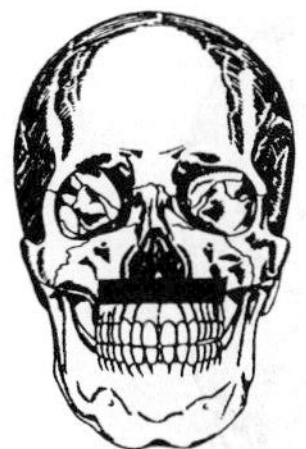

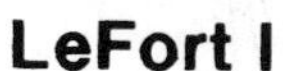

LeFort I
(Transverse fracture)

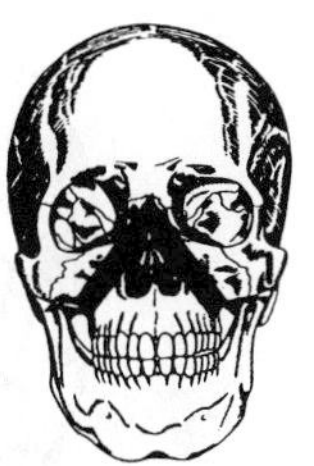

LeFort II
(Pyramidal fracture)

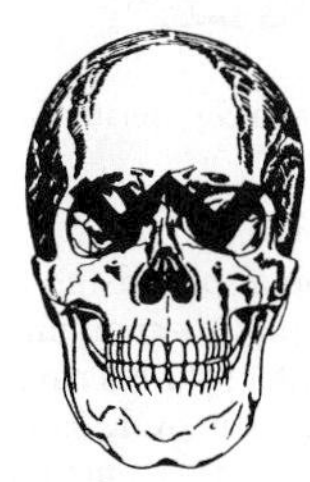

LeFort III
(Craniofacial disjunction)

FIG. 3

b) Maxilla (Figure 3)–pass orogastric tube if maxillofacial fracture suspected.
   1) LeForte I–transverse.
   2) LeForte II–pyramidal.
   3) LeForte III–craniofacial dysjunction.
   4) On exam will likely have significant facial swelling.
   5) Midface will be unstable to bimanual exam.
   6) Treatment–ORIF within 7-14 days.
   7) Complications.
      (a) Maxillary retrusion (LeForte I).
      (b) "Dish face" deformity (LeForte II/III).
      (c) Malocclusion.

c) Zygoma (Tripod) fracture (Figure 4).
   1) On exam–periorbital edema and ecchymosis, depressed cheek, tenderness, step off, proptosis or enophthalmos, infraorbital nerve hypesthesia, trismus.

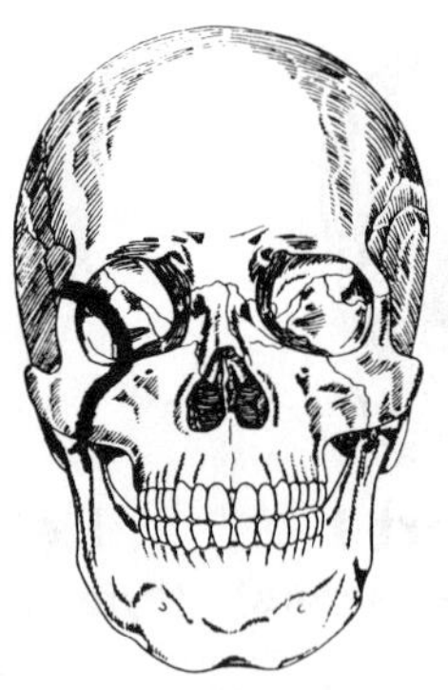

FIG. 4 Fracture of Zygomatic Complex

2) Treatment.
   (a) Non-displaced–no treatment.
   (b) Displaced–comminution or zygomatic-frontal suture separation.
      i. Present–ORIF.
      ii. Absent–reduction only.
3) Complications–sinusitis, diplopia, enophthalmos, blindness, superior orbital fissure syndrome (compromised cranial nerves III, IV, VI), orbital apex syndrome (compromised cranial nerves II, III, IV, VI), persistent infraorbital nerve anesthesia.

d) Orbital.
   1) Exam–diplopia, enophthalmos, periorbital edema, ecchymosis, infraorbital nerve hypesthesia.
   2) Treatment–to correct entrapment, prevent enophthalmos–ORIF with/without bone grafting.
   3) Operative complications–visual loss (rare), orbital hemorrhage (1%), infection (3-4%), infraorbital neuralgia (rare), ectropion (1%), persistent diplopia (2-50%), persistent enophthalmos (15-22%).

(3) Lower third–mandible.
   a) Symptoms–malocclusion, trismus, pain.
   b) Exam–tenderness, edema, ecchymosis, laceration, displacement, instability on bimanual exam, mental nerve hypesthesia.
   c) Radiologic–Panorex series.
   d) Management–as soon as conveniently possible.
      1) Closed reduction.

(a) Maxillomandibular fixation (MMF)–85-95% may be treated in this way.
(b) External fixation rare.
2) ORIF–helps minimize time in MMF.
e) Complications.
1) Malocclusion.
2) Temporal-mandibular joint (TMJ) pain.
3) Nonunion.
f) Complications of MMF.
1) Weight loss and feeding problems.
2) Airway compromise and poor pulmonary toilet.
3) Poor oral hygiene.
4) Social and communication problems.
g) Special cases.
1) Children–avoid open reduction and internal fixation–tooth buds; early mobilization important, especially for condylar fractures.
2) Edentulous mandible.
(a) Thin mandible with no teeth makes accurate reduction, fixation, and subsequent bony union a challenge.
(b) May do closed reduction with splints and MMF.
(c) ORIF may be necessary.

I. Trauma in pregnancy.

1. *Diagnosis.*
a. **Initial assessment.**
(1) Patient position–keep patient on left side (unless spinal injury suspected) to avoid inferior vena cava compression by gravid uterus; if the patient is supine, elevate right hip and manually displace uterus to left.
(2) Primary survey–support physiologic hypervolemia liberally with crystalloid and blood administration (the pregnant patient can lose up to 35% of her blood volume before tachycardia, hypotension, and other signs of hypovolemia occur; thus, the fetus may be in severe jeopardy while the mother appears stable); vasopressors should be avoided.
b. **Secondary assessment.**
(1) Assessment of uterine irritability, fundal height and tenderness, fetal heart tones, fetal movement.
(2) Uterine contractions, vaginal bleeding.
(3) Ruptured membranes suggested by fluid in vagina with pH of 7.0 to 7.5.
(4) Cervical effacement and dilatation, fetal presentation, station.
2. Management.
a. Monitoring.
(1) Patient–monitor while on left side.

(2) Fetus–continuous monitoring with ultrasonic Doppler cardioscope to diagnose fetal distress (inadequate accelerations, late decelerations).
(3) Routine radiographs of mother should be performed–fetal survival depends on maternal well-being.

b. Definitive care.
(1) Initial management directed at resuscitation and stabilization of the pregnant patient–the fetus' life is totally dependent on the integrity of the mother's.
(2) DPL–open technique, above uterus.

3. Specific injuries.
a. Uterine rupture–uterus is protected during first trimester but thereafter becomes progressively more vulnerable; may present with minimal symptoms or with shock; radiographic evidence includes extended fetal extremities, abnormal fetal position, free intraperitoneal air; suspicion mandates surgical exploration.
b. Abruptio placenta (placental separation from uterine wall)–leading cause of fetal death after blunt trauma; presents with vaginal bleeding, premature labor, fetal distress and demise, abdominal pain, uterine tenderness and rigidity, expanding fundal height, maternal shock, disseminated intravascular coagulation.
c. Pelvic fractures–additional hemorrhagic complications due to engorged pelvic veins.

J. Pediatric trauma.

1. General.
a. Trauma is the leading cause of death in the pediatric patient.
b. Most frequent mechanism is blunt injury, with motor vehicle accidents accounting for > 50%.
c. Basic management is similar as for adults, with some differences outlined below.

2. Special considerations in initial management.
a. Airway–young infants are obligate nose breathers (clear nasal obstruction), trachea is short (avoid bronchial intubation), trachea is small (intubate with uncuffed tubes of appropriate size), cricothyroidotomy almost never indicated (use needle jet insufflation if needed).
b. Shock.
(1) Recognition of shock (normal vitals are age-related).
a) Tachycardia–≥ 120-160.
b) Cool extremities.
c) Hypotension–systolic blood pressure < 80-100.
(2) Fluid replacement.
a) Initial bolus of lactated Ringer's solution–20 cc/kg over 10 min, may repeat once.
b) Blood–give 20 cc/kg whole blood or 10 cc/kg PRBC after above measures fail.

(3) Acid-base disturbances–usually can be corrected with ventilation, give bicarbonate for pH < 7.2.
(4) Venous access–after percutaneous lines placed; cut-down options are saphenous, cephalic (elbow and upper arm), external jugular.
(5) Thermoregulation–maintain temperature at 36-37°C by use of overhead heaters and thermal blankets.

3. Specific injuries.
   a. **Chest trauma.**
      (1) Pneumothorax/hemothorax–poorly tolerated.
      (2) Flail chest–especially sensitive.
      (3) Bronchial injuries, diaphragmatic rupture–more prone.
      (4) Great vessel injury–less prone.
      (5) Because of increased chest wall compliance, significant intrathoracic injuries may exist without rib fractures.
   b. **Abdominal injuries**–the evaluation of blunt abdominal injury in the child differs from the adult in that hemoperitoneum is not an absolute indication for surgery. Consequently, CT scan is preferable to peritoneal lavage in the diagnosis of abdominal injury.
      (1) CT scan indicated for: stable vital signs, suspected intra-abdominal injury, slowly declining hematocrit, requirement for continued fluid resuscitation, neurologic impairment, multiple injuries requiring general anesthesia, multiple bleeding sources, hematuria.
      (2) Routine liver enzymes in all patients with blunt trauma; SGOT > 200, SGPT > 100 correlates well with CT demonstrable hepatic injury.
      (3) Majority of splenic and hepatic injuries stop bleeding with conservative (non-operative) therapy.
      (4) If DPL used, use 10 cc/kg lactated Ringer's solution as lavage fluid.
      (5) Criteria for surgical exploration:
         a) Continued hemodynamic instability.
         b) Multiple, large devitalized tissue fragments noted on CT scan.
         c) Persistent bleeding (transfusion requirement > 50% of calculated blood volume over 24 h).
         d) Splenic injury with known pre-existing splenic disease (mononucleosis, leukemia, etc.).
         e) Pneumoperitoneum or peritoneal signs.
         f) Inability to provide continuous surgical intensive care observation or lack of adequate surgical support.
   c. Extremity trauma–potential for injury to growth plate.
   d. Depending on type of injury, suspicion of child abuse.

APPENDIX

I. PENETRATING CHEST TRAUMA

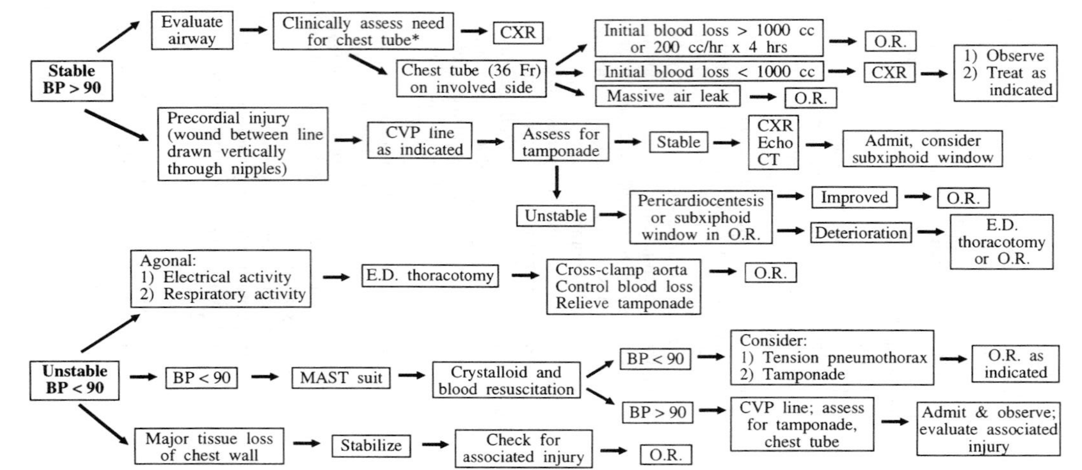

* 1) Tension pneumothorax; 2) Sucking chest wound; 3) Hemothorax

II. BLUNT CHEST TRAUMA

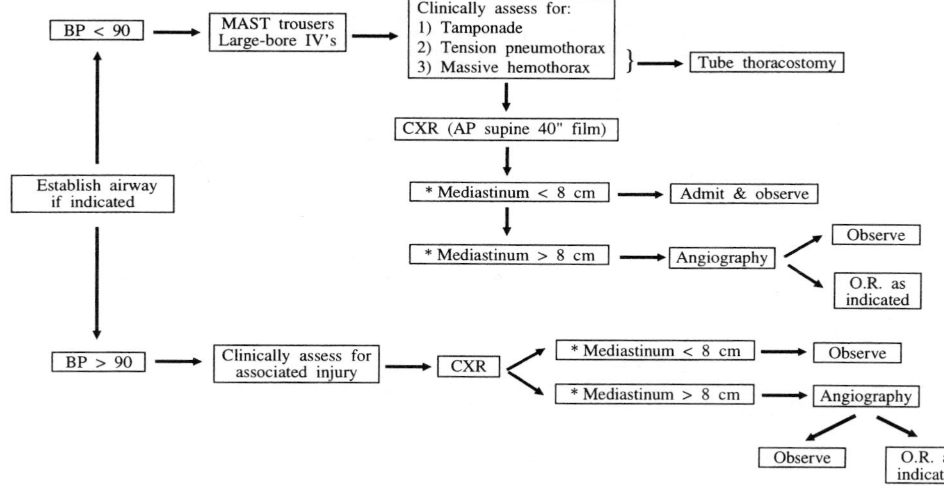

See above for complete list of chest radiographic signs that are indications for angiography.

III. PENETRATING ABDOMINAL TRAUMA

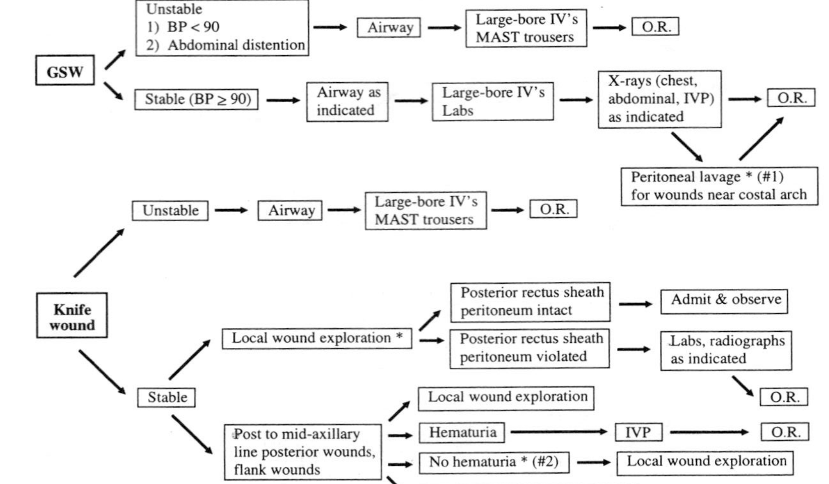

* Consider peritoneal lavage:
1) For wounds near costal arch below 4th ICS.
2) In lieu of exploration.

IV. BLUNT ABDOMINAL TRAUMA

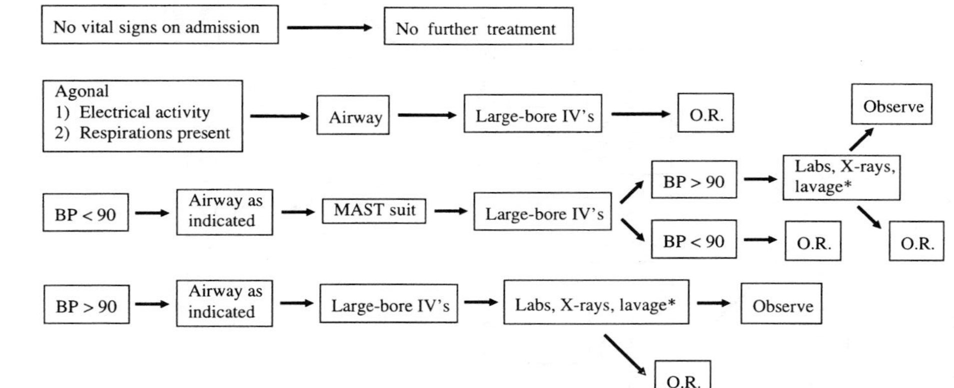

* Indications:
1) ETOH intoxication
2) Drug intoxication
3) Head injury
4) Cord injury
5) Equivocal exam
6) Significant trauma on both sides of diaphragm

V. PENETRATING EXTREMITY TRAUMA

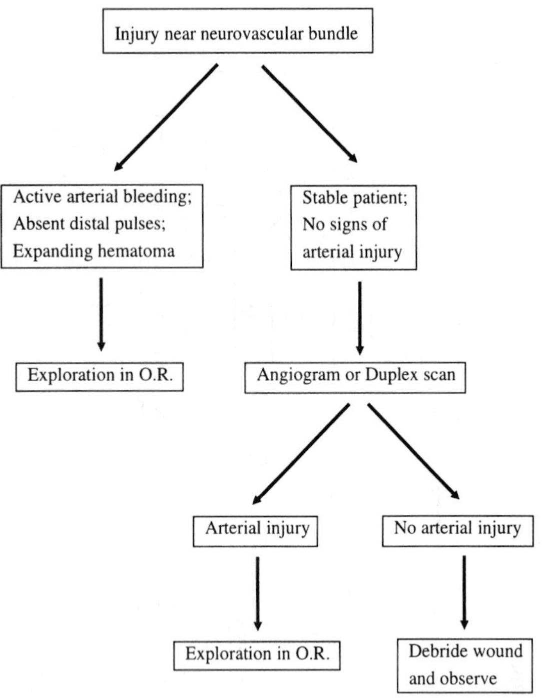

VI. PENETRATING NECK TRAUMA

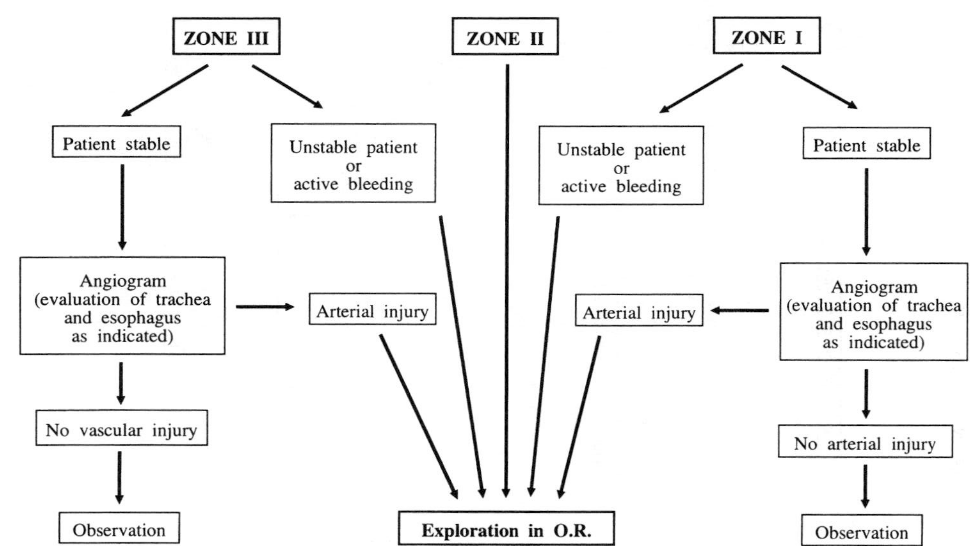

VII. BLUNT NECK TRAUMA

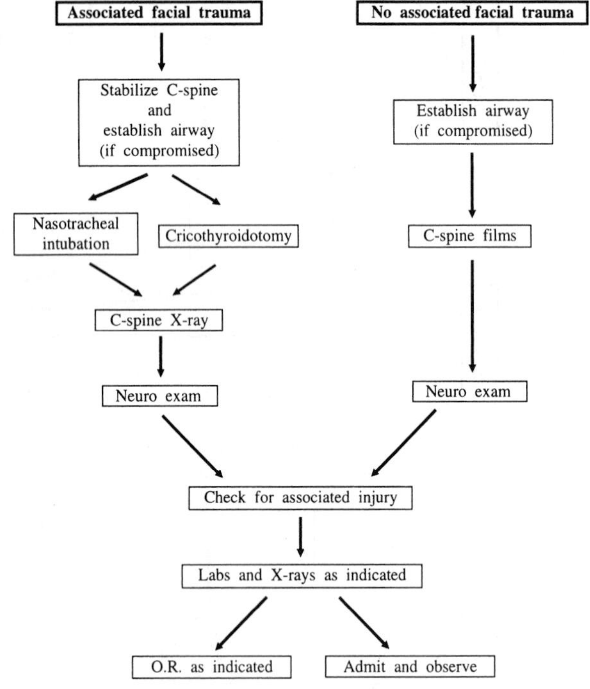

16

Burn Care

Michael J. Goretsky, M.D.

I. INDICATIONS FOR HOSPITAL ADMISSION

A. Some burn injuries may be managed on an outpatient basis. The following guidelines are based upon the American Burn Association Injury Severity Grading System.

B. Indications for admission to burn unit.

1. Full-thickness burns of > 10% TBSA.
2. Partial-thickness burns > 25% in an adult; > 20% in a child.
3. Involvement of the face, hands, feet, or perineum.
4. Electrical, chemical, or inhalation injury is present.
5. High-risk patient–age > 65, < 3 years; pre-existing medical problems, multitrauma.
6. Suspicion of abuse or neglect.

II. INITIAL MANAGEMENT

This is directed toward resuscitation, stabilization, and thorough evaluation of injuries.

A. History.

1. Associated with burn (i.e., unconscious, arrest, jumped from house).
2. Burn agent–flame, scald, chemical, electrical.
3. Open *vs.* closed space.
4. Time of burn.
5. Pre-hospital treatment administered and vital signs during transport.
6. Past medical history–allergies, immunizations, current medications, or medical problems.

B. Airway/Breathing.

1. Ensure adequate airway–prophylactic endotracheal/nasotracheal intubation for significant inhalation injury, extensive (> 60%) burns, deep facial burns, supraglottic obstruction, facial fracture, closed head injury with unconsciousness.
2. Inhalation injury–major contributor to mortality.

a. Carbon monoxide (CO) poisoning–CO displaces oxygen (affinity is 200X higher for hemoglobin and cytochromes), binds hemoglobin forming carboxyhemoglobin. Poor oxygen delivery results, and carboxyhemoglobin levels > 50% are potentially lethal.
   (1) Diagnosis–signs/symptoms of hypoxia, serum carboxyhemoglobin level > 10% (non-smokers) or > 20% (smokers) is diagnostic. Levels of 40-50% are not uncommon in survivors with aggressive care. Oxygen saturations are normal despite high levels of carboxyhemoglobin.
   (2) Treatment–100% O_2 reduces half-life of CO from 250 min to 50 min. Follow with carboxyhemoglobin levels, continue to treat until level 10-15%. Persistent metabolic acidosis despite adequate volume resuscitation implies CO poisoning of cellular respiration.

b. Results from exposure to carbon monoxide, chemical irritants, and toxic gases. Rarely due to thermal injury (exception is superheated steam). Suspect inhalation injury if:
   (1) Closed space injury (e.g., house fire).
   (2) Presence of facial burns, singed nasal hairs, bronchorrhea, carbonaceous sputum, wheezing and rales, tachypnea, progressive hoarseness, and difficulty clearing secretions.

c. Upper airway–obstruction may occur within the ensuing 48 h (maximal edema approximately 24 h).

d. Lower airway–pulmonary edema and chemical tracheobronchitis due to noxious gases.

e. Diagnosis.
   (1) Upper–direct laryngoscopy. Look for carbon deposits, airway edema, oropharyngeal burns.
   (2) Lower–fiberoptic bronchoscopy. Findings of airway edema, carbon deposits in tracheobronchial tree, and mucosal erythema and necrosis.
   (3) ^{133}Xenon scan–evaluates the lower respiratory tract by washout of radioisotope. Incomplete washout by 90 seconds indicates lower airway involvement.

f. Treatment–O_2 supplementation, ventilatory assistance, aggressive pulmonary toilet, O_2 saturation monitor, arterial line for serial ABGs, bronchodilators, and bronchioalveolar lavage to remove debris. Systemic corticosteroids and prophylactic antibiotics are *contraindicated.*

C. Burn evaluation—totally expose patient and remove any burned clothing and constricting jewelry, examine with suspicion of associated injuries.

1. Depth.
   a. First degree–epidermal layer involved, basal layer intact, painful, pink, no blisters.
   b. Second degree (partial thickness)–partial dermal layer in-

volved, painful, white to pink, blebs and blisters may be present. If partial thickness burn is deep, then most epidermal appendages are destroyed and spontaneous re-epithelialization is markedly delayed. (Similar to third degree injury.)

c. Third degree (full thickness)–entire dermal layer involved (all dermal appendages destroyed); insensate, white, black, or red in color; dry and leathery (inelastic) texture.
d. Fourth degree–underlying fascia, muscle, and/or bone involved.
e. The estimate of TBSA burn injury is the sum of second- and third-degree burns.
f. Epithelialization occurs in partial-thickness burns from epithelial cells surrounding hair follicles or sweat glands (skin appendages) and from the wound edges.

2. Size estimation–rule of 9s–9% head and neck, 9% each upper extremity, 18% each lower extremity, 18% anterior trunk, 18% posterior trunk, 1% perineum.
   a. Children have a larger head and trunk proportionally and smaller lower body.
   b. For final size calculation, use Lund-Browder chart, which is more accurate for patients of any age.
   c. Calculate total body surface area (TBSA) = 71.84 X weight (kg) X height (cm), or use standard nomogram (see "Reference data").

D. Fluid resuscitation.

1. Access.
   a. Two large-bore ($\geq$ 18-ga.) peripheral catheters–burned area can be used if necessary.
   b. Central venous access–more suitable than peripheral catheters.
   c. CVP or pulmonary catheters to be used in patients with cardiac or pulmonary disease, questionable fluid status, or hemodynamic instability. Catheters are changed every 48-72 h.
   d. In children, recommend femoral or jugular insertion sites.
2. Formulas for fluid resuscitation.
   a. Parkland formula is the most widely used. The basic formula is lactated Ringer's solution at 4 ml/kg/% burn, with half the total volume given over the first 8 h (calculated from the time of burn), and the other half over the following 16 h (Table 1).
   b. Remember to include allowance for basal fluid requirements–especially important in children.
   c. Initial K^+ supplementation is not required, although large amounts will be needed in the anabolic phase of healing.
   d. Colloid may be given as early as 12 h after injury and usually consists of albumin infused at a constant rate. Fresh frozen plasma may be given if coagulation defects are present.

   e. Hypertonic saline appears to replenish intravascular fluid (from intracellular source) more quickly, improves cardiac contractility while decreasing total IV fluid volume and edema–its use remains controversial. We add 1 ampule of bicarbonate to each liter of lactated Ringer's solution during first 8 h of resuscitation.
   f. Blood should not be used for initial resuscitation.
   g. Avoid fluid boluses but adjust IV rate as needed. Remember, resuscitation formulas only serve as a guideline for IV fluid administration. Adjust based on physiologic response.
3. Goals of resuscitation.
   a. Adequate urine output–best indicator of resuscitation fluid status. Goal is to maintain urine output (adults 0.5 ml/kg/h, children 1 ml/kg/h).
   b. Normal mentation.
   c. Well-perfused extremities (warm, good capillary refill).
   d. Normal arterial pH and lactate levels.
   e. Mixed venous O_2 saturations ≥ 70%.
4. Inadequate volume restoration is manifested by oliguria, tachycardia, and persistent or worsening base deficit.

E. Initial procedures.

1. Foley catheter–required for accurate urine output measurements during resuscitation in patients with ≥ 20% TBSA burn.
2. NG tube–gastric ileus occurs frequently after burns. Also a useful route for oral medications.
3. Nasojejunal feeding tube–placed under fluoroscopy beyond the ligament of Treitz, with immediate initiation of enteral feedings.
4. Escharotomy–may be required for burns to extremities and chest to prevent compartment syndrome and respiratory compromise.
   a. Compartment syndrome–loss of motor and sensory nerve function, diminished pulses, decreased capillary refill, pressure ≥ 30 mm Hg by direct measurement.
      (1) Incise the lateral and medial aspects of the extremity. The incision must be carried out across the joint and into normal skin.
      (2) If symptoms are unrelieved, fasciotomy may be required.
   b. Circumferential chest burns–reduce compliance of chest wall, but escharotomies are rarely needed. Escharotomies should be performed if there are increased peak pressures, increased PCO_2, and decreased compliance.

F. Initial tests.

1. Baseline weight.
2. Labs–CBC, electrolytes, arterial blood gas with carboxyhemoglobin, coagulation studies.

TABLE 1
Resuscitation Calculations

RESUSCITATION	
Calculated resuscitation and basal requirements.	(4 ml × ____kg × ____% burn) + (1500 ml × BSA [cm^2]) = ml/24 h. (____________________) + (____________________) = ____ml/24 h.
Resuscitation fluid per 8 h.	1st 8 h = ______CC, ______ml/h. 2nd 8 h = ______CC, ______ml/h. 3rd 8 h = ______CC, ______ml/h.
MAINTENANCE	
Basal fluid requirement: 1500 ml/m^2	Total body surface area = ______m^2 24 h = ______ml. Hour = ______ml/h.
Evaporative water loss.	Adults: (25 + % burn) m^2 = ml/h. Children: (35 + % burn) m^2 = ml/h. Calculated evaporative loss: (______ + ______% burn) ______m^2 = ml/h; ______ml/24 h.
Total maintenance fluids: basal requirement & evaporative loss.	24 h = ______ml. Hour = ______ml.

3. Chest radiograph and EKG (for history of cardiac problems or electric burns).
4. Urinalysis.

G. Medications.

1. Tetanus prophylaxis–unless received booster within last 5 years.
2. Ulcer prophylaxis–may use sucralfate (Carafate® 1 g PO qid) or H_2 blocker (ranitidine 50 mg IV q 8 h), with antacids 30 ml q 2-4 h per NG to titrate gastric pH > 5.0.
3. Fungal prophylaxis–nystatin 15 ml swish and swallow and 15 ml per NG tid.
4. Multivitamins in tube feedings.
5. Hemoglobinuria/myoglobinuria–treat myoglobin based on urine color. If tea-colored or reddish, increase urine output to > 1 ml/kg/h by increasing IV rates, if no improvement may give mannitol 12.5 g IV, and alkalinize urine with 1 ampule $NaHCO_3$ in IV fluids to keep urine pH > 7.0. If not adequately treated, renal failure can occur.
6. Prophylactic antibiotics are contraindicated.

III. PATHOPHYSIOLOGIC CHANGES ASSOCIATED WITH BURNS

A. Edema—maximal at 18-24 h, due to:

1. Generalized increase in microvascular permeability–involves nonburned tissue if burn is > 30%.
2. Generalized impairment in cell membrane function ≥ increased intracellular volume drawn in by increased intracellular Na^+ concomitant with loss of K^+.

B. Hemodynamic.

1. Initial hypodynamic state with decreased cardiac output/contractility and increased vascular resistance. This usually resolves with adequate resuscitation.
2. By day 2-3 a hyperdynamic state exists with increased cardiac function and decreased vascular resistance.

C. Metabolic—wound, central nervous system, and stress hormone induced hypermetabolism.

1. Begins at 48 h post burn.
2. Caloric needs increased 1.3 to 2X normal.
3. Characterized by increased oxygen consumption, heat production, elevated body temperature, hypoproteinemia due to catabolism and wound exudate, gluconeogenesis, and hyperglycemia.
4. Gradually returns to normal after wound is closed and the inflammation is resolved.

D. Immunocompromise.

1. All aspects of the immune function are depressed including cellular-mediated immunity (T cells), humoral mediated immunity (B cells), opsonization due to decreased complement and antibodies, decreased phagocytosis and bactericidal ac-

tivity by macrophages and neutrophils, and loss of natural barrier function of the skin.

2. Predisposes the patient to infections and multiple organ failure.

IV. BURN WOUND CARE

A. Goals of burn wound care.

1. Cover wound.
2. Decrease infection.
3. Allow for optimal re-epithelialization of partial thickness burns.
4. Burns (2nd or 3rd degree) that do not heal by 2-3 weeks produce significantly more scarring; thus, these wounds require excision and grafting for best cosmetic and functional results.
5. The mortality of large burns has been reduced by the expeditious excision of the burn wound followed by coverage with autograft or allograft.

B. Topical agents—decrease wound sepsis, but do not prevent colonization of eschar.

1. Bacitracin ointment–useful for partial-thickness burns and facial burns.
2. Silver sulfadiazine (Silvadene®)–broad spectrum, includes *Candida.* Intermediate eschar penetration but less than mafenide acetate. Nonpainful on application. Apply bid. *Contraindicated* in patients with glucose-6-phosphate dehydrogenase deficiency.
3. Mafenide acetate (Sulfamylon®) (not used frequently)–broad spectrum, but little fungicidal activity. Penetrates eschar well, but pain on application. Carbonic anhydrase inhibitor, absorption can cause hyperchloremic metabolic acidosis. Apply bid.
4. Silver nitrate 0.5%–applied as wet dressing, poor eschar penetration. May result in Na^+, K^+, Ca^{++}, Mg^{++} depletion. May cause methemoglobinemia.

C. Local care.

1. First-degree burns–minor care, symptomatic pain control.
2. Partial-thickness burns–initial wash with antiseptic soap (e.g., chlorhexidine gluconate), remove debris, unroof vesicles. Apply topical agents (bacitracin).
3. Deep partial-thickness, full-thickness burns–initially treat as for partial-thickness burns. If no healing after 2 weeks–graft.

D. Early excision and grafting—excise eschar in layered fashion to the point of capillary bleeding; perform within 2-7 days of admission for obvious deep 2nd and 3rd degree burns. Graft immediately or cover temporarily with homograft or biologic dressing. May excise and then graft the next day (decreases operative blood loss). *Advantages*–early removal of eschar and coverage; improved joint function; shortened hospitalization; earlier mobilization and rehabilitation; improved immune status and decreased wound sepsis.

E. Grafting—decreases evaporation pain, protects neurovascular tissue and tendons.

1. Partial thickness wounds should heal spontaneously by day 14.
2. Without immediate physiologic coverage, fascial dessication and subsequent infection may occur.
3. Sheet *vs.* mesh graft–sheet grafts are optimal for cosmetic appearance but do not expand to cover large surface area. Mesh grafts are better for non-optimal recipient beds. Sheet grafts are preferred for hands, feet, and face.
4. Grafts usually 0.010 – 0.014 inches thick–thicker grafts have less scarring but slightly increased risk of graft failure and increased scarring of donor sites.
5. Types of grafting material.
   a. Autograft (from self)–optimal. Split thickness *vs.* full thickness, sheet *vs.* mesh.
   b. Allograft (same species; i.e., cadaver). Indications for use of allograft:
      (1) Insufficient autologous skin available.
      (2) Temporary wound coverage prior to autologous grafting.
      (3) Speeds epithelialization.
      (4) Prevents infection.
   c. Xenograft (different species; i.e., porcine)–used infrequently due to the establishment of skin banks.
   d. Skin substitutes.
      (1) Cultured keratinocytes–trend is towards decreased use (needs a dermis).
         a) For use in large burns with little donor skin available.
         b) Poor resistance to infection.
         c) Fragile, easily scars.
         d) Variable take.
         e) Place on dermal allografts.
      (2) Dermal substitutes–cover wound until autograft available.
         a) Dermal allograft.
         b) Collagen/GAG.
         c) Polyglactin acid (Vicryl®) mesh.
      (3) Skin substitutes (bilayer material).
         a) Both dermal and epidermal components.
         b) Improved take in recent reports.
         c) Still not as good as STAG.
6. Priorities–graft hands, feet joints, extremities, and face first, then trunk.
7. Graft care.
   a. Donor site–covered with topical antimicrobial (bacitra-

cin, silver sulfadiazine), biologic dressing such as calcium alginate (Kaldostat®), or occlusive dressing.

b. Graft site.
   (1) Wet–dressings irrigated with antibiotic solution to be kept constantly damp.
   (2) Dry–nonstick gauze (Adaptic®) then pressure dressing over graft.

c. Nonadherence of graft is due to avascular or infected graft bed, hematoma, seroma, or graft movement.

V. SUPPORTIVE CARE

A. Nutrition—start early. Metabolic rate is proportional to burn size up to 40-50% TBSA burn and may be 1.3X to 2X usual. Total body O_2 consumption and water loss proportional to burn size.

1. Nutrient needs.
   a. Caloric needs based on Harris-Benedict equation using a multiplier (see "Nutrition").
   b. Indirect calorimetry is often used.
2. Route.
   a. Enteral (nasoduodenal) preferred, start during first 12 h post-injury–decreased infection and complication rates, decreased cost.
   b. If intravenous, *must* change IV site every 48-72 h. Catheter is used for all infusions, including TPN. Parenteral nutrition is associated with an increased rate of sepsis in burn patients.

B. Physical and Occupational Therapy (PT/OT)—aggressive PT/OT is necessary to prevent contracture and maintain function.

1. Positioning of limbs and joints begins Day 1.
2. Splinting required to prevent contractures.
3. Active exercise program with stretching greatly superior to passive range of motion.
4. Involve OT early for long-term rehabilitation planning.

C. Analgesia—use methadone for pain management, with IV morphine for acute pain.

VI. MANAGEMENT OF INFECTION IN BURN INJURY

A. Pneumonia—most common infection.

1. Early pneumonia most commonly gram-positive organisms.
2. Later pneumonia (> 7 days after hospitalization) most commonly gram-negative organisms.
3. More common in intubated patients, although can occur in non-intubated patients.

B. Pathogenesis—in untreated burn wound, surface bacteria proliferate, migrate through nonviable tissue, pause at the subeschar space, and, when microbial invasiveness "outweighs" host defense capability, invade viable tissue with microvascular involvement and systemic dissemination (burn wound sepsis). Avascularity and ischemia of full-thickness burn wound allows microbial proliferation and prevents delivery of systemic antibiotics and cellular components of host defense.

C. Clinical signs.

1. Conversion of a partial to full-thickness injury.
2. Rapidly spreading ischemic necrosis.

D. Diagnosis of invasive burn wound sepsis.

1. Cultures of burn wound surface do *not* accurately predict progressive bacterial colonization or incipient burn wound sepsis. Qualitative and quantitative correlation are poor between flora on the surface of the burn wound and bacterial colonization of the deep layers of the eschar.
2. Bacterial growth is best monitored by semi-quantitative burn wound biopsy–calculate precise number of organisms per gram of tissue. If biopsy cultures reveal $> 10^5$ organisms/g tissue or if there is 100-fold increase in the concentration of organisms/g tissue within a 48-h period, then the organisms have escaped effective control by the topical chemotherapeutic agent, and burn wound sepsis is incipient. (Note: false-positive results often occur.)
3. Wound colonization of dead tissue must be differentiated from invasion of viable tissue.
   a. Best evaluated by clinical diagnosis.
   b. Biopsy will find organisms in viable subeschar tissue on histologic examination.
   c. Microvascular invasion connotes possible hematogenous dissemination and mandates systemic antibiotic therapy.
4. Wound–often dry, crusted, black, or violaceous color. May be unchanged.
5. Clinical picture of sepsis–fever, hypoxia, mental status changes, leukocytosis, new onset ileus, tachypnea, thrombocytopenia, hypotension, oliguria, acidosis, tachycardia, hyperglycemia. Bacteremia occurs late in burn sepsis.

E. Bacteriology of nosocomial burn infection.

1. Know your hospital's flora and antibiotic sensitivities of species.
2. Most common pathogens–*Staphylococcus aureus*, Group A streptococcus (less common), *Pseudomonas aeruginosa*, other gram-negative rods, *Enterococcus*, *Candida albicans*.

F. Prevention of burn infection.

1. Dressing change bid and topical agents.
2. Strict handwashing.

G. Treatment of burn infection.

1. Remove *all* devitalized tissue.
2. Surgically drain closed-space abscesses.
3. Apply diffusible topical agent.
4. Empiric antibiotic therapy–broad-spectrum. Always cover

initially for *Pseudomonas* sp. Rarely needs anaerobic coverage. Specific antibiotic therapy upon bacteriologic identification will require larger doses than usual (especially aminoglycosides) to provide adequate tissue levels. Our routine "triple" antibiotic therapy is Nafcillin, Piperacillin, and Amikacin.

5. Clysis of antibiotic solution under infected burn eschar.

H. Nonbacterial infection.

1. Viral infection–usually heals with time. Virucidal agent recommended for systemic involvement.
2. Fungal infection–topical application of nystatin effectively clears fungi and yeast, and may be used prophylactically prior to eschar excision. Amphotericin B is used for systemic involvement. Severe fungal infection may require aggressive debridement.

VII. ELECTRICAL INJURIES

A. Tissue destruction—most severe at the points of entry and exit (the points at which the electrical current is most concentrated). Deep tissue damage often greatly exceeds skin injury–usually not obvious at the time of initial injury. Electrical resistance of tissues (least to most)–nerve, blood, and blood vessel, muscle, skin, tendon, fat, bone.

B. Treatment.

1. CPR–high-voltage currents usually cause cardiac standstill, whereas low-voltage (<440 volts) usually produces ventricular fibrillation.
2. Protection against neurologic damage caused by fractures of the spine–place in C-spine collar and on long back board to immobilize the entire spine. Tetanic contraction of muscle may cause fractures of the cervical and lumbosacral spine and long bones; therefore, perform screening radiographs. Frequent examinations.
3. Fluid resuscitation–cannot be calculated from % of skin burns. Give sufficient volume to establish urine output of 1.5 ml/kg/h.
   a. High incidence of muscular and blood injury causes hemoglobinuria/myoglobinuria. Hence, larger fluid requirements. If increased fluid resuscitation is not successful, then mannitol (25 g/h) and $NaHCO_3$ are necessary to prevent precipitation of myoglobin/hemoglobin in the renal tubules. Mannitol is continued until the urine color clears.
   b. Progressively severe metabolic acidosis occurs with electrical injuries and massive tissue destruction. Use IV sodium bicarbonate to correct base deficit.
4. Early debridement of grossly necrotic tissue; amputation may be needed if unable to control acidosis.

5. Immediate extremity fasciotomy is frequently required; check compartment pressures.

VIII. CHEMICAL INJURIES

A. Major problem—failure to recognize ongoing destruction of tissue.

B. Initial management—dilution with copious amounts of water, not neutralization of the chemical burn, as the heat of neutralization can extend the injury (may need to irrigate ≥ 1 h for alkali burns).

1. Avoid hypothermia.
2. Special precautions.
   a. Lithium–remove particles prior to irrigation.
   b. Hydrofluoric acid–apply 10% calcium gluconate cream in most cases. Can inject calcium gluconate subcutaneously for severe burns.
   c. Phenol–irrigation must be vigorous (shower) because absorption increases when spread over large area.
   d. Tar/asphalt–use medisol, bacitracin, or other petroleum-based product.

IX. OUTPATIENT AND CLINIC TREATMENT

A. Patients that do not meet admission criteria—can be treated as outpatients.

B. Treatment.

1. Tetanus prophylaxis.
2. Wounds washed with mild soap.
3. Debris and blisters should be debrided.
4. Apply antibiotic ointment (bacitracin, neosporin, polysporin), nonstick porous gauze (Adaptic®), and wrap with gauze.

C. Follow-up care.

1. Dressing care bid–wash with mild soap (to remove debris and fibrinous exudate) and reapply dressing.
2. Vigorous range of motion exercises.
3. Return to clinic and/or physical therapy as needed.

D. Deep partial- or full-thickness burns—the patient may be treated as an outpatient until excision and grafting is required.

1. If wound is not re-epithelialized by 2 weeks, it should undergo excision and grafting.
2. Longer healing time increases scarring.

E. Scarring problems—the patient should be fitted for pressure garments and wear them 23 h a day until wounds no longer blanche.

F. Moisturizing cream—use on healing skin.

G. Hyperemic healed wounds that blanch—the patient should vigorously massage-pressure the wound daily to help prevent scarring.

H. Sun exposure to graft or burn—should be avoided because it may cause hyperpigmentation.

I. Pruritis—treat with moisturizing cream, oral Benadryl®, or Vistaril® prn.

X. COMPLICATIONS OF BURN INJURY

A. Gastrointestinal.

1. Adynamic ileus–especially large burns. Gastric and colonic involvement. Generally resolves within 24 h with IV hydration and NG suction. May be early signs of sepsis.
2. Ulcers–"Curling's ulcer"–occurs anywhere in the GI tract; mostly in stomach, duodenum, and jejunum. Etiology unknown, but thought to be due to hypovolemia, hypoperfusion, not necessarily related to burn size. Incidence is very rare with early antacids and H_2 blockers and with early enteral feeding. Initial non-operative management and indications for surgical intervention are essentially the same as those for hemorrhage from peptic ulcer disease (see "GI Bleeding").
3. Acalculous cholecystitis–uncommon, but diagnose with HIDA scan or ultrasound. Treat with antibiotics, and either percutaneous drainage or cholecystectomy.

B. Ocular.

1. Keep eyes moist using artificial tears or ointments.
2. Corneal abrasions–associated with facial burns. Treatment includes topical antibiotics, and release and grafting of ectropion.
3. Cataracts (especially with electrical injury).

C. Cutaneous.

1. Wound contracture–result of scarring (prevented by massage and pressure garment). May result in cosmetic or functional problems. May limit range of motion, especially if it extends across a joint. Contracture may be released surgically with grafting or Z-plasty. As children grow, contractures will become more pronounced because the scars do not grow; multiple releases may be required.
2. Hypertrophic scar.
   a. Occurs with wounds that take > 2 weeks to heal, but increased incidence with deep burns and extended exposure of ungrafted burn wound, with maximal scarring at 3-6 months after injury.
   b. Treatment.
      (1) Pressure-fitted pressure masks, garments, and massage are used for 1st year to reduce scar formation.
      (2) Resurface with graft later.
      (3) Cosmetic treatment often disappointing.
   c. Keloids–variant of hypertrophic scarring beyond original wound. Difficult to treat, but steroid injections have been used. Often recur after excision.

D. Miscellaneous.

1. Heterotopic calcification.
   a. Elbows most common joint.
   b. May be related to overvigorous OT/PT.
2. Chondritis–secondary to *S. aureus* and *Pseudomonas* ear and joint infection.
3. Hyperpigmentation–avoid sun exposure for at least 1 year. Use sun-blocking agents (>15 SPF).

17

Acute Abdomen

Patricia A. Abello, M.D.

An acute abdomen is defined as the rapid onset of abdominal pain, with or without associated symptoms such as nausea and vomiting, in patients who have been previously well. When patients present with signs and symptoms consistent with acute abdomen, the importance of making an *early* accurate diagnosis cannot be overemphasized. The recovery rate from acute abdominal disease decreases proportionately with delay in diagnosis and treatment.

I. PHYSIOLOGY OF ABDOMINAL PAIN

A. Visceral pain—diffuse and ill-defined. Pain from stimulation of visceral afferents results from contraction or spasm, stretching or distention against resistance, and chemical irritation. Usually colicky in nature.

1. Visceral pain is usually experienced in the midline, corresponding to the anatomic location of visceral afferent nerve plexuses. The foregut, including stomach, duodenum, pancreas, gallbladder, and liver, has pain transmitted to the celiac plexus, resulting in epigastric pain. The midgut has pain transmitted to the superior mesenteric plexus, causing periumbilical pain; hindgut pain is transmitted to the inferior mesenteric plexus near the bifurcation of the aorta, characteristically producing pain in the hypogastrium.
2. Pain may be referred to a distant body region (e.g., inflamed gallbladder causes both right upper quadrant as well as shoulder pain). Involves complicated misinterpretation of visceral afferent impulses that cross the nerve cells of the corresponding somatic dermatome level within the CNS.
3. Visceral efferent fibers control the organ response to the noxious stimulus–sympathetic and parasympathetic.
   a. Sphincter spasm (sympathetic), decrease in gut motility (parasympathetic), and decrease in organ secretion (parasympathetic). Responses producing diaphoresis, nausea, vomiting, and reflex hypotension. Severe somatic pain also may produce autonomic responses.

4. Visceral organs may be burned, crushed, or cut without eliciting pain.

B. Parietal pain—abdominal pain secondary to parietal peritoneal irritation; perceived through segmental somatic fibers. Reflex involuntary muscle wall rigidity may result from irritation of segmental sensory nerves. Hyperaesthesia of the skin may result from ipsilateral peritoneal irritation. Usually a dull, steady ache.

1. ***Rebound tenderness*—** elicited by stretching the inflamed parietal peritoneum during examination. Does *not* require deep palpation with rapid release; may be elicited with simple percussion or coughing or straining or other subtle change of intra-abdominal pressure

C. Generalized pain—sudden flooding of the peritoneal cavity by pus, blood, or acrid fluid resulting in generalized peritonitis. May produce somatic as well as autonomic responses.

D. Nausea and vomiting.

1. Non-specific complaint; its relationship to abdominal pain important in separating pain of inflammation from mechanical obstruction.
2. Severe irritation of the nerves of the peritoneum or mesentery–ulcer perforation, gangrenous appendicitis, ovarian cyst torsion, pancreatitis (celiac plexus involvement), intestinal strangulation.
3. Obstruction of an involuntary muscular tube–biliary duct, ureter, uterine canal, intestine, appendix. Occurs secondary to peristaltic contraction and muscle stretching; hence, colic comes in spasms with vomiting at its peak.
    a. Character of vomitus may aid in establishing level of intestinal obstruction.
4. Action of absorbed toxins on medullary centers–may contribute to vomiting in intestinal obstruction or pancreatitis.

II. HISTORY

A. Pain.

1. Location of pain–localization of pain may give clues to etiology, but abdominal pain may be referred to a site remote from the source of pathology. Diffuse pain suggests two possibilities: visceral pain or uncontained peritonitis.
2. Character of pain–sharp, dull, burning, constant, intermittent.
3. Intensity of pain–nagging, mild, severe, "worst ever".
4. Onset of pain–acute *vs.* insidious.
5. Radiation of pain–back, flank, shoulder, hip, groin.
    a. Biliary colic–to right scapula.
    b. Renal colic–to ipsilateral testicle or groin.
    c. Pancreatitis–to the back.
6. Exacerbating or ameliorating factors–food, medication, ac-

tivity, deep breathing or coughing, vomiting, defecation, change in position.

7. Associated complaints–respiratory, GI, genitourinary, systemic.

B. Nausea, vomiting, and anorexia.

1. Frequency and onset of vomiting–in intestinal obstruction, related to the site of obstruction. The more proximal the obstruction, the more frequent the vomiting and the earlier the onset. Vomiting may not occur with colonic obstruction, especially if there is a competent ileocecal valve.
2. Character of vomitus.
   a. Bilious–nonspecific.
   b. Food–upper obstruction.
   c. Retching–torsion of viscus.
   d. Feculent (succus entericus)–pathognomonic of intestinal obstruction (unusual in colonic obstruction). Feculence is caused by overgrowth of bacteria in stagnant small bowel contents, *not* regurgitation of feces.
3. Relationship of pain to vomiting–in acute appendicitis, nausea and vomiting rarely occurs before the onset of pain.
4. Acute appetite loss–frequently significant, important complaint in acute appendicitis. Characteristically precedes onset of pain.

C. Bowel function.

1. Diarrhea–gastroenteritis, appendicitis in children, early in partial or complete small bowel obstruction due to evacuation of bowel distal to site of obstruction, acute diverticulitis.
2. Constipation or obstipation–obstruction, paralytic ileus, acute appendicitis.
3. Change in stool color.
   a. Blood and/or mucus–intussusception in children; colitis, proctitis in adults.
   b. Acholic stools–biliary tract obstruction or dysfunction.
   c. Melenic stools–upper GI bleed; usually not associated with acute abdominal pain.

D. Menstruation and sexual history—ectopic pregnancy, pelvic inflammatory disease, ovarian cysts or torsion, Mittleschmerz.

E. Thorough review of systems.

1. Cardiopulmonary.
   a. Pneumonia, emphysema, or myocardial ischemia may present with severe abdominal complaints.
   b. Recent upper respiratory infection symptoms may precede onset of acute mesenteric adenitis, especially in children.
2. Neuromuscular.
   a. Herpes zoster.
   b. Fractures, tumors, or osteomyelitis of the spine.
   c. Tabes dorsalis.

3. Genitourinary.
   a. Unilateral flank or abdominal pain radiating to the ipsilateral testicle or groin with or without hematuria suggests renal or ureteral stone.
   b. Pneumaturia–enterovesical fistula, most commonly due to colonic diverticular disease, frequently associated with pelvic abscess.
4. Vascular.
   a. Autoimmune diseases or vasculitis.
   b. Dissection, rupture, or expansion of abdominal aortic aneurysm.
5. Hematologic.
   a. Sickle cell crisis or sickle-associated splenic infarct.
   b. Lymphoma or leukemia.
6. Endocrine/metabolic.
   a. Acute diabetic ketoacidosis may present as acute abdomen.
   b. Porphyria.
   c. Addisonian crisis.
7. Psychiatric.

F. Past medical history—may suggest etiology of abdominal pain.
1. Previous abdominal surgeries.
2. History of peptic ulcer disease.
3. Documented diverticular disease.
4. Known gallstones or renal stones.
5. Previous episode of similar complaints.

G. Current medications.
1. Steroids–may mask severity of condition owing to blunted inflammatory response. Patients taking steroids may have intra-abdominal catastrophe with relatively benign exam.
2. Analgesics, antipyretics, and antibiotics–may mask pain and fever.

III. PHYSICAL EXAMINATION

A. General appearance.
1. Level of discomfort.
2. Nutritional status.
3. Hydration status.

B. Attitude in bed.
1. Still, resists movement, may have knees bent or drawn up–peritonitis.
2. Restless, cannot find comfortable position–colic.
3. Writhing–consider mesenteric vascular event.

C. Temperature—a subnormal, normal, or elevated temperature can accompany an acute abdomen.
1. 95-96°F (core)–severe shock of toxemia.
2. Normal temperature–common in non-inflammatory process.

3. 99-100°F (oral)–early inflammatory process, usual finding with acute appendicitis.
4. 104-105°F–suspect intra-abdominal abscess or urinary source.

D. Pulse.

1. Tachycardia is common and may be due to fever, hemorrhage, dehydration, pain, anxiety.
2. Bradycardia can be seen with advanced sepsis or metabolic disturbances (i.e., hypothyroidism.)

E. Respiratory rate.

1. Tachypnea is common.
2. Respiratory alkalosis can be present as early finding in sepsis.
3. Kussmaul breathing with diabetic ketoacidosis.

F. Blood pressure.

1. Hypertension may be associated with severe pain.
2. Hypotension–hemorrhage, sepsis, volume depletion.

G. Cardiopulmonary exam.

1. Cardiac murmur, rub or gallops may be significant in cardiac disease presenting as abdominal pain (myocardial infarction, congestive heart failure, acute rheumatic heart disease, pericarditis, etc.).
2. Pulmonary consolidation, effusion, or pleural rub may be significant in pulmonary disease presenting as abdominal pain (pneumonia, pleuritis, infarct, etc.).

H. Abdominal examination.

1. Observation, inspection.
   a. Scaphoid, flat, obese, distended.
   b. Movement with respiration–note limitation of movement indicating rigidity of the abdominal muscles or diaphragm.
   c. Have patient indicate the exact point of maximal pain.
   d. Inspect all potential sites for hernias, especially the inguinal and femoral region.
2. Auscultation.
   a. Absent or hypoactive bowel sounds–peritonitis or ileus.
   b. High-pitched bowel sounds with rushes, hyperactive–obstruction.
   c. Aortic and renal artery bruits–absence of a bruit never excludes the presence of an aortic aneurysm.
3. Palpation/percussion–gentleness is essential.
   a. Evaluate presence and extent of muscular rigidity.
   b. Palpate four quadrants of abdomen, costovertebral angles to assess tenderness (mild, moderate, severe), abdominal masses, abnormal pulsations, hernial orifices. Begin *away* from point of maximal pain. Have patient's legs flexed and relaxed. Conversation or other diversion may be useful in the examination of the anxious patient or young child.
   c. Signs of peritoneal irritation.

(1) Percussion ("rebound") tenderness.
(2) Pain with coughing, Valsalva, or sudden movement.
(3) Rigidity–"involuntary guarding."
    a) Pain worsens when rigidity is overcome in abdominal disease.
    b) Muscular rigidity/resistance may be slight, even in the presence of serious peritonitis with fat, flabby abdominal wall, severe toxemia, and elderly patients.
(4) "Obturator sign"–pain with flexion and internal rotation of the hip. Positive with inflammation of obturator internus muscle (e.g., appendicitis).
(5) "Psoas sign"–pain on passive extension of hip (stretching the psoas muscle). Positive with irritation of psoas/iliopsoas muscle (retrocecal appendix).
(6) "Rovsing's sign"–pain in the right lower quadrant when pressure is applied to the left lower quadrant. May be present with peritoneal irritation of acute appendicitis.
(7) "Cutaneous hyperaesthesia"–may be tested by pin prick or light touch. Nearly always indicates parietal peritoneal inflammation. Most commonly caused by appendicitis; occurs in lower abdominal wall.
(8) Palpation of the flank to detect renal disease (perinephric abscess, inflamed kidney) or retrocecal appendix (both affect quadratus lumborum muscle).
(9) Liver percussion.
    a) Normal dullness is detected from the 5th rib to the costal margin along the right vertical nipple line and from the 7th to 11th rib in the midaxillary line.
    b) Loss of liver dullness (with new resonance) occurs with free air in the peritoneum (must be in the absence of abdominal distention).
(10) Fluid wave.
    a) Indication of free fluid in peritoneal cavity.
    b) Most commonly associated with ascites from liver disease. When a patient with known ascites presents with abdominal pain, fever, and/or leukocytosis, consider spontaneous bacterial peritonitis.

I. Examination of the pelvic cavity.

1. Suprapelvic palpation and percussion.
2. Rectal examination–extremely important and informative.
    a. Look for localized tenderness, fluctuance, induration, masses, occult or gross blood.
    b. Digital examination of stomas if present.
3. Bimanual pelvic examination.

a. Bleeding–menses, threatened abortion, endometritis, trauma.
b. Discharge–venereal disease, pelvic inflammatory disease.
c. Appearance of cervix on speculum exam–cyanosis of pregnancy, blood from os, purulent discharge.
d. Presence of adnexal mass or tenderness–tuboovarian abscess, ectopic pregnancy, etc.
e. Uterine size and contour–consider pregnancy, fibroids, etc.
f. Cervical motion tenderness–classically present in pelvic inflammatory disease, but may be caused by any source of inflammation in the pelvis.

4. Check for signs of bladder distention–percuss bladder size, catheterize if necessary to ensure empty bladder, especially in elderly.

IV. LABORATORY EXAMINATION

A. **WBC**—degree of leukocytosis and differential. *Note*: The absence of leukocytosis *never* excludes an inflammatory abdominal diagnosis.
B. **Hematocrit**—anemia, chronic (micro- or macrocytic) or acute. Hemoconcentration may indicate hypovolemic state.
C. **Platelet count**—thrombocytopenia consistent with severe sepsis.
D. **Electrolytes**—indicative of volume status, may demonstrate GI losses from diarrhea or protracted vomiting (e.g., hypochloremic hypokalemic metabolic alkalosis or "contraction alkalosis"). Hyperglycemia in diabetic ketoacidosis, or sepsis-induced glucose intolerance.
E. **Arterial blood gas (ABG)**—metabolic acidosis or alkalosis. Metabolic acidosis and generalized abdominal pain in the elderly is ischemic colitis until proven otherwise.
F. **Urinalysis**—check for RBCs, WBCs, casts.
G. **Serum βHCG**—mandatory in all women of child-bearing age to 45.
H. **Liver function tests**—bilirubin (direct and total), alkaline phosphatase elevation in biliary obstruction; elevated transaminases in hepatocellular injury.
I. **Amylase elevation**—seen in pancreatitis, although relatively non-specific. May be elevated in mesenteric ischemia, perforated duodenal ulcer, ruptured ovarian cyst, renal failure. Lipase more sensitive.

V. RADIOLOGIC EVALUATION

A. **Upright chest radiograph**—look for pneumonia, free air under the diaphragms; pleural effusion may suggest subdiaphragmatic inflammatory process.

B. Abdominal flat and upright (or left lateral decubitus) radiograph—look for bowel distension and air fluid levels consistent with ileus or obstruction; bowel gas cut off *vs.* air through to rectum. Localized ileus ("sentinel loop") may indicate location of inflammatory process (i.e., pancreatitis). Abnormal calcifications (e.g., chronic pancreatitis, 20% of gallstones, renal calculi). Pneumatosis, air in biliary tree are ominous signs of dead gut. May see mass effect from tumor or abscess. Left lateral decubitus may detect free air in patients in whom upright CXR cannot be obtained.

C. Ultrasonography—of value in visualizing the hepatobiliary tree, pancreas, vascular structures, kidneys, pelvic organs, and intra-abdominal fluid collections.

D. CT scan—helpful in cases of acute abdominal pain without clear etiology. Useful in the evaluation of abdominal aortic aneurysm. Better definition than ultrasound.

E. Contrast studies.

1. Upper GI studies.
   a. Water-soluble contrast may be helpful in demonstrating a suspected but questionable perforation.
   b. Useful in discerning the point of obstruction in small bowel obstruction. Must rule out colonic obstruction first (see below) to avoid inspissated barium above colonic obstruction.
2. Lower GI series.
   a. Useful in discerning the point of obstruction in cases of colonic obstruction.
   b. Avoid if colonic inflammatory process (i.e., diverticulitis) is suspected.
   c. Air enema is diagnostic and often therapeutic in intussusception in children.
3. Intravenous pyelogram–for diagnosis of ureteral stone or obstruction.
4. Angiography–diagnosis of mesenteric ischemia.

VI. OTHER PROCEDURES

A. Endoscopy.

1. EGD–primary usefulness in evaluation of GI bleeding, or evaluation of epigastric pain in non-acute setting.
2. Sigmoidoscopy or colonoscopy.
   a. Evaluation of colonic obstruction.
   b. Diagnosis and potential therapy for nonstrangulated sigmoid volvulus.
   c. Decompression of severely dilated colon secondary to adynamic ileus.
   d. Diagnosis of ischemic colitis, pseudomembranous enterocolitis, ulcerative or Crohn's colitis.

B. Paracentesis and/or peritoneal lavage.

1. Diagnosis of spontaneous bacterial peritonitis in cirrhotic

patients. Considered diagnostic if absolute neutrophil count $\geq$ 500.

2. Diagnostic peritoneal lavage may be useful bedside test in diagnosis of mesenteric infarction in critically ill patients.

C. Culdocentesis—valuable in the diagnosis of ruptured ectopic pregnancy.

D. Laparoscopy.

1. Greatest value is in diagnosis and treatment of suspected gynecologic causes of acute abdomen.
2. Useful in suspected appendicitis in woman of child-bearing age (highest negative exploration rate). May also perform appendectomy laparoscopically if appendicitis is found.
3. The role of laparoscopy in the evaluation of acute abdomen is changing as laparoscopic instruments and techniques improve.

VII. DIFFERENTIAL DIAGNOSIS OF ACUTE ABDOMEN

A. Inflammatory.

1. Perforated viscus.
   a. Stomach, duodenum–ulcer.
   b. Bowel–diverticulum, appendix, carcinoma, traumatic small bowel injury.
   c. Gallbladder.
2. Primary peritonitis (peritonitis without obvious etiology).
   a. Gram-positive organisms (*Pneumococcus, Streptococcus*) formerly most common; gram-negatives are increasing, especially in females.
   b. Tuberculosis–"doughy" abdomen.
   c. Cirrhotics with ascites may develop spontaneous bacterial peritonitis (SBP) and have minimal symptoms.
3. Gastroenteritis, colitis–viral or bacterial.
4. Inflammatory bowel disease.
5. Diverticulitis.
6. Meckel's diverticulitis.
7. Pancreatitis–alcoholic, biliary, viral, thiazide-induced, steroid-related, hyperlipidemia, hypercalcemia.
8. Hepatitis.
   a. Viral–mimics cholecystitis.
   b. Alcoholic.
9. Hepatic abscess–look for other primary septic focus.
10. Splenic abscess.
11. Mesenteric lymphadenitis.
12. Foreign body perforation of bowel.
13. Gynecologic.
    a. Pelvic inflammatory disease.
    b. Fitz-Hugh-Curtis syndrome (gonococcal perihepatitis).
    c. Endometritis.
    d. Toxic shock syndrome.
    e. Ruptured ovarian cyst.

B. Mechanical.

1. Intestinal obstruction.
   a. Small bowel–adhesions, hernia, neoplasm, volvulus, intussusception, gallstone ileus, Meckel's band, inflammatory mass.
   b. Gastric outlet obstruction–peptic ulcer disease (pyloric channel), gastric carcinoma.
   c. Colon–neoplasm, hernia, diverticulitis, volvulus.
2. Biliary obstruction.
   a. Cholelithiasis with impacted or "ball-valve" cystic duct stone.
   b. Choledocholithiasis.
   c. Cholangitis.
      (1) Neoplasm.
      (2) Choledochal cyst.
      (3) Choledocholithiasis.
3. Solid viscera (rare).
   a. Acute splenomegaly–various hematologic disorders.
   b. Acute hepatomegaly–pericarditis, congestive heart failure, Budd-Chiari.
4. Omental torsion–rare.
5. Gynecologic.
   a. Torsion of ovarian cyst or uterine fibroid.
   b. Ectopic pregnancy.
      (1) Symptoms of early pregnancy–delayed menses, nausea, vomiting, breast tenderness.
      (2) Increased uterine size, but less than anticipated by last menstrual period.
      (3) Pain and cramping.
      (4) Adnexal mass, cervical motion tenderness.
      (5) βHCG may not be positive.
      (6) Hypovolemic shock due to hemorrhage in 10% of cases.

C. Vascular.

1. Intraperitoneal bleeding.
   a. Traumatic rupture of liver, spleen, mesentery.
   b. Delayed splenic rupture.
   c. Ruptured ectopic pregnancy.
   d. Ruptured abdominal aortic aneurysm–sudden onset of new back pain in an individual with atherosclerotic risk factors.
   e. Ruptured splenic or hepatic aneurysm–rare.
2. Ischemia.
   a. Mesenteric thrombosis or embolus.
      (1) Usually other signs of peripheral atherosclerosis.
      (2) Atrial fibrillation, valvular heart disease, history of myocardial infarction predispose to embolization.
      (3) Pain out of proportion to exam.
      (4) Metabolic acidosis is a late finding and usually indicates intestinal gangrene.

(5) Short segment involvement may result in self-limiting episodes and late intestinal stricture formation.

3. Splenic infarction–common in sickle cell patients.

VIII. COMMON CONDITIONS MIMICKING THE ACUTE ABDOMEN

A. **Pneumonia**—pain may be localized in the RUQ or LUQ if lower lobes involved.
B. **Angina or myocardial infarction**—epigastric pain, "heart burn".
C. **Obstructive uropathy** (urethral and prostatic).
D. **Acute hepatitis**—RUQ pain, vomiting.
F. **Sickle cell crisis**—diffuse pain.
F. **Leukemia**—diffuse pain.
G. **Radiculopathy from spinal cord tumors, compression fracture of spine, hip fracture.**
H. **Cystitis**—suprapubic pain and tenderness.
I. **Prostatitis**—rectal and buttock pain.
J. **Pyelonephritis**—costo-vertebral angle tenderness.
K. **Ureteral obstruction.**
   1. Calculus or neoplasm.
   2. Pain, nausea, vomiting out of proportion to exam.
L. **Toxins**—lead poisoning, venoms, tetanus, petroleum distillates, aspirin in children.
M. **Abdominal wall hematoma**—swimmers, gymnasts, or following severe effort.
N. **Psychogenic**—may have ingested foreign body causing psychogenic pain without trauma to the GI tract, or may have true perforation, hemorrhage, or obstruction.
O. **Pericarditis.**
P. **Herpes zoster** (shingles).
Q. **Diabetic ketoacidosis.**
R. **Systemic lupus erythematosus** (SLE).
S. **Uremia.**
T. **Torsion of the testes.**
U. **Acute intermittent porphyria.**

IX. INITIAL TREATMENT AND PRE-OPERATIVE PREPARATION

A. **Prompt, timely work-up**—in first 4-6 h.
B. **Diet**—NPO until diagnosis is firm and treatment plan is formulated.
C. **IV fluids**—should be based on expected fluid losses; large volumes may be required.
D. **Hemodynamic monitoring**—may be required in cases where fluid status and cardiac status are in question or when septic shock is present.
E. **Nasogastric intubation**—for bleeding, vomiting, signs of obstruction, or when urgent or emergent laparotomy is planned in a patient who has not been NPO.

F. Foley catheter—to monitor fluid resuscitation.

G. Decisions.

1. Immediate surgery.
   a. If yes, what is the timing of operative intervention (does the patient need time for resuscitation)?
   b. What incision should be used?
   c. What are the likely findings?
   d. Develop primary operative plan.
   e. Consider alternative diagnosis and plans.
   f. Use appropriate pre-operative antibiotics based on suspected pathology.
2. Admit and observe for possible operation.
   a. Serial examinations every 2-4 h during the first 12-24 h in cases without definite diagnosis; minimal use of narcotics and sedatives to avoid masking physical signs and symptoms (although this is controversial); monitor vital signs frequently.
   b. Serial lab exams may be useful; repeat CBC with differential every 4-6 h.
3. No operation–develop treatment plan for further diagnostic work-up or non-operative therapy.

18

Gynecological Causes of Acute Abdomen

Scott C. Hobler, M.D.

The term *acute abdomen* describes a syndrome in which there is an abrupt onset of abdominal pain usually associated with inflammation, perforation, obstruction, infarction, or rupture of an intraabdominal organ. Although operative therapy is not required in all cases, delay in diagnosis and treatment can have serious and potentially fatal consequences.

The acute abdomen in the female patient poses difficult diagnostic challenges and is associated with a high rate of diagnostic inaccuracies. This is principally related to the fact that abdominal pain in this group can arise from a gastrointestinal, urinary, systemic, or a genital source. This chapter principally focuses on the gynecological causes of the acute abdomen.

I. CAUSES OF THE ACUTE ABDOMEN IN WOMEN

Five to 10% of cases of acute abdominal pain in women are attributable to a gynecological cause. The following represents the diagnosis and incidence of the various causes of the acute abdomen in females of reproductive age presenting to the ER:

Diagnosis	Percentage of Cases
Non-specific Abdominal Pain	48%
Appendicitis	22%
Pelvic Inflammatory Disease (PID)	14%
Urinary Tract Infection	12%
Ovarian Cysts	4%
Ectopic Pregnancy	1%

II. DIAGNOSTIC FEATURES OF GYNECOLOGICAL DISEASE

A. Age—the age of the patient influences the likelihood of a particular disease process being present. The following represents common causes of the acute abdomen in females along with their incidence relative to the patient's age:

Diagnosis	Age < 20	Age 20-30	Age 30-40	Age > 40
Appendicitis	50%	20%	15%	15%
PID	34%	44%	18%	14%
Ovarian Cyst	18%	38%	14%	30%
Ectopic Pregnancy	4%	54%	38%	4%

B. Pain—the onset, character, location, and duration of abdominal pain are all important in assessing a female patient with an acute abdomen. The location of the pain is influenced by the level of innervation of the pelvic organs which is as follows:

Ovary	T10	Lower Abdomen
Fallopian Tubes	T11-T12	Lower Abdomen
Uterus	T10-L1	Lower Abdomen
Uterine cervix	T11-S4	Sacrum and Buttocks

1. Pain associated with PID, ovarian cysts, and ectopic pregnancies are commonly bilateral.
2. Gynecological causes of pain do not typically radiate to other sites and do not typically migrate over time.
3. Pain outside the abdomen (back and shoulder tip) is more commonly seen with gynecological causes of the acute abdomen than with appendicitis.

C. Associated symptoms—gynecologic pathology often can be associated with GI symptoms (nausea/vomiting, anorexia, or changes in bowel movements) or genitourinary symptoms (frequency, urgency, or dysuria).

III. EVALUATION OF THE FEMALE PATIENT

The key to arriving at the appropriate diagnosis in the female patient is a thorough and systematic examination, keeping in mind the characteristics of gynecological disease already mentioned.

A. History.

1. Description of the pain–duration, onset, character, and location.
2. Gynecological history.
   a. Menstrual history–LMP, regular vs. irregular menses, abnormal flow.
   b. Abnormal bleeding.
   c. Vaginal discharge.
   d. Possibility of pregnancy–nausea, tender breasts, fatigue, frequency.
   e. Contraceptive history.
   f. Sexual history.
   g. Previous gynecological history.
3. Medical and surgical history.

B. Physical examination.
1. General appearance.
2. Abdominal exam–focal *vs.* diffuse, +/- mass, +/- peritoneal signs.
3. Pelvic exam–includes manual, speculum, and rectal exam.

C. Laboratory data.
1. Depend on the clinical status.
2. Should include CBC, renal, βHCG, Gram stain of cervix, urinalysis.

D. Radiographic studies.
1. Radiographs–supine abdominal film, erect chest radiograph, and lateral decubitus.
2. Ultrasound–pelvic ultrasound has become a very helpful noninvasive diagnostic tool in the evaluation of pelvic pathology.

E. Invasive studies.
1. Culdocentesis–needle aspiration of the posterior cul de sac through the posterior vaginal fornix using an 18-ga. spinal needle. May provide valuable information in evaluating possible intra-abdominal bleeding (e.g., ectopic pregnancy).
2. Laparoscopy–when the diagnosis of an acute abdomen is in question and there is no clear indication for laparotomy, diagnostic laparoscopy may provide a definitive diagnosis and means of treatment.

IV. GYNECOLOGICAL CAUSES OF THE ACUTE ABDOMEN

A. Pelvic inflammatory disease (PID) (see "Abdominal Pain in Pregnancy").
1. Clinical presentation.
   a. History–many patients are asymptomatic. Lower abdominal pain (bilateral) is a frequent complaint (89%) and is described as constant and dull. Other less specific complaints include fever/chills, vaginal discharge, and nausea.
   b. Physical examination–can vary markedly depending on the extent of disease. Common objective findings:
      (1) Fever.
      (2) Bilateral lower abdominal pain.
      (3) Vaginal discharge.
      (4) Cervical motion tenderness (Chandelier's sign).
      (5) Additional findings–may include bilateral lower abdominal masses or fullness and/or rectal tenderness.
2. Right upper quadrant pain or pleuritic pain develops in 5-10% of cases and represents perihepatic inflammation (Fitz-Hugh-Curtis syndrome).
3. Laboratory studies.
   a. Leukocytosis (> 10,000 in 68% of cases).
   b. (−) βHCG
   c. Possible Gram stain showing *N. gonorrhea.*

4. Pelvic ultrasound–often useful when the diagnosis is unclear, and particularly useful in the presence of an adnexal mass. Tubo-ovarian abscess is represented by a complex adnexal mass in 94% of cases and cystic mass in 6%.
5. Laparoscopy–if the diagnosis is uncertain, diagnostic laparoscopy may be indicated in selected patients.
6. Therapy–the choice of therapy takes into account the patient's clinical status and suspected diagnosis. The range of therapy from ambulatory treatment to emergent laparotomy is representative of the spectrum of this disease. Because this disease is typically seen during the reproductive years, every effort should be made to minimize the chance of infertility.
7. Ambulatory management–is reserved for selected patients (asymptomatic, good chance of follow-up). Associated with a high rate of recurrence.
8. Recommended therapy.
   a. Cefoxitin 2 g IM + Probenecid 1 g PO (or Ceftriaxone 250 mg IM).
   b. Doxycycline 100 mg PO bid x 10-14 days (or tetracycline 500 mg PO qid).
9. Inpatient management–many believe that any patient with PID should receive inpatient therapy because of the high rate of recurrence in the outpatient group. Hospitalization is indicated in the following conditions: Poor follow-up, N/V, fever, + βHCG, failure of outpatient treatment, abdominal mass, peritonitis, uncertain diagnosis.
10. Therapy.
   a. Bed rest, NPO, IV fluids.
   b. IV antibiotics.
      (1) Cefoxitin 2 g IVPB q 6 h (or clindamycin 900 mg IVPB q 8 h).
      (2) Doxycycline 100 mg IVPB q 12 h (or gentamicin 2 mg/kg load followed by 1.5 mg IVPB q 8 h).
11. Surgical management–operative intervention is indicated in the following situations:
   a. Ruptured tubo-ovarian abscess (5-10% mortality).
   b. Septic shock.
   c. Failure to respond to inpatient therapy.
   d. The standard surgical therapy in the past was TAH BSO, which carries the lowest morbidity and mortality. The current trend is toward more conservative procedures aimed at preserving reproduction (e.g., unilateral adenectomy).

B. Hemorrhage from ovarian cysts—acute abdominal pain can arise from several benign ovarian pathologies.

1. Corpus luteum cysts.
2. Ovarian endometrioma.
3. Follicular cysts.
4. The pain that is seen with these conditions is frequently due to the expansion of the ovarian capsule or peritoneal irritation

secondary to hemorrhage or rupture of these structures. The vast majority of follicular and corpus luteum cysts can be managed expectantly, and most resolve within 4 to 8 weeks without medical or surgical intervention.

5. Corpus luteum cysts–formed following hemorrhage into the corpus luteum with subsequent resorption of blood. A corpus luteum is termed a corpus luteum cyst if it is > 3 cm.
   a. History–pain typically begins at or after ovulation. Typically occurs in the lower abdomen and is typically bilateral (unilateral pain may be present). Abnormalities in menstrual cycle may be seen.
   b. Physical exam.
      (1) Typically febrile.
      (2) Bilateral lower abdominal pain.
      (3) Adnexal mass may be palpable.
      (4) Diffuse pelvic tenderness.
      (5) Rupture with hemoperitoneum is more frequent on the right side (67%). Blood loss may be significant enough to require operative intervention. When bleeding occurs it may be difficult to differentiate from ectopic pregnancy.
   c. Laboratory test–a pregnancy test in this group of patients is very helpful in differentiating from ectopic pregnancy. A (-) βHCG in an ovulating female with blood in the pelvis is highly suggestive of a ruptured corpus luteum cyst.
   d. Pelvic ultrasound–when the patient is stable, a pelvic ultrasound may be valuable. Classic findings:
      (1) Free fluid in the cul de sac.
      (2) Presence of complex or cystic adnexal mass.
      (3) Presence of an intrauterine gestational sac rules out ectopic pregnancy.
   e. Management–the majority of functional cysts resolve spontaneously within 4 to 8 weeks and as a result are best managed conservatively. In the absence of hemorrhage or torsion an interval ultrasound in 4-6 weeks is all that is needed to assess for cyst regression. When there is significant hemorrhage or torsion is present, operative intervention is indicated. After confirmation that the bleeding is secondary to an ovarian cyst, cystectomy is the operative treatment of choice.

C. **Ovarian endometrioma—**acute abdominal pain can result from rupture of or leaking of old blood from an ovarian endometrioma. Leakage can cause an intense chemical peritonitis and may be associated with a low-grade fever. Contents of the endometrioma may pool in the cul-de-sac and cause rectal discomfort with defecation. This condition is typically associated with pelvic endometriosis and history of pelvic pain associated with menses.

D. **Ectopic pregnancy—**defined as a fertilized ovum implanted outside the uterine cavity. Extrauterine sites include the fallopian tubes (99%), ovary (1%), uterine cervix, and abdominal cavity. The incidence has been increasing since the 1970s and parallels the rise in PID. Approximately 2% of pregnancies are ectopic. Remains the leading cause of maternal mortality. The arterial supply to the fallopian tube is derived from the ovarian and uterine artery, which provides a rich blood supply that can result in significant hemorrhage with a tubal pregnancy.

1. Risk factors include a history of PID, presence of IUD, previous pelvic surgery, previous ectopic pregnancy, prior tubal ligation, and Progestin-only contraceptives.
2. History–presenting complaints.
   a. Amenorrhea or abnormal uterine bleeding (50-80%).
   b. Abdominal pain (usually unilateral) (90-100%).
   c. Symptoms of early pregnancy (10-25%).
   d. Shoulder pain occurs in 25% of women with ectopic pregnancies as a result of diaphragmatic irritation from hemoperitoneum.
3. Physical examination–physical exam may be non-specific and as a result a high index of suspicion is required. Pelvic exam reveals adnexal mass in 1/3 of patients and is typically tender. The uterus is slightly enlarged in 1/3 of cases.
4. Diagnostic studies.
   a. Pregnancy test–ectopic pregnancies produce low levels of HCG and require a sensitive test for detection. Currently the enzyme-linked immunoassay urine pregnancy test (ICON) is used. Serial pregnancy tests may be useful.
   b. Culdocentesis–a simple test that can diagnose intraperitoneal bleeding. (+) test = > 0.5 cc of non-clotting blood with Hct > 15%.
   c. Ultrasound–transvaginal ultrasound can identify intrauterine pregnancies and effectively rule out ectopic pregnancies. Fetal heart activity outside the uterus is diagnostic of ectopic pregnancy. Free fluid in the cul de sac is not uncommon.
   d. Laparoscopy–helpful if the diagnosis is uncertain after the above tests. If the history is classic or culdocentesis is positive, diagnostic laparoscopy is not indicated.
5. Management–surgery is the mainstay of therapy for diagnosed or suspected ectopic pregnancy. The stability of the patient, the size of the ectopic pregnancy, and the patient's desire for future fertility affect the therapeutic approach.
   a. Hemodynamically unstable–immediate exploratory laparotomy.
   b. Hemodynamically stable.
6. Surgical options–laparoscopic partial or complete salpingectomy or salpingostomy with removal of the ectopic pregnancy and preservation of the tube.
7. Medical options–methotrexate has been used as an alternative to surgical therapy in selected patients with success. Those

selected patients include those with the following: Ectopic < 3 cm, intact tubal serosa, desire for future fertility, no active bleeding, stable or rising HCG, no hepatic or renal dysfunction.

E. **Ovarian torsion—**unusual but important cause of acute abdominal pain. Occurs most commonly during the reproductive years, but may occur at any age. Occasionally torsion may be intermittent with spontaneous resolution. Torsion more frequently occurs on the right. Most cases of torsion are produced by ovarian enlargement by a functional cyst or neoplasm (50-60% of cases). The most common neoplasm leading to torsion is the benign cystic teratoma and fibroma.
   1. History–acute onset of unilateral lower quadrant abdominal pain. Associated nausea/vomiting in two-thirds of patients. Intermittent pain may precede the event.
   2. Physical exam–low-grade fever may occur, but significant fever is unlikely. Tenderness to palpation noted but peritoneal signs are uncommon. Pelvic exam reveals unilateral tenderness. Mass may or may not be present. Interval pelvic exam may reveal ovarian or adnexal swelling secondary to developing edema.
   3. Diagnostic studies.
      a. (-) βHCG.
      b. Pelvic ultrasound–typically shows an enlarged ovary that is uniformly echogenic.
      c. Diagnostic laparoscopy–indicated if the diagnosis is uncertain and there is a high degree of suspicion for torsion.
   4. Management–the key to successful management of torsion is early diagnosis so as to prevent infarction of the ovary or adnexa. Most patients with torsion present with signs and symptoms that are severe enough to demand operative intervention. At operation, the first step is to determine ovarian and adnexal viability. The surgical treatment of torsion is then based on the presence or absence of infarction.
      a. Infarction present–salpingo-oophorectomy.
      b. No infarction:
         (1) Untwist the pedicle.
         (2) Perform cystectomy.
         (3) Stabilize the ovary.

F. **Midcycle ovulatory pain (Mittelschmerz)—**pain associated with intraperitoneal bleeding associated with ovulation. The associated pain is highly variable. Pain is described as sharp, sudden, and localized to one quadrant. Pain usually subsides over several hours. Ovulatory pain in the anticoagulated patient may be more severe because of increased bleeding from the follicle.

19

The Surgical Abdomen During Pregnancy

Scott M. Berry, M.D.

In uncomplicated early pregnancy, nausea, emesis, and anorexia may mimic surgical disease. The number of radiographic studies obtained must be limited in these patients; thus, the history of present illness assumes greater importance. Firm pre-operative diagnosis is correct in only 50% of pregnant patients, but is unnecessary for exploration to proceed. Diagnostic and therapeutic delay is the major cause of maternal and fetal morbidity and mortality.

I. PHYSIOLOGIC ALTERATIONS DURING PREGNANCY

A. Cardiovascular.

1. Total blood volume is increased 25-40%.
2. Plasma volume is increased 50%.
3. Red cell mass remains unchanged or may increase up to 15%.
4. These changes lead to the physiologic anemia of pregnancy.
5. Cardiac output is increased by 30-50%.
6. Blood flow is redistributed to the placenta, uterus, skin, kidneys, and mammary glands.
7. Progesterone and prostacyclin reduce systemic vascular resistance.

B. Pulmonary.

1. Functional residual capacity is decreased 20%.
2. Oxygen consumption is increased 15%.
3. Thus, hypoxic early if hypoventilation occurs.

C. Hematologic.

1. The pregnant patient is hypercoagulable.
2. Increased levels of factors VII, VIII, X, and fibrinogen.
3. Fibrinolytic activity of the plasma is depressed.
4. Reduction in the velocity of venous blood returning from the lower extremities and a rise in venous pressure in the lower extremities.

5. Overall a 5- to 6-fold increased incidence of deep vein thrombosis in the gravid patient.

D. Renal.

1. The glomerular filtration rate and renal plasma flow is increased by 30-50%.
2. Blood urea nitrogen and creatinine are 25% lower than for non-gravid females.
3. The renal calices, pelves, and ureters dilate.
4. The urinary stasis may explain why a higher incidence of pyelonephritis is associated with bacteruria than in non-pregnant women with bacteruria.

E. Fetal hemoglobin.

1. Fetal hemoglobin is oxygen avid.
2. A maternal PaO_2 of 60 mm Hg saturates fetal hemoglobin 100%.
3. Raising maternal PaO_2 above this does not provide more oxygen to the fetus.
4. If maternal PaO_2 falls below 60 mm Hg, fetal hemoglobin saturation falls dramatically.
5. Fetal PaO_2 is 10-33 mm Hg and depends upon uterine blood flow provided maternal PaO_2 is greater than 60 mm Hg.

II. RADIOGRAPHS AND THE PREGNANT PATIENT

The maternal and fetal mortality of surgical disease is the mortality of diagnostic and therapeutic delay. In general, radiographic studies that are deemed necessary to document a life-threatening condition in the pregnant patient should be performed without delay. Many studies have shown no increase in the incidence of abortions or malformations with exposures less than 0.05 Gy delivered at any time during pregnancy (Tables 1 & 2).

III. COMPLICATIONS OF PREGNANCY

The incidence of non-obstetric surgery in pregnant patients is approximately 1 per 500 deliveries. It should be remembered that pregnancy-specific causes of abdominal pain occur in 1 per 100-300 deliveries and are thus far more common than general surgical causes of abdominal pain.

A. Ectopic fetus—occurs in 1 out of 200 pregnancies.

1. Greater than 90% occur in the uterine tube, 3% in the ovary, and the remainder in the peritoneum or cervix.
2. Risk factors–salpingitis, tubal ligation, tubal repair, IUD, prior ectopic pregnancy.
3. Lower abdominal pain in 97%.
4. Abnormal uterine bleeding in 86%.
5. Temperature elevation rare; if present, it suggests other diagnoses.
6. Serum pregnancy test positive in 96%.
7. Ultrasound diagnostic in only 84%.
8. Shoulder pain and fecal urgency suggest rupture.

TABLE 1
Acceptable Levels of Fetal Radiation Exposure

Trimester of Pregnancy	Acceptable Exposure	Overexposure Malformations
Implantation	<0.1 Gy	>0.1 Gy abortion is likely
1st	<0.1 Gy	Retardation, microcephaly, retinal degeneration
2nd	<0.15 Gy	Stunted growth, microcephaly, mental retardation
3rd	<0.15 Gy	Dermal and hematologic cancer

TABLE 2
Average Radiation Exposure of Selected Studies

Study	Exposure
Chest Radiograph PA and Lateral	0.0001-0.0003 Gy
KUB Flat and Upright	0.0001-0.0004 Gy
Intravenous Pyelogram	0.004-0.1 Gy
Voiding Cysto-Urethrogram	0.004-0.008 Gy
Barium Enema	0.003-0.005 Gy
Upper GI	0.003-0.005 Gy
Small Bowel Follow-Through	0.004-0.006 Gy
CT Abdomen	0.02-0.03 Gy
CT Chest	0.02-0.03 Gy
HIDA Scan	0.005-0.007 Gy
Nuclear Bleeding Scan	0.001-0.005 Gy
Feeding Tube Placement	0.001-0.01 Gy
V/Q Scan	0.0002 Gy
ERCP	0.0004-0.004 Gy

9. 5% of tubal pregnancies will hemorrhage > 500 ml; 85% of ovarian pregnancies will hemorrhage > 500 ml.

B. Ruptured ovarian cysts.

1. May present early in pregnancy.
2. Most can be managed expectantly.
3. Ill-defined, bilateral lower abdominal pain.
4. Gastrointestinal symptoms are not prominent.
5. Pelvic ultrasound will reveal pelvic fluid.
6. Intrauterine gestation sac excludes ectopic pregnancy.
7. When hemorrhage necessitates ovary resection, progesterone replacement may be tried with variable fetal salvage.

IV. NON-OBSTETRIC GYNECOLOGIC DISEASE

Sexually transmitted diseases (STD) can have profound effects on maternal and neonatal outcome. Pelvic inflammatory disease (PID) must be considered in every woman of reproductive age with low abdominal pain. Gonorrhea affects 0.3-3% of gravidas, syphilis 0.2-2%, and chlamydia up to 12% of gravidas.

A. Pelvic inflammatory disease.

1. Usually bilateral.
2. Usually asymptomatic.
3. Salpingitis occurs when infection ascends to the adnexae during the first trimester, after which chorion-decidua fusion obliterates the uterine cavity.
4. *Neisseria gonorrhea.*
   a. A strong association between gonococcal infection and septic spontaneous abortion.
   b. Treatment with Ceftriaxone 125-250 mg IM or Spectinomycin 2 gm IM.
5. *Chlamydia trachomatis.*
   a. Cultured from 2-24% of gravidas.
   b. The most common bacterial STD in women.
   c. Urethritis, cervicitis, and salpingitis.
   d. Causes neonatal conjunctivitis and pneumonias.
   f. Treatment with erythromycin or amoxicillin 500 mg po every 6 h for 1 week.

B. Tubo-ovarian abscess.

1. A frequent complication of acute salpingitis.
2. The abscess may be confined to the tube, but more commonly involves the entire tube and ovary complex.
3. Tubo-ovarian abscess is unilateral in 70% of cases.
4. Polymicrobial in almost 100% of cases.
   a. *Streptococcus* sp. (18%),
   b. *Escherichia coli* (37%).
   c. *Haemophilus influenzae* (11%).
   d. *Peptostreptococcus* sp. (18%).
   e. *Bacteroides* sp. (48%).
5. *Chlamydia trachomatis* and *Neisseria gonorrhea* are usually not present in the abscess, but can be recovered from the cervix in 30% of cases.
6. Pelvic and cervical motion tenderness are present in 90%.
7. Nausea and vomiting occur in up to 40% of cases.
8. Pelvic ultrasound shows a complex adnexal mass in 95%.
9. Unruptured abscess should be treated with clindamycin and Claforan®.
10. 25% of patients fail antibiotic therapy; most will lose their pregnancy not as a result of the surgical procedure itself, but rather because of the unresponsive abscess. The exception is the first trimester patient who has the corpus luteum-containing ovary resected.

C. Leiomyoma can degenerate, bleed, and torse during pregnancy.

1. Exquisite pain and tenderness.
2. The patient may be in labor.

3. White blood cell count often is elevated.
4. The patient may have emesis at the onset, but usually have a paucity of gastrointestinal symptoms.
5. Ultrasound can show the leiomyoma, but may not differentiate infarcted or torsed leiomyomas from non-pathologic ones.

D. Ovarian torsion.

1. Usually the ovary is enlarged by a cyst or neoplasm.
2. Can be intermittent with periods of remission of symptoms.
3. The pain may be colicky or constant and progressive.
4. Temperature elevation is not prominent; if present, other diagnoses should be considered.
5. Ultrasound usually can demonstrate the torsion.
6. Operation may allow salvage of the ovary and pregnancy.

E. Ovarian cancer.

1. Occurs in 1 in 18,000-20,000 pregnancies.
2. Epithelial carcinomas are most common.
3. Germ cell tumors are the next most common type.
4. When symptomatic during early pregnancy it is usually due to torsion; when symptomatic late in pregnancy it is usually due to rupture or hemorrhage of the tumor.
5. Large tumors can obstruct delivery and may make cesarian section necessary.
6. When > 5 cm and persistent into the second trimester, surgical exploration is mandatory.
7. 2-5% of ovarian tumors discovered during pregnancy are malignant compared to 20% in non-pregnant patients.
8. Pregnancy does not adversely affect the maternal prognosis.

V. GENERAL SURGICAL DISEASE

A. Features present most frequently in patients with surgical disease.

1. Acute onset of pain.
2. Pain less than 48 h duration.
3. Pain followed by vomiting.
4. Guarding on physical exam.
5. Age greater than 65.
6. Prior surgery.
7. The most common disease sent home is appendicitis, the second most common is bowel obstruction.
8. The most common diagnostic error is a pre-operative diagnosis of acute appendicitis with operative findings consistent with acute salpingitis.

B. Acute appendicitis occurs in 1:1500 pregnancies.

1. The most common extrauterine complication for which laparotomy is performed.
2. Accounts for 60% of laparotomies during pregnancy.
3. The incidence is equally distributed throughout trimesters.
4. Anorexia, which is present in greater than 90% of people

with appendicitis between 15-60 years of age, is present in only 60% of pregnant patients with appendicitis.

5. Nausea and vomiting are variable.
6. Right-sided abdominal pain is the only constant finding.
7. Rebound and guarding become less prevalent in the second and third trimesters and may be present in only 50-60% of patients in the first trimester.
8. Temperature < 100°F in 25-50% of patients.
9. Tachycardia in < 25%.
10. The normal range for a WBC count during pregnancy is 10,000-16,000/ml blood; over 90% of pregnant women with appendicitis are within this range.
11. If appendicitis cannot be ruled out in the gravida, patient should undergo appendectomy.
12. Fetal mortality for ruptured appendicitis is > 75%; for negative laparotomy is 1-5%.
13. During the first trimester a lower midline incision should be made because of the high incidence of non-appendiceal pathology.
14. In the second and third trimesters, a muscle splitting incision should be made over the point of maximal tenderness.
15. A fresh abdominal incision is no contraindication to labor, and dehiscence is rare.
16. Perforation with peritonitis (10% of gravidas with appendicitis) is an indication for cesarean section.
17. The incidence of premature labor and fetal death is 38% when the baby is left *in utero*. Cesarean delivery does not increase the incidence of complications in the mother when peritonitis is present.

C. Acute cholecystitis occurs in roughly 1 in 2000 pregnancies.

1. During pregnancy there is an increase in the resting volume of the gallbladder, an increased residual volume after emptying, an increase in the content of cholesterol in bile, and a decrease in the circulating bile salt pool.
2. Right upper quadrant pain is invariably present.
3. Murphy's sign is present in only 5% of gravidas.
4. Nausea and vomiting are variable.
5. Laboratory evaluation is seldom helpful.
6. Jaundice occurring during pregnancy is due to hepatitis in 45% of cases, benign cholestasis of pregnancy 20%, and common duct stones only 7% of the time.
7. Ultrasonic evaluation retains 95% sensitivity in gravidas.
8. HIDA scan can be performed; pregnancy is relative contraindication to this study.
9. Management should be conservative and will be successful in 85% of patients.
10. Operation should be performed when clinical condition does not respond rapidly to antibiotics.

11. When cholecystitis is uncomplicated, maternal morbidity and mortality of acute cholecystitis is not affected by pregnancy.
12. Fetal loss from operation for acute cholecystitis is about 15% during the first trimester and 5% during the second and third trimesters
13. If gangrene or perforation occurs, maternal mortality approaches 15%; fetal mortality is in the range of 60%.
14. Performing cholangiography is debatable; if the pregnancy is at least in the second trimester, most recommend single-shot cholangiography.

D. **Pancreatitis** occurs in 1 in 3000 pregnancies.
1. Most authorities would now remove pregnancy from the long list of etiologic agents leading to pancreatitis.
2. Usually due to gallstones.
3. Alcoholic pancreatitis is rare.
4. Management is conservative: > 90% resolve within 3 days.
5. When unresponsive, most surgeons would opt for endoscopic sphincterotomy, which will be successful in greater than 90% of patients.
6. Radiation exposure to the fetus can be limited to less than 0.0004 Gy by lead apron.
7. Definitive cholecystectomy can then be performed after delivery or, if necessary, during the second trimester.

E. **Bowel obstruction** occurs in 1 of 4000 pregnancies.
1. 60% are due to adhesions.
2. 25% are due to volvulus.
3. 5% are due to intussusception.
4. 3% are due to hernias.
5. < 1% are due to neoplasms.
6. Greatest risk during their first pregnancy after abdominal surgery.
7. Three periods of greatest risk.
   a. In the 4th and 5th months when the uterus changes from a pelvic to an abdominal organ leading to traction on previously formed adhesions.
   b. In the 8th and 9th months when the fetal head descends into the pelvis.
   c. During delivery when a sudden change in the intraabdominal anatomy occurs.
8. Concealed placental abruption is the most common diagnostic error.
9. Abdominal pain, vomiting, and obstipation in non-pregnant patients with small bowel obstruction is unchanged by pregnancy.
10. Obstruction presents with acute onset of pain in 85% of patients.
11. Vomiting may be present in as few as 25%.
12. Diarrhea may occur in up to 20%.

13. Distention can be difficult to assess, and bowel sounds may be normal.
14. 60% have a leucocyte count within the normal range.
15. Abdominal films are not only indicated, but requisite.
16. Fever, tachycardia, oliguria, and hypotension occur late, usually signifies compromised bowel, and portends to near 100% fetal mortality.
17. Early surgery should be the rule, as the pre-operative diagnosis of strangulation is only accurate in 50% of cases.
18. The incision should be vertical and sufficient to afford good exposure without undue manipulation of the uterus.
19. The only reason to disturb the pregnancy is if adequate exposure to resolve the problem cannot be attained.
20. Only sigmoid volvulus should be managed non-operatively. Colonoscopic detorsion with or without rectal tube may suffice as a temporizing measure. Recurrence rates are high, so definitive therapy should be planned.
21. Maternal mortality for bowel obstruction is 10-15%; fetal mortality is 33-50%.
22. Maternal hypovolemia and hypoxia are most often responsible for fetal death.

F. **Peptic ulcer** is rare in pregnancy.
1. When perforation occurs, management should be the same as for non-pregnant patients.
2. Non-operative management for perforation has not been reported in pregnant patients.
3. Consideration should be given to the length of the procedure, as limiting general anesthetic time will decrease the chances of premature labor.
4. Vagotomy and pyloroplasty or Graham patch seem the best choices.
5. Most bleeding ulcers can be managed endoscopically to completion of pregnancy, then the appropriate surgical therapy can be undertaken.
6. When recurrent bouts of hypotension occur with bleeding episodes, aggressive surgical therapy should be undertaken. Because the uterus cannot autoregulate during hypotensive episodes, the fetus becomes hypoxic. Episodes of hypoxemia will certainly be of greater risk to the fetus than will a single general anesthetic for definitive surgical therapy.

G. **Colorectal cancer** occurs in 1 of 50,000-100,000 pregnancies.
1. Delay in diagnosis is common because pregnancy may mimic some of the early signs of colon cancer (distention, constipation, and anorexia).
2. 75% of these cancers are discovered because of rectal exam done during pregnancy or at the time of delivery.
3. Severe constipation, weight loss, anorexia, abdominal pain, distention, rectal bleeding, and occult fecal blood can and should be evaluated in the pregnant patient by colonoscopy.

4. Carcinoembryonic antigen is of little use during pregnancy.
5. Management should be as for non-pregnant patients.
6. Resectable lesions should be operated expeditiously unless fetal maturity is shortly forthcoming.
7. With metastatic disease, surgery should be delayed until after delivery, unless colostomy is necessary.
8. Cesarean section may be indicated for large lesions occurring below the pelvic brim; otherwise type of delivery is dictated by the usual obstetric indications.
9. Pregnancy does not seem to affect long-term maternal outcome.

VI. UROLOGIC DISEASE

A. Bacteruria occurs in 4-7% of gravidas.

1. Usually asymptomatic.
2. 20-40% of pregnant patients with bacteruria will develop pyelonephritis.
3. Gravidas should receive 7-10 days of antibiotics for bacteruria.

B. Urolithiasis occurs in approximately 1 of 1500 pregnancies.

1. Most prevalent during the 2nd and 3rd trimesters.
2. Ultrasound is diagnostic in roughly 50% of cases.
3. Limited excretory urogram can be performed.
4. Initial management should be conservative, as 50-80% of stones will pass spontaneously.
5. If conservative management fails, internal urinary stents can be placed under ultrasonic guidance. If stents cannot be passed from below, ultrasound-guided percutaneous nephrostomy tube placement under local should be considered. Internal stents should be changed every 8 weeks.
6. Nephrolithotomy should not be undertaken because of prolonged anesthetic requirements and ionizing radiation exposure.
7. Extracorporeal shockwave lithotripsy has not been approved for use during pregnancy.

20

GI Bleeding

Betty J. Tsuei, M.D.

I. HISTORY

A history and physical exam can often elucidate the cause of GI bleeding. In addition to the routine questions, particular attention should be paid to the following areas.

A. Initial presentation of bleeding, including type of bleeding and estimation of volume of blood loss.

1. Hematemesis (bright red or coffee-ground emesis)–usually indicates an upper GI source proximal to the ligament of Treitz. Massive pulmonary, upper airway, or nasopharyngeal hemorrhage may be mistaken for GI bleeding.
2. Hematochezia (bloody stool)–often a lower GI source, but may also occur with brisk upper GI bleeding.
3. Melena (black tarry stool)–frequently an upper GI source.
4. Occult blood–may be either an upper or lower GI source.

B. Bowel habits—recent change in bowel habits (new onset of constipation or diarrhea), change in stool color, consistency or size.

C. Associated abdominal pain.

1. Painless bleeding may occur with varices, angiodysplasia, diverticulosis, or carcinoma.
2. Epigastric pain may be associated with ulcer disease, gastritis, or esophagitis.
3. Crampy abdominal pain associated with diverticulitis, inflammatory bowel disease, partially obstructing colon cancer, or colitis.
4. Pain out of proportion to abdominal tenderness and associated with lower GI bleeding is the hallmark of bowel ischemia.
5. Severe, acute, sudden onset of pain usually indicates a perforated viscus.

D. Risks and precipitating factors.

1. Ulcerogenic agents–steroids, aspirin or salicylates, nonsteroidal anti-inflammatory agents, alcohol and tobacco use.

2. Severe stress–major trauma or massive burns.
3. GI instrumentation–nasogastric intubation, colonoscopy, esophagogastroduodenoscopy.
4. Severe vomiting or retching (Mallory-Weiss tear of the gastro-esophageal junction).
5. Blunt or penetrating trauma.

E. Systemic complaints.

1. Fevers and chills–inflammatory or infectious etiology.
2. Weight loss, anorexia, fatigue–common symptoms associated with malignancies.
3. Dizziness, orthostatic symptoms–indicate large acute volume loss or severe anemia.

F. Past history.

1. Prior episodes of GI bleeding–including severity (how much blood was transfused), frequency, diagnostic and therapeutic interventions performed.
2. Prior surgeries–GI, vascular, ENT.
3. Prior GI complaints.
4. Significant medical history–cardiac, vascular, pulmonary, diabetes, cirrhosis, anti-coagulation therapy, blood dyscrasias.

G. Social history—drug and alcohol use.

II. PHYSICAL EXAMINATION

A. General appearance—may be pale, diaphoretic, or anxious, with moderate to severe hemorrhage.

B. Vital signs.

1. Blood pressure–watch for hypotension or orthostatic changes (postural drop in systolic BP > 20 mm Hg).
2. Pulse–tachycardia or orthostatic changes (postural increase of > 20 bpm).
3. Temperature–may be elevated with infection.
4. Respirations–may be shallow and rapid with significant blood loss.

C. Skin—jaundice, palmar erythema, spider angiomata associated with cirrhosis, and portal hypertension are commonly seen with variceal bleeding. (Other signs of portal hypertension include gynecomastia, atrophic testicles, and asterixis.) Significant ecchymosis or petechia may be noted if there is a contributory coagulopathy or thrombocytopenia.

D. Head and neck—pale or dry mucous membranes, evidence of oro-pharyngeal bleeding.

E. Abdomen.

1. Distension, caput medusa, jaundice on inspection.
2. Bowel sounds (usually increased with upper GI bleeding).
3. Localization of abdominal tenderness.
4. Palpation of masses, ascites, hepatosplenomegaly.

F. Rectal exam—stool, hemorrhoids, rectal mass, anal fissure or fistula.

III. LABORATORY EVALUATION

A. **Type and crossmatch**—6 units of packed RBCs. This should be done immediately and should be available at all times.

B. **Hemoglobin/hematocrit**—underestimate the volume of acute blood loss because equilibration has not occurred. Hypochromia and microcytosis suggest chronic blood loss; macrocytosis suggests nutritional abnormalities due to alcohol abuse.

C. **Platelet count**—thrombocytopenia is the usual defect present in coagulopathies secondary to massive hemorrhage. Also found in cirrhotics due to hypersplenism.

D. **PT/PTT**—screen for coagulation defects. Check fibrinogen and fibrin split products to identify a dilutional coagulopathy after massive transfusion.

E. **Renal profile**—renal failure, electrolyte disturbances secondary to volume loss, or emesis may be identified. Increased BUN can be due to the increased protein absorbed from blood in the GI tract as well as to a state of dehydration.

F. **Liver function studies**—assessment of hepatic dysfunction.

G. **Chest radiographs and abdominal films**—to check for free air, pulmonary infiltrate, and splenic or hepatic enlargement.

IV. INITIAL MANAGEMENT

A. Assess magnitude of hemorrhage.

B. Stabilize hemodynamic status.

1. Two large bore IVs (14- to 16-ga. if possible).
2. Begin resuscitation with crystalloid (Lactated Ringer's solution).
3. Type-specific blood used if further resuscitation required after 2 L of crystalloid.
4. Place Foley catheter.
5. Place nasogastric tube–can help differentiate an upper from lower GI source. Saline lavage should be used to remove blood from the stomach until the returning fluid is clear. An upper GI source can be present with clear NG return in up to 20%. Return of bilious fluid without blood suggests a bleeding site beyond the ligament of Treitz.

C. Monitor for continued blood loss.

1. Vital signs frequently, urine output hourly.
2. Frequent lab tests to assess the adequacy of transfusion and correction of coagulopathies. The hematocrit should be maintained above 28-30, especially in elderly patients with cardiovascular disease.
3. CVP or pulmonary artery monitoring in unstable patient.

V. DIAGNOSTIC PROCEDURES

A. **Nasogastric tube**—see above.

B. **Endoscopy**—most useful in localizing sources of bleeding;

therapeutic interventions also may be instituted at the same time.

1. Esophagogastroduodenoscopy (EGD)–for upper GI source has 95% diagnostic accuracy if used within the first 24 h. Esophagitis, varices, Mallory-Weiss tears, gastritis, and peptic ulcer disease can be identified. The stomach must first be lavaged clear if possible. EGD may be used for sclerotherapy of varices or cauterization of bleeding vessels.
2. Anoscopy/sigmoidoscopy/colonoscopy–diverticular disease, angiodysplasia, carcinoma may be found if bleeding permits an accurate exam. Lack of an adequate bowel prep often renders these tests inconclusive, but, at minimum, rigid sigmoidoscopy can exclude a rectal source of bleeding.

C. Angiography.

1. Requires brisk bleeding (> 0.5 cc/min) to identify the source.
2. Can be used for therapeutic interventions such as selective vasopressin or embolization.

D. Technetium labelled red blood cell scan.

1. Very sensitive (requires 0.1 cc/min bleeding) and less invasive than angiography, but far less specific.
2. May identify the location of bleeding but not the source.

E. Radiographic contrast studies—rarely useful and interfere with other diagnostic procedures.

VI. NONSURGICAL TREATMENT

A. Sclerotherapy—used for bleeding varices during EGD.

B. Electrocautery—of bleeding vessels in peptic ulcer disease. This is useful in high-risk patients and can be performed at the time of the diagnostic study.

C. Vasopressin infusion.

1. Can be given systemically or by selective arterial infusion.
2. Selective infusion may be initiated at the time of the diagnostic angiogram and may minimize the systemic effects of the drug.
3. Recent myocardial infarction or significant coronary artery disease are relative contraindications to this form of therapy. Simultaneous infusion of nitroglycerin may help to reduce risks of infarction.
4. Dosage:
   a. Loading–20 U over 20-30 min.
   b. Infusion–0.2-0.4 U/min.

D. Embolization—usually reserved for upper GI sources of bleeding, as there is a high risk of ischemia with infarction or perforation with colonic embolization.

VII. SURGICAL THERAPY

A. Peptic ulcer disease (see "Peptic Ulcer Disease").

1. Conservative measures as above.
2. Nasogastric suctioning and prophylactic measures to keep

gastric pH > 5–H_2 receptor blockers, antacids, or cytoprotective agents (Carafate®).

3. Surgery should be performed if the patient requires 6 or more units of blood during a 24-h period, or if there is rebleeding on maximal medical therapy.

B. Esophageal varices (see "Cirrhosis").

1. Sclerotherapy.
2. Vasopressin.
3. Sengstaken-Blakemore tube if bleeding continues.
4. Portosystemic shunt if conservative treatment fails.
5. Orthotopic liver transplant has become an alternative in select patients with severe hepatic dysfunction.

C. Mallory-Weiss tear—mucosal tear at the gastroesophageal junction. Occurs after violent retching or emesis. Most stop spontaneously with supportive measures alone.

D. Diverticulosis (see "Diverticulosis").

1. 70% of lower GI bleeding, can occur anywhere.
2. Surgery for a blood loss exceeding 5 units in 24 h.
3. 60% stop spontaneously; 25% rebleed.
4. Surgical options should be considered after the second significant bleed. For persistent hemorrhage, resect the segment of colon involved with diverticuli. If question exists, subtotal colectomy with ileoproctostomy is the procedure of choice.

E. Angiodysplasia.

1. Occurs throughout GI tract, commonly in the right colon.
2. Surgical treatment for massive acute bleeding or chronic intermittent bleeding.

F. Carcinoma—elective surgery following adequate bowel prep is preferred.

21

Intestinal Obstruction

Gregory B. Strothman, M.D.

I. DEFINITIONS

A. **Ileus**—mechanical or functional intestinal obstruction; most common usage of the word is to connote failure of aboral passage of bowel contents due to dysfunctional motility of the bowel, as in "adynamic" or "paralytic ileus".

B. **Mechanical obstruction**—complete or partial physical blockage of the intestinal lumen (85% small bowel, 15% large bowel).

C. **Simple obstruction**—one obstructing point.

D. **Closed loop obstruction**—both the afferent and efferent limbs of bowel are occluded, as in volvulus; may be accompanied by strangulation.

E. **Strangulated**—circulation to the obstructed intestine is impaired; more likely in closed loop than simple obstruction secondary to sustained increased intraluminal pressure.

II. ETIOLOGY

A. Small bowel obstruction (SBO).

1. ***Adhesions***—the most common cause of SBO. Approximately 80-90% of SBOs in patients with prior abdominal surgery are due to adhesions or internal herniation through a surgically created defect.
2. ***Hernias***—the second most common cause of obstruction overall, but the most common cause in patients without prior abdominal surgery.
3. ***Other causes of SBO.***
   a. **Extrinsic.**
      (1) Carcinomatosis or tumor encasement from non-small bowel source.
      (2) Intra-abdominal abscess.
      (3) Hematoma.
      (4) Malrotation with Ladd's bands or midgut volvulus.
      (5) Annular pancreas (duodenal obstruction).

(6) Endometriosis.
(7) Superior mesenteric artery (SMA) syndrome–compression of third portion of the duodenum by the SMA in thin patients with severe acute weight loss.

b. **Intrinsic.**
(1) Small bowel neoplasms.
(2) Congenital lesions.
a) Small bowel atresia, stenosis, or webs.
b) Small bowel duplications, or mesenteric cysts.
c) Meckel's diverticulum or other remnants of the omphalo-mesenteric duct.
(3) Inflammatory lesions.
a) Regional enteritis, Crohn's disease.
b) Radiation enteritis, stricture.

c. **Intraluminal obstruction.**
(1) Meconium ileus.
(2) Gallstone ileus–more common in elderly.
(3) Intussusception.
(4) Foreign bodies–bezoars, barium, worms.

4. Other conditions that mimic the clinical picture of SBO.
a. Colonic obstruction–right colonic obstruction near ileocecal valve may be indistinguishable from SBO.
b. Adynamic ileus (see II.C. below).
c. Vascular insufficiency.
(1) Mesenteric embolism.
(2) Non-occlusive mesenteric ischemia.
(3) Mesenteric thrombosis–due to severe dehydration, disseminated intravascular coagulation, polycythemia, atherosclerosis.
d. Hirschsprung's disease involving small bowel.

B. Colonic obstruction—in general, colon obstruction produces less fluid and electrolyte disturbance than mechanical SBO.

1. ***Extrinsic.***
a. Volvulus–sigmoid 60-80%; cecal 20-40%.
b. Adhesions.
c. Hernia–particularly sliding type.
d. Endometriosis.

2. ***Intrinsic.***
a. Carcinoma of the colon–most common cause (60%) of colonic obstruction.
b. Inflammatory lesions.
(1) Ulcerative colitis.
(2) Diverticulitis.
(3) Radiation enteritis.
c. Congenital lesions–imperforate anus.

3. ***Intraluminal obstruction.***
a. Meconium ileus.
b. Intussusception.
c. Fecal impaction, foreign bodies, barium.

4. Other conditions that may mimic colonic obstruction.
   a. Adynamic ileus–see below.
   b. Hirschsprung's disease.
   c. Focal ischemic colitis.

C. Adynamic ileus.

1. ***Metabolic.***
   a. Hypokalemia.
   b. Hypomagnesemia.
   c. Hyponatremia.
   d. Ketoacidosis.
   e. Uremia.
   f. Porphyria.
   g. Heavy metal poisoning.
2. Response to localized inflammatory process within or adjacent to the peritoneal cavity–appendicitis, cholecystitis, diverticulitis, abscess, pyelonephritis.
3. Sepsis.
4. ***Diffuse peritonitis***—bacterial or chemical.
5. ***Retroperitoneal process.***
   a. Retroperitoneal hematoma.
   b. Pancreatitis.
   c. Spinal or pelvic fracture.
6. ***Drugs.***
   a. Narcotics.
   b. Antipsychotics.
   c. Anticholinergics.
   d. Ganglionic blockers.
   e. Agents used to treat Parkinson's disease.
7. ***Neuropathic disorders.***
   a. Diabetes.
   b. Multiple sclerosis.
   c. Scleroderma.
   d. Lupus erythematosus.
   e. Hirschsprung's disease.
8. ***Post-operative ileus following intra-abdominal surgery.***
   a. Small bowel motility usually returns within 24-48 h.
   b. Gastric motility usually returns by 48 h.
   c. Return of colonic motility may take 3-5 days.
9. ***Ogilvie's syndrome.***
   a. Colonic pseudo-obstruction of uncertain etiology.
   b. Associated with pelvic retroperitoneal processes, long-term debilitation, chronic disease, immobility, narcotics, prolonged bed rest, and polypharmacy.
   c. Usually manifested by moderate to marked segmental cecal dilatation. Cecal diameter > 12 cm significantly increases risk of perforation.
   d. Treatment of choice is decompression with gentle enemas. If unsuccessful or if marked cecal dilatation is already pres-

ent, colonoscopic decompression is indicated. Rarely, cecostomy or right hemicolectomy is needed for perforation, ischemia, or unsuccessful colonoscopic decompression.

III. DIAGNOSIS OF INTESTINAL OBSTRUCTION

A. History.

1. ***Age.***
   a. Neonate–consider meconium ileus, Hirschsprung's disease, malrotation, intestinal atresias.
   b. 2-24 months–consider intussusception, Hirschsprung's disease.
   c. Young adults–hernia, inflammatory bowel disease.
   d. Adults–hernia, neoplasms, diverticular disease.
   e. Elderly–neoplasms, diverticular disease, hernia, Ogilvie's syndrome.
2. ***Nausea, vomiting, obstipation***—in proximal obstruction, bilious vomiting may occur early and the patient may have little abdominal distension. He/she may continue to pass stool and flatus as the bowel distal to the obstruction is evacuated. In distal bowel obstruction, the patient may initially complain of obstipation and distension prior to the onset of vomiting feculent material (secondary to bacterial overgrowth of small bowel contents). Blood in the vomitus suggests strangulation or associated lesion. Obstipation and failure to pass gas from the rectum are characteristic of complete obstruction. These are evident only after bowel distal to the obstruction has been evacuated.
3. ***Pain***—in proximal obstruction, pain is typically crampy and referred primarily to the periumbilical region. It is due to distension of the bowel lumen secondary to continued peristalsis against the obstruction and may subside after a long period secondary to inhibited bowel motility. In distal obstruction, pain is usually referred to the lower abdomen. When crampy abdominal pain is succeeded by continuous severe pain, strangulation and peritonitis should be suspected. If there is immediate torsion and vascular compromise of a bowel segment, obstruction and ischemia can occur early.
4. ***Past surgical history***—prior operative procedures, particularly pelvic and lower abdominal procedures, implicate adhesions or internal herniation as the cause of the obstruction. Sudden cessation of colostomy or ileostomy output signals mechanical obstruction.
5. ***Past medical history.***
   a. History of severe atherosclerosis, cardiac arrhythmias, prior myocardial infarction, chronic congestive heart failure, and atrial fibrillation may suggest intestinal ischemia.
   b. Previous history of inflammatory bowel disease or diverticulitis may suggest mechanical obstruction.

   c. Gallstone ileus should be considered in a patient with known gallstones or history of recurrent biliary colic, especially in patients > 70.
6. ***Medications.***
   a. Digitalis–possible intestinal ischemia.
   b. Narcotics–adynamic ileus.
   c. Anticholinergics, ganglion blockers, antipsychotics, drugs for Parkinson's disease suggest adynamic ileus.
   d. Diuretics–consider hypokalemia as the source of adynamic ileus.
   e. Polypharmacy–consider Ogilvie's syndrome (see above).
7. ***Review of systems.***
   a. Recent weight loss–consider neoplasm first, also chronic intestinal ischemia.
   b. If severe acute weight loss from other cause, consider superior mesenteric artery syndrome (see above).

B. Physical exam.

1. ***Vital signs.***
   a. Fever–usually absent in uncomplicated obstruction. If present, consider inflammatory process or strangulation.
   b. Tachycardia–may be secondary to dehydration and hypovolemia, but if associated with leukocytosis and localized tenderness, it is one of the cardinal signs of strangulation.
   c. Orthostatic hypotension–often associated with dehydration and "third space" losses as fluid is sequestered in obstructed bowel.
2. ***Abdominal exam.***
   a. Distension–minimal in proximal obstruction, but marked in prolonged distal obstruction.
   b. The presence of surgical scars from prior operations should always be noted.
   c. Mild tenderness is common; however, localized tenderness and guarding suggest peritonitis and the likelihood of strangulation or perforation.
   d. Mass–may be palpable due to a fixed distended loop of bowel or due to a carcinoma or inflammatory mass that is the cause of the obstruction. A careful exam for the presence of inguinal, femoral, umbilical, or incisional hernia is mandatory.
   e. Bowel sounds–initially active with intermittent rushes and borborygmus, but decrease with time. In adynamic ileus, bowel sounds are usually absent.
3. ***Rectal exam.***
   a. Rectal vault is usually empty with established obstruction.
   b. Fecal impaction can be ruled out.
   c. Guaiac positive stool suggests an alimentary mucosal lesion, as may occur with cancer, intussusception, or mesenteric infarction.

d. Extrinsic pelvic masses as well as intrinsic colon lesions can be diagnosed.

C. Laboratory evaluation.

1. ***WBC*** – usually normal in uncomplicated SBO. Elevated with strangulation or if the source of obstruction is inflammatory. Markedly elevated late with mesenteric infarction.
2. ***Hematocrit*** – is often increased due to hemoconcentration. Anemia in the presence of clinical low SBO or colonic obstruction often is characteristic of colon carcinoma.
3. ***Electrolyte abnormalities*** – especially hypokalemia (see above).
4. ***Alkalosis*** – usually develops in proximal SBO or pyloric obstruction because vomiting results in loss of hydrogen and chloride via gastric acid and fluid.
5. ***Acidosis*** – usually occurs late in the course of bowel infarction; a normal pH does not rule out bowel infarction.
6. ***Amylase*** – may or may not be elevated in SBO.

D. Radiographs—essential to confirm clinical diagnosis and define more accurately the site of obstruction.

1. ***Upright chest radiograph*** – sensitive for detection of free air under the diaphragm.
2. ***Abdominal flat and upright radiographs*** (left lateral decubitus if the patient is unable to stand)–characteristic features of intestinal obstruction are dilated bowel loops, usually containing air-fluid levels proximal to the point of obstruction with little or no gas distally. Air-fluid levels are not normally seen in an upright radiograph of the abdomen in persons with normal bowel motility. Gas may still be visualized distally with partial obstruction, early in the course of complete obstruction, or if air has been introduced from below during rectal exam or enema.
   a. Small bowel can be distinguished from large bowel by the presence of **Valvulae conniventes** (also known as plicae circulares), which traverse the entire diameter of the bowel as opposed to haustral markings of the colon, which only extend 1/2 to 2/3 the diameter of the bowel.
   b. Air fluid levels in the upright projection can be seen with both ileus and obstruction. In obstruction they are usually more pronounced, and a "step-ladder" pattern is often seen progressing down the abdomen.
   c. Fluid-filled loops of bowel appear as areas of increased density without gas and can easily be overlooked.
   d. In colonic obstruction or ileus, if the cecal diameter is > 12 cm, the patient is at increased risk for perforation; emergency decompression of the colon should be considered. When the cecum is acutely dilated to 12-14 cm, the wall tension exceeds perfusion pressure, and focal areas of necrosis may occur. These may progress even though the cecum is decompressed by non-operative means.

e. Sigmoid volvulus–appears as a large dilated loop of bowel that resembles a "bent inner tube" or the symbol "omega" with the apex in the LLQ and the convexity in the RUQ.
f. Cecal volvulus–a large, dilated, ovoid, air-filled cecum is usually visualized in the upper abdomen as the hypermobile cecum has rotated upward and to the left around ileocolic vessels.

3. ***Contrast enema*** — most commonly used to rule out obstruction of the colon.
   a. Useful when the diagnosis is uncertain.
   b. Must be done with low pressure. The objective is identifying the site of obstruction, not defining mucosal detail. Free barium in the peritoneum from perforation of the colon has a very high mortality. If any question of a perforation exists, use water-soluble contrast.
   c. Will show the point of colonic obstruction, but care must be taken not to force barium beyond a partial obstruction and thereby create complete obstruction (controversial).
   d. In unclear cases of suspected distal SBO, barium enema should be done prior to upper GI series.
      (1) To rule out colonic obstruction with fluid-filled proximal colon indistinguishable from SBO on plain radiographs.
      (2) Reflux through the ileocecal valve will often visualize a collapsed terminal ileum, confirming the diagnosis of SBO.
   e. Hydrostatic or air contrast barium enema may be used if intussusception is suspected–to make the diagnosis, and to attempt a reduction. In children with intussusception, up to 60-70% reduce with enema alone. Hydrostatic reduction should not be attempted in adults because of the high frequency of underlying mucosal lesions as the lead point for the intussusception.
   f. In sigmoid or cecal volvulus, a "bird's-beak" pattern is demonstrated at the site of the volvulus.
4. ***Upper GI series with small bowel follow-through.***
   a. Useful if the diagnosis is uncertain or for demonstrating a partially obstructing lesion.
   b. In cases of uncertain diagnosis, barium enema should be done *first* to rule out colonic obstruction.

IV. TREATMENT

A. Resuscitation.

1. Rehydration–rapid volume repletion with normal saline until adequate urine output (½ cc/kg body weight/h) is established.
2. Correction of electrolyte abnormalities–patients often have hypochloremic, hypokalemic metabolic alkalosis, and normal saline with added potassium is the fluid of choice. (KCl is added only after urine output is established.)
3. Foley catheter to monitor urine output.

B. Nasogastric suction—to prevent vomiting with aspiration.
   1. Prevents further gaseous distension from swallowed air and partially decompresses the bowel.
   2. The stomach must be empty in preparation for and during induction of anesthesia. Anesthesia relaxes the esophageal sphincters, allowing free regurgitation of both gastric and small bowel contents (which may rapidly refill the stomach).

C. Small bowel intubation—with "long tube" (i.e., Miller-Abbott or Cantor tube). Use of a long tube as therapy for mechanical intestinal obstruction is generally inappropriate because it may delay operation for a complete mechanical obstruction. Only major indications for long-tube therapy:
   1. Resolving partial obstruction.
   2. Partial obstruction in the immediate post-operative period. About 50-60% of cases will resolve with a long tube.
   3. Partial small bowel obstruction or obstruction due to inflammation that is expected to resolve with non-operative therapy, or due to carcinomatosis or radiation enteritis. These seldom strangulate and are often very difficult operative procedures, with high complication and recurrence rates.

D. Peri-operative antibiotics—coverage of gram-negative aerobes and anaerobes is indicated because of bacterial overgrowth in the obstructed lumen and the possibility of small or large bowel resection. If necrotic bowel or abscess is found, a full treatment course rather than peri-operative prophylaxis is given.

E. Operative treatment of SBO—SBO is a surgical emergency and should be treated by laparotomy with few exceptions.
   1. Patients with localized peritoneal signs, leucocytosis, fever, and tachycardia with SBO should be assumed to have ischemic or necrotic bowel and should be taken to the O.R. as soon as they are hemodynamically stable.
   2. Patients with complete obstruction but without signs of vascular compromise should be resuscitated and operated upon urgently (as soon as possible within 6-8 h of admission).
   3. Patients with an uncertain diagnosis or those who continue to pass flatus or stool, indicating either a very early complete obstruction or a partial obstruction, can be treated conservatively while a diagnostic evaluation is in progress. Intestinal obstruction due to an acute exacerbation of Crohn's disease treated conservatively may permit resolution of the obstruction.
   4. Lysis of all adhesions or resection of the involved segment of bowel is recommended. Intestinal bypass may be necessary in cases of advanced malignancy.
   5. In obstruction due to radiation injury, lysis of adhesions should be limited. Radiation-injured bowel may be "revascularized" through adhesions.
   6. In cases of extreme bowel distension preventing easy abdominal closure, the intraluminal fluids can be carefully milked back into the stomach. A long intestinal tube is useful if it has

passed through the ligament of Treitz prior to surgery. Otherwise it is difficult to manipulate through the duodenum. Intentional enterotomy is not recommended because of a high likelihood of fecal contamination, late leakage, abscess, or fistula.

7. It is important to determine whether a segment of bowel is viable. The general criteria are color, motility, and arterial pulsation. If in question, the bowel segment should be completely released and placed in a warm saline-moistened sponge for 15-20 minutes and then re-examined. If normal color and peristalsis are evident, the bowel may be returned safely. Any nonviable bowel should be resected. Intravenous fluorescein and a Wood's lamp can be helpful in determining viability, as can Doppler examination of the involved segment. If there is any question of bowel viability, a second-look laparotomy can be performed at 24-48 h.

F. Operative treatment of colonic obstruction.

1. ***Obstructing carcinoma.***
   a. **Right colonic obstruction**–usually treated by resection and primary anastomosis when there is no gross contamination, massive edema, shock, or long-standing peritonitis. Otherwise should undergo decompressive ileostomy and mucous fistula.
   b. **Left colonic obstruction.**
      (1) Primary resection with creation of colostomy and mucous fistula or rectal pouch (2-stage procedure) is usually indicated. In extremely debilitated/unstable patients without perforation or abscess, an initial diverting colostomy allows decompression and stabilization prior to resection and colostomy closure at later dates (3-stage procedure). [*Mucous fistula* is the term used to describe a stoma created from the proximal end of the remaining distal bowel after a segment has been resected. A rectal pouch is created by leaving the distal divided end of rectosigmoid colon within the abdomen after sigmoid resection. This procedure is done if there is insufficient length to bring the bowel to the abdominal wall as a mucous fistula.]
      (2) There are data that support resection with primary anastomosis using on-table bowel preparation, but this is controversial.
   c. Patients with peritonitis secondary to an ischemic colon should be treated with resection of the involved bowel, end colostomy and mucous fistula or rectal pouch.
2. ***Obstructing diverticulitis***–(see "Colonic Diverticulitis").
3. ***Sigmoid volvulus.***
   a. Initial treatment–non-operative decompression via sigmoidoscopy and placement of a long, soft, well-lubricated rectal tube past the point of obstruction. This usually re-

sults in reduction (80% of cases) of the volvulus with immediate passage of stool and flatus. Mucosal inspection is then done to evaluate bowel viability.

b. Because of high frequency of recurrence (> 50% in first year), many authors recommend elective sigmoid resection after the first episode if the patient is a reasonable operative risk.

c. If volvulus cannot be reduced, strangulation should be suspected and immediate resection carried out.

4. ***Cecal volvulus***—always treated operatively. Resection is indicated for vascular compromise, but cecopexy or cecostomy is adequate in other cases.

G. Paralytic ileus—treated by NG suction and IV fluids. Electrolyte imbalances are corrected, especially hypokalemia. Long tubes or colonoscopic decompression should be employed for extreme distension. It most commonly occurs after surgery, and is transient (2-3 days). If persistent and without obvious etiology, mechanical obstruction or extrinsic process must be excluded.

H. Post-operative care.

1. Nasogastric decompression until bowel activity is re-established.
2. If post-operative course prolonged (> 5 days), parenteral nutrition should be considered.

V. RESULTS OF SURGICAL TREATMENT OF BOWEL OBSTRUCTION

A. Recurrent SBO—occurs in 10% of patients treated by enterolysis, and this incidence increases with each subsequent enterolysis.

B. Multiple adhesive SBOs requiring enterolysis—patients with this condition may benefit from plication of the bowel in an organized position to promote the formation of adhesions in a non-obstructed pattern.

1. Transmesenteric plication–seromuscular stitches are used to plicate adjacent bowel loops.
2. Intra-operative oral placement of a Leonard tube or a Baker tube through a gastrostomy or high jejunostomy. Tube is left in place 12-14 days to maintain an adequate intestinal lumen while healing occurs.

C. Mortality of operation.

1. SBO–0-5% (4.5-31% if gangrene has occurred).
2. Colonic obstruction.
   a. 1-5% in diverticulitis.
   b. 5-10% in carcinoma.
   c. 40-50% if bowel necrosis has occurred with volvulus.

22

Neurosurgical Emergencies

JEFFREY LARSON, M.D.

Neurosurgical emergencies represent clinical conditions in which rapid evaluation and appropriate intervention may significantly decrease morbidity and mortality. Early assessment of altered level of consciousness and any focal neurologic deficit, as well as prompt initial management are essential, particularly in the head-injured patient.

It must be stressed that conditions leading to central, uncal, upward cerebellar, and tonsillar herniation syndromes can be rapidly fatal, literally within a few minutes. This chapter provides the basic principles necessary for the early care of the patient with an acute neurosurgical problem.

I. APPROACH TO THE UNCONSCIOUS PATIENT

A. **Unconsciousness** requires either or both bilateral hemispheric dysfunction and depression of the reticular activating system (RAS) in the upper brainstem.

B. **Etiologies.**

1. ***Structural causes of coma***—may originate for multiple reasons, including traumatic, vascular (both ischemic and hemorrhagic), neoplastic, infectious, congenital, and inflammatory factors.
   a. **Supratentorial mass**—leads to compression of diencephalon and eventually the brainstem. Initial depression of level of consciousness followed by rostral to caudal deterioration is characteristic. Symmetric deterioration suggests central herniation, whereas asymmetric decline suggests uncal herniation.
   b. **Infratentorial mass**—leads to direct compression of RAS and is characterized by extremely sudden onset of coma. Deterioration is typically caudal to rostral, with hemodynamic instability, abnormal respiratory pattern, and cranial nerve palsies common.

2. ***Toxic/metabolic causes of coma*** – may be due to electrolyte or endocrine imbalance; self-induced, accidental, or iatrogenic intoxication; CNS or systemic infection; nutritional deficiencies; inherited metabolic disorders; global hypoxia or ischemia; seizure (e.g., post-ictal state or non-convulsive status epilepticus); or organ failure (e.g., uremic and hepatic encephalopathy). Note that onset of coma is more gradual with a symmetric neurologic exam and preserved pupillary responses. Asterixis, tremor, myoclonus, and acid/base disturbances are characteristic of toxic/metabolic causes.
3. ***Pseudocoma*** – includes psychiatric causes, such as catatonia and conversion reaction, as well as "locked-in" syndrome due to ventral pontine infarction. Note that in psychiatric causes, objective findings are absent, and active lid closing, normal pupillary response, physiologic reflexes, and normal motor tone and responses are detectable.

C. History.

1. Important features include abrupt *vs.* subacute *vs.* insidious onset; presence of lucid interval; recent neurologic complaints; and spatial progression of neurologic deficits.
2. Look for factors in past medical and surgical histories, allergies, social and sexual habits, occupational exposure, and travel that could explain decline.
3. A medication history is essential, especially regarding psychotropics, sedatives, and opiates.

D. Physical examination.

1. ***General.***
   a. Vital signs.
   b. Respiratory pattern.
   c. External evidence of trauma or intravenous drug abuse.
   d. Nuchal rigidity.
2. ***Level of consciousness.***
   a. Awake and alert–eyes open, responsive to verbal stimuli.
   b. Lethargic–sleepy, but easily arousable to full waking state.
   c. Obtunded–sleeps unless continually stimulated, but can be fully aroused with effort.
   d. Stupor–responds to vigorous physical stimuli, but cannot be fully aroused to waking state.
   e. Coma–totally unarousable.

Best Eye Opening	Best Verbal	Best Motor	Points
–	–	Obeys	6
–	Oriented	Localizes	5
Spontaneous	Confused	Withdraws to pain	4
To speech	Inappropriate	Decorticate	3
To pain	Incomprehensible	Decerebrate	2
None	None	None	1

3. ***Glasgow Coma Scale (GCS).***
   a. Not a neurologic examination, but a reproducible measure of level of consciousness. Ranges from 3 to 15 points.
4. ***Children's Coma Scale (CCS).***
   a. For age < 4 years.
   b. Ranges from 3 to 15.

Best Eye Opening	Best Verbal		Best Motor	Points
–	–		Obeys	6
–	Smiles, oriented to sound, follows objects, interacts		Localizes	5
	Crying	*Interaction*		
Spontaneous	Consolable	Inappropriate	Withdraws to pain	4
To speech	Inconsistently consolable	Moaning	Decorticate	3
To pain	Inconsolable	Restless	Decerebrate	2
None	None	None	None	1

5. ***Evaluation of brainstem.***
   a. Response to visual threat (CN II, VII).
   b. Pupillary responses (CN II, III).
   c. Corneal reflexes (CN V, VII).
   d. Extraocular movements (CN III, IV, VI). Look for conjugate *vs.* dysconjugate gaze; gaze deviation; roving eye movements.
   e. Oculocephalic reflex ("doll's eyes") (CN VI, VIII). Test only if cervical spine cleared.
   f. Oculovestibular reflex (CN VI, VIII). Known as "cold calorics" test (see "Brain Death").
   g. Gag reflex (CN IX, X).
   h. Response to central pain using supraorbital or sternal pressure. Tests general integrity of motor and sensory tracts in brainstem. Use only if not obeying commands.
6. ***Motor examination.***
   a. Check tone, bulk.
   b. Test strength, if possible.
   c. Decorticate posturing–indicates level of lesion above red nucleus.
   d. Decerebrate posturing–indicates levels of lesion above lateral vestibular nucleus but below red nucleus. Results from loss of inhibition to extensor muscles.
7. ***Sensory examination.***
   a. Difficult to assess in unconscious patient.
   b. Check whether patient withdraws to pin-prick or nailbed pressure.
8. ***Reflexes.***
   a. Check superficial and deep tendon reflexes.

b. Check presence or absence of pathologic reflexes (Babinski, Hoffman's).
c. Check sphincter for tone and for clonus.

II. INITIAL MANAGEMENT OF THE HEAD-INJURED PATIENT

A. Initial management of the head-injured patient, particularly if GCS < 12, should include mild hyperventilation and a bolus of mannitol (1g/kg).

B. Obtain a CT scan of the head as soon as possible.

C. Circulation—optimize hemodynamic status with fluids and vasopressors, if necessary. Brain injury rostral to the medulla is rarely a primary cause of systemic hypotension except in very young children.

D. Treat remediable causes of coma immediately.

1. Hypoglycemia–25 g glucose IVP (50 ml of 50% dextrose). Always give unless it is certain that glucose is normal.
2. Opiate intoxication–naloxone 1 amp (0.4 mg) IVP.
3. Also give thiamine 100 mg IVP to prevent Wernicke-Korsakoff syndrome, which can be caused by large infusion of glucose.

E. Laboratory studies.

1. CBC, renal profile, Ca^{++}, Mg^{++}, PO_4, arterial blood gas, osmolarity, coagulation profile, toxicology screen, ETOH level, type and screen, urinalysis.
2. Consider hepatic profile, ammonia level, thyroid function tests, endocrine panel, blood cultures if febrile.

F. Control seizures, if necessary.

1. *Lorazepam 1.5-2.0 mg or diazepam 5-10 mg IVP. Also load with longer-acting phenytoin.*
2. *See management of status epilepticus.*
3. *Consider EEG if suspect nonconvulsive status epilepticus.*

G. Pan-culture if febrile.

1. Consider lumbar puncture if no evidence of increased intracranial pressure and head CT is normal(Table 1).
2. Consider empiric treatment of infections.

H. Normalize pH if necessary.

I. Normalize temperature if necessary.

J. Protect eyes with lacrilube or artificial tears.

K. Sedation as needed; generally the less, the better. Generally a Fentanyl drip is used up to a maximum of 100 μg/h to maintain the neurologic examination while keeping the patient safe.

L. Treat coagulopathy with fresh frozen plasma, vitamin K, cryoprecipitate, and platelets as needed.

III. TRAUMATIC LESIONS

A. Epidural hematoma.

1. Seen in about 1% of head trauma patients.

TABLE 1

CSF Findings in Various Pathologic Conditions (Adult Values)

Condition	Opening Pressure (cm H_2O)	Appearance	Cells (per mm^3)	Protein (mg %)	Glucose (% serum)	Miscellaneous
Normal	7-18	Clear, colorless	0 PMN, 0 RBC, 0 mono	15-45	50	
Acute purulent meningitis	Frequently increased	Turbid	Few-20 K (WBCs mostly PMNs)	100-1000	<20	Few cells early or if treated
Viral meningitis and encephalitis	Normal	Normal	Few-350 (WBCs mostly monos)	40-100	Normal	PMN early
Guillain-Barre'	Normal	Normal	Normal	50-1000	Normal	Protein ↑, frequently IgG
Polio	Normal	Normal	50-250 (monos)	40-100	Normal	
TB meningitis	Frequently increased	Opal, yellow, fibrin clot	50-500 (monos)	60-700	<20	PMN early, (+) AFB culture, (+) Ziel-Neelson stain
Fungal meningitis	Frequently increased	Opalescent	30-300 (monos)	100-700	<30	(+) India ink for cryptococcus
Traumatic (bloody) tap	Normal	Bloody, supernatant colorless	RBC:WBC as in peripheral	Slight ↑	Normal	Blood ↓ in succeeding tubes, xanthochromia takes hours
Subarachnoid hemorrhage	Increased	Bloody Supernatant xanthochromic	Early ↑ RBCs Late ↑ WBCs	50-400 100-800	Normal	RBCs disappear in 2 weeks, xanthochromia may persist for weeks
Multiple sclerosis	Normal	Normal	5-50 (monos)	Normal-800	Normal	Usually ↑ gamma globulins (oligoclonal)

2. Classic presentation is brief loss of consciousness, followed by lucid interval, then progressive obtundation, ipsilateral pupillary dilatation, and contralateral hemiparesis (seen in 60%). Other presentations include headache, nausea, vomiting, seizure, unilateral hyperreflexia, and positive Babinski sign.
3. Usual etiology is laceration of middle meningeal artery by fracture of squamous portion of temporal bone, but can also be produced by a dural sinus tear.
4. On CT, seen as lenticular, biconcave mass overlying brain with high attenuation.
5. Optimally treated, has a 5-10% mortality.

B. Subdural hematoma.

1. Twice as common as epidural hematomas.
2. Source of bleeding usually venous, but can also be arterial.
3. Two types.
   a. Tearing of bridging veins from acceleration/deceleration. Often presents with a lucid interval followed by later deterioration secondary to mass effect.
   b. Laceration of parenchyma and cortical vessels. Usually presents with coma, localizing signs, and severe underlying brain injury.
4. On CT, seen as crescent-shaped mass overlying convexities with high density. Usually less dense than epidural hematoma due to dilution of blood in CSF.
5. Classified as acute from 0-48 h, subacute from 2 days - 3 weeks, and chronic beyond 3 weeks.
6. If evacuated in OR in < 4 h, 30% mortality. If > 4 h elapses, 90% mortality. Also much worse outcome if post-operative ICP ≥ 20.

C. Hemorrhagic contusions.

1. Most commonly found in temporal, frontal, and occipital lobes.
2. Will typically "blossom" with continued hemorrhage and edema 24-72 h after presentation.
3. Generally managed medically with usual maneuvers to lower ICP, but if medical therapy fails, region of contused brain can be resected depending on its location.
4. Patients with an isolated temporal lobe contusion can herniate and die without evidence of increased ICP because of local temporal swelling.

D. Diffuse axonal injuries.

1. Result from "shearing" of white matter tracts from rotational forces at time of impact.
2. Can be visualized on MRI or CT as punctate hemorrhages in centrum semiovule, corpus callosum, or brainstem.
3. Generally not associated with elevations in ICP.
4. If brainstem affected, prognosis for functional neurologic recovery extremely poor.

E. Skull fractures.

1. Can be open, closed, linear, compound, or depressed.
2. "Racoon's eyes" diagnostic of fracture of floor of anterior fossa.
3. Basilar skull fracture usually diagnosed clinically without benefit of CT, in presence of Battle's sign (retroauricular hematoma), CSF otorrhea, or CSF rhinorrhea.
4. Criteria to elevate depressed skull fracture:
   a. > 8-10 mm depression.
   b. Deficit related to underlying brain.
   c. CSF leakage secondary to dural laceration.
   d. Open, depressed skull fractures.

IV. MANAGEMENT OF INTRACRANIAL HYPERTENSION

A. ICP Monitoring.

1. ICP Monitoring is indicated for those patients in whom a neurological examination cannot be followed.
   a. Motor examination is abnormal flexion or worse.
   b. Intracranial pathology may necessitate monitoring if managed non-surgically.
   c. Patients with significant intracranial pathology who lose their neurological examination iatrogenically, either from anesthesia or sedation.

B. Critical Pathway for the Treatment of Established Intracranial Hypertension.

1. A critical pathway, developed by a consensus of the Brain Trauma Foundation, is presented in Figure 1.
2. The absolute value defining unacceptable intracranial hypertension is unclear. Although a general threshold of 20–25 mm Hg has been presented, such pressures may be too high in some situations.
3. General maneuvers to control intracranial hypertension
   a. Control of body temperature.
   b. Seizure prophylaxis.
   c. Elevation of the head of the bed.
   d. Avoidance of jugular venous outflow destruction.
   e. Sedation and pharmacologic paralysis.
   f. Maintenance of adequate arterial oxygenation.
   g. Complete volume resuscitation to a cerebral perfusion pressure (CPP) or 70mm Hg or more.
4. When a ventricular catheter is being used to ICP monitoring, cerebrospinal fluid drainage should be used first for ICP elevations.
5. Persistent intracranial hypertension despite using general maneuvers and ventricular drainage when possible to decrease ICP requires additional treatment.
   a. Aggressive use of mannitol, limited by serum osmolarity levels of 320 mOsm/l. The patient's volume status should be closely observed during mannitol administration and

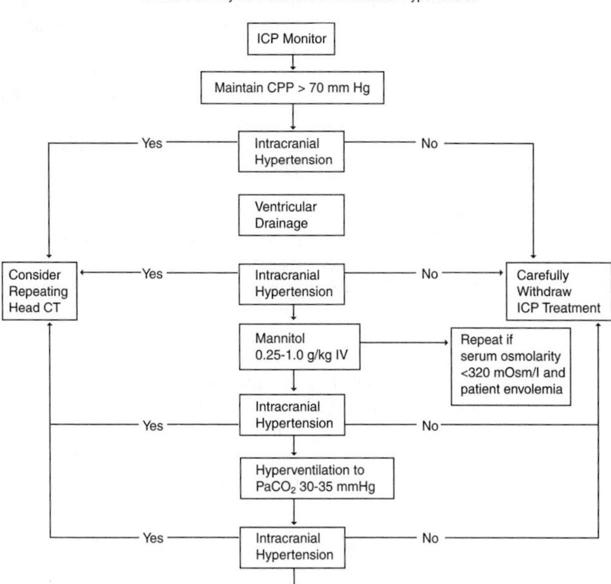

FIG. 1 Recommendation of the Brain Trauma Foundation consensus

envolemia to mild hypervolemia maintained by careful fluid replacement.

b. If mannitol administration is ineffective in controlling the ICP, the level of ventilation may be increased to obtain $PaCO_2$ levels of 30–35 mm Hg. If available, measurement of cerebral blood flow (CBF) or jugular venous (SjO_2) saturation should be considered when hyperventilation is increased.

6. For intracranial hypertension refractory to the above techniques, second tier therapies should be considered when it is the physician's opinion that the patient may benefit if ICP control can be accomplished. Second-tier therapy includes both treatment modalities that have been proven to be effective in improving outcome but have very significant complication rates (e.g., barbiturates) as well as therapies that appear to be effective in lowering ICP but which remain unproven in

terms of their influence or outcome or complication rate. These latter modalities include hypothermia, hyperventilation to $PaCO_2 < 30$ mm Hg, decompressive crainectomy, and hypertensive therapy. The Brain Trauma Foundation consensus suggests that the precise indications for employment and methods of application of second tier therapies in an individual patient are left to the discretion of the managing physician.

C. Second Tier Therapy: Barbiturates.

1. Dosing of pentobarbital.
   a. Loading:
      (1) 2.5 mg/kg over first hour in 4 divided doses (while pharmacy is mixing dose).
      (2) 7.5 mg/kg over the next 3 hours IV continuous infusion.
   b. Maintenance: 1.5 mg/kg/hr and titrate as needed for ICP > 20 mm Hg.
2. All patients require ICP monitoring, daily CT scans and a Swan-Ganz catheter during barbiturate therapy.
3. The endpoint of therapy is either ICP control or pharmacological toxicity.
   a. Serum barbiturate level is not important for therapy.
   b. EEG is *not* necessary.
4. Major toxicity–cardiosuppression
   a. Hypotension must be avoided at all times. May require pressors.
   b. Use cardiac output from Swan-Ganz catheter to detect first signs of compromise.
5. Sepsis.
   a. May not mount a leukocytosis or fever when in barbiturate coma.
   b. Signs.
      (1) Falling platelets.
      (2) Hyperglycemia.
      (3) Coagulopathy.
      (4) Hypotension.
      (5) Rising CO, falling SVR.
   c. Cultures from multiple sites required as surveillance.

V. SPINE AND SPINAL CORD INJURIES

A. General considerations.

1. These injuries are usually due to severe cervical spine fractures and/or subluxations. Because of its greater mass and greater inherent stability, the thoracolumbar spine is not as frequently affected.
2. Not all spine injuries are associated with paralysis. More than half of patients with spinal injuries have a normal motor, sensory, and reflex examination.
3. Any patient sustaining an injury above the clavicle or a head

injury resulting in unconsciousness should be suspected of having an associated cervical spine injury unless proven otherwise.

B. Assessment.

1. General assessment.
   a. Examination must be carried out with patient in neutral position on back-board and cervical spine immobilized.
   b. Other associated injuries must be ruled out, including head injury.
   c. The paralyzed patient's abdominal exam is unreliable, so a diagnostic peritoneal lavage is generally required.
2. Mechanical assessment.
   a. Log-roll patient, so entire spine can be visualized.
   b. Look for any open wounds, "step-off" deformities, prominence of spinous processes.
   c. Palpate for any regions of tenderness.
3. Neurologic assessment.
   a. Complete *vs.* incomplete spinal cord lesion.
      (1) If patient has any neurologic deficit, this is most important part of assessment.
      (2) Distinction between complete and incomplete injury determines prognosis and urgency of subsequent treatment.
      (3) Any preservation of motor or sensory function below level of injury indicates incomplete injury. Sparing of pin-prick and fine-touch sensation in sacral dermatomes indicates incomplete injury ("sacral sparing"). Preservation of any voluntary control of sphincter tone also indicates sacral sparing, thus incomplete injury.
      (4) Preservation alone of anal wink and bulbocavernosus reflexes does not constitute sacral sparing.
   b. Sensory/motor function.
      (1) Determine level of lesion by assessing sensory and motor function.
      (2) See motor chart (Table 2) and sensory dermatome diagram (Figure 2).
      (3) Check sphincter tone and presence or absence of superficial, deep tendon, and pathologic reflexes.
      (4) Injuries at C4 or higher impair ventilation, and patients require blind or fiberoptically-guided nasal intubation.
4. Spinal shock.
   a. May occur immediately after spinal cord injury, particularly complete injury.
   b. Due to abrupt loss of sympathetic tone.
   c. Characterized hemodynamically by hypotension and bradycardia. Extremities warm due to dilated peripheral vessels ("cold nose, warm feet").

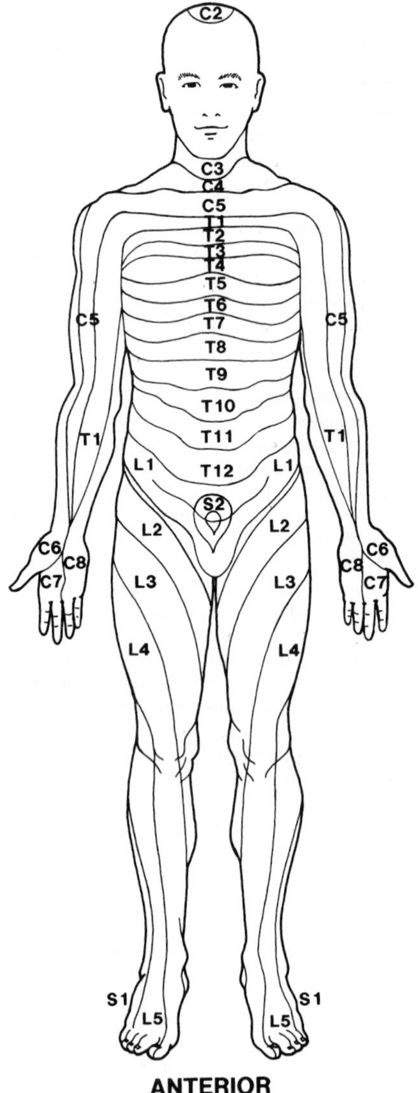
C2
C3
C4
C5
T1
T2
T3
T4
T5
T6
T7
T8
T9
T10
T11
T12
C5
C5
T1
T1
L1
L1
S2
L2
L2
C6
C8
C7
C6
C8
C7
L3
L3
L4
L4
S1
L5
S1
L5
ANTERIOR

FIG. 2

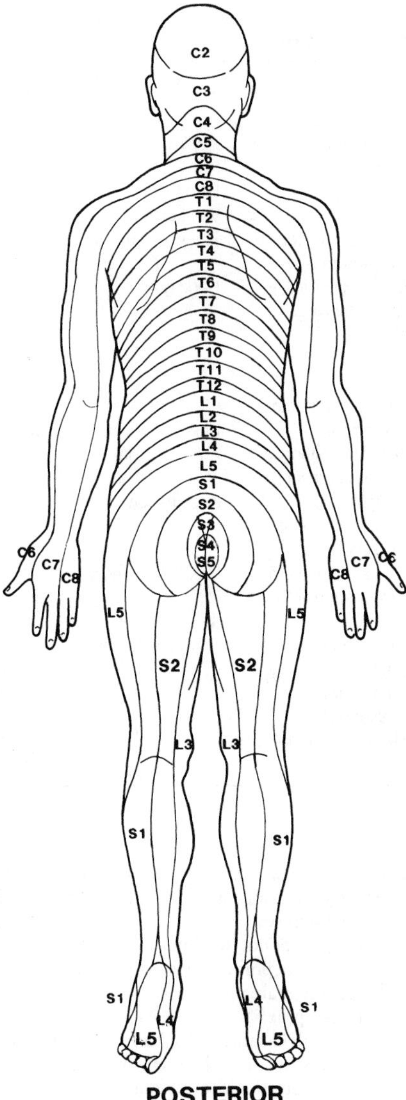

POSTERIOR

FIG. 2 (*continued*)

TABLE 2
Motor Level Assessment

Segment	Muscle	Action to Test	Reflex
C1-3	Neck muscles		
C4	Diaphragm, trapezius	Inspiration	
C5	Deltoid		
C5-6	Biceps	Elbow flex	Biceps
C6	Extensor carpi radialis	Wrist extension	Supinator
C7	Triceps, extensor digitorum	Elbow extension	Triceps
C8	Flexor digitorum	Hand grasp	
T1	Hand intrinsics		
T2-T12	Intercostals		
T7-L1	Abdominals		Abdominal cutaneous
L2	Iliopsoas, adductors	Hip adduction	
L3-4	Quadriceps	Knee extension	Quadriceps
L4-5	Medial hamstrings, tibialis anterior	Ankle dorsiflex	Medial hamstrings
L5	Lateral hams, posterior tibialis, peroneals	Knee flexion	
L5-S1	Extensor digitorum, extensor hallicus longus	Great toe extension	
S1-S2	Gastrocnemius, soleus	Ankle plantar flex	Ankle jerk
S2	Flexor digitorum, flexor hallucis		
S2-4	Bladder, lower bowel		Anal wink and bulbocavernosus

d. Characterized neurologically by flaccid paralysis, absent sensory function, flaccid sphincter, absent pathological and normal reflexes.

e. Usually responds to fluid resuscitation, but vasopressors (e.g., neosynephrine) are occasionally needed.

5. Radiographic evaluation.

   a. Cervical spine.

      (1) Lateral C-spine–all 7 cervical vertebrae and C7/T1 inter-space must be seen. Best obtained while pulling down on shoulders. Swimmer's view may be necessary.

      (2) Assess alignment, presence of fractures, soft tissue swelling.

      (3) AP cervical and odontoid views are needed to fully

clear C-spine. Should only be obtained once patient is stabilized.

(4) Tomograms, oblique views, lateral flexion/extension films, CT, MRI, or myelography may be needed to completely clear the cervical spine.

(5) Lateral flexion/extension films should be obtained in patients with posterior neck pain only (i.e., with no neurologic deficit) to rule out ligamentous instability.

b. Thoracolumbar spine.

(1) AP and lateral views needed.

(2) Assess alignment and presence of fractures.

(3) Must be cleared before removing back-board and allowing flexion at waist.

c. Emergency MRI or CT-myelogram mandatory in patient with *incomplete injury* whose examination cannot be explained by plain CT or plain radiographs alone. Soft tissue injury such as epidural hematoma or traumatic herniated disc must be ruled out. These patients would be taken to surgery emergently to decompress cord and preserve or improve neurologic function. Patients with *complete* injury do not need emergent surgery.

C. Treatment.

1. Neurosurgical consultation mandatory.
2. Immobilization.
   a. Semi-rigid cervical (Philadelphia) collar and spine board are sufficient for pre-hospital care and initial evaluation.
   b. Every attempt should be made to clear TLS spine as soon as possible so back-board can be removed, thus preventing pressure sores.
3. Realignment.
   a. Every effort is made to achieve realignment and closed reduction as soon as possible in the cervical spine with Gardner-Wells tongs and weight in both complete and incomplete injuries, as well as in intact patients.
   b. If a closed reduction is not possible in an incomplete injury, emergent open reduction is necessary to decompress the cord and/or roots. An emergent open reduction in a complete injury is not necessary.
4. Stabilization.
   a. Generally is not necessary emergently, but is done as expediently as possible to minimize medical complications of recumbency.
   b. Stabilizing devices may be external (e.g., halo, SOMI® brace, hip spica cast) or internal (e.g., plates, screws, rods).
   c. Choice of devices to use depends on type of injury, location of instability, and medical condition of patient.
5. Medications–immediate treatment with high-dose methylprednisolone (i.e., 30 mg/kg bolus at presentation, followed by 23-h drip at 5.4 mg/kg/h) is now standard of care.

6. IV fluids–limit to maintenance fluids unless more needed for spinal shock.
7. Airway–nasal intubation or tracheostomy often required for high cervical injuries.
8. Effective nursing care with attention to skin, bowel training, and bladder training is absolutely essential in long-term care of these patients.
9. Every attempt should be made to start rehabilitation as soon as possible.

D. Spinal Cord Injury Without Radiographic Abnormality (SCIWORA).

1. SCIWORA is defined as objective signs or symptoms of myelopathy as a result of trauma in patients where there is no radiographic abnormality.
2. SCIWORA results from nondisruptive and self-reducing intersegmental deformation of the spinal column, with injury to the spinal cord.
3. SCIWORA is more frequent in children and young adults when the spinal column is excessively malleable due to:
   a. Horizontal orientation of the facet joints.
   b. Anterior wedging of the vertebral bodies.
   c. More elastic ligaments and joint capsules.
4. Age-related properties of SCIWORA: persons < 12 years of age.
   a. 30% of spinal injuries.
   b. 70% complete injuries.
   c. Poor prognosis for complete recovery.
5. Age-related properties of SCIWORA: persons > 12 years of age.
   a. 12% of spinal injuries.
   b. Complete injuries rare.
   c. Excellent prognosis for complete recovery.
6. Treatment does not affect the final outcome of SCIWORA. Outcome is directly related to the degree of initial injury.
7. SCIWORA is a diagnosis of exclusion; treat as an unstable spine injury (Figure 3: Treatment algorithm for SCIWORA).

VI. OTHER NEUROSURGICAL EMERGENCIES

A. Subarachnoid hemorrhage (SAH).

1. Characterized by sudden onset of "worst headache of life," nuchal rigidity, photophobia, and sometimes loss of consciousness.
2. Seen on non-contrast CT in about 90% of cases if scanned within 48 h. Regions of high density found in subarachnoid spaces, particularly around basilar cisterns. Often accompanied by acute hydrocephalus.
3. Etiologies.
   a. Trauma–most common cause of SAH.
   b. Aneurysm–75-80% of cases of spontaneous SAH.

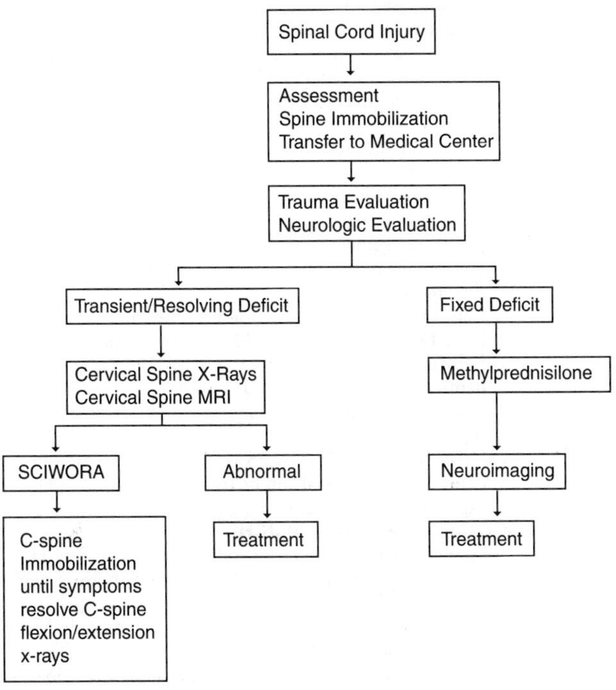

c. Arteriovenous malformation (AVM)–approximately 5% of cases of spontaneous SAH.
d. Unknown etiology–approximately 15% of cases of spontaneous SAH.

4. If CT negative in cases in which index of suspicion is high, lumbar puncture is obligatory to look for red cells in CSF and xanthochromia.
5. Initial medical management.
   a. Control of blood pressure. Should use IV labetalol, esmolol, or sodium nitroprusside. Hypertension can contribute to rebleeding.
   b. Avoid over-treatment of blood pressure if patient's baseline is hypertension.
   c. Prophylaxis for seizures with anticonvulsant such as phenytoin.
   d. Prevention of vasospasm with calcium channel blocker, nimodipine.

e. CSF drainage with intraventricular catheter (IVC) if patient develops acute hydrocephalus.
f. Intubate if patient becomes lethargic.
g. Treat elevated ICP, if necessary, with hyperventilation, osmotic diuretics, and CSF drainage.
h. Consider steroids (controversial).
i. Cerebral angiogram (4-vessel) obligatory to rule out aneurysm. In patients with aneurysm, 20% will have multiple aneurysms.
j. MRI useful for subacute SAH and in those cases in which angiogram is negative.

6. Surgical management.
   a. For vast majority of ruptured aneurysms, direct clipping is the procedure of choice.
   b. Endovascular balloon occlusion is becoming a more accepted form of therapy for difficult aneurysms.
   c. Early surgery (within 48-72 h after SAH) is favored in patients in good medical and neurologic condition, large amounts of subarachnoid blood, and intracerebral hemorrhage with mass effect.
   d. Delayed surgery (10-14 days after SAH) is favored in patients in poor medical and neurologic condition and those experiencing effects of vasospasm.

B. Intracerebral hemorrhage (ICH).

1. Defined as hemorrhage within brain matter itself. ICH accounts for approximately 10% of all strokes, both ischemic and hemorrhagic.
2. Seen easily on non-contrast CT scan as region of high density within brain parenchyma.
3. Location of hemorrhage on CT often suggests etiology of bleeding. For example, basal ganglia, thalamic, pontine, and cerebellar ICHs are likely hypertensive in origin.
4. Causes.
   a. Hypertension.
   b. Arteriovenous malformation (AVM).
   c. Aneurysm.
   d. Hemorrhage into brain tumor, either primary or metastatic.
   e. Arteriopathies such as amyloid angiopathy, fibrinoid necrosis, or lipohyalinosis.
   f. Coagulation or clotting disorders, either as result of primary illness or iatrogenic (e.g., as complication of use of Coumadin®, thrombolytic agents, or aspirin).
   g. Trauma (unusual).
   h. Hemorrhage into infarct.
   i. Sympathomimetic abuse (e.g., cocaine).
   j. Other vascular malformations, such as venous angioma, cavernous malformation, or capillary telangiectasia.
5. Initial medical management is similar to that of subarachnoid hemorrhage.

6. Surgical management.
   a. Advisability of surgery depends on cause, patient's neurologic condition, and location of hemorrhage.
   b. Aneurysms should generally be clipped; AVMs can be either surgically resected or embolized.
   c. Hypertensive hemorrhages generally can be managed medically, but if the patient begins to deteriorate, can be evacuated stereotactically, endoscopically, or through an open procedure.

C. Carotid dissection.

1. Often seen in setting of trauma, but can be spontaneous.
2. Suspect in those cases in which a lateralizing sign (e.g., hemiparesis) cannot be explained by an intracranial CT finding.
3. Diagnosed by angiography. Characterized by "string sign" or "double lumen sign." Can be bilateral.
4. Most dissections will heal with recanalization and so are treated with anticoagulation (IV heparin followed by Coumadin®) to prevent clot propagation and emboli.
5. Medical failures can be managed by direct repair with interposition vein graft or carotid ligation with or without extracranial-intracranial bypass.

D. Vertebral dissection.

1. Associated with cervical spine fractures.
2. Consider angiography if fracture extends into foramen transversarium.

E. Status epilepticus.

1. Defined as recurrent seizures occurring too frequently for consciousness to be regained between seizures or any seizure that lasts longer than 30 min.
2. Most common scenario is a patient with known seizure disorder with low anticonvulsant levels for any reason.
3. Permanent CNS injury results if seizures are not controlled within 60 minutes. Can be fatal.
4. Management involves control of seizures.
   a. Intubate if airway compromised or if seizures persist unabated.
   b. Lorazepam 0.02 mg/kg (1.4 mg/70 kg) IVP over 2 minutes. Repeat if ineffective q 2-3 min x 3 doses total. Alternatively, may use diazepam 10 mg IVP (at rate of < 2 mg/min) q 20 min if necessary x 3 doses total.
   c. Simultaneous loading with phenytoin.
      (1) If patient not on phenytoin, give 18 mg/kg (1200 mg/70 kg) IV at rate < 50 mg/min.
      (2) If patient on phenytoin, give 500 mg IV at rate < 50 mg/min.
   d. Persistent seizure activity.
      (1) Continue phenytoin 8 mg/kg at rate < 50 mg/min, followed by:

a) Phenobarbital drip at 100 mg/min up to 20 mg/kg (1400 mg/70 kg), or:
b) Diazepam infusion of 100 mg in 500 ml D5W at 40 ml/min.

(2) If seizures still continue:
a) Initiate induction of pentobarbital coma with IV dose of 10-15 mg/kg followed by maintenance drip of 1 mg/kg/h.
b) Consider calling anesthesiologist and placing the patient under general inhalation anesthesia and neuromuscular junction blockade.
c) As temporizing measure, may give paraldehyde 5 ml in 500 ml D5W at 50 cc/hr and titrating to stop seizures or lidocaine 2-3 mg/kg IVP at < 50 mg/min, followed by infusion of 100 mg in 250 ml D5W at 1-2 mg/min.

F. Compressive spinal epidural metastases.

1. Spinal epidural metastases present in up to 10% of all cancer patients at some time during disease; 5-10% of malignancies present with cord, conus, or cauda equina compression.
2. Usual route of spread is hematogenous via spinal epidural veins (Batson's plexus), but can be arterial or perineural.
3. Usual location is epidural, but can be intradural (2-4%) and even intramedullary (1-2%).
4. Back pain is usually first symptom. Radicular pattern of pain, paresthesia, and weakness often follows. Symptoms exacerbated by recumbency, movement, neck flexion, straight leg raising, coughing, sneezing, or straining.
5. If cord compression develops, patient experiences quadriplegia or paraplegia, sensory loss (manifested as a sensory level on exam), loss of reflexes acutely, and bowel or bladder dysfunction.
6. If symptoms involve perineum and lower extremities symmetrically, conus medullaris lesion is most likely. If perineum and lower extremities involved asymmetrically, cauda equina lesion more likely.
7. Patients presenting with acute neurologic deterioration should be given dexamethasone (100 mg IVP) stat, and plain films of the entire spine should be obtained. An emergency MRI or CT-myelogram should also be obtained. Neurosurgical consultation is mandatory.
8. Most patients are treated initially with local radiation therapy (XRT). Surgery indicated if XRT fails, for tissue diagnosis, for unstable spine, or if compression is due to bone rather than tumor.
9. Key point is that back pain in cancer patients represents metastatic disease until proven otherwise.

G. Brain death.

1. Criteria established by Cincinnati Society of Neurologists and Neurosurgeons. These may vary in different locations.

a. Absence of brainstem function.
   (1) Pupillary light reflex absent.
   (2) Corneal reflex absent.
   (3) Oculocephalic reflex ("doll's eyes") absent.
   (4) Oculovestibular reflex (cold water calorics) absent.
      a) With head of bed at 30°, 60 cc of ice water flushed into each ear with eyes held open.
      b) Intact response is slow deviation of eyes toward flushed ear and fast nystagmus toward opposite ear. Remember COWS: *c*old–*o*pposite/*w*arm–*s*ame, which indicates direction of fast nystagmus depending on temperature of water used.
   (5) Oropharyngeal (gag) reflex absent.
   (6) No spontaneous respirations for 3 min in normocarbic state.
b. No response to central pain stimulation (supraorbital notch pressure).
c. The presence of monosynaptic spinal withdrawal reflexes does not rule out brain death.

2. Conditions to rule out.
   a. Hypothermia as cause of coma.
   b. Remediable endogenous or exogenous intoxication, especially metabolic factors, barbiturates, paralytics, benzodiazepines.
   c. Hypotension.
   d. Nonconvulsive status epilepticus.
3. Two clinical examinations 6 h apart meeting criteria of 1 and 2 confirm brain death. The brain death examination is not reliable in setting of hypoxic or ischemic brain damage for 24-48 h after correction of insult, as brain stem dysfunction as result of hypoxia or ischemia often resolves during this period.
4. At this institution, no further laboratory tests, such as angiography, EEG, or cerebral blood flow studies, are mandatory.

23

Orthopedic Emergencies

David J. Shelley, M.D.
Joel I. Sorger, M.D.

I. FRACTURE ASSESSMENT

As part of the basic trauma evaluation, the patient should be carefully examined for fractures, dislocations, ligamentous injuries, neurovascular injuries, and intra-articular lacerations. Systematic inspection and palpation of every bone and joint should be carefully carried out. The following characteristics should be evaluated in every fracture:

A. Open fracture *vs.* closed fracture.

B. Degrees of soft tissue injury.

C. Neurovascular status.

D. Location.

1. Intra-articular *vs.* extra-articular.
2. Metaphyseal *vs.* diaphyseal.

E. Fracture configuration:

Pattern	Mechanism
transverse	tension
oblique	compression
spiral	torsion
butterfly	bending
comminuted	high energy

F. Displacement.

G. Angulation.

H. Rotation.

I. Length.

II. ORTHOPEDIC EMERGENCIES IN THE TRAUMA PATIENT

A. Open fractures—The type of open fracture influences the plan of treatment, the subsequent clinical course, and the overall prognosis for the injury.

1. ***Classification:***

Grade	Wound	Energy	Contamination	Soft Tissue Injury
I.	<1 cm	low	clean	minimal stripping
II.	>1 cm	moderate	moderate	moderate strip
III.	>10 cm	high	severe	extensive strip
IIIA.	Adequate soft tissue coverage			
IIIB.	Soft tissue defect requiring reconstructive procedure			
IIIC.	Soft tissue defect and associated vascular injury			

* Special grade III injuries include: (1) Farm injuries; (2) Traumatic amputations; (3) Segmental open fractures; (4) High-velocity gunshot wounds; (5) Associated neurovascular injury; (6) Open fractures over 8 h old.

2. ***Treatment.***
   a. Wound cultures.
      (1) Pre-operative culture to evaluate initial wound contamination.
      (2) Post-irrigation culture to assess residual bacterial flora.
   b. Antibiotics–reduce the rate of infection in open fractures.
      (1) Cefazolin–1 g q 6 h.
      (2) Gentamicin–2.5 mg per kg q 12 h.
      (3) Penicillin–2 million units q 4 h. Required in farm injuries for clostridial coverage.
   c. Tetanus prophylaxis–(see "Trauma").
   d. Fracture stabilization.
      (1) Betadine®-soaked gauze to minimize further wound contamination.
      (2) Preliminary splinting or traction.
         a) Prevents further soft tissue injury.
         b) Immobilization decreases pain.
         c) Facilitates patient transport.
         d) Helps maintain perfusion to extemity.
      (3) Secondary stabilization–definitive fracture stabilization: open reduction internal fixation (ORIF), external fixation, or skeletal traction.
   e. Irrigation and debridement.
      (1) Meticulous removal and excision of foreign and nonviable tissue within 6 h of injury.
      (2) Reduces bacterial contamination of wound.
      (3) Serial debridement indicated every 36-48 h to reevaluate and prepare for wound closure.
   f. Wound management.
      (1) Preliminary evaluation of all wounds is performed in the Emergency Room, and a photograph is taken to document soft tissue injury.
      (2) Secondary evaluation of wound is performed in the operating room, and serial photographs are taken to document extent of soft tissue and bony injury.

(3) Definitive care must provide for coverage of bone, tendons, hardware, and neurovascular bundle.
(4) Primary wound management–wound left open (standard treatment).
(5) Secondary wound management–no grade II or grade III open fractures are closed on initial debridement; all are taken back to OR in 48 h for debridement and coverage/closure.
   a) Delayed primary closure (common in grade I and grade II injuries).
   b) Delayed skin graft (split or full-thickness) or muscle flap (frequent in grade II and grade III).
   c) Healing by secondary intention (occasional grade I or grade II).

g. Relative indications for immediate amputation.
   (1) Complete anatomic disruption of posterior tibial nerve in adults.
   (2) Crush injuries with warm ischemia time > 6 h.
   (3) Serious associated multitrauma.
   (4) Severe ipsilateral foot trauma.
   (5) Anticipated protracted course in soft tissue coverage and bony reconstruction.
   (6) Crush injury to both muscles and skin with complete neurovascular injury (MESS Score >7 and Grade IIIB or C injuries).
   (7) Intact neurovascular system with severe muscular deficit and bone loss such that reasonable function is unlikely.
   (8) Insensate limb with intact vascular system and limited motor function.

B. Compartment syndrome.

1. Definition–compartment syndrome is characterized by increased pressure within a closed space that causes irreversible ischemic damage to the contents of that space.
2. Pathophysiology.
   a. Any condition that increases the content of a compartment or reduces the space of a compartment can lead to the development of an acute compartment syndrome:

Decreased space	Increased pressure
external compression	hemorrhage
cast or dressing	fractures
MAST trousers	reperfusion/burns 2° to capillary permeability

   b. Pressure within the compartment continues to rise until capillary perfusion pressure is exceeded. This results in arterial shunting leading to muscle and nerve ischemia, which causes irreversible damage if untreated.

c. Palpable pulses are invariably present in an acute compartment syndrome unless there is an associated vascular injury. Pressure within a compartment is rarely elevated enough to obstruct the major artery traversing that compartment.
d. One must clinically distinguish between compartment syndrome, vascular injury, and neuropraxia. Each of these diagnoses requires different therapeutic intervention. Keep in mind that any of these injuries may coexist with each other.

3. Diagnosis.
   a. Subjective findings–pain disproportional to level of injury.
   b. Objective findings.
      (1) Early.
         a) Pain on palpation of swollen compartment.
         b) Increased pain with passive stretch of compartment musculature.
      (2) Late.
         a) Hypoesthesia in the distribution of the nerve traversing the compartment.
         b) Muscle weakness.
4. Compartment pressure monitoring.
   a. Devices.
      (1) Stic catheters (Stryker®, Ace®)–hand-held device that allows physician to measure compartment pressures. Quick and simple to use.
      (2) Arterial line setup–readily accessible in most emergency rooms and all surgical intensive care units.
   b. Measurements.
      (1) Measurement of all compartments of the affected limb is mandatory.
      (2) Low threshold to measure compartment pressures in obtunded, neurologically impaired, or multitrauma patients.
5. Indications for fasciotomies (Figure 1)–There is not a universally accepted threshold for fasciotomy, but compartment pressures > 30 mm Hg appear to be the most commonly recognized standard. These numbers must be evaluated with regard to the patient's mean arterial pressure because compartment syndrome may be present with compartment pressures < 30 mm Hg in hypotensive patients. However, clinical findings are most important.
6. Treatment–release elevated compartment pressure with compartment fasciotomies.
   a. Hand.
      (1) Commonly occurs secondary to crush injuries with associated metacarpal or carpal fractures.
      (2) Symptoms and clinical findings are secondary to effect on intrinsic muscles.
      (3) Treatment requires release of intrinsic compartments.

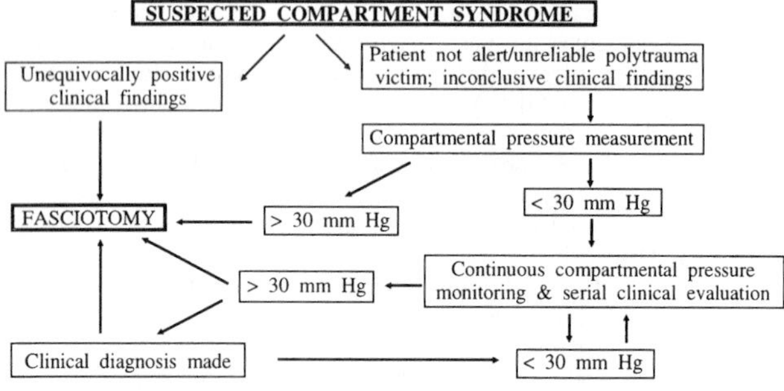

FIG. 1

b. Wrist.
   (1) Occasionally occurs with fracture of the distal radius or perilunate dislocations.
   (2) Clinical findings are consistent with median and ulnar nerve compression.
   (3) Compartment decompression requires fracture reduction, release of transverse carpal ligament, and exploration of carpal tunnel and Guyon's canal.

c. Forearm.
   (1) Occasionally occurs with fractures of the radius and ulna.
   (2) Forearm contains 3 compartments: superficial flexor, deep flexor, and extensor.
   (3) Fasciotomies require volar and dorsal incision to release all compartments.

d. Thigh.
   (1) Trauma to thigh with/without femoral fracture.
   (2) Three compartment release: anterior, posterior, and obturator.

e. Leg.
   (1) Compartment syndrome commonly occurs as a complication of tibial shaft and tibial plateau fractures.
   (2) Tibial compartments.
      a) Anterior.
      b) Lateral.
      c) Superficial posterior.
      d) Deep posterior.
   (3) Fasciotomy techniques.
      a) Subcutaneous fasciotomies–never indicated.
      b) Fibulectomy–historic interest only.
      c) Single incision–rarely indicated.
      d) Double incision–standard of care (Figure 2). Employs two vertical incisions separated by a skin

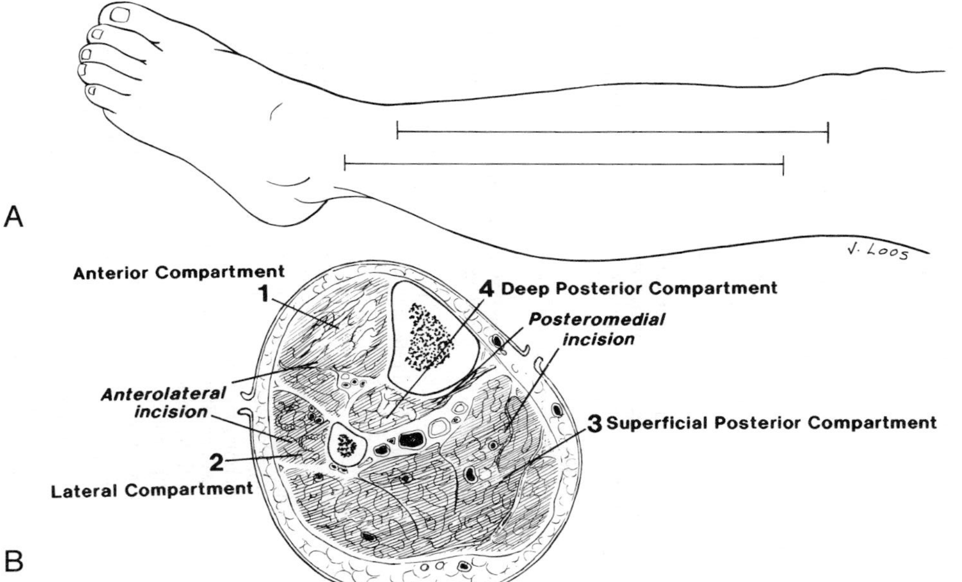

FIG. 2 A, Double-incision technique for performing fasciotomies of all four compartments of the lower extremity. **B,** Cross-section of lower extremity showing a position of anterolateral and posteromedial incisions that allows access to the anterior and lateral compartments (1 & 2) and the superficial and deep posterior compartments (3 & 4).

bridge of 7 cm. First incision is centered between the anterior and lateral compartments; the second incision is 1-2 cm behind the posterior medial border of tibia. The underlying fascia over each compartment is then released. The skin is left open, and the patient is brought back to the OR in 48-72 h for delayed primary wound closure *vs.* STSG.

C. Dislocations—pure dislocations and fracture dislocations represent an orthopedic emergency owing to the associated risk of neurovascular compromise, acute compartment syndrome, chondrolyis, and development of avascular necrosis. It is critical to carefully document the neurovascular status of the limb prior to and following successful reduction maneuvers. After reduction, check stability of joint and ROM, and document where a redislocation occurs. Reduction of all dislocations requires adequate IV sedation. Dislocations frequently found in trauma patients are outlined below.

1. Hip dislocations.
   a. Hip dislocations and fracture dislocations frequently result from loading the hip joint through 3 mechanisms:
      (1) Flexed knee striking stationary object (dashboard).
      (2) Axial loading of foot with extended ipsilateral knee (floor-board).
      (3) Lateral compression through greater trochanter.
   b. Diagnosis.
      (1) Posterior dislocations (90%)–classically present with an adducted, flexed, and internally rotated position of the hip.
      (2) Anterior dislocations (10%)–classically present with an extended and externally rotated position of the hip.
      (3) Hip dislocations are frequently associated with fractures of the acetabulum and femoral head.
   c. Reduction–Allis reduction maneuver uses traction applied in line with deformity and countertraction to stabilize the pelvis. Reduction is evident with an audible and palpable "clunk". It is important to test the stability of reduction by performing range of motion of the hip. Radiographs are required to confirm concentric reduction and to rule out intra-articular loose fragments.
   d. Complications.
      (1) Avascular necrosis of femoral head (2-11%)–incidence is increased with prolonged delay between dislocation and reduction.
      (2) Osteoarthritis.
      (3) Sciatic nerve injury (8-19%).
      (4) Heterotopic ossification.
2. Ankle.
   a. Ankle dislocations almost exclusively occur with fracture dislocations. These fractures are clinically unstable and require preliminary stabilization with splinting followed by ORIF.

b. Complications.
   (1) Post-traumatic arthritis.
   (2) Neurovascular compromise.
   (3) Open fracture.
c. Reduction–longitudinal traction and manipulation reversing the injury force followed by a well-molded splint.

3. Shoulder.
   a. Most commonly dislocated joint in body.
   b. To rule out dislocation, shoulder A/P, axillary, and scapular lateral radiographs are required.
   c. Mechanisms.
      (1) Anterior dislocation (90%)–combination of abduction, external rotation, and extension.
      (2) Posterior dislocation (10%)–axial loading of adducted and internally rotated arm and direct force to anterior shoulder. Historically associated with electro-convulsive therapy and seizures.
   c. Complications.
      (1) Recurrent instability (younger > older).
      (2) Neurovascular injury (axillary nerve common especially in the elderly).
      (3) Osteoarthritis.
      (4) Rotator cuff tear.
      (5) Avascular necrosis (secondary to chronic dislocation).
   d. Reduction.
      (1) Modified Stimson technique–patient is prone with arm hanging over edge of table, and gentle downward traction is applied. Gentle scapular rotation may facilitate reduction.
      (2) Traction/counter-traction–gentle longitudinal traction is applied along the axis of the arm while counter-traction is applied to the axilla. Avoid internal and external rotation due to the associated risk for fracture.
4. Knee.
   a. Associated with complex ligamentous knee injuries.
   b. Immediate reduction critical to vascular status and peroneal nerve function.
   c. Arteriogram indicated for all posterior knee dislocations (even those with good distal pulses) to rule out popliteal artery injury (40-50% incidence).
5. Elbow.
   a. Mechanism–the elbow is a highly constrained joint, but dislocations are not uncommon. The exact mechanism is not completely understood.
   b. Incidence.
      (1) Greatest among 10- to 20-year-old population.
      (2) Posterior (most common).
      (3) Anterior (rare).
   c. Complications.
      (1) Heterotopic ossification.

(2) Flexion contraction.
(3) Vascular injury (brachial, radial).
(4) Nerve injury (median, ulnar, radial, anterior interosseous).

d. Reduction—performed with elbow in semiflexed position with longitudinal traction applied to the forearm and counter-traction applied to the humerus. Post-reduction radiographs should be obtained out of plaster to check concentric reduction and rule out intra-articular fracture.

D. Spinal trauma (see "Neurosurgical Emergencies").

E. Intra-articular laceration.

1. Associated with open fractures and joint penetration by foreign objects.
2. Surgical emergency because of the associated risk for septic arthritis due to contamination introduced at the time of injury.
3. Common locations.
   a. Knee.
   b. Elbow.
   c. Hand.
4. Diagnosis—accurate diagnosis requires clinical exam and intra-articular injection of sterile saline. Enough saline to distend the joint capsule must be injected. An open joint laceration is indicated by the extrusion of saline through the laceration.
5. Treatment
   a. Intra-operative irrigation and debridement.
   b. Antibiotics.

F. Pulseless extremity.

1. Encountered frequently in trauma patients with vascular injuries and occasionally in those with dislocations and complex fractures.
2. Treatment.
   a. Fracture or dislocation reduction should be attempted, as pulses may return.
   b. Vascular repair.
      (1) Acute repair within 6 h of the time of vascular injury is critical to limb survival.
      (2) Compartment syndrome common after revascularization.
      (3) In general, fracture reduction and fixation is performed prior to vascular repair. If ischemia time precludes this, intra-arterial shunts may be used to restore blood flow temporarily during fixation.

III. COMMON FRACTURES

A. Pelvic fractures.

1. Evaluation—secondary assessment of the following conditions.
   a. Fracture stability.

b. Fracture pattern.
c. Soft tissue injury.
d. Neurologic deficits.

2. Physical examination.
   a. Inspection.
      (1) Rule out open fracture (rectal and vaginal exam).
      (2) Hemorrhage, hematoma, contusions.
      (3) Leg length discrepancies.
      (4) Rotational abnormalities.
   b. Palpation.
      (1) Rotational stability–axial loading of anterior iliac spines to assess if pelvis opens or closes.
      (2) Vertical stability–push and pull evaluation to determine vertical migration.
3. Radiographic assessment.
   a. Primary assessment–AP: overview of pelvic injuries used to assess pubic rami, iliac wing, pubic symphysis, sacroiliac joints, and acetabulum. Sacral fractures are commonly missed with AP views.
   b. Secondary assessment (order based on initial screening AP):
      (1) Inlet view–used to assess posterior displacement of sacro-iliac (SI) joints, sacrum, iliac wing, and rotational deformities of sacrum and ilium.
      (2) Outlet view–used to assess vertical displacement and to evaluate sacral foramina.
      (3) Judet view–used to assess acetabular fractures.
         a) Obturator oblique–visualizes anterior column and posterior wall.
         b) Iliac oblique–visualizes posterior column and anterior wall.
      (4) CT scan–used to evaluate acetabulum and posterior structures of pelvis.
4. Associated injuries.
   a. Hemorrhage–frequently result in the loss of several units of blood secondary to bleeding from fracture sites, arterial and venous vessels.
   b. Urologic–associated injuries to bladder, urethra, and genitals (see "Urologic Problems").
   c. Gastrointestinal–open fractures and parenchymal injuries are common because of the the close anatomic relationship of these structures. Open fractures with GI contamination require immediate diverting colostomy. Wounds are managed with serial wet to dry dressing changes. There is a very high associated morbidity and mortality rate associated with these injuries (50% mortality).
   d. Neurologic–commonly involves sciatic and sacral nerves.
5. Indications for external fixation.
   a. Resuscitation–if pelvic ring is disrupted, then may aid with tamponade hemorrhage.

   b. Rotationally unstable fracture.
   c. Adjunct to traction in unstable fractures (type C).
6. Indications for ORIF.
   a. Anterior ring fixation (rotationally unstable type B).
   b. Posterior fixation (vertically unstable type C).
      (1) Displaced SI joint or fracture dislocation (C1.3).
      (2) Failure to obtain reduction in extra-articular SI joint; vertically unstable fracture (C1.3).
      (3) Multi-trauma with unstable pelvis (type C).
      (4) Open posterior fracture with no rectal or perineal injury.
   c. Anterior and posterior fixation.
      (1) Displaced unstable posterior injury with disruption of pubic symphysis.
      (2) Displaced unstable posterior injury with displaced or unstable pubic rami fractures.
   d. Anterior fixation with external fixation.
      (1) Pubic symphysis disruption with unstable posterior injury or severe posterior soft tissue injury.
      (2) Unstable pubic rami fracture with unstable posterior injury or severe posterior soft tissue injury.

B. Acetabular fractures.

1. Anatomy.
   a. Anterior column–iliac crest to pubic symphysis; includes anterior wall.
   b. Posterior column–descends from superior gluteal notch through acetabulum, including inferior pubic rami, obturator foramen, posterior wall of acetabulum, and ischial tuberosity.
   c. Acetabular fossa–medial wall and teardrop.
2. Indications for non-operative management.
   a. Displacement < 2-5 mm in dome depending on fracture location and patient factors.
   b. Low anterior column fracture.
   c. Low transverse fracture.
   d. Minimal posterior column displacement.
3. Indications for operative management.
   a. Most displaced acetabular fractures, especially those involving the acetabular dome.
   b. Retained bone fragments large enough to cause incongruity.
   c. Unstable posterior wall fracture.
   d. Displaced fractures of both columns (floating acetabulum).
   e. High transverse or T fractures.
   f. Femoral head fracture with associated acetabular fracture.

C. Femoral shaft fractures—usually the result of major trauma. Most fractures are sustained by young adults during high-energy injuries such as vehicular accidents, falls, or gunshot wounds. Patients must therefore have a complete physical exam to evaluate for associated injuries. Radiographic assessment must include an AP pelvis view.

1. Treatment.
   a. A large number of complex associated factors are evaluated in determining the appropriate treatment of different femoral shaft fractures.
      (1) Open *vs.* closed.
      (2) Fracture location.
      (3) Comminution.
      (4) Associated injuries and fractures.
      (5) Bone quality (degree of osteoporosis).
   b. Treatment modalities.
      (1) Intramedullary (IM) nailing.
         a) Treatment of choice for appropriate femoral shaft fractures.
         b) Advantages include earlier post-operative mobilization and fewer pulmonary complications.
      (2) Traction–treatment of choice in pediatric femoral shaft fractures in children younger than 10 years of age.
      (3) Plating.
      (4) External fixator.
      (5) Casting.
2. Complications.
   a. Neurovascular injury (peroneal).
   b. Shortening and malrotation.
   c. Nonunion.
   d. Stiffness.
   e. Infection.
   f. Compartment syndrome.

D. Ankle fractures.

1. Evaluation.
   a. Neurovascular exam–may need intervention for vascular injury or compromise.
   b. Rule out open fracture.
   c. Assess soft tissue swelling and skin compromise.
   d. Radiographic evaluation–AP, lateral, and mortise views.
   e. Preliminary fracture stabilization.
2. Treatment.
   a. Non-operative treatment.
      (1) Closed reduction is obtained by reversing the mechanism of injury and holding this reduction with a well-molded splint.
      (2) Splints are used for acute fracture stabilization to allow for soft tissue swelling.
      (3) Stable fractures typically require treatment in a cast for 6 weeks; unstable fractures require longer immobilization.
   b. Operative treatment.
      (1) Anatomic reduction of the fracture is the goal.

(2) Operative treatment is recommended for the following indications.
    a) Failure to obtain satisfactory closed reduction.
    b) Displaced, unstable, or open fractures.
    c) Multi-trauma.
    d) Patient factors (compliance, age, associated medical problems, etc.).

E. Distal radius fractures.

1. Fracture characteristics.
   a. Common fracture of the upper extremity.
   b. Involve both intra- and extra-articular injury patterns.
   c. Most fractures can be managed by closed reduction and casting.
2. Evaluation.
   a. Neurovascular status–trauma to adjacent nerves and arteries can lead to ischemia and possible carpal tunnel syndrome.
   b. Associated injuries–the energy of impact dissipates at fracture site, but there may be the following associated injuries.
      (1) Ligamentous injuries of wrist.
      (2) Carpal fractures.
      (3) Distal radial ulnar joint disruption.
      (4) Proximal ulna fracture.

F. Clavicle fracture.

1. Superficial location makes the clavicle one of the most commonly fractured bones in the body. Most clavicle fractures heal uneventfully with conservative treatment.
2. Treatment.
   a. Nondisplaced–sling and swath.
   b. Displaced–figure-8 bandage.
   c. ORIF–limited indications.
      (1) Open.
      (2) Skin tenting.
      (3) Neurovascular injuy.
      (4) Some distal fracture types.

G. Humeral shaft fractures.

1. Most humeral shaft fractures can be managed non-operatively with an expected union rate of 90-100%. These fractures are initially stabilized in a coaptation splint and are later changed to Sarmiento fracture brace at approximately 14 days after injury. Most closed treatments of humeral shaft fractures require patient cooperation and gravity/dependency for alignment.
2. Indications for ORIF.
   a. Open fracture.
   b. Multitrauma.
   c. Pathologic fracture.
   d. Vascular injury–supracondylar fracture.
   e. Malreduction or failure of conservative treatment.
   f. Floating elbow (humeral, radial, and ulnar fractures).

   g. Post-reduction radial nerve palsy.
3. Complications.
   a. Nonunion.
   b. Malunion.
   c. Radial nerve palsy.
   d. Volkmann's ischemic contracture–supracondylar fractures.

24

Malignant Skin Lesions

Khang N. Thai, M.D.

I. PREMALIGNANT TUMORS

A. Actinic (Solar) keratosis.

1. 20% give rise to squamous cell carcinoma.
2. Appear on sun-exposed areas.
3. Often multiple.
4. Therapy–biopsy, followed by electrodesiccation and curettage or cryotherapy. Topical 5-FU is usually reserved for widespread lesions.

B. Leukoplakia.

1. Found on mucous membranes (vulva, mouth, rectum).
2. Therapy–cryotherapy or excision, cessation of predisposing factors (i.e., chewing tobacco).

C. Bowen's disease—squamous cell carcinoma *in situ*.

1. Erythematous, sharp, irregular outline with crusting center; multiple lesions often present.
2. When seen on penis, vulva, or oral cavity, termed Erythroplasia of Queyrat.
3. Approximately 5% become invasive carcinoma.
4. Excision is most widely accepted treatment.
5. Bowen's disease of non-exposed areas is associated with a high incidence of visceral malignancy.

II. CARCINOMA

Both basal cell carcinoma (BCC) and squamous cell carcinoma (SCC) are the most common skin malignancies in the Caucasian population. They comprise approximately one-third of all cancers in the United States. The principal cause of BCC and SCC is sunlight exposure, although other etiological factors include chemical carcinogens (i.e., arsenic and hydrocarbons), human papillomavirus, cigarette smoking, chronic irritation or ulceration (e.g., Marjolin's ulcer), and immunosuppression. Clinical diagnosis of these lesions can be difficult because there are a variety of benign lesions that can mimic the appearance of BCC and SCC. In addition, certain congenital as well as hereditary lesions may predispose to the development of skin cancer. If there is any doubt, a biopsy *must* be performed.

A. Predisposing lesions.

1. ***Keratoacanthoma*** — benign lesion usually found in elderly population as a single, raised 1-2 cm lesion with a characteristic horn-filled crater. Spontaneous involution can occur within months.
2. ***Parakeratosis*** — characterized by disseminated annular plaques with horny border. Approximately 13% of parakeratosis may transform into BCC or SCC.
3. ***Nevus sebaceous*** — usually present at birth and remain fairly quiescent throughout childhood. Location usually on the scalp or face. Characteristically has well-circumscribed, slightly raised, hairless, yellowish plaque, which often progresses into a more verrucous, nodular lesion at the time of puberty. About 10% undergo malignant degeneration into BCC.

B. Basal cell carcinoma.

1. Men:women–2:1.
2. 60-75% of skin malignancies; outnumbers squamous cell carcinoma 4:1.
3. Occur on face and other sun-exposed areas, with older, fair-skinned individuals at highest risk; 25% occur in non-sun-exposed areas.
4. Locally invasive–rarely metastasizes; usually slow-growing.
5. Five histologic types.
   a. Noduloulcerative BCC.
      (1) Most common type (50%-54%); the most common location is on the head.
      (2) Waxy or pearly nodular lesion with an ulcerated center appearance.
   b. Sclerosing or morphea-form BCC.
      (1) Single, flat, indurated, yellow, waxy, ill-defined macule. Patient often depicts it as "enlarging scar" that cannot be accounted for by previous trauma.
      (2) Histology shows a dense, fibrous connective stroma in which small focal areas of basaloid cells are found.
      (3) Seen on the head and neck.
      (4) Accounts for about 2% of all BCC.
      (5) High recurrence rate.
   c. Superficial BCC.
      (1) Raised, pinkish, scaling, usually flush with the skin.
      (2) Accounts for about 9% to 11% of all BCC.
      (3) May have thread-like border in appearance and may contain shallow ulcer or crusting, or atrophic scarring.
      (4) Can be misdiagnosed as eczema or fungal infection.
      (5) Found on trunk and arms.
   d. Pigmented BCC.
      (1) Dark brown or black due to melanin-containing property.

(2) Often confused with melanoma, and can be extremely difficult to differentiate from seborrheic keratosis and nodular melanoma.
(3) Uncommon, accounts for about 6% of all BCC.

e. Fibroepithelial BCC.
(1) Characterized as a flesh-colored papule without surrounding inflammatory changes.
(2) Occurs primarily on the trunk.

6. Diagnosis.
a. Excisional biopsy performed if lesion is small.
b. Can do incisional biopsy if lesion is large or is in aesthetically important location.
c. Punch biopsy (6-mm) needs to include normal epithelium for accurate diagnosis.
d. Shave biopsies will not allow determination of depth in cases of malignant melanoma.
e. Avoid injecting local anesthetic agent into or beneath the lesions since this will alter the histology of the specimen.
f. In planning the incision, remember that a re-excision may be indicated. Therefore, the incision should be placed such that future procedure can also include the previous scar.

7. ***Treatment.***
a. Simple excision–with 2-4 mm margin, with larger margins for larger lesions. Cure rates range from 85% to 95%
b. Moh's micrographic surgery–series of excisions with histologic control of margins.
(1) Good for ill-defined lesions and recurrent disease.
(2) Used in aesthetically important locations.
(3) Cure rate via this method is about 99%.

c. Radiation treatment.
(1) Equal cure rates to surgery (92%).
(2) Requires multiple visits, but often has aesthetic results equal to surgery.
(3) Reserved for cases where surgery is not possible.

d. Electrodesiccation and Curettage (EDC).
(1) Most common method of treatment; cure rate is 96% to 100%.
(2) Best reserved for small tumors less than 2 mm in diameter.

e. Cryosurgery.
(1) Acceptable modality of treatment when indicated. In experienced hands, the cure rate can be as high as 97.4%.
(2) Indications.
a) Nodular or ulcerated carcinomas.
b) Lesions with well-defined borders.
c) Lesions overlying bony or cartilaginous structures.
d) Facial areas such as eyelid, tip of nose.
e) Poor surgical candidates.

(3) Absolute contraindications.
   a) Patients with abnormal cold intolerance (i.e., cryoglobulinemia, cryofibrinogenemia).
   b) Morpheaform or sclerosing BCC.

(4) Complications include marked edema, long period (4-6 weeks) of morbidity, permanent pigment loss, hyperpigmentation, neuropathic changes.

8. Follow-up–every 3 months for 1 year, then every 6 months.

C. Squamous cell carcinoma.

1. Usually secondary to chronic skin damage.
2. Prevalence only one-fourth that of BCC.
3. Other predisposing conditions–solar keratosis, xeroderma pigmentosa, leukoplakia, radiation exposure, arsenic exposure. More common in fair-skinned people.
4. Histologically, consists of irregular masses of squamous epithelium that proliferate downward to the dermis layer. Cellular differentiation dictates the grade of the tumor. Other factors such as changes in size and shape of the cells, hyperchromasia, keratinization, and degree of mitotic figures influence the prognosis.
5. Clinical appearance can be smooth, verrucous, papillomatous, or ulcerative. However, all advanced stage SCC have features of induration, inflammation, and ulceration.
6. Marjolin's ulcer–squamous cell carcinoma arising in chronic wounds (burns, osteomyelitis, chronic vascular ulcers, decubitus ulcers); usually very aggressive.
7. Squamous cell carcinoma has a more rapid course than does basal cell carcinoma. It has a cell cycle of only 50.2 h.
8. May metastasize to regional lymph nodes and distant organs such as bone, brain, and lung.
9. Treatment.
   a. Excision with 5-10 mm margin.
   b. Consider node dissection if nodes are palpable or in cases of Marjolin's ulcers.
   c. Mohs' chemosurgery–best for lesions of the eyelids, ears, and nasolabial folds.
   d. Radiation offers similar cure rates as surgery, but is usually reserved for unresectable lesions.

D. Kaposi's sarcoma.

1. A neoplasm of vascular endothelial cells.
2. Characterized by the presence of bluish-red nodules, edema, and hemosiderin deposition.
3. During the AIDS epidemic, the incidence of Kaposi's sarcoma has increased markedly,

E. Other non-melanoma skin tumors.

1. Cutaneous horns.
   a. Hard, keratotic growths extending from normal-looking skin and resembling a miniature animal horn.
   b. Dominant feature is a keratotic mass approximately 1- to

1.5 times as long as it is wide. Histologically, they are very advanced actinic keratoses.
    c. Superficial excision usually is adequate.
    d. About 10% of cutaneous horns have an underlying SCC.
2. Merkel cell tumor of the skin.
    a. Otherwise known as trabecular carcinoma or neuroendocrine carcinoma.
    b. Arise in the dermis, locally very aggressive, have tendency to metastasize early to regional lymph nodes.
    c. Lesions may occur anywhere in the body except the trunk.
    d. Three distinct types based on clinical and pathologic features.
        (1) Trabecular-cell: most favorable prognosis.
        (2) Intermediate-cell: most frequent, characterized by diffuse architectural pattern with multiple mitoses, lymphocytic infiltrates, and necrotic areas.
        (3) Small-cell: most aggressive form, always associated with metastases < 2 years.
    e. Immunoperoxidase studies aid in the diagnosis.
    f. Surgical excision, with or without lymph node dissection, is the treatment of choice.
    g. Cure rates very low (58% at best).
3. Dermatofibrosarcoma Protuberans.
    a. Characterized clinically by raised, hard fibrous appearance, which usually begins as a plaque-like thickening or small nodule.
    b. Typically occurs in patients 20- to 40-years old.
    c. High propensity to recur.
    d. Treatment of choice is by Mohs' micrographic surgery.

F. Syndromes associated with BCC and SCC.

1. Basal cell nevus (Gorlin's syndrome).
    a. Primary features.
        (1) Multiple basal cell carcinomas scattered throughout the body.
        (2) Cystic formation of the jaws and other skeletal abnormalities, including bifid ribs, scoliosis, brachymetacarpalism.
        (3) Overdeveloped supraorbital ridges, broad nasal root, and hypertelorism.
        (4) Calcification of the falx cerebri.
        (5) Occasional neurologic abnormalities, including mental retardation and medulloblastomas.
2. Xeroderma pigmentosum.
    a. Characterized by intolerance of skin and eyes to ultraviolet.
    b. Manifested early in life as persistent erythema, pigmentation, freckling, premature aging of skin, and multiple epithelial neoplasm.
    c. Inherited as an autosomal recessive trait.
    d. Treatment with retinoids is indicated in this syndrome, but

not yet approved by FDA.

3. Epidermodysplasia verruciformis.
   a. Characterized by wart-like, lichenoid, and flat-topped lesions on the face, neck, hand, feet, and trunk.
   b. Histological features similar to verruca plana.
   c. Viral infection has been implicated in etiology.
   d. Has tendency to degenerate into SCC.
4. Bazex syndrome.
   a. Consisting of follicular atrophoderma with multiple BCC, hypotrichosis, hypohidrosis.
   b. Inheritance is probably X-linked dominant.

III. MALIGNANT MELANOMA

A. Incidence—2% of *all* malignancies and about 5% of skin cancer; incidence is increasing at a rate of 3-5% annually. Accounts for about 75% of deaths from skin cancer. Projected incidence by the year 2000 will be 1 out of 75.

B. Affected age—rare prior to puberty.

C. White:black—20:1.

D. Risk factors.

1. Patients with a previous melanoma have been found to have an increased (3-5%) risk of having a second melanoma.
2. Fair complexion, especially people with fair or red hair, light skin, blue eyes, and a propensity to sunburn carry a higher risk for developing melanoma.
3. Sunlight exposure, especially a history of blistering sunburn. Stronger correlation between occasional or recreational sunlight than with lifetime exposure.
4. Benign nevi have not been shown to function as a precursor, but the number of nevi has been found to increase the risk for developing melanoma.
5. Familial history predisposes an increased risk up to 5-10% of patients with relatives who have the disease. Hereditary factor is even stronger in patients with relatives who have dysplastic nevus syndrome.
6. Chromosomal alterations have been implicated. Four distinct genes are located on chromosomes 1p, 6q, 7, and 9.
7. Dysplastic nevus syndrome, also known as familial atypical mole and melanoma syndrome (FAM-M) has been shown to be precursors of melanoma.

E. Distribution of Melanoma—females tend to develop lesions in the appendages, whereas males develop lesions in the head and neck and the trunk.

F. Disease pathogenesis.

1. Serves as a mode to categorize melanoma.
2. Histologic growth pattern occurs in two phases.
   a. **Radial growth**—comprises lesions in which the cancerous melanocytes are contained within the epidermis and papillary dermis. Cell growths in this phase are defined in terms

of biologic neoplastic development. Very little, if any, risk for metastatic potential.

b. **Vertical growth**–the direction of growth is perpendicular to that of radial phase. The tumor has a more aggressive pattern, characterized by rapid invasions of deeper structures. Very high propensity for metastases. Pigmentation also changes to dark nodule.

G. Morphologic classification.

1. Superficial spreading.
   a. Most common type –comprises about 70-75%.
   b. May develop anywhere in the body, but has tendency to occur on the upper back in both genders and on the lower extremities in females.
   c. Horizontal growth, with irregular margins, multicolored with shades of brown; average size approximately 2 cm.
2. Lentigo maligna (Hutchinson's freckle).
   a. Accounts for approximately 4-10% of all cases.
   b. Older age group.
   c. Sun-exposed areas (i.e., face, neck, dorsum of hands).
   d. Lesions are usually flat and large.
   e. Carries the best prognosis because of a very slow, indolent radial growth phase.
3. Nodular.
   a. Accounts for approximately 15-30% of all cases.
   b. Vertical growth only, hence a very rapid progression.
   c. Clinically has dark brown or black color with grayish/bluish cast and regular borders.
   d. These lesions are amelanotic in about 5% of all cases.
   e. Often occurs in middle-aged men and has predilection toward the trunk and head areas.
4. Acral lentiginous.
   a. Comprises about 2-8% of cases in Caucasians; prevalence much higher in other races.
   b. Palms, soles, subungual areas, mucous membranes.
   c. Average age at diagnosis is about 60 years old.
   d. Usually diagnosed late.
   e. Characteristically have a flat outline with irregular borders. Average size is about 3 cm in diameter.
   f. Early pre-invasive intradermal phase, making it more aggressive than other subtypes.
5. Desmoplastic melanoma.
   a. Also known as neurotropic melanoma, a rare variant of melanoma.
   b. Produce mucin.
   c. Have a high tendency to infiltrate the adventitia of blood vessels and perineural invasion with spreading along the nerves.
   d. Often recur locally after excision.
   e. Frozen-section for adequate margin is indicated.

f. Adjuvant radiotherapy post excision may decrease the risk of local recurrence.

H. Diagnosis.

1. Clinical features of melanoma:
   a. A–Asymmetry of lesion.
   b. B–Border irregularity.
   c. C–Color variegation.
   d. D–Diameter of lesion. Risk increases with lesions > 6 mm.
2. Any pigmented lesion that undergoes a change in size, configuration, or color should be biopsied.
3. Tumor markers: S-100 protein and HMB-45 may aid in the diagnosis of difficult cases.
4. Differential diagnosis:
   a. Junctional nevi.
   b. Compound nevi.
   c. Lentigo.
   d. Seborrheic keratosis.
   e. Hemangioma.
   f. Blue nevi.

I. Biopsy techniques.

1. Excisional biopsy.
   a. Recommended for lesions < 1.5 cm in diameter.
   b. A narrow margin of skin 2-3 mm should be included with specimen.
   c. Longitudinal axis of elliptical excision should be oriented to facilitate possible wider re-excision.
2. Incisional biopsy.
   a. Performed in areas where maximum skin preservation is essential.
   b. Does not affect survival rate.
   c. Frozen section not indicated, except in desmoplastic melanoma.
3. Punch biopsy.
   a. Lesions > 1.5 cm in diameter.
   b. Performed on most raised area, or the darkest area of lesion.
4. Electrodesiccation/electrocoagulation/Mohs' micrographic surgery. *Has no role in the management of melanoma.*

J. Prognostic factors.

1. Clark's levels of invasion (Figure 1).
   a. Level I–all tumor cells above basement membrane.
   b. Level II–into papillary dermis.
   c. Level III–to junction of papillary and reticular dermis.
   d. Level IV–into reticular dermis.
   e. Level V–into subcutaneous fat.
2. Breslow classification.
   a. Thickness ≤ 0.75 mm–over 90% cure rate.
   b. Thickness 0.75-1.65 mm–higher metastatic risk if lesion on back, arms, neck, or scalp (BANS).
   c. Thickness 1.65-4.0 mm–increased risk for regional disease.

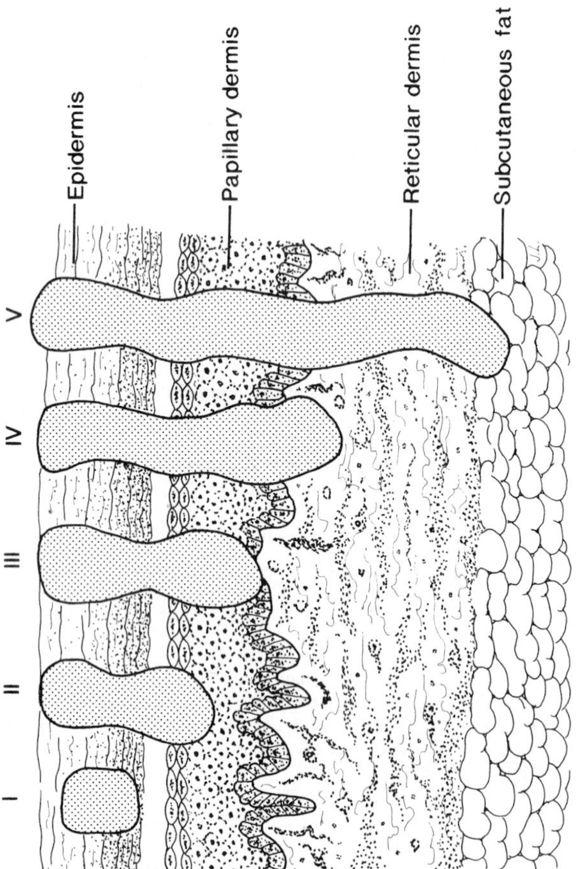

FIG. 1 Clark's Levels of Invasion

d. Thickness > 4.0 mm–80% chance of occult distant metastases.

K. Work-up.

1. Complete physical exam with attention to regional nodes as well as abdomen (looking for organomegaly or masses).
2. Complete search for other lesions in the body.
3. CXR and liver function test.
4. CT of chest and abdomen in patients with lesions > 2 mm thick or in patients with palpable nodes, as these lesions have a higher rate of metastasis.

L. Treatment.

1. Excisional biopsy is the treatment of choice for suspicious lesions–Do *not* perform shave biopsies, curettage, or electrocoagulation of lesions suspected of being melanoma.
2. Acceptable skin margins are 1-3 cm for most lesions. The following are current recommendations.
   a. Thin melanoma (< 1 mm thick)–1 cm margin.
   b. Intermediate (1-4 mm)–2 cm margin.
   c. Thick (> 4 mm thick)–3 cm margin.
3. Lymph node dissection (controversial)–regional lymph node dissection if nodes are palpable.
4. For subungual melanomas–partial amputation.
5. Chemotherapy–used for disease beyond regional nodes, but is strictly palliative.
6. Immunotherapy–has shown some success in metastatic disease.

M. Follow-up treatment.

1. First year–every 3 months.
2. Second year–every 4 months.
3. Third-fifth year–every 6 months.
4. > 5 years–annually.
5. Components of each visit.
   a. Complete physical examination.
   b. Chest radiograph.
   c. Liver function test, including serum lactate dehydrogenase (useful marker for distant metastases).

N. Common sites of metastases.

1. Lymph nodes, skin, subcutaneous–59%.
2. Lung–36%.
3. Liver–20%.
4. Brain–20%.
5. Bone–17%.
6. GI tract–7%.

O. Management of lymph nodes.

1. Elective lymph node dissection (ELND).
   a. Offers theoretical advantage of treating melanoma nodal metastases at an early stage.
   b. Does *not* benefit patients with thin melanomas (< 1 mm

thickness), since these lesions are associated with 95% cure rate with wide local excision.

c. Intermediate-thickness melanomas (1-4 mm) have an increased risk of occult regional metastases (60%), but relatively low risk for distant metastases (< 20%). Therefore, these lesions might benefit from ELND.
d. Thick melanomas (> 4 mm) carry high risk (> 60%) for regional nodal micro-metastases and a high risk (> 70%) for distant metastases. Therefore, ELND should be deferred until regional nodal invasions are clinically evidenced.
e. Currently, ELND is performed with wide local excision when there are palpable lymph nodes.
f. Morbidity of ELND–wound infection (5-19%), fistula, lymphocele, or seroma (3-23%), lymphedema.

2. Sentinel node biopsy.
   a. A new technique allows identification of nodal metastases within regional basin at the time of initial resection.
   b. Performed by injecting vital blue dye (patent blue V, or isosulfan blue) intradermally.
   c. Sentinel nodes can be identified in about 80% of cases.
   d. This technique has a 5% false-negative rate.

25

Head and Neck Malignancies

Michael A. Helmrath, M.D.

Approximately 67,000 head and neck cancers are diagnosed annually in the United States. The relative frequency by site is 40% in the oral cavity, 25% in the larynx, 15% in the oropharynx, 7% in the salivary glands, and 13% other sites. The male:female ratio is 3:1, and the average age is in the sixth decade. Risk factors include heavy tobacco and alcohol exposure. Some studies have shown an association with syphilis, human papilloma virus, and neglect of oral hygiene. Pathologically, invasive carcinomas are classified as well differentiated, moderately differentiated, poorly differentiated, or undifferentiated. Immunohistochemical techniques can distinguish SCC (squamous cell carcinoma) from malignant melanoma and lymphomas. Regional metastasis to cervical lymph nodes is common, whereas distant metastasis occurs late (most commonly to liver, lung, and bone). The tumors initially appear as a white plaque (leukoplakia), a velvety red area (erythroplakia), or an ulcer. Common symptoms include non-healing lesion, bleeding, otalgia, facial pain or mass, hoarseness, and dysphagia. Physical exam includes inspection and digital examination of the neck, oral cavity, tonsils, and base of the tongue. The oropharynx, hypopharynx, and larynx can be visualized by indirect laryngoscopy. Ultrasound, CT, or MRI may be helpful and should be obtained prior to biopsy to avoid misinterpretation caused by manipulation of tissues. Fine needle aspiration (FNA) may be helpful but requires an experienced cytopathologist for interpretation. Patients with persistent adenopathy after 2 weeks of antibiotics should be evaluated by FNA. Excisional biopsy is not recommended.

I. STAGING

Head and neck cancers are staged according to the TMN system of the AJCC.

Stage grouping:

Stage I T1, N0, M0
Stage II T2, N0, M0

Stage III	T3, N0, M0, or T1-3, N1, M0
Stage IV	T4, N0 or N1, M0
	Any T, N2, or N3, M0
	Any T, any N, M1 (evidence of metastasis)
Primary oral tumor (T):	
Tis	Carcinoma *in situ*
T1	Tumor <2 cm
T2	Tumor >2 cm
T3	Tumor >4 cm
T4	Tumor invasion
Regional lymph nodes (N):	
N0	No nodal metastasis
N1	Metastasis ipsilateral node <3 cm
N2	Metastasis ipsilateral or contralateral 3-6 cm
N3	Metastasis in a node >6 cm

II. NECK DISSECTION

A. Lymph node groups.

Level I	Submental and submandibular.
Level II	Upper jugular group.
Level III	Middle jugular group.
Level IV	Lower jugular group.
Level V	Posterior triangle group.
Level VI	Anterior compartment group.

B. Radical neck dissection—removal of all ipsilateral cervical lymph nodes (level I-V). Dissection from the inferior border of the mandible to clavicle, posteriorly to the anterior border of the trapezius muscle, and anteriorly to the lateral border of the sternohyoid muscle. Depth is to the fascia overlying the anterior scalene and levator scapulae muscles. The spinal accessory nerve, internal jugular vein and sternocleidomastoid muscle are removed.

C. Modified radical neck dissection—excision of all lymph nodes (levels I-V) with preservation of the spinal accessory nerve, internal jugular vein, and sternocleidomastoid muscle.

III. CARCINOMA OF THE LIP

A. Usually SCC arising at the skin-vermilion junction.

B. Exposure to sunlight and tobacco increase risk; men:women–15:1.

C. If < 1 cm in diameter, local excision is usually curative.

D. Patients with larger lesions or palpable nodes should have surgical excision with neck dissection.

E. 5-year survival is 90% for lesions without lymph node metastases.

F. Radiation also has a high cure rate, but generally reserved for unresectable lesions.

G. Invasion of mental nerve is associated with nodal involvement and a 35% 5-year survival.

IV. TONGUE

A. Most common intraoral malignancy.

B. Intraoral glossectomy can be performed for patients with lesions limited to the anterior or middle third of the oral tongue.

C. Lesions < 1 cm have minimal incidence of nodal metastasis, lesions larger than 1 cm have a 20% incidence of metastasis and therefore require a supraomohyoid neck dissection.

D. Tumors of the posterior oral tongue with extension are best treated by a transcervical excision combined with an *en bloc* neck dissection.

V. CARCINOMA OF THE OROPHARYNX

A. Oral cavity.

1. Represent about 10,000 cancer deaths/year.
2. 95% of malignancies are squamous cell carcinoma.
3. 75% present in an advanced state.
4. Treatment.
    a. T1 and T2 lesions are treated with primary surgical excision and supraomohyoid neck dissection.
    b. Staged bilateral neck dissection if lesion crosses the midline.
    c. Radiation is recommended for T3 and T4 lesions, for smaller lesions away from mandible, or for recurrence of disease.
5. 5-year disease-free survival is 30-40%.

B. Buccal mucosa and hard palate.

1. Usually SCC.
2. Radiotherapy is effective in reducing the incidence of local recurrence.
3. Ipsilateral neck dissection advised.

VI. CARCINOMA OF THE NASOPHARYNX

A. Uncommon.

B. Increased incidence among Chinese.

C. Lymphoid and epidermoid elements.

D. Symptoms.

1. Respiratory obstruction.
2. Palsies of CN's III, IV, V, VI if cavernous sinus is invaded.
3. Horner's syndrome if cervical sympathetic chain is compressed.

E. Treatment.

1. Radiation for primary and metastatic disease.
2. 5-year survival–25-30%.

VII. SALIVARY TUMORS

A. Pathology.

1. Benign.
    a. Pleomorphic adenoma (mixed tumor).
        (1) Account for 75% of parotid neoplasms.

(2) Most frequent in middle-aged women.
(3) 10% recurrence rate with surgical treatment.

b. Papillary cystadenoma lymphomatosum (Warthin's tumor).
(1) More common in males.
(2) 10-15% bilateral.

c. Hemangioma–most common salivary tumor in children.

2. Malignant.
   a. Mucoepidermoid carcinoma–most common parotid malignancy.
   b. Malignant mixed tumor–second most common.
   c. Adenoid cystic carcinoma.
   d. Papillary adenocarcinoma–rare.
   e. Epidermoid carcinoma.
   f. Acinic cell adenocarcinoma–rare.
   g. Lymphoma–usually in parotid or submaxillary gland.

B. Parotid tumors.

1. Approximately 2/3 of malignant salivary tumors arise in parotid gland; however, most parotid tumors are benign. Tumors are more common in superficial lobe.
2. Cranial nerve VII (facial nerve).
   a. Courses and subdivides within substance of gland.
   b. If patient has CN VII paralysis, then tumor is probably malignant.
3. Formal lobe resection (not enucleation) should be performed even for benign tumors because of high recurrence rate.
4. Perform ipsilateral neck dissection for palpable nodes.

C. Submandibular gland tumors.

1. Not as common (10% of malignant salivary tumors), but are more frequently malignant.
2. Lymph nodes more commonly involved than in parotid gland tumors.

D. Minor salivary gland tumors.

1. Majority are mixed tumors.
2. > 50% are malignant.
3. Represent 10% of malignant salivary tumors.

VIII. CARCINOMA OF THE HYPOPHARYNX

A. Incidence—Three times more common than carcinoma of larynx.

B. Related to tobacco use, alcohol use, and Plummer-Vinson syndrome.

C. Usually well-differentiated.

D. Symptoms.

1. Dysphagia–aspiration pneumonia.
2. Palpable cervical lymph node.

E. Treatment.

1. Wide resection of larynx and hypopharynx with *en bloc* radi-

cal neck dissection has become standard treatment, using a jejunal free-graft to restore pharyngeal continuity.

2. Less radical operations are currently being evaluated.

IX. CARCINOMA OF THE LARYNX

A. Men:women—10:1.

B. Supraglottic (above true vocal cords)–45%.

C. Glottic (involving vocal cords)–50%.

D. Subglottic (below vocal cords)–< 5%.

E. Symptoms—hoarseness, respiratory obstruction, dysphagia (a late symptom).

F. Treatment.

1. Supraglottic.
   a. If small, radiation is primary therapy.
   b. More advanced lesions are treated with combination radiation and surgery; partial or total laryngectomy may be necessary.
   c. Radical neck dissection indicated if nodes are palpable.
2. Glottic.
   a. Radiation for early lesions (more likely than surgery to preserve voice).
   b. Partial *vs.* total laryngectomy for larger lesions (with neck dissection if nodes are palpable).
3. Subglottic.
   a. Usually presents in a more advanced state.
   b. Total laryngectomy with neck dissection (regardless of clinical node status) with hemithyroidectomy is standard treatment.
4. Overall 5-year survival of patients with laryngeal carcinoma treated with total laryngectomy is 50-65%.

26

Diseases of the Breast

Rebeccah L. Brown, M.D.

I. ANATOMIC AND PHYSIOLOGIC CONSIDERATIONS

A. Relevant anatomy.

1. Modified sweat gland of ectodermal origin that lies cushioned in fat and is enveloped by superficial and deep layers of superficial fascia of the anterior chest wall.
2. Each mammary gland consists of 15-20 lobules, which are drained by lactiferous ducts that open separately on the nipple.
3. Fibrous septae (Cooper's ligaments) interdigitate the mammary parenchyma and extend from the deep pectoral fascia to the superficial layer of fascia within the dermis. These provide structural support to the breast and hold it upward.
4. Base of breast extends from the second to the sixth rib. Medial border = lateral margin of sternum. Lateral border = midaxillary line. Axillary tail of Spence pierces the deep fascia and enters the axilla.
5. Divided into 4 quadrants–upper outer (UOQ), lower outer (LOQ), upper inner (UIQ), and lower inner (LIQ).

B. Lymphatic drainage—of importance during mastectomy and axillary node dissection.

1. ***Axillary nodes***—75% of drainage from ipsilateral breast; contains about 40-50 nodes. Axillary nodes secondarily drain to supraclavicular and jugular nodes.
2. ***Levels of axillary nodes.***
   a. **Level I**–lateral to pectoralis minor. Includes external mammary, subscapular, axillary vein, and central nodal groups.
   b. **Level II**–deep to insertion of pectoralis minor muscle on the coracoid process. Includes central nodal groups. Borders of level I and II axillary nodes include the latissimus dorsi muscle laterally, the axillary vein superiorly, and the pectoralis minor muscle medially.

c. **Level III**—medial to pectoralis minor and extending up to apex of axilla. Includes central nodal groups.

3. ***Internal mammary nodes***—account for 20% of drainage; contains about 4 nodes per side, with one node in each of first 3 interspaces and another in the fifth or sixth interspace. Drains UIQ and LIQ.
4. ***Interpectoral (Rotter's) nodes***—lie between pectoralis major and pectoralis minor muscles.
5. ***Abdominal and paravertebral nodes***—account for 5% of drainage.

C. Associated nerves (of surgical importance).

1. ***Intercostobrachial nerve***—traverses the axilla from chest wall to supply cutaneous sensation to upper medial arm. Sacrificing this nerve results in hypoesthesia or anesthesia of upper medial arm.
2. ***Long thoracic nerve (of Bell)***—arises from roots of C5, C6, and C7. Courses close to chest wall along medial border of axilla to innervate serratus anterior muscle. Injury results in a "winged" scapular deformity.
3. ***Thoracodorsal nerve***—arises from posterior cord of brachial plexus (C5, C6, C7). Courses along lateral border of axilla to innervate latissimus dorsi muscle.
4. ***Lateral pectoral nerve***—arises from lateral cord of brachial plexus. Innervates both pectoralis major and minor muscles.

D. Relevant physiology.

1. Phases of breast development depend on mammotropic effects of pituitary and ovarian hormones.
   a. **Estrogen**—promotes ductal development and fat deposition.
   b. **Progesterone**—promotes lobular-alveolar development and prepares breast for lactation.
   c. **Prolactin**—involved in milk production.
   d. **Oxytocin**—involved in milk ejection.
2. Menopause—cessation of ovarian hormonal stimulation results in involution of breast tissue with atrophy of lobules, loss of stroma, and replacement with fatty tissue.

II. HISTORY

A. Age.

1. Fibroadenoma is most common breast lesion in females younger than 30 years of age.
2. Risk for breast cancer increases with increasing age. Rare in patients younger than 30 years of age ($< 1\%$). Over 70% of all cases occur in patients older than 50 years of age.

B. Mass—determine when first noted, how first noted, tender or nontender, change in size over time, and relation to menstrual cycle.

C. Nipple discharge—determine nature of discharge, unilateral or bilateral, from single or multiple duct orifices, spontaneous or induced, association with mass.

1. Bloody–intraductal papilloma or invasive papillary cancer. Discharge should be sent for cytology.
2. Milky (galactorrhea)–pregnancy, lactation, pituitary adenoma, acromegaly, hypothyroidism, stress, drugs (oral contraceptives, antihypertensives, certain psychotropic drugs). Evaluation may include urine or serum pregnancy tests, prolactin levels.
3. Serous–normal menses, oral contraceptives, fibrocystic change, early pregnancy.
4. Yellow–fibrocystic change, galactocele.
5. Purulent–superficial or central breast abscess.

D. Breast pain—may be associated with menstrual irregularity, as a pre-menstrual symptom, with administration of exogenous ovarian hormones during or after menopause, or with fibrocystic change. Rarely a symptom of breast cancer.

E. Gynecologic history (see "Breast Cancer" in this chapter).

F. Past medical history—prior history of benign breast disease (i.e., fibrocystic change), breast cancer, radiation therapy to the breast or axilla.

G. Past surgical history—prior history of breast biopsy, lumpectomy, mastectomy, axillary node dissection, hysterectomy, oophorectomy, adrenalectomy.

H. Family history of breast disease—especially in mother, sisters, or daughters.

I. Constitutional symptoms—anorexia, weight loss, dyspnea, cough, chest pain, hemoptysis, bony pain.

III. PHYSICAL EXAMINATION

A. Inspection—Examine with patient seated with arms at her side; seated with arms raised over head; seated with hands on hips; and supine. Note breast size, shape, contour, symmetry, skin coloration, skin dimpling, edema, erythema, "peau de orange", excoriation, nipple inversion or retraction, or nipple discharge.

B. Palpation.

1. With patient in the sitting position, support the patient's arm and palpate each axilla to detect axillary adenopathy. The supraclavicular fossae and cervical region should also be palpated. Note node size and mobility.
2. Palpation of the breast is performed with the patient in the supine position with the arms stretched above the head and with the arms at her side. Identify any masses, noting location, size, shape, consistency, tenderness, skin dimpling, and mobility. 4 "Ds" to distinguish a true lump from a lumpy area–dominant, discrete, dense, and different. Carcinoma is typically firm, nontender, poorly circumscribed, and relatively immobile.
3. Nipples should be palpated to identify any discharge.

C. Emphasize breast self-examination (BSE)—should be performed approximately 5 days after completion of menses in the premenopausal female and monthly in the post-menopausal female.

D. Recommended follow-up.

1. BSE on monthly basis beginning at age 20-25. Majority of breast masses are found by patients themselves.
2. Physician exam every 1-3 years, depending upon risk factors.

IV. RADIOGRAPHIC STUDIES

A. Indications for mammography.

1. Screening (current American Cancer Society recommendations).
   a. Baseline mammogram for women ages 35-39 years.
   b. Mammogram every 1-2 years for women ages 40-50 years.
   c. Annual mammogram for women older than 50 years.
2. Metastatic adenocarcinoma without known primary.
3. Nipple discharge without palpable mass.

B. Mammographic findings suggestive of malignancy.

1. Irregularly marginated stellate or spiculated mass.
2. Architectural distortion with retraction and spiculation.
3. Asymmetric localized fibrosis.
4. Fine microcalcifications with a linear, branched, or rod-like pattern, especially when focal or clustered. Increased likelihood of cancer with increased number of microcalcifications.
5. Increased vascularity.
6. Altered subareolar duct pattern.

C. Ultrasonography—useful for distinguishing between cystic and solid masses. Effective for lesions greater than 0.5 cm in diameter. Value of ultrasonography is limited, however, since needle aspiration provides both diagnosis and treatment for most cystic masses.

V. EVALUATION OF BREAST MASS

A. Needle aspiration—for palpable cystic lesions. Send fluid for cytology if serosanguinous or grossly bloody. Excisional biopsy indicated when (1) needle aspiration produces no cyst fluid, and solid mass is diagnosed, (2) cyst fluid is blood-tinged or grossly bloody, (3) cyst fluid is withdrawn, but mass fails to resolve completely, (4) mass reappears in same area after more than 2 aspirations, and (5) cyst fluid reaccumulates within 2 weeks after initial aspiration.

B. Fine needle aspiration (FNA) biopsy—for palpable solid masses, especially if clinical suspicion for malignancy is high. Use 20- to 22-ga. needle with 10-cc syringe, with or without local anesthetic. Make multiple passes at different angles through the mass while aspirating on syringe. Immediately fix in 95% ethanol. Accuracy rates approach 90%.

1. Non-diagnostic cytology–excisional biopsy.
2. Diagnostic cytology–discuss cancer treatment options.

C. **Excisional biopsy**—*definitive* method for tissue diagnosis. Majority of procedures performed on outpatients, usually under local anesthesia.

1. Non-palpable lesion–requires prior mammographic localization with a needle or hook wire. Post-biopsy radiograph of specimen should be obtained to confirm adequacy of biopsy.
2. Biopsy incisions should be placed with deliberation–transversely oriented, curvilinear incisions in upper hemisphere of the breast; radial incisions in lower hemisphere of the breast, circumareolar incisions to be used only for masses just beneath the areola. Incision should be made so that subsequent mastectomy can incorporate biopsy site. *All* breast biopsies should be performed with the assumption that the lesion is malignant.
3. Sharp dissection should be used, with little or no electrocautery because steroid hormone receptors are heat-labile.
4. The entire mass and a surrounding 1 cm rim of normal tissue should be excised to fulfill requirements for "lumpectomy", thus avoiding need for re-excision if pathology reveals malignancy. The specimen should be properly oriented, labeled, and sent fresh (unfixed) on ice for pathology. The specimen should be processed for hormone receptor analysis and flow cytometry.
5. Deep parenchymal sutures to close dead space should be avoided because they act as nidus for infection and distort breast architecture, yielding a poorer cosmetic result. Fibrin quickly fills dead space and restores normal breast contour. A simple subcuticular closure of skin is all that is necessary.

VI. BENIGN BREAST DISEASE

A. **Fibrocystic change**—encompasses a wide spectrum of clinical and histological findings, including cyst formation, breast nodularity, stromal proliferation, and epithelial hyperplasia. May represent an exaggerated response of normal breast stroma and epithelium to circulating and locally produced hormones and growth factors.

1. Incidence greatest around age 30-40 years, but may persist into 8th decade.
2. Usually presents with breast pain, swelling, and tenderness, which may be associated with focal areas of nodularity, induration, or gross cysts. Frequently bilateral. Varies with menstrual cycle. Sustained symptoms may reflect anovulatory cycles.
3. Not associated with increased risk of breast cancer unless biopsy specimen reveals ductal or lobular hyperplasia with atypia.
4. *Treatment.*
   a. Rule out carcinoma by aspiration or excisional biopsy of

any discrete mass that persists without change over several menstrual cycles.

b. Frequent breast examinations (BSE and physician).
c. Baseline mammogram for ages 35-39 and annual mammogram for women older than 40 to identify any new or changing lesions.
d. Avoid xanthine-containing products (coffee, tea, chocolate, cola drinks) and nicotine.
e. **Danazol,** a weak androgen, 50-200 mg po BID for severe symptoms. Must be continued for 2-3 months to see a potential effect. 50% recurrence within 1 year of discontinuing drug. Side-effects include amenorrhea, body fat redistribution, weight gain, hirsutism, deepening of the voice, acne, and liver dysfunction.
f. **Tamoxifen** 20 mg po qd for severe symptoms. Antiestrogenic–binds estrogen receptors. Administer 4- to 6-week course, then discontinue to assess for continued symptoms.

B. Fibroadenoma.

1. Most common breast lesion in women under age 30.
2. Round, well-circumscribed, firm, rubbery, mobile, nontender mass 1-5 cm in diameter. Lesions > 5 cm are referred to as **giant fibroadenomas,** which must be differentiated from cystosarcoma phyllodes. Usually solitary, but may be multiple and bilateral. Hormonally dependent; may increase in size with normal menses, pregnancy, lactation, and use of oral contraceptives.
3. ***Treatment***—excisional biopsy to remove the tumor and establish the diagnosis, or may be followed clinically if static in young patient.

C. Cystosarcoma phyllodes—rare variant of fibroadenoma.

1. May occur at any age, but most common in 5th decade.
2. Presents as a large, bulky mass; overlying skin is red, warm, and shiny, with venous engorgement. The tumor itself is smooth, well-circumscribed, and freely mobile, with a median size of 4-5 cm; characterized by rapid growth.
3. May be considered a low-grade malignancy. Contains both mesenchymal and stromal components. Most are benign, but a few develop true sarcomatous potential. Metastases are infrequent.
4. High rate of local recurrence after simple excision or enucleation.
5. ***Treatment***—wide local excision with at least 1 cm margins for smaller tumors; simple mastectomy for larger tumors.

D. Intraductal papilloma—benign, solitary polypoid lesion involving epithelium-lined lactiferous duct.

1. Presents as bloody nipple discharge in pre-menopausal women. Fluid should be sent for cytology.
2. Major differential diagnosis is between intraductal papilloma and invasive papillary carcinoma.

3. Treatment–excision of involved duct after localization by physical examination.

E. Fat necrosis.

1. Presents as an ecchymotic, tender, firm, ill-defined mass, often accompanied by skin or nipple retraction, which is almost impossible to differentiate from carcinoma by physical exam or mammography.
2. History of antecedent trauma may be elicited in about 50% of patients. Pain is characteristic.
3. ***Treatment***—excisional biopsy to rule out carcinoma.

F. Mammary duct ectasia (plasma cell mastitis).

1. Subacute inflammation of ductal system characterized by dilated mammary ducts with inspissated secretions and marked periductal inflammation, and infiltration of plasma cells.
2. Occurs at or after menopause. History of difficult nursing may be elicited.
3. Presenting symptoms include noncyclical breast pain (mastodynia) associated with nipple retraction or discharge, and subareolar masses.
4. Benign lesion; difficult to differentiate from carcinoma clinically or radiographically. Excisional biopsy is indicated to rule out carcinoma. Multiple biopsies may be required owing to the diffuse nature of the lesion. Curative treatment usually requires subareolar duct excision.

G. Galactocele.

1. Occurs after cessation of lactation secondary to an obstructed lactiferous duct filled with inspissated milk and desquamated epithelial cells.
2. Presents as round, well-circumscribed, mobile, tender subareolar mass associated with milky yellow or greenish-yellow nipple discharge.
3. ***Treatment***—needle aspiration; excision indicated if cyst cannot be aspirated or cyst becomes infected.

H. Mastitis and breast abscess.

1. Common in lactating females, possibly due to inspissation of milk, obstruction, and secondary infection. May develop generalized cellulitis of breast tissue (mastitis) or abscess.
2. Progression from mastitis to abscess formation occurs in 5-10% of cases.
3. Most common etiologic organisms in lactating females are *Staphylococcus aureus* and *Staphylococcus epidermidis*; less commonly *Streptococcus* and diphtheroid organisms.
4. Most common etiologic organisms in nonlactating females are *S. aureus* and anaerobes such as *Bacteroides* and *Peptostreptococcus.*
5. ***Treatment.***
   a. Local measures–application of heat, ice packs, or use of mechanical breast pump on affected side.

b. Broad-spectrum antibiotics.
c. Incision and drainage if fluctuant and not improved with appropriate antibiotic therapy.
d. Recurrent infection best treated by excision of diseased subareolar ducts.

4. Differential diagnosis of mastitis includes inflammatory carcinoma. When incision and drainage performed, biopsies of abscess cavity should be sent in all patients.

I. Mondor's disease (thrombophlebitis of superficial thoracoepigastric vein).

1. Presents as acute pain over superolateral breast or axilla, often related to local trauma.
2. Finding of palpable cord is diagnostic.
3. ***Treatment***—reassurance, heat, and analgesics.

J. Gynecomastia—breast hypertrophy in males.

1. Physiologic.
   a. Newborns–due to exposure to maternal estrogens.
   b. Pubertal (ages 13-17)–may be bilateral or unilateral; usually regresses with adulthood; treated with reassurance.
   c. Senescent (> age 50)–due to male "menopause" with relative estrogen increase; frequently unilateral; breast tissue is enlarged, firm, and tender; usually regresses spontaneously within 6-12 months.
2. Drug-induced–associated with use of estrogens, digoxin, thiazides, phenothiazines, phenytoin, theophylline, cimetidine, antihypertensives (reserpine, spironolactone, methyldopa), diazepam, tricyclics, antineoplastic drugs, marijuana. Treatment is discontinuation of offending drug.
3. Pathologic–associated with cirrhosis, renal failure, malnutrition, hyperthyroidism, adrenal dysfunction, testicular tumors, hermaphroditism, hypogonadism (e.g., Klinefelter's syndrome).
4. Any dominant or suspicious mass should be biopsied to rule out carcinoma, especially in the senescent male.

BREAST CANCER

I. EPIDEMIOLOGY

A. Frequency—Most common non-skin cancer in U.S. women: 12% (about 1 in 9) will develop breast cancer during their lifetime and 3.5% will die of the disease.

B. Incidence—increases with increasing age.

C. Leading cause of death in U.S. women 40-55 years of age.

D. Age-adjusted incidence—appears to be increasing but age-adjusted death rate appears to be decreasing–may be related to earlier detection and/or improved therapy.

II. RISK FACTORS

A. Sex—female: male ratio for breast cancer is 100-150:1.

B. Age—risk increases with increasing age. The risk that breast cancer will develop in a white American female in a single year increases from 1:5900 at age 30 to 1:290 at age 80.

C. Mother and/or sister(s) with breast cancer—2-3 x increased risk. Risk decreases with more distant affected relatives. Overall risk depends on number of first-degree relatives with breast cancer, their ages at diagnosis, and whether the disease was unilateral or bilateral.

1. If premenopausal breast cancer–20-30% risk.
2. If premenopausal, bilateral breast cancer–50% risk.

D. Genetic predisposition–accounts for less than 3% of all breast cancers. Breast cancer invariably develops in patients with Li-Fraumeni syndrome, a rare disorder involving a germline mutation in the tumor suppressor gene *P53*. Gene located on chromosome 17q known as BRCA-1 may be responsible for early-onset (familial) breast cancer.

E. Prior history of breast cancer–5 x increased risk in contralateral breast.

F. History of breast biopsy regardless of underlying pathology.

G. Atypical ductal or lobular hyperplasia identified on breast biopsy–approximately 5 x increased risk.

H. Coexistence of positive family history of breast cancer and atypical ductal or lobular hyperplasia on biopsy–9 x increased risk.

I. Non-invasive carcinoma (ductal or lobular carcinoma *in situ*).

J. Early menarche (< 12 years of age) or late menopause (> 55).

K. Cumulative duration of menstruation. Increased risk in those who menstruate for > 30 years.

L. Nulliparity or age > 30 years at first delivery.

M. Exogenous hormone use–use of postmenopausal estrogen replacement increases risk of breast cancer by about 40%. However, there is no statistically significant increase in risk associated with the use of oral contraceptives.

N. Exposure to low-dose ionizing radiation between ages 13 and 30.

O. Alcohol consumption, especially before age 30.

III. CLINICAL PRESENTATION

A. Non-palpable, suspicious lesion on mammogram—requires needle localization biopsy or stereotactic fine needle biopsy for diagnosis.

B. Palpable mass—most common presentation; majority detected by patient on routine self-exam; typically non-tender, firm, irregular, relatively immobile, most commonly located in upper outer quadrant of breast (approximately 50%); may be multifocal, multicentric, or bilateral.

C. Skin changes—skin dimpling (tethering of Cooper's ligaments), nipple retraction or inversion, erythema, warmth, edema, "peau de orange" (dermal lymphatic invasion), ulceration, eczema/excoriation of superficial epidermis of nipple (as in Paget's disease).

D. **Nipple discharge—**bloody; most commonly due to intraductal papilloma, but invasive papillary carcinoma must be ruled out.

E. **Metastatic spread—**to lungs, bone, brain, liver, and lymph nodes; may present with anorexia, weight loss, cachexia, dyspnea, cough, hemoptysis, bony pain (especially vertebral), pathologic fractures.

IV. TNM CLASSIFICATION

Tumor (T)

T0	No evidence of primary tumor.
TIS	Carcinoma *in situ*—ductal or lobular, or Paget's disease of nipple without tumor.
T1	Tumor 2.0 cm or smaller.
T2	Tumor greater than 2.0 cm but less than 5.0 cm.
T3	Tumor greater than 5.0 cm.
T4	Tumor of any size with direct extension to chest wall or skin.
T4a	Extension to chest wall.
T4b	Edema (including "peau de orange"), ulceration of skin of breast, or satellite skin nodules confined to same breast.
T4c	Both T4a and T4b.
T4d	Inflammatory carcinoma—characterized by diffuse, brawny induration of skin, with erysipeloid edge, usually without underlying palpable mass.

Regional Lymph Nodes (N)

N0	No regional lymph node metastases.
N1	Metastases to moveable ipsilateral axillary lymph nodes.
N2	Metastases to ipsilateral axillary lymph nodes fixed to one another or to other structures.
N3	Metastases to ipsilateral internal mammary lymph nodes.

Distant Metastasis (M)

M0	No distant metastasis.
M1	Distant metastasis—includes supraclavicular, cervical, or contralateral internal mammary lymph nodes.

V. STAGING

Stage 0	TIS	N0	M0
Stage I	T1	N0	M0
Stage II			
Stage IIa	T0	N1	M0
	T1	N1	M0
	T2	N0	M0
Stage IIb	T2	N1	M0
	T3	N0	M0
Stage III			
Stage IIIa	T0	N2	M0

	T1	N2	M0
	T2	N2	M0
	T3	N1,2	M0
Stage IIIb	T4	Any N	M0
	Any T	N3	M0
Stage IV	Any T	Any N	M1

VI. PATHOLOGY

A. Growth patterns.

1. May be broadly divided into epithelial tumors arising from cells lining ducts or lobules *vs.* non-epithelial tumors arising from supporting stroma (i.e., angiosarcoma, malignant cystosarcoma phyllodes, primary stromal sarcomas). Non-epithelial tumors are much less common.
2. May be non-invasive (ductal or lobular carcinoma *in situ*) or invasive (infiltrating ductal or lobular carcinoma). Non-invasive refers to the absence of invasion of the basement membrane.
3. May be multifocal (disease within same quadrant as dominant lesion), multicentric (disease in distant quadrant(s) within the same breast), or bilateral (disease in both breasts).

B. Common histologic types of breast cancer.

1. Non-invasive.
   a. **Ductal carcinoma *in situ* (DCIS)**—proliferation of malignant epithelial cells completely contained within breast ducts; more common than lobular carcinoma *in situ*; average age at diagnosis is mid-50s; approximately 80% of DCIS lesions are non-palpable and detected by screening mammography; occasionally may present with palpable mass; clustered microcalcifications may be seen on mammography; tends to be multicentric (35%); occult invasive carcinoma may co-exist with *in situ* lesion in 11-21% of cases; risk for subsequent invasive ductal carcinoma is approximately 25-30% and usually occurs within 10 years of diagnosis; size and extent of DCIS appears to correlate with incidence of multicentricity and synchronous invasive foci as well as risk for progression to invasive carcinoma. *Considered a premalignant lesion.*
   b. **Lobular carcinoma *in situ* (LCIS)**—proliferation of malignant epithelial cells completely contained within breast lobules; the average age of diagnosis is mid-40s; two-thirds of women with LCIS are pre-menopausal at diagnosis; estrogens are hypothesized to play an important role in the pathogenesis of LCIS; does not form a palpable mass; no mammographic findings; usually discovered incidentally upon biopsy for another abnormality; identified in approximately 4% of biopsy specimens obtained for benign disease; tends to be bilateral and multicentric; LCIS identified in contralateral breast in 50-90% of cases;

risk for subsequent invasive carcinoma (usually ductal) is approximately 20% in the ipsilateral breast and about the same in the contralateral breast; invasive carcinoma usually occurs more than 15 years after diagnosis. *Considered a marker for increased risk of invasive disease.*

2. Invasive.
   a. **Infiltrating ductal carcinoma**—most common breast malignancy (80%); originates from ductal epithelium and infiltrates supporting stroma; less common forms include medullary carcinoma, colloid carcinoma, tubular carcinoma, and papillary carcinoma.
   b. **Invasive lobular carcinoma**—accounts for 8-10% of all invasive breast malignancies; originates from lobular epithelium and infiltrates supporting stroma; does not form microcalcifications; more apt to be bilateral; may have slightly better prognosis.
   c. **Paget's disease of the nipple**—accounts for 1-3% of all breast malignancies; usually associated with intraductal carcinoma (DCIS) or invasive carcinoma just beneath the nipple; malignant cells invade across epithelial-epidermal junction and enter epidermis of the nipple; results in eczematous change in the nipple with crusting, scaling, erosion, or discharge, with or without associated breast mass.
   d. **Inflammatory breast carcinoma**—accounts for 1-4% of all breast malignancies; most rapidly lethal malignancy of the breast; poorly differentiated; characterized by dermal lymphatic invasion on pathological exam; presents as diffuse induration, erythema, warmth, edema, "peau de orange" of the skin of the breast, with or without palpable mass; axillary lymphadenopathy is almost always present; distant metastases common at time of diagnosis (17-36%).
3. Staging more important than histology in determining prognosis.
4. Other prognostic indicators include nuclear and histologic grade, presence or absence of estrogen and progesterone receptors, DNA content, and proliferative fraction (S-phase). Aneuploid tumors with high S-phase fraction tend to be more aggressive and carry poorer prognosis than diploid tumors with low S-phase fraction.

VII. SURGICAL TREATMENT OPTIONS

A. Wide local excision (WLE) / lumpectomy / segmental mastectomy.

1. Breast-conserving therapy.
2. Major objectives.
   a. Complete excision of tumor with tumor-free margins.
   b. Good cosmetic result.
3. Usually accompanied by axillary node dissection (through a separate incision) and radiation therapy to the whole breast

(approximately 5000 rads over 5-week period beginning 2-4 weeks post-operative), often with "boost" of radiation to tumor bed.

4. Eligibility criteria.
   a. Tumor size 4 cm or less.
   b. Appropriate tumor size to breast size ratio.
   c. No fixation of tumor to underlying muscle or chest wall.
   d. No involvement of overlying skin.
   e. No multicentric cancer (unless immediately juxtaposed).
   f. No fixed or matted axillary nodes.
5. For best cosmetic results, curvilinear incisions should be used in the upper quadrants, and radial incisions should be used in the lower quadrants.

B. Subcutaneous mastectomy.

1. Removes breast tissue only, sparing nipple-areolar complex, skin, and nodes.
2. Not a cancer operation–leaves 1-2% of breast tissue behind. Rarely, if ever, indicated.

C. Simple mastectomy (total mastectomy).

1. Removes breast tissue, nipple-areolar complex, and skin.
2. No axillary node dissection is performed.
3. Often performed for DCIS or LCIS.

D. Modified radical mastectomy (MRM).

1. Removes breast tissue, pectoralis fascia, nipple-areolar complex, skin, and axillary lymph nodes in continuity. Spares pectoralis major muscle.
2. ***Patey*** modification–preserves pectoralis major, but sacrifices the pectoralis minor in order to remove Levels I, II, and III axillary lymph nodes.
3. ***Auchincloss*** modification–preserves both pectoralis major and pectoralis minor. Preservation of pectoralis minor limits high axillary node dissection (Level III), but this does not appear to be clinically significant in most cases.

E. Radical mastectomy (Halsted) (RM).

1. Removes breast tissue, nipple-areolar complex, skin, pectoralis major and minor, and axillary lymph nodes in continuity.
2. Leaves bare chest wall with significant cosmetic and functional deformity.
3. Of historical interest only; clinical trials comparing modified radical mastectomy with radical mastectomy reveal no significant difference in disease-free survival, distant disease-free survival, or overall survival.

VIII. SURGICAL TREATMENT BY STAGE

A. Stage 0.

1. DCIS–total ipsilateral mastectomy *vs.* WLE plus radiation therapy (XRT). General agreement that axillary node dissection is not required for DCIS. Overall 5-year survival rate of

95-100% independent of whether treated by total mastectomy or WLE plus XRT.
2. LCIS–close observation *vs.* bilateral total mastectomy. Axillary node dissection is not required.
3. Clinically occult invasive carcinoma–MRM *vs.* WLE with axillary node dissection plus XRT.
4. Paget's disease–total mastectomy *vs.* MRM.

B. Stages I and II—represent approximately 85% of breast cancers.

1. Current treatment recommendations–MRM *vs.* WLE with axillary node dissection plus XRT.
2. Clinical trials have shown WLE with axillary node dissection plus XRT to be equivalent to MRM in terms of disease-free survival, distant disease-free survival, and overall survival.
3. WLE with axillary node dissection plus XRT offers breast conservation with clinical outcome equivalent to MRM.
4. Tumor-free margins are essential when WLE is performed.
5. Addition of XRT to WLE with axillary node dissection improves disease-free survival (e.g., decreased local-regional recurrence) but does not improve distant disease-free survival or overall survival in node-negative patients.
6. Adjuvant chemotherapy is indicated for node-positive patients and high-risk node-negative patients.
7. Factors associated with high risk of recurrence.
   a. Age < 35 years.
   b. Tumor size greater than 2 cm.
   c. Poor histologic and nuclear grade.
   d. Absence of estrogen and progesterone receptors.
   e. Aneuploid DNA content.
   f. High proliferative fraction (S-phase).
   g. Overexpression of epidermal growth factor receptor (EGF-2).
   h. Presence of cathepsin-D.
   i. Amplification of *c-erb* B-2 oncogene.
8. Lobular carcinoma–use of mirror-image biopsy or total mastectomy for the contralateral breast is controversial.
9. 5-year survival rates for Stages I and II breast cancer are approximately 80% and 60%, respectively.

C. Stages III and IV.

1. Multi-modality therapy including surgery, radiation therapy, and systemic therapy is usually employed.
2. Surgical therapy must be individualized based on extent of tumor and technical ease of resection. Role of breast conservation has not been specifically defined. Mastectomy (total or MRM) remains the mainstay of surgical therapy.
3. Pre-operative chemotherapy and local radiation therapy is under investigation as potential treatment for inflammatory breast carcinoma.
4. Goal of multi-modality therapy is control of local-regional

and distant disease. Even with aggressive therapy, however, most of these patients will die as a result of distant metastatic disease.

5. 5-year survival rates for Stages III and IV breast cancer are approximately 20% and 0%, respectively.

IX. CHEMOTHERAPY AND HORMONAL THERAPY

A. Surgery and radiation therapy—used to achieve local-regional control; chemotherapy and hormonal therapy are used to achieve systemic control.

B. Indications for chemotherapy or hormonal therapy— adjuvant therapy for node-positive patients and high-risk node-negative patients, and palliation for metastatic disease.

Nodes	Menopause	Size	Therapy
Positive nodes	pre-menopausal	any	CMF,CAF,AC
	pre-menopausal	any	CMF,CAF,AC
	post-menopausal	any	CMF,CAF,AC
	post-menopausal	any	tamoxifen
Negative Nodes	pre- or post-menopausal	<1 cm	none
	pre- or post-menopausal	1-2 cm	±CMF,CAF,AC
	pre- or post-menopausal	≥2 cm	CMF,CAF,AC
	pre- or post-menopausal	≥1 cm	tamoxifen

C = cyclophosphamide, M = methotrexate, F = 5-fluorouracil, A = adriamycin

1. Palliation for metastatic disease.
   a. Decision to offer systemic therapy for metastatic disease should be based on the extent and rate of progression of metastatic disease, hormone receptor status, degree and progression of symptoms, and the patient's ability to tolerate therapy without significant toxicity.
   b. Chemotherapy tends to have a shorter time to response (4-6 weeks *vs.* 8-12 weeks), better overall response rate (40-60% *vs.* 25-35%), shorter mean duration of action (8-12 months *vs.* 14-18 months), and increased toxicity compared to hormonal therapy.
   c. Chemotherapy should be considered for patients with hormone receptor negative tumors, aggressive metastatic disease, and the ability to tolerate side-effects of cytotoxic drugs.
   d. Hormonal therapy should be considered for patients with hormone receptor positive tumors and relatively indolent metastatic disease. Tamoxifen is the treatment of choice for most of these patients.

C. Cytotoxic chemotherapy.

1. Combination chemotherapy more effective than single-agent chemotherapy.
2. Associated with higher toxicity than hormonal therapy. May be poorly tolerated by elderly or debilitated patients.
3. Pre-menopausal patients tend to have better response to cytotoxic chemotherapy, whereas post-menopausal patients

tend to have better response to hormonal therapy. Difference in response is based on more aggressive nature of tumors in pre-menopausal patients (i.e., hormone receptor negative, aneuploid, high S-phase fraction), which increases likelihood of response to cytotoxic agents.

D. Hormonal therapy.

1. Indications.
   a. Adjuvant therapy for hormone receptor positive, pre- or post-menopausal, node-positive or high-risk node-negative patients.
   b. Palliative therapy for relatively indolent metastatic disease in pre-menopausal or post-menopausal patients with hormone receptor positive tumors.
2. Response to hormonal therapy depends on the status of hormone receptors.

Hormone Receptor Status

ER+,PgR+	ER+,PgR−	ER−,PgR+	ER−,PgR−
78%	34%	45%	10%

3. ***Tamoxifen*** is therapeutic agent of choice.
   a. Competitive antagonist of estrogen. Binds to estrogen receptors and prevents binding of estrogen.
   b. As effective as any other form of hormonal therapy, including oophorectomy.
   c. If chemotherapy is used, tamoxifen therapy should start after completion of chemotherapy.
   d. Tamoxifen therapy should be continued for at least 2 years.
   e. Role of tamoxifen prophylactically in patients at high risk for breast cancer is under investigation.
4. Alternatives to tamoxifen.
   a. Progestation agents (progestins).
   b. Luteinizing hormone-releasing (LHRH) analogues.
   c. Aminoglutethimide–aromatase inhibitor; decreases circulating levels of estrogen by blocking the peripheral conversion of androstenedione to estrogen (medical adrenalectomy).
   d. Anti-progestins–new class of drugs being evaluated in clinical trials.
   e. Oophorectomy–only indication is in the treatment of metastatic breast cancer in pre-menopausal, hormone receptor positive patients. Tamoxifen, however, has been shown to be equally effective and should be used first.

XI. BREAST CANCER AND PREGNANCY

A. Incidence of breast cancer detected during pregnancy—2 per 10,000 gestations, accounting for 2.8% of all breast cancers.

B. **Diagnosis** is more difficult and frequently delayed due to breast engorgement, tenderness, and increased nodularity.
C. **Suspicious masses detected during pregnancy** should undergo fine-needle aspiration or excisional biopsy.
D. **If malignancy is identified,** subsequent treatment decisions are influenced by specific trimester of pregnancy. Goal of treatment is cure of breast cancer without injury to fetus.
   1. Studies have demonstrated that termination of pregnancy in hopes of decreasing hormonal stimulation of tumor has no added benefit.
   2. For cancer detected during 1st and 2nd trimesters, modified radical mastectomy is the treatment of choice. Immediate breast reconstruction should not be performed, however, since a symmetric result is impossible until the postpartum appearance of the contralateral breast is known.
   3. Breast conservation therapy is complicated by fact that XRT is contraindicated in pregnancy. For cancer detected during 3rd trimester, wide local excision and axillary node dissection may be safely performed with XRT delayed until after delivery.
   4. For those requiring adjuvant chemotherapy, studies have shown no increased risk of fetal malformation for chemotherapy administered during the 2nd and 3rd trimesters. There is, however, an increased incidence of spontaneous abortion and congenital malformation associated with chemotherapy administered during the 1st trimester.

XII. MALE BREAST CANCER

A. Approximately 1% of that in women.
B. **Increased risk may be associated with hyperestrogenic states**—i.e., Klinefelter's syndrome, liver disease, use of exogenous estrogens (metastatic prostate cancer, transvestites). Low-dose radiation also implicated.
C. **Usually diagnosed at a later age than in women.** Mean age at diagnosis 60-65 years.
D. **Delay in diagnosis** may result in more advanced stage at presentation and worse prognosis.
E. **Infiltrating ductal carcinoma**—most common histologic type of breast cancer in males. Lobular carcinoma occurs very rarely.
F. **Because there is scant breast tissue in males,** pectoralis major muscle is more often involved.
G. **Node-negative disease**—prognosis similar to that in women. Node-positive disease–significantly worse prognosis than in women.
H. **Treatment**—depends on stage and local extent of tumor.
   1. If underlying pectoralis major muscle is involved, a radical mastectomy should be performed. Otherwise, MRM is procedure of choice.

2. Post-operative XRT may be considered because of local aggressiveness of these tumors. Improves local control, but does not affect survival.
3. Adjuvant chemotherapy or hormonal therapy should be offered to node-positive or high-risk node-negative patients. Since greater than 80% of male breast cancers are hormone receptor positive, tamoxifen may play an important role.

XIII. BREAST RECONSTRUCTION FOLLOWING MASTECTOMY

A. **Evidence**—There is no evidence to suggest that breast reconstruction following mastectomy compromises adjuvant chemotherapy, increases incidence of local recurrence, or delays diagnosis of recurrence on chest wall.

B. **Significantly improves patient's concept of body image.**

C. **Timing**—May be performed immediately or may be delayed until after completion of adjuvant chemotherapy or XRT. Recent trend is toward immediate reconstruction.

D. **Types of reconstructive procedures.**
1. Prosthetic breast implant–filled with silicone or saline; inserted subpectorally; disadvantage–presence of foreign body.
2. Myocutaneous flap reconstruction–more complicated procedure, but better long-term cosmetic results.
   a. Transverse rectus abdominus flap (TRAM)–based on superior mesenteric artery and vein; entire contralateral rectus abdominus muscle is transposed with transverse ellipse of skin and subcutaneous tissue from lower abdomen.
   b. Latissimus dorsi flap–based on thoracodorsal artery and vein.
   c. Free rectus abdominus flap–thoracodorsal or anterior serratus vessels are anastomosed to inferior epigastric vessels to maintain blood supply to flap.
   d. Greater omentum pedicle flap covered with a skin graft.
   e. Gluteus maximus free flap.
3. Nipple-areolar reconstruction may be performed as a secondary procedure following prosthetic breast implant or myocutaneous flap reconstruction. Typically delayed 6-12 weeks to allow reconstructed breast to attain its final shape and position.

E. **Complications of breast reconstruction.**
1. Infection.
2. Tissue loss–especially flap loss due to vascular compromise.
3. Poor cosmetic result.
4. Slippage of prosthetic implant or capsular contraction.

27

Thyroid

Scott M. Berry, M.D.

I. INTRODUCTION

A. Diseases of the thyroid gland are among the most common endocrine disorders seen by clinicians. They fall into three broad categories.

1. Hypofunction.
2. Hyperfunction.
3. Enlargements.
   a. Diffuse.
   b. Nodule.

B. Diffuse enlargement for any reason, regardless of functional status, is termed *goiter.*

II. THYROID FUNCTION TESTS

A. Clinical manifestations.

1. Hyperthyroidism is suggested by weight loss, irritability, heat intolerance, thinning hair, palpitations, tachycardia.
2. Hypothyroidism is suggested by weight gain, lethargy, coarse hair, cold intolerance, thick skin, slowed muscle reflexes, constipation, and slowed mentation.

B. The initial work-up of a patient suspected of hypo- or hyperthyroidism should consist of serum TSH, T_4, and T_3 radioiodine uptake. T_4 multiplied by T_3RU gives the free T_4 index (FT_4I, the level of circulating T_4 that has been corrected for changes in transport protein levels):

	Pituitary failure	Hypothyroid	Hyperthyroid
FT_4I	Low	Low	High
TSH	Low	High	Low

III. SURGICAL THYROID DISEASE

Surgeons are called upon to manage three types of thyroid disease: 1) enlargement causing compression; 2) certain types of hyperthyroidism; and 3) thyroid nodules.

A. Compression.

1. Dyspnea, dysphagia, tracheal or esophageal deviation clinically or radiographically are indications for surgical debulking of the goiter.
2. Chest and neck radiographs along with thyroid function tests should be obtained.
3. Compression symptoms suggest substernal extension of thyroid. CT scan of neck and chest may be indicated.

B. Hyperthyroidism.

1. Surgical management is indicated for Graves' disease, toxic multi-nodular goiter, and toxic solitary nodule. In all 3 entities the medical control of thyrotoxicosis is crucial if thyroid storm is to be prevented.
   a. Propylthiouracil (PTU)–300-600 ng/day 6-8 weeks preoperative.
   b. Propranolol–40-480 mg/day 6-8 weeks pre-operative.
   c. SSKI or Lugol's–1-2 drops TID 1 week pre-operative.
2. Graves' disease–total thyroidectomy will cure Graves' disease, with 100% postoperatove hypothyroidism; leaving a 6-8 g remnant will cure 96% of patients, with post-operative hypothyroidism in 20-30%.
3. Toxic multinodular goiter–bilateral subtotal lobectomies.
4. Toxic solitary nodule–lobectomy.
5. ***Thyroid storm***—can be induced in hyperthyroid patient by any stress, especially surgery.
   a. Symptoms–hyperpyrexia, tachycardia, numbness, irritability, vomiting, diarrhea, and proximal muscle weakness. Cause of death is usually high-output cardiac failure.
   b. Treatment–mechanical cooling, oxygen and volume resuscitation, 100 mg hydrocortisone IVPB to prevent adrenal insufficiency, propranolol 1-2 mg IVP followed by 50-100 μg/min IV drip to control symptoms, IV sodium iodide (1-2.5 g), and q 2 h glucose management with D_{50} for blood sugars < 100. PTU therapy should begin during acute management.

C. Nodules.

1. 4-8% of the U.S. population have palpable nodules.
2. 20-30% of these nodules are malignant. The differential diagnoses include the following.
   a. Adenoma.
   b. Cyst.
   c. Thyroiditis.
   d. Graves' disease.
   e. Teratoma.
   f. Metastasis to thyroid.
   g. Thyroid carcinoma.
3. Most metastatic tumors to thyroid are breast, lung, kidney, and melanoma.
4. Clinical characteristics that suggest malignancy:

a. Male gender.
b. Age < 15, > 60 years.
c. History of head and neck radiation.
d. Family history of thyroid cancer.
e. Rapidly enlarging nodule.
f. Single nodule.
g. History of thyroiditis.
h. Hoarseness.
i. Cervical adenopathy.

5. Physical exam–stand behind the patient and have them swallow some water to help palpate thyroid masses. Thyroid masses move with swallowing because of the tracheal attachment. Note size, consistency, tenderness, and nodularity of the gland.
6. Thyroid function tests, thyroid scanning with ^{123}I, and ultrasound will not differentiate benign from malignant lesions.
7. Fine needle aspiration is the single most useful test in evaluating thyroid nodules.
   a. Insert 20- to 22-ga. needle.
   b. Apply suction and fan needle.
   c. Release suction, then remove needle.
   d. Expel contents onto slide and fix.
   e. Results.
      (1) 7% non-diagnostic.
      (2) Reliable for all cancers except follicular; because the cytology of follicular adenoma and follicular carcinoma are the same, determination of capsular or vascular invasion is necessary to differentiate the two.
      (3) Surgical excision is necessary for follicular neoplasms.
      (4) Intermediate lesions have a 20-60% malignancy rate.
      (5) Positive cytology is diagnostic except in follicular neoplasms.
      (6) There is a 20% false-negative rate; thus, if malignancy is suspected clinically, negative cytology should never delay or deter surgical excision.
8. Thyroid cancer is the most common endocrine malignancy in the U.S.–4/100,000 population.
   a. Papillary carcinoma–70%. Slow-growing, 60% multicentric, male:female 1:3, 80-90% of post-radiation cancers of the thyroid, spread by lymphatics (50% have positive nodes at diagnosis). Presence of nodes does *not* affect prognosis.
      (1) Lobectomy with isthmusectomy unless tumor is > 3 cm, male > 40, female > 50, distant metastasis or angioinvasion. Total thyroidectomy is then indicated because of poor prognosis.
      (2) 85% 10-year survival.
   b. Follicular carcinoma–10%. More aggressive, unifocal, male:female 1:3, angioinvasive, metastasis to lung and bone.

   (1) Total thyroidectomy is indicated.
   (2) 40% 10-year survival.

c. Mixed papillary-follicular carcinoma behaves and is treated like papillary carcinoma.

d. Hürthle cell tumor–5%. Intermediate, unifocal, male:female 2:1, spread by lymphatics.
   (1) Thallium scan for metastatic localization.
   (2) Does not take up ^{131}I, so surgery is only chance for cure; total thyroidectomy is indicated.
   (3) 60% 10-year survival.

e. Lymphoma–5%. Usually intermediate lymphomas, usually affects females, may have history of Hashimoto's; rapid enlargement, compressive symptoms common.
   (1) Chemotherapy and radiotherapy sensitive.
   (2) Surgery for diagnosis and compressive symptoms.
   (3) 80% 5-year survival if confined to gland, 40% if tumor has spread.

f. Medullary thyroid cancer–7%. Aggressive tumors, 90% sporadic, 10% in association with MEN-II; amyloid stroma histologically, 95% produce calcitonin, 85% produce carcinoembryonic antigen (CEA). Sporadic form is unifocal, occurs around 45 years of age, and carries a worse prognosis. Familial form is multifocal, occurs around 35 years of age, and carries a better prognosis. C-cell hyperplasia is the precursor to medullary thyroid cancer in MEN-II.
   (1) Does not concentrate ^{131}I.
   (2) Thallium, MIBG, DMSA are used to localize metastatic disease if calcitonin begins to rise.
   (3) All patients with medullary thyroid cancer should be screened for pheochromocytoma (MEN-II), which should be resected first.
   (4) Total thyroidectomy is indicated.

g. Anaplastic carcinoma–3%. Very aggressive, 30% develop in a well-differentiated carcinoma. Must differentiate from lymphoma.
   (1) Chemotherapy and radiation may improve 5% survival.
   (2) Mean survival 2-4 months.

D. Post-operative care.

1. Position patient with elevated head of bed, provide cool misted oxygen.
2. Hypocalcemia–calcium is checked post-operatively, then q 8 h x 24 h, then q day.
3. Hypothyroidism.
   a. Synthroid® replacement 1 μg/lb to prevent hypothyroidism and suppress TSH (a growth factor for well-differentiated cancers–papillary, follicular, mixed and Hürthle cell).
   b. Hold Synthroid® prior to post-operative iodine scan (per-

formed 2-3 months post-operatively) so TSH will be elevated and residual or metastatic tissue will have maximal stimulation for iodine uptake.

c. Liothyronine (Cytomel®–75 μg/day) is given as thyroid replacement in the interim, then discontinued 2 weeks before scan.

4. Have tracheostomy tray available in case of airway compromise.

E. Complications.

1. Vocal cord paralysis due to recurrent laryngeal nerve damage 1% if nerve visualized, 4% if nerve is "avoided".
2. Hypoparathyroidism in total thyroidectomy–1-2% permanent, 10-20% temporary.
3. Hypothyroidism–100% in total thyroidectomy, 20-30% if 6-8 g of tissue are left.
4. Pneumothorax–infrequent.
5. Wound hematoma–if this occurs and patient has respiratory distress, open the wound at the bedside.

28

Parathyroid

SCOTT M. BERRY, M.D.

I. PRIMARY HYPERPARATHYROIDISM

A. One or more glands elaborate inappropriately increased amounts of parathyroid hormone (PTH) relative to the serum calcium level.

B. Occurs in 1:1000 population, recently diagnosed more frequently because of availability of routine serum calcium determinations.

C. Three histologic patterns.

1. Single adenoma–90% of cases. A rim of normal parathyroid tissue around the adenoma distinguishes adenoma from hyperplasia.
2. Hyperplasia–10% of cases. No rim of normal tissue and lack of stromal fat. All 4 glands are involved. The hyperparathyroidism of MEN syndromes is due to hyperplasia.
3. Parathyroid carcinoma–< 1% of cases. Exceptionally high calcium or palpable neck mass should raise suspicion. Excision with thyroid lobectomy indicated. Radical neck dissection for recurrent disease. Recur locally 30%; distant metastasis to lung, liver, and bone in 30%.

D. Clinical presentation.

1. 70% are asymptomatic.
2. "Stones"–nephrolithiasis or nephrocalcinosis, but never both. Present in 10-20% of patients, usually calcium phosphate. Calcium oxalate less common.
3. "Bones"–bone pain, arthralgias, and muscular aches.
   a. Present in 20% of symptomatic patients.
   b. Cortical resorption with medullary bone sparing secondary to increased turnover.
   c. Osteitis fibrosa cystica is a condition in which resorption leads to "Brown cysts" in the bone. Predisposes to fractures.
4. "Groans"–peptic ulcer disease and pancreatitis. Present in 20% of symptomatic patients.

5. "Psychic overtones"–fatigue, depression, anxiety, irritability, lack of concentration, and sleep disturbances.
   a. Present in 40% of symptomatic patients.
   b. No relationship of PTH or calcium levels to the severity of symptoms.
   c. Surgery improves all symptoms except anxiety.

E. Physical exam.

1. Usually not helpful in diagnosis.
2. If a mass is palpable, suspect thyroid pathology or parathyroid carcinoma.

F. Laboratory exam.

1. Hypercalcemia, hypophosphatemia, and hypercalcuria are the classic hallmarks of hyperparathyroidism.
2. With the availability of PTH assay, the diagnosis is made when PTH levels are elevated relative to the serum ionized calcium level, which need not be markedly elevated and may fall into the upper limit of normal.
   a. The N terminal of PTH confers the biologic effect–half-life is minutes.
   b. C terminal is inactive, but better for determining hyperparathyroidism–half-life is 1-2 h.
   c. Elevated PTH levels may occur with renal failure and do not necessarily imply hyperparathyroidism.
   d. The humoral hypercalcemia of malignancy (hypercalcemia without bone metastasis) is mediated by PTH-like molecules that are not picked up on serum PTH assays, except with ovarian cancer, which may produce intact PTH.
3. Serum phosphorus is low in primary hyperparathyroidism, high in secondary hyperparathyroidism.
4. Chloride is high secondary to renal HCO_3 wasting (direct effect of PTH).
   a. Chloride to phosphorus ratio of > 33 is diagnostic of primary hyperparathyroidism.
   b. "Poor man's" parathyroid hormone assay.
5. Malignancy with or without bone metastasis is the cause of > 50% of hypercalcemia (hematologic, lung, pancreas, bone, ovary, breast, and prostate).
6. Other causes of hypercalcemia.
   a. Endocrine disorders–hyperthyroidism, adrenal insufficiency, pheochromocytoma.
   b. Vitamin D toxicity.
   c. Lymphomas with ectopic vitamin D_3 production.
   d. Granulomatous disease–sarcoidosis, tuberculosis, histoplasmosis, coccidioidomycosis, leprosy.
   e. Drugs–thiazides, lithium, milk alkali syndrome.
   f. Immobilization.
7. Only 20% of hypercalcemia is caused by hyperparathyroidism.
8. The serum calcium may be intermittently normal with hyperparathyroidism, so 3 separate determinations should be made.

G. Radiographic exam—may show subperiosteal resorption in the classic distribution on the radial aspect of the 2nd and 3rd phalanges, distal phalangeal tufts, and distal clavicles.

1. Solitary bone cysts (Brown tumors).
2. Intravenous pyelogram may show urolithiasis or nephrocalcinosis.

H. Medical treatment of hypercalcemic crisis.

1. Symptoms include anorexia, nausea, vomiting, polyuria, polydipsia, abdominal pain, lethargy, bone pain, and muscular weakness.
2. If untreated may progress to dehydration, oliguria, acute tubular necrosis, and delirium within hours.
3. Rapid rehydration with normal saline to restore urine output.
4. Following rehydration, begin forced diuresis with furosemide drip (10-20 mg/h).
5. Steroids may be useful in hypercalcemic crisis due to malignancy.
6. Etridonate disodium 7.5 mg/kg IV daily for 3 days followed by 5-20 mg/kg PO daily inhibits bone metabolism in hypercalcemia of malignancy. This should not be used in renal failure patients.
7. Mithramycin may be used as a last resort. If used improperly, can lead to aplastic anemia (25 μg/kg over 4 h IVPB).
8. Dialysis can be used to lower serum calcium emergently.
9. Surgery is treatment for the hypercalcemia of hyperparathyroidism, but only after hydration with adequate urine output is established.

I. Surgical indications.

1. Parathyroid carcinoma.
2. Asymptomatic patients with the following conditions.
    a. Persistent calcium elevation 1-1.6 mg/dl above normal.
    b. Calciuria > 400 mg/d.
    c. Decreased bone density > 2 standard deviation points from normal for age, sex, and race.
    d. Creatinine clearance decrease by 30% below normal for age, sex, and race.
3. Symptomatic patients.
    a. Urolithiasis or nephrocalcinosis.
    b. Peptic ulcer disease.
    c. Pancreatitis.
    d. Musculoskeletal symptoms.
4. With single adenoma, resection is curative.
5. For hyperplasia, 3.5 gland resection or 4 gland resection with 0.5 gland reimplanted in the forearm or sternocleidomastoid muscle is indicated.
6. For parathyroid carcinoma, wide excision including involved structures is indicated.
7. Initial exploration is successful in 90-95% of cases without preoperative localization studies.

8. Ectopic locations.
   a. Thymic–substernal–20%.
   b. Posterior neck–5-10%.
   c. Intrathyroid–5%.
   d. Carotid sheath–1%.
   e. Anterior mediastinum–1-2%.
9. If initial exploration fails, localization studies are indicated.
   a. Ultrasound–80% accuracy for glands as small as 3 mm. Will not detect mediastinal tumors.
   b. CT scan/MRI–will detect mediastinal tumors > 2 cm.
   c. Thallium-technetium subtraction scan–80% accuracy.
   d. Arteriography–50% accuracy.
   e. Selective venous sampling for PTH–70% accuracy.

J. Post-operative care.

1. Tracheostomy tray to bedside in case of hematoma causing airway compromise.
2. Recurrent laryngeal nerve palsy 1-3%–only 10% of these are permanent.
3. Hypocalcemia is common and occurs almost immediately.
   a. Serum calcium in PACU, then q 8 h x 24 h, then q AM.
   b. Symptoms–anxiety, hyperventilation, Chvostek's and Trousseau's signs, acral and circumoral paraesthesias.
   c. Some advocate treating only symptomatic hypocalcemia.
   d. Treat hypocalcemia with oral calcium carbonate 1 g PO q 6 h, or IV calcium gluconate for severe hypocalcemia (< 7.0).
   e. Vitamin D supplementation may be necessary for refractory hypocalcemia.

II. SECONDARY HYPERPARATHYROIDISM

A. Hyperparathyroidism secondary to malfunction of another organ system.

B. Usually occurs in patients with chronic renal failure, but may also be due to osteogenesis imperfecta, Paget's disease, or multiple myeloma.

1. Pathophysiology in renal failure is increased phosphate because of poor renal excretion leading to decreased serum calcium, decreased gut absorption of calcium due to decreased renal l-hydroxylation of vitamin D_2, and decreased renal clearance of PTH breakdown products.
2. Clinically manifests as psychiatric disorders, headache, muscle weakness, weight loss, fatigue, renal osteodystrophy (bone resorption with pathologic fractures), and soft-tissue calcifications (vessels, tendons, joint sheaths).

C. Treatment is directed at underlying disorder–phosphate-binding antacids, oral calcium, and vitamin D, increased calcium dialysate for chronic renal insufficiency patients.

D. Surgery is indicated for uncontrolled symptoms–either 3.5 gland parathyroidectomy or 4 gland parathyroidectomy with implantation of minced glands into sternocleidomastoid or forearm muscles marked by a surgical clip.

III. TERTIARY HYPERPARATHYROIDISM

A. **Persistent hyperparathyroidism and hypercalcemia** following successful renal transplant or resolution of underlying disorder.

B. **Occurs in up to 30% of patients who have pretransplant hyperparathyroidism.**

C. **Pathophysiology**—irreversible parathyroid gland hyperplasia with autonomous PTH production.

D. **Surgery**—indicated for symptomatic patients or patients unresponsive to medical management 6 months post-transplant–either 3.5 gland or 4 gland parathyroidectomy with implantation of minced glands into muscle.

29

The Adrenal Gland

Michael A. Helmrath, M.D.

I. EMBRYOLOGY

A. Cortex.

1. Derived from mesoderm of the urogenital ridge.
2. During fetal development the cortex has a thick inner "fetal zone" and a thin outer neocortex. During development the inner zone produces steroids, which are converted into estrogens by the placenta.
3. At mid-gestation the adrenal is larger than the kidney.
4. The inner zone involutes shortly after birth, and only the outer cortex persists.

B. Medulla (ectoderm).

1. At the 20th week of gestation, cells from the neural crest invade the cortex to form the medulla.
2. Neuroblasts also arrive and form sympathetic ganglia.

II. ANATOMY (Figure 1).

A. Inner medulla surrounded by outer cortex. Cortex is divided into three layers, with each producing different hormones.

1. Zona Glomerulosa–aldosterone.
2. Zona Fasciculata–androgens, cortisol.
3. Zona Reticularis–estrogens, androgens, cortisol.

B. Vascular supply.

1. Arterial supply–inferior phrenic, renal, and aorta.
2. Venous drainage is the IVC on the right, and the renal vein on the left.

III. PHYSIOLOGY

A. The hypothalamic-pituitary-adrenal axis—Corticotropin-releasing hormone (CRF) is released from the anterior hypothalamus, which stimulates the anterior pituitary gland to secrete adrenocorticotropic hormone (ACTH).

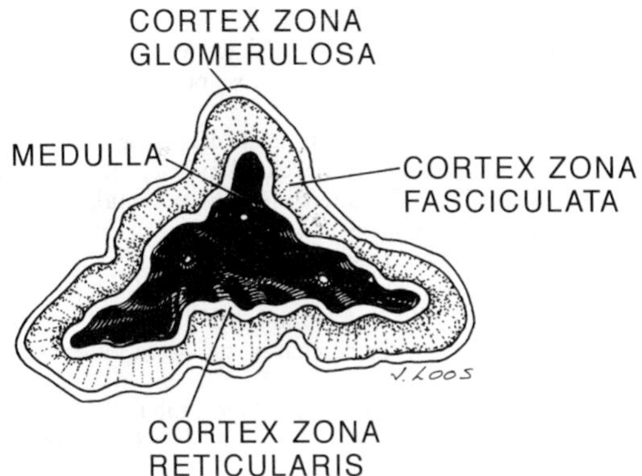

FIG. 1

1. ACTH and melanocyte-stimulating hormone (MSH) derive from a large precursor molecule (POMC).
2. ACTH stimulates the adrenal gland to secrete cortisol and mineralocorticoids.

B. The adrenal cortex gland makes three classes of hormones—glucocorticoids, mineralocorticoids, androgens.

1. All cortical hormones are derived from cholesterol.
2. Hormones circulate in bound and unbound forms.
3. Free steroid hormones enter the cytosol and bind with receptors; then, the complex enters the nucleus to bind to DNA and activate mRNA synthesis.

C. Cortisol.

1. 75% bound to transcortin (increases with pregnancy or exogenous estrogens), 15% bound to albumin, 10% unbound (active form).
2. Circadian rhythm–highest in AM, lowest in PM.
3. Metabolized by the liver (90 min half-life).
4. Metabolites, 17-hydroxy/ketosteroids, cleared by kidneys.
5. Effects of cortisol.
   a. Increased gluconeogenesis, proteolysis, lipolysis.
   b. Increased free fatty acids, triglycerides.
   c. Increased glycogen deposition in the liver.
   d. Decreased glucose uptake peripherally.
   e. Anabolic in the liver, catabolic peripherally.
   f. Immunosuppressant.
   g. Anti-inflammatory (stabilizes lysosomal membranes).
   h. Decreased wound healing.
   i. Increased bone reabsorption.

D. Adrenal sex steroids.

1. Androgens from the adrenal guide fetal development of the external genitalia, vas deferens, prostate, and epididymis (Wolffian system).
2. Postnatally, androgens stimulate deepening of voice, phallus growth, development of skeletal muscle, and body hair.
3. Estrogen from the adrenal in females stimulates breast and vaginal development.

E. Mineralocorticoid—aldosterone.

1. From the zona glomerulosa.
2. Degraded by the liver (15 min half-life).
3. Secretion from the adrenal is stimulated by angiotensin II and K+ increase.
4. Aldosterone acts on the distal renal tubule to increase Na+ reabsorption with loss of K+ and H+ (sodium-potassium pump).

F. Physiology of the adrenal medulla.

1. Tyrosine is converted into L-dopa, then dopamine, then norepinephrine, then epinephrine.
   a. 80% of catecholamines are stored as epinephrine, 20% as norepinephrine.
   b. Release is under sympathetic control. The medulla receives preganglionic sympathetic innervation from the splanchnic plexus.
   c. Activity of catecholamines.
      (1) Increase glycogenolysis.
      (2) Increase gluconeogenesis.
      (3) Increase glucagon secretion.
      (4) Decrease glucose uptake.
2. The medulla receives blood rich in glucocorticoids from the cortex, which influences catecholamine secretion.
3. Systemic catecholamine receptors.
   a. Alpha receptor affinity–NE > EPI > ISO.
   b. Alpha-1–cause vasoconstriction, pupillary dilatation, uterine contractions.
   c. Alpha-2–causes norepinephrine release at synapses and platelet aggregation.
   d. Beta receptor affinity–ISO > EPI > NE
   e. Beta-1–cardiac stimulation, lipolysis, intestinal relaxation.
   f. Beta-2–bronchodilation, vasodilation, uterine relaxation.
4. Catecholamines are cleared by the urine, by peripheral enzymatic degradation, and by uptake at nerve endings.
   a. The monoamine oxidase (MAO) system of the liver, kidney, intestine, and stomach clears norepinephrine.
   b. Metabolites of catecholamines: normetanephrine, metanephrine, vanillylmandelic acid (VMA), and methoxyhydroxyphenylglycol (MHPG).

IV. DISEASES OF THE ADRENAL CORTEX

A. Cushing's syndrome.

1. Described in 1932 by Harvey Cushing.
2. Hypercortisolism either from over-production of cortisol independently from the adrenal or secondary to increased ACTH from the pituitary or an ectopic site.
3. Affects women 9 times as often as men.
4. ***Symptoms***—centripetal obesity, moon facies, buffalo hump, acne, purple striae, hirsutism, weakness, menstrual irregularity, increased blood pressure, glucose intolerance, pancreatitis, peptic ulcer disease.
5. Causes of hypercortisolism.
   a. Pituitary–Hypercortisolism from a pituitary adenoma with increased secretion of ACTH is called Cushing's disease. This is the most common cause of hypercorticolism (60-70%).
   b. Adrenocortical–adrenal adenomas cause 10-20% of Cushing's syndrome. Of these cases, 10% are bilateral.
   c. Ectopic ACTH production–an additional 10-15% of hypercorticalism originates from ectopic ACTH production. This patients do not appear "cushingoid"; rather, they are cachectic from their underlying cancer. Etiologies include the following.
      (1) Lung (small cell) 50%.
      (2) Pancreatic 10%.
      (3) Thymoma 10%.
   d. Diagnosis is based on very high ACTH levels, as well as increased cortisol and 17-ketosteroid levels.
   e. Adrenocortical carcinoma–rare cause of Cushing's syndrome. Aggressive tumor with poor prognosis. Most are secretory (60%) and many are palpable at presentation (50%).
6. ***Diagnosis*** (See algorithm below).
   a. Cortisol levels–serum increased in 80%.
   b. Can screen by checking urinary free cortisol levels.
   c. A more accurate test is a 24-h urinary free cortisol level.
   d. Urinary levels of 17-hydroxycorticosteroids.
   e. Low-dose dexamethasone suppression test–dexamethasone is stronger suppressant to ACTH secretion than cortisol. 2 mg dose given night before. Morning cortisol (or 17-hydroxycorticosteroid) is low in normal individuals, not suppressed in Cushing's syndrome (from any etiology).
   f. Tests to localize the cause.
      (1) ACTH–high in pituitary disease, extremely high if from an ectopic site, low in adrenal disease.
      (2) High-dose dexamethasone suppression–given over 24 h. Will only suppress pituitary adenomas (50% of adenomas). If cortisol not suppressed, suspect ectopic ACTH production or an adrenal adenoma.

(3) Metyrapone stimulation test–inhibits the enzymatic production of cortisol, causing increase in ACTH and urinary excretion of cortisol precursors in normal individuals. In hypercortisolism from a pituitary abnormality (adenoma), ACTH increases as well as cortisol precursors. In hypercortisolism from primary adrenal abnormality, no change in precursors is noted.

(4) CRH–administration of CRH should cause a slight increase in cortisol levels. With Cushing's disease, levels are markedly increased. With ectopic ACTH secretion or adrenal adenomas, there is no change.

7. ***Treatment.***
   a. Pituitary–trans-sphenoidal hypophysectomy for tumors < 1 cm allows pituitary function to be preserved in many cases. Transfrontal resection for tumors extending outside the sella turcica. Radiation is used if the tumor is unresectable. Bilateral adrenalectomy was used in the past for unresectable disease. Pharmacologic therapy occasionally used pre- or early post-operatively to control cortisol levels.
   b. Adrenal–adrenalectomy curative for adrenal adenomas. Posterior approach is associated with decreased morbidity. If cancer is a possibility, an anterior approach is indicated. Must cover with steroids peri-operatively (hydrocortisone IV). Contralateral adrenal function may take weeks to recover. For bilateral adrenal hyperplasia, bilateral adrenalectomy is indicated.
8. Cushing's syndrome in children.
   a. Most common cause is a neoplasia; the majority are malignant.
   b. Affects females more than males (3:1).

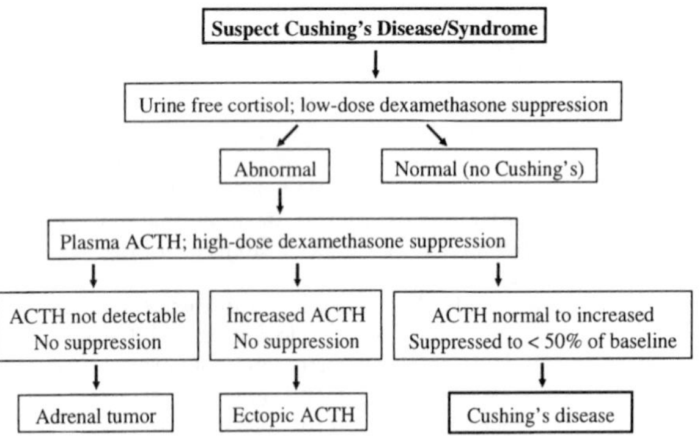

c. Cushing's disease and ectopic ACTH production are rare in children.

9. Nelson's syndrome–complication found in 10% of patients after bilateral adrenalectomy. ACTH and MSH levels are increased, causing an increase in skin pigmentation.

B. Conn's syndrome—low renin hyperaldosteronism.

1. Surgical cause of hypertension, although hypertension is not as severe as seen in renovascular hypertension.
2. Diagnosis.
   a. Suggested by hypertension, hypokalemia, metabolic alkalosis (40% of hypertensive patients with hypokalemia have Conn's syndrome).
   b. Serum renin and aldosterone levels (to distinguish from renovascular hypertension).
   c. 24-h urine collection for aldosterone.
   d. Sometimes a high-sodium diet or an IV infusion of $Na+$ is used to further elevate the aldosterone level to make the diagnosis (95% sensitivity).
3. Differential diagnosis of decreased renin and increased aldosterone.
   a. Adrenocortical adenoma.
   b. Bilateral adrenal hyperplasia.
   c. Adrenal carcinoma.
   d. Aldosterone-secreting ovarian tumor.
4. 80% are single adrenal adenomas; 15% are bilateral adrenal hyperplasia. These must be distinguished, since only 20% of patients with hyperplasia are cured surgically. CT/MRI can distinguish bilateral/unilateral disease.
5. To distinguish adenomas from hyperplasia, check renin/aldosterone levels 2 h after being in a recumbent position, then after walking 4 h:
   a. Adrenal hyperplasia: increase in renin and aldosterone after walking.
   b. Adenoma: decreased renin/aldosterone.
   c. 18-hydroxycorticosterone levels increased with adenomas, normal with hyperplasia.
6. Management.
   a. Non-operative therapy–spironolactone opposes the action of aldosterone. Can cause gynecomastia and hyperkalemia. Treatment of choice for bilateral adrenal hyperplasia.
   b. For adenomas, adrenalectomy on the affected side is curative.

C. Adrenogenital syndromes.

1. Definition–syndrome of salt wasting and ambiguous genitalia arising from enzymatic deficiencies of cortisol synthesis.
   a. Low cortisol allows ACTH levels to rise, stimulating the adrenal gland to produce more cortisol precursors.

b. Androgens cause virilization (increased phallus size, muscle mass, body hair) in males, usually presenting at puberty. Males can present in infancy with salt wasting and hypertension.
c. Females present at birth with ambiguous genitalia (fused labia, enlarged clitoris) but normal internal reproductive organs.
d. When children present later, they often have an early period of rapid growth followed by premature closure of growth plates (short stature).

2. 21-Hydroxylase deficiency.
   a. Most common enzymatic deficiency in these patients (94%).
   b. Common in Eskimos.
   c. Presentation–virilizing in females, precocious sexual development in males. A complete lack of the enzyme presents with salt wasting (40%).
   d. Diagnosed by low cortisol levels and increased 17-hydroxyprogesterone.
   e. Treatment–aldosterone and cortisol replacement.
3. 11-Hydroxylase deficiency.
   a. 5% of individuals with adrenogenital syndrome.
   b. Present with hyperpigmentation, virilization, hypertension, and low cortisol.

D. Adrenal neoplasms associated with increased sex steroids.

1. Virilizing tumors.
   a. Females more often affected (2:1).
   b. Usually present after the first year of life as clitoral enlargement, increased pubic hair in girls, enlarged phallus, hirsutism in males.
   c. Tumors secrete androgen precursors.
   d. These slow-growing tumors must be excised because they do not suppress with dexamethasone.
2. Feminizing adrenal tumors.
   a. Rare tumors that present with bilateral gynecomastia, rapid growth, and increased bone age in young males (20-40 years).
   b. Diagnosed by increased 17-ketosteroids, estrogens.
   c. Women present with precocious puberty and an abdominal mass.
   d. Half are benign.

E. Adrenocortical insufficiency (Addison's disease).

1. Bilateral adrenal cortical destruction.
   a. Chronic steroid use with suppression of the adrenal gland is the most common etiology.
   b. Most common non-iatrogenic etiology–idiopathic. Presumed to be autoimmune mediated (associated with hyperthyroidism, diabetes mellitus).

c. Females more often affected (2:1).
d. Tuberculosis found in 20% of patients.
e. Metastatic carcinomas (lung) can cause Addison's disease.

2. Clinical presentation.
   a. Fatigue, weight loss, anorexia, nausea/emesis, abdominal pain, diarrhea, hyperpigmentation.
   b. Decreased Na+, increased K+, azotemia, hypoglycemia, increased calcium.
3. Diagnosis.
   a. Can present in "Addisonian crisis" with fever, abdominal pain, hypotension, vomiting, lethargic.
   b. Can occur after stopping steroids, stress, infection, hemorrhage, Waterhouse-Friderichsen syndrome.
   c. Cortisol levels low.
4. Treated acutely with 100 mg hydrocortisone, then chronic replacement.

F. Adrenocortical carcinoma.

1. Rare tumor with very poor prognosis.
2. Males = females, usually in 40s.
3. Most (75%) are functional.
4. Presentation: abdominal pain, mass, anemia, fever, virilization, feminization.
5. Diagnosis.
   a. Assess if functional: urine cortisol, serum ACTH, low-dose dexamethasone test.
   b. Most are > 5 cm, seen on CT.
   c. T2 MRI images can distinguish carcinoma from adenomas.
   d. Chest radiographs, CT liver to rule out metastatic disease.
   e. Malignant *vs.* benign–histologically can be difficult to distinguish. Likely malignant if large, metastatic, local invasion.
6. Treatment.
   a. 60% are metastatic at diagnosis.
   b. *En bloc* resection (often includes nephrectomy).
   c. Non-surgical.
      (1) Most patients benefit from debulking.
      (2) Mitotane improves symptoms, but has many side-effects and often requires steroid replacement.
      (3) Radiation/chemotherapy have no proven roles.
7. Results–25% 5-year survival. 40% if localized disease.

V. PHEOCHROMOCYTOMA

A. Clinical presententation—hypertension, headaches, and palpitations.

1. Equally affects males, females, age 20-50.
2. Hypertension (50-70%) usually sustained. Episodes can be elicited by physical exertion and emotional stress and can last 15-30 min.

3. Episodes also associated with consumption of foods rich in tyramine: beer, wine, cheese.
4. Nonfunctioning tumors are rare.
5. 10-20% of pheochromocytomas are:
   a. Malignant.
   b. Extra-adrenal in location.
   c. Multiple.
   d. Associated with other conditions (MEN II, neurofibromatosis 1).
   e. In children.
6. Associated conditions.
   a. MEN IIa–medullary carcinoma of the thyroid, parathyroid hyperplasia, pheochromocytoma. Autosomal dominant, with all affected individuals developing MTC. 50% develop parathyroid hyperplasia or pheochromocytomas.
   b. MEN IIb–MTC, pheochromocytomas, mucosal neuromas, ganglioneuromatosis. Rare syndromes, autosomal dominant or sporadic.
   c. Neurocutaneous disorders–5-10% of patients with pheochromocytomas have neurofibromatosis. Also associated with tuberous sclerosis, Sturge-Weber syndrome, and von Hippel-Lindau syndrome.
7. Pheochromocytoma in pregnancy.
   a. Associated with a 50% fetal mortality.
   b. If condition unknown, 60% maternal mortality. If known, 18% mortality.
   c. Can cause hypertensive crisis up to 48 h postpartum.
   d. Can be excised if diagnosed before third trimester or alpha blockade can be initiated and the child carried to term.
   e. Child should be delivered by C-section and the tumor excised immediately.
8. Pheochromocytoma in childhood.
   a. Males most commonly affected.
   b. 10% of pheochromocytomas in individuals < 20 years.
   c. 40% bilateral, and more often extra-adrenal.
   d. Presents with sweating, hypertension, polyuria, polydypsia.
9. Malignant pheochromocytomas.
   a. 10-20% are malignant.
   b. Females affected (3:1).
   c. Hypertension, symptoms more consistent if malignant.
   d. Associated with extra-adrenal pheochromocytomas.
   e. Associated with increased dopamine levels.
   f. Malignancy determined by demonstration of metastases or local invasion since difficult to determine histologically.
   g. Should always be resected, even if only to debulk.

10. Extra-adrenal pheochromocytomas.
    a. 90% of pheochromocytomas are found in the adrenal, 98% are within the abdomen.
    b. Other locations–bladder, Organ of Zuckerkandl (anterior aorta), carotid body (chemodectoma), or sympathetic ganglia.
    c. Organ of Zuckerkandl most common site. Difficult to excise from anterior border of aorta. Suspect if only norepinephrine elevated.

B. Clinical presentation.

1. Hypertension (usually sustained, but can be episodic), headache, sweating, palpitations, chest pain, anxiety, fever, abdominal pain.
2. Suspect in cases of refractory hypertension, hypertension in children, or pregnancy.

C. Diagnosis.

1. Increased urinary levels of norepinephrine, epinephrine, metanephrines, normetanephrines, VMA–found in 90% of patients.
2. Catecholamines may be elevated in essential hypertension.
3. Stimulation tests.
    a. Glucagon–used if blood pressure is normal. Has few side-effects. A 3-fold increase of catecholamines is diagnostic.
    b. Clonidine suppression test–central alpha agonist that decreases catecholamine release. In patients with pheochromocytomas, catecholamine levels are unchanged.
4. Localization.
    a. 97% can be diagnosed with CT scan. Should be done without contrast to prevent a dye-induced hypertensive crisis.
    b. MRI–especially with T2-weighted images. Can better distinguish anatomic extension. Can also distinguish medullary and cortical neoplasms as well as malignancy from benign processes (adenoma).
    c. MIBG–norepinephrine analog. Taken up by adrenergic vesicles throughout the body. Can locate even extra-adrenal pheochromocytomas. 10% false negatives, 1-2% false positives.
    d. If above methods to localize pheochromocytoma are unsuccessful, can attempt venous sampling.

D. Surgical treatment.

1. Pre-operative preparation.
    a. Alpha blockade (phenoxybenzamine, phentolamine, metyrosine) should be started 2 weeks prior to surgery to control hypertension and restore the blood volume.
    b. Beta blockade–may begin only after alpha blockade. Beta blockade alone can worsen CHF and HTN by blocking epinephrine induced vasodilation. Only used if hypertensive.

c. With alpha blockade, will not see increased hypertension intra-operatively with manipulation of the pheochromocytoma.
d. Without alpha blockade, increased risk of post-operative hypotension.

2. Anesthesia management.
a. Reverse Trendelenburg position can increase venous capacitance.
b. Nipride or phentolamine (short-acting alpha blocker) for intra-operative blood pressure control. Norepinephrine may be necessary post-operatively for hypotension.
c. Lidocaine often necessary to control catecholamine induced arrhythmias.
d. Arterial line, CVP, Foley catheter for monitoring.
e. Halothane associated with less cardiac stimulation.
f. Sedate pre-operatively.

3. Technical aspects.
a. Anterior approach used because of risk of multiple primary tumors, bilateral disease, malignancy, ectopic location.
b. Remove with capsule intact to decrease risk of recurrence.
c. Manipulate as little as possible.
d. Identify and ligate veins early to prevent hypertensive episodes.

E. Prognosis.
1. Normal life expectancy.
2. 10-30% recur.

F. Paraganglionoma.
1. Nonfunctional medullary neoplasm.
2. Presents as an abdominal mass.
3. First rule-out functional mass, then excise.
4. 50% have recurrence or metastatic disease.
5. 75% 5-year survival.

VI. METASTATIC DISEASE TO THE ADRENAL

A. Most frequent site of metastatic disease (by weight).

B. Most common—breast, lung, kidney, pancreas.

C. Can cause Addison's disease, though masked by other symptoms of end-stage cancer.

D. 40% bilateral.

E. Best diagnosed by CT. Can be resected in certain circumstances.

VII. ADRENAL IMAGING

A. Noninvasive techniques.
1. Urography–adrenal tumors > 2 cm will displace the kidney. < 50% of adrenal tumors can be imaged in this manner.
2. Ultrasonography–must be 2-3 cm to visualize.
3. CT–effective in imaging masses 1.0 cm and greater.

4. MRI–allows imaging without radiation or intravenous contrast exposure.
5. Radionuclide imaging–MIBG (^{131}I-metaiodobenzylguanidine) scintigraphy can effectively demonstrate intra- and extra-abdominal pheochromocytomas. Can also be used therapeutically in cases of unresectable tumors.

B. Invasive techniques.

1. Arteriography–especially helpful in pheochromocytoma imaging because of their vascularity. Infusion of contrast can induce a hypertensive crisis.
2. Venography–selective catheterization allows location of tumors with contrast injection as well as venous sampling to determine function of adrenal mass.

VIII. INCIDENTAL ADRENAL MASSES (Figure 2)

A. Frequency—0.6% of abdominal CTs.

B. With history of carcinoma—must rule out metastatic disease.

C. Most incidental masses are benign cortical adenomas.

D. Check functional status if indicated by history, physical.

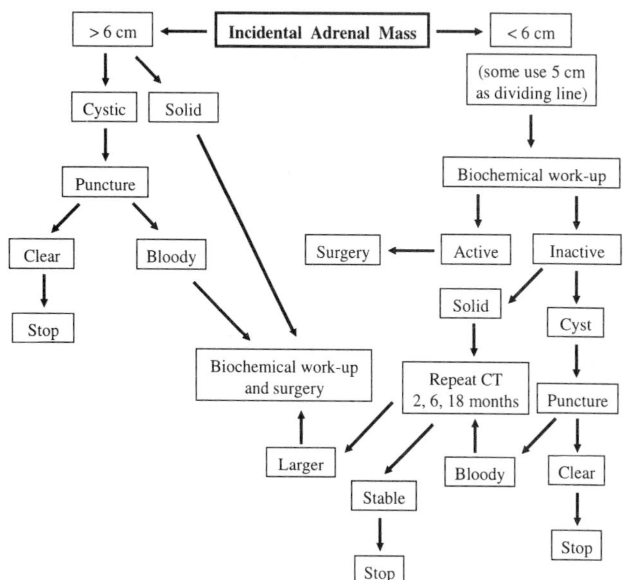

FIG. 2

E. **If cystic**—FNA. If clear, follow. If bloody, requires further evaluation.
F. **MRI,** with T2 images, can give additional information.
G. **If > 5 cm**—check functional status, then excise.
H. **If < 3.5 cm and non-functional**—follow with CTs at 2, 6, 18 months.
I. **If functional**—excise.
J. **3.5-5.0 cm**—debatable.

30

Miscellaneous Endocrine Disorders

Michael A. Helmrath, M.D.

I. APUD CELL (*A*MINE *P*RECURSOR *U*PTAKE AND *D*ECARBOXYLATION) CONCEPT

A. **A group of cells** (presumed neuroectodermal origin) that have similar biochemical characteristics.

B. **Provides a *theoretical* framework** for understanding the normal and pathologic biosynthesis of over 40 polypeptides by gastrointestinal (bowel, pancreas) system, thyroid, parathyroid, adrenal medulla, carotid body, and neural cells.

C. **Symptoms**—from overproduction of these polypeptides.

D. **All tumors may be multihormonal.** Predominant symptoms are related to the most biochemically potent):

Tumor	Site	Predominant Hormone	Symptoms
Carcinoid	Appendix, ileum Other GI sites, broncial tree Often	Bradykinin; serotonin	Flushing, diarrhea, cramping
Gastrinoma	Pancreas, duodenum Ectopic	Gastin	Severe peptic ulcer disease, diarrhea, abdominal pain
Insulinoma	Pancreas (β-cell)	Insulin	Symptoms of hypoglycemia often misdiagnosed as neurologic or psychiatric
Glucagonoma	Pancreas (α-cell) (50% in tail)	Glucagon	Migratory necrolytic erythema, anemia, mild diabetes, glossitis, thrombosis

Tumor	Site	Predominant Hormone	Symptoms
VIP-oma	Pancreas (D-cell), (80%) 10-20% extra-pancreatic	Vasoactive intestinal polypeptide (VIP)	**W**atery **d**iarrhea, **h**ypokalemia, **a**cholorhydria (WDHA syndrome)
Somato-statinoma	Pancreas (D-cell)	Somatostatin	Mild diabetes, steatorrhea, indigestion, often incidental finding (e.g., at time of cholecystectomy)

II. CARCINOID TUMORS

A. Most common GI APUD-oma, most common tumor of small bowel; all potentially malignant tumors of enterochromaffin cell origin.

B. Can originate from foregut (including bronchial tree, pancreas, gallbladder), small bowel, or large bowel.

1. Bronchial and metastatic small bowel carcinoids most likely to cause **carcinoid syndrome.**
2. Appendix: most common site (41%), followed by small bowel (20%), rectum (16%) [overall 85-90% in the GI tract]; lungs and bronchial tree (10%), larynx, thymus, kidney, ovary, prostate, skin (5%).
3. Except for appendiceal and rectal carcinoid, lesions tend to be multicentric.
4. Survival depends on growth rate and the presence or absence of metastases.

C. Hormone production.

1. Serotonin predominates; may also produce kallikrein, substance P, and others.
2. Large bowel tumors are rarely hormonally active.
3. Hormones may be deactivated by the liver prior to entering systemic circulation.

D. Symptoms.

1. Mechanical obstruction due to tumor or secondary desmoplastic reaction; occasionally rectal bleeding from rectal carcinoid.
2. ***Carcinoid syndrome*** requires elaboration of active hormone by tumor *outside* portovenous drainage.
3. Most common symptoms of the syndrome and probable cause.:
   a. Flushing (94%)–kallikrein (bradykinin).
   b. Diarrhea (78%)–serotonin.
   c. Cramping (51%)–serotonin.
   d. Valvular heart lesions (50%)–serotonin.
4. Other symptoms can include telangectasias, wheezing, edema.

E. Diagnosis.

1. Most are found during surgery for intestinal obstruction or appendectomy; pre-operative search unusual, but angiography, endoscopy, barium studies, and CT scan can all be useful; bronchial lesions diagnosed by chest radiograph and/or bronchoscopy.
2. ***5-HIAA*** (hydroxyindoleacetic acid) levels > 10 mg in 24-h urine is diagnostic of hormonally active tumor, if the patient is not on phenothiazines (false negatives) and is not eating serotonin-containing foods (e.g., pineapple, chocolate, bananas, walnuts, avocados).
3. Bronchial carcinoids may cause elevated **5-HTP** (hydroxytryptophan) levels with normal 5-HIAA values.

F. Treatment—surgical resection is the most likely chance for cure. *Always* consider lesions to be *malignant.*

1. Appendiceal carcinoid < 1.5 cm–simple appendectomy.
2. Appendiceal carcinoid either > 1.5 cm, at base of cecum, serosal with invasion, or local nodal disease requires right hemicolectomy.
3. Treatment of small bowel carcinoids–resection including mesenteric nodes. There is a high incidence of other primary tumors.
4. Rectal carcinoids locally excised unless > 2 cm, locally invasive, or nodal disease, in which case abdominoperineal resection is recommended, or low anterior resection if possible.
5. Often multicentric; thus, careful exploration is necessary; all gross disease should be resected to reduce hormone production.
6. Bronchial carcinoids are resected as indicated based on location.
7. If pre-operative diagnosis is made (e.g., carcinoid syndrome), the patient should be prepared for surgery with hydration, serotonin antagonists, and possibly α- and/or β-adrenergic blockers to avoid extreme response to tumor manipulation (see "Adrenal Gland" section VI).

G. Treatment—medical (symptomatic treatment).

1. Anti-hormonal measures–serotonin antagonists (methysergide, cyproheptadine, ketanserin); treats only GI symptoms, not flushing.
2. Anti-secretory measures–somatostatin analogue (Sandostatin®) has alleviated both flushing and GI symptoms in clinical trials.
3. Chemotherapy–variable results in small series; most common regimens include streptozotocin and 5-FU; some add doxorubicin; most respond poorly.
4. Some reports of long-term remission with hepatic artery embolization for liver metastases.

H. Prognosis (5-year survival).

1. Overall–65-80%.

2. Localized disease–up to 95%.
3. Regional nodal disease–approximately 65%.
4. Distant metastases–20%.
5. Appendix highest survival (99%); lungs and bronchi next (96% local disease, 87% all stages).

III. GASTRINOMA (Zollinger-Ellison Syndrome)

A. Location—85% are located in the gastrinoma triangle (Figure 1); 15-20% duodenal or ectopic (splenic hilum, gastric wall, mesentery, liver). More than 50% are malignant, over half of those are metastatic at time of diagnosis (to lymph nodes, liver, spleen, peritoneum, mediastinum). Very slow-growing tumors; prolonged survival if ulcers are controlled. Of patients with peptic ulcer disease, 0.1-1.0% have a gastrinoma. Duodenal tumors are usually solitary, and 75% are benign; benign tumors elsewhere tend to be multicentric, and the head of the pancreas is most common.

B. Clinical presentation—severe peptic ulcer disease with atypical location of multiple ulcers, often resistant to medical therapy. Associated complications (bleeding, perforation, outlet obstruction) are common.

1. Diarrhea–may be the only symptom in up to 40% of pa-

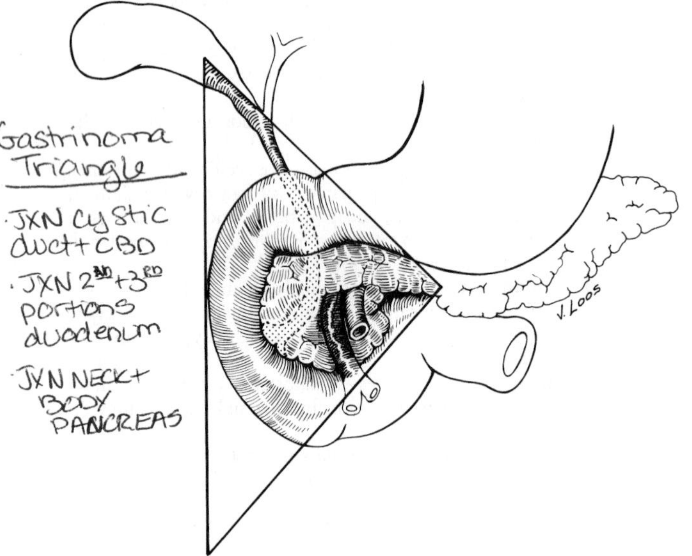

FIG. 1 The Gastrinoma Triangle

tients. Secondary to acid secretion, inactivated enzymes, and gastrin-stimulated increased motility.

2. Abdominal pain–present in > 90% of patients. May become malnourished and dehydrated.
3. Associated with parathyroid and pituitary tumors (MEN-I) in 25% of patients.

C. Diagnosis—elevated fasting **gastrin** levels (> 500 pg/ml) in a patient with *increased* gastric acid (differential diagnosis: gastrinoma, retained antrum, gastric outlet obstruction, renal failure, short bowel syndrome); if gastric acidity is *decreased,* elevated **gastrin** is secondary (chronic gastritis, gastric carcinoma, pernicious anemia, vagotomy, H_2 blockers or omeprazole).

1. If gastrin above normal (20-150 pg/ml) but < 500, need provocative test (off H_2 blockers at least 24-48 h).
2. Secretin stimulation (positive in ≥ 90% of cases; peak usually at 2-5 minutes)–test of choice.

Measure serum gastrin
⇓
Secretin 2 U/kg IV bolus
⇓
Serum gastrin at 2, 5, 10, 20, 30 minutes after infusion
⇓
Positive test if gastrin increased 100-200 pg/ml above baseline

3. ***Calcium stimulation*** (may cause arrhythmias, need to monitor)–80% sensitive, 50% specific.

Monitor patient
⇓
Ca^{++} gluconate 5 mg/kg/h infusion x 3 h
⇓
Serum gastrin every 30 minutes
⇓
Positive is 300-400 pg/ml rise above baseline

4. Acid output measurement.
   a. **Basal acid output (BAO)** > 15 mEq/h or > 100 mmol HCl/12 h suggests gastrinoma.
   b. **Maximal acid output (MAO)** with pentagastrin stimulation shows minimal increase over BAO with gastrinoma. BAO/MAO ratio usually > 0.6 with gastrinoma, since parietal cells are already maximally stimulated endogenously.
   c. Acid outputs less accurate than secretin stimulation test.
5. Gastrin levels > 5000 pg/ml, or presence of α-HCG in serum suggests metastatic disease.
6. Always check serum Ca^{++} to screen for MEN-I.

D. Localization—often not possible pre-operatively because of small tumors. Duodenal tumors can sometimes be identified endoscopically.

1. ***Transhepatic portal venous sampling/mapping***—up to 90% success in some hands, but others report much poorer results.
2. ***CT scan***—20-80% success; various series, most on lower end of range. Angiography, ultrasound < 25% successful.
3. ***Intra-operative ultrasound*** is very successful, and when combined with thorough palpation of the pancreas, can locate the majority of gastrinomas.
4. Radiolabeled octreotide scan may aid in localization.

E. Treatment.

1. High-dose H_2 blockade often controls secretory and peptic ulcer disease symptoms, but breakthrough acid secretion can occur with time; some patients never respond.
2. ***Omeprazole*** (Prilosec®) (H^+-K^+ ATPase inhibitor) provides better control of acid secretion at doses up to 60 mg BID.
3. All patients with Zollinger-Ellison syndrome should be explored to attempt curative resection (20% of patients are cured with complete resection).

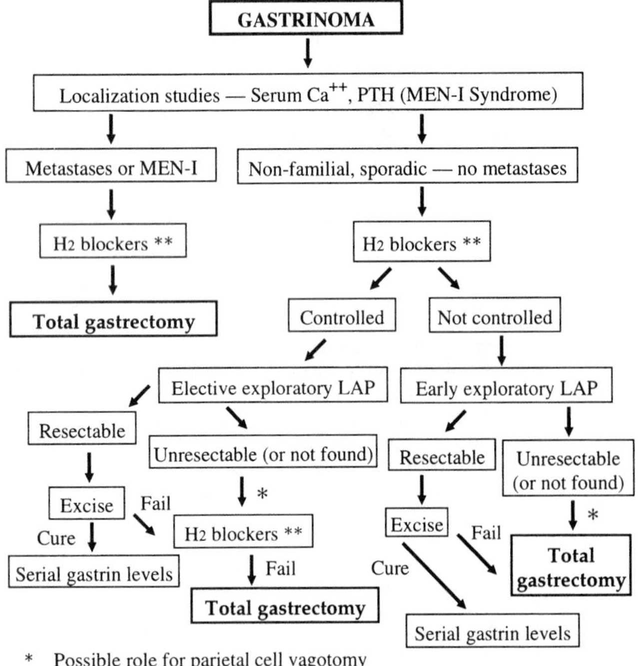

* Possible role for parietal cell vagotomy
** Or omeprazole

4. Some authors report good symptomatic results with tumor debulking combined with parietal cell vagotomy and H_2 blockade when unresectable.
5. Classic surgical approach in the past: total gastrectomy; cures the symptoms, but late deaths still occur due to metastatic disease; variable nutritional consequences following gastrectomy.

IV. INSULINOMA

A. Functional β-cell tumor of pancreatic islet; second most common endocrine tumor of pancreas. 10% malignant, 10% multiple (includes nesidioblastosis), 4-10% associated with MEN-I; multiple lesions associated with MEN-I over 50% of the time. Tumors are small (60-70% < 1.5 cm), equally distributed through pancreas, up to 90% solitary and benign, usually are resectable. Insulin is produced as proinsulin which is cleaved into C-peptide and insulin.

B. Clinical.

1. Symptoms of **hypoglycemia** (primarily neurologic) with reactive epinephrine release. Usually brought on by fasting or exercise; often occurs in the AM; patients are often obese due to learned habit of frequent ingestion of sweets to alleviate the symptoms.
2. Hypoglycemic symptoms of diplopia, blurred vision, confused behavior, amnesia, weakness, focal or generalized seizures, paralysis, coma. Adrenergic symptoms of sweating, hunger, tremor, and palpitations.
3. With repeated attacks, permanent neurologic damage can occur; often initially confused with neuropsychiatric problems; mean of 33 months from onset of symptoms to diagnosis.

C. Diagnosis.

1. ***Whipple's Triad*** strongly suggests diagnosis (95% accurate with up to 72-h fast).
   a. Symptoms of hypoglycemia with fasting.
   b. Blood glucose < 50 mg/dl at time of symptoms.
   c. Symptoms relieved by glucose.
2. Some use insulin/glucose (I/G) ratio > 0.30 during fast as diagnostic, or insulin > 6 μU/ml.
3. Measure insulin antibodies, urinary sulfonylureas, and **proinsulin/C-peptide** (both *low* with self-administered human insulin) to search for factitious hyperinsulinemic hypoglycemia.
4. Most useful (although rarely necessary) suppression test may be the euglycemic (administer *both* insulin and glucose to maintain euglycemia) **C-peptide suppression test** (positive if C-peptide does not decrease).
5. Provocative tests (tolbutamide test, calcium gluconate infu-

sion) are less reliable than 72-h fast; both tests risk severe side-effects; not recommended by most authors.

6. Malignant tumor is suggested by very high proinsulin level and/or presence of HCG in serum.

D. Localization—generally proceeds with ultrasound ⇒ CT scan (or MRI) ⇒ **p**ercutaneous **t**ranshepatic **p**ortal **v**ein **s**ampling (**PTPVS**).

1. ***Angiography*** with subtraction techniques can be up to 90% successful; shows localized, dense tumor blush on capillary phase; false-positive results can occur (accessory spleens, inflamed lymph nodes); test is invasive.
2. ***CT scan, ultrasound*** in general are less than 50% successful in localizing these small tumors, but if positive, save patient from angiography.
3. ***PTPVS*** has variable but encouraging results when other methods fail; but is tedious, costly, uncomfortable, requires skilled angiographer; safe and useful in selected cases.
4. ***Intra-operative ultrasound*** is extremely accurate (and should be available), as is intra-operative bimanual pancreatic palpation.

E. Treatment—surgical resection is goal, with up to 90% success (cure).

1. Pre-operative maintenance of glucose levels with frequent meals and/or glucose infusion; frequent intra-operative glucose measurements.
2. Mobilize and palpate entire gland, even if single tumor localized pre-operatively (Kocher maneuver and mobilization of pancreatic tail and spleen).
3. Enucleate small tumors near surface; pancreatic resection for others, including Whipple procedure if necessary for tumor located in head; frozen section to confirm pathology. *Caution* should be used with enucleation in tail or deep in head due to possible damage to pancreatic duct.
4. If no tumor is found–intra-operative ultrasound.
   a. Biopsy or resection of pancreatic tail–if frozen section reveals nesidioblastosis (adenomatosis), 75-80% resection is thought to provide best control of symptoms with the least morbidity; may require subsequent medical therapy.
   b. Do not blindly resect head of pancreas.
5. Metastatic disease should be treated by debulking as much tumor mass as possible.
6. ***Medical treatment***—for patient who cannot tolerate general anesthesia, for control of symptoms pre-operatively, or to treat metastatic disease.
   a. **Diazoxide**–inhibits insulin release, decreases peripheral glucose utilization; multiple side-effects may preclude use (edema, hirsutism, nausea, bone marrow depression, hyperuricemia); diuretic may control edema.

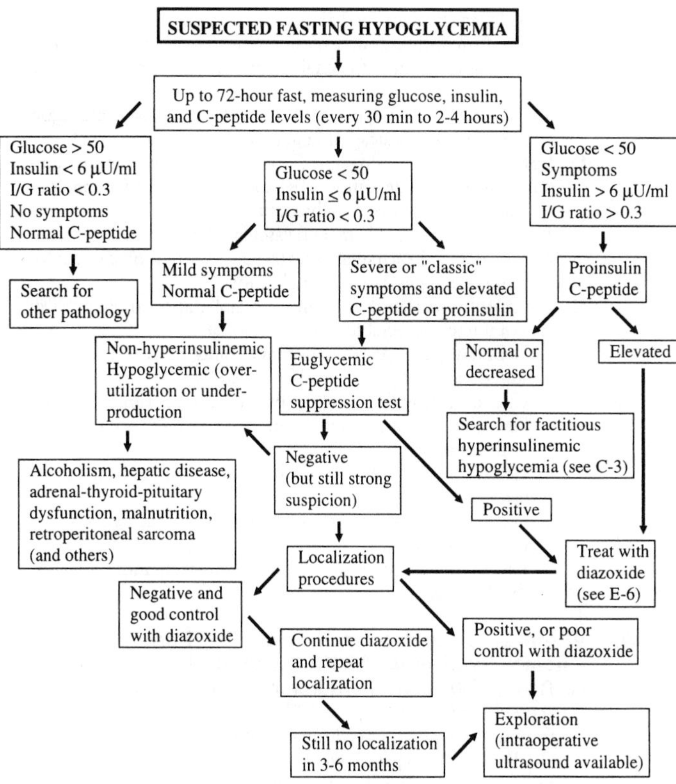

b. **Streptozotocin** with 5-FU to treat malignant insulinoma; 50-66% achieve partial remission, 17-33% with complete remission; up to 95% experience nausea and vomiting, sometimes severe; renal tubular, hepatic toxicity also possible.

V. GLUCAGONOMA

A. Rare α-cell pancreatic islet tumor— < 100 reported cases.

B. Clinical—see chart in section I; mean age 55.

C. Diagnosis.

1. Skin lesions are best clue–migratory annular erythematous eruptions, superficial necrosis ("**migratory necrolytic erythema**").

2. Mild, easily controlled diabetes.
3. Confirm with elevated plasma glucagon. *Note:* Levels may also be elevated with renal failure, liver failure, and severe stress.
4. Provocative test (arginine infusion: elevates plasma glucagon in patient with glucagonoma) is rarely needed.

D. Localization—arteriography, CT scan, selective venous sampling can all localize tumor; MRI appears best for liver metastases; ultrasound is occasionally useful.

1. Most are bulky (> 3 cm) and vascular, therefore easier to find.
2. 50% in tail, 50% malignant, 50% metastatic at time of exploration (to nodes, liver, adrenal, spine).

E. Treatment—surgical excision if possible; approximately 30% are completely resectable.

1. Debulking unresectable primaries and metastases has resulted in prolonged survival.
2. Chemotherapy for recurrent or unresectable tumors can relieve the symptoms; DTIC and 5-FU/streptozotocin have both been used.
3. Hepatic artery embolization has been used for liver metastases.
4. Somatostatin analogue (**Sandostatin**®) has been effective in treating symptoms.
5. Rash is treated with zinc, high-protein diet, and control of the diabetes.

VI. VIPoma (Verner-Morrison Syndrome, Pancreatic Cholera Syndrome, WDHA Syndrome)

A. Rare (< 100 cases) syndrome due to production of vasoactive intestinal polypeptide (VIP: normally a neurotransmitter) from a pancreatic islet cell tumor (70%), extrapancreatic tumor (10-20%, includes ganglioneuroblastoma, adrenal medulla, pulmonary sites), or possibly islet cell hyperplasia (10-20%). About 50-60% are malignant, most are metastatic at the time of diagnosis; extrapancreatic tumors are *rarely* malignant.

B. Clinical: WDHA—2-10 L/day of **w**atery **d**iarrhea, resulting in dehydration, **h**ypokalemia, acidosis; associated with **a**chlorhydria (hypochlorhydria more common) due to suppressive action of VIP on gastric acid secretion.

1. Up to 20% of patients will exhibit spontaneous flushing similar to carcinoid syndrome.
2. Hyperglycemia/hypercalcemia occur in 50-75% of VIPoma patients for unclear reasons.
3. Occasionally associated with MEN-I.

C. Diagnosis—presence of WDHA syndrome (with associated electrolyte abnormalities) with low gastric acid secretion and elevated VIP levels.

1. VIP is invariably elevated, but assay is difficult and requires a reliable lab.

2. Pancreatic polypeptide (PP) may be elevated with pancreatic VIPomas.

D. Localization—use CT and/or ultrasound first; 80% will be body or tail; if unsuccessful, use angiography; transhepatic venous sampling may prove helpful in difficult cases.

E. Treatment.

1. Vigorous pre-operative fluid resuscitation, then surgical resection.
2. If no tumor is found, some authors feel subtotal pancreatectomy is indicated if tumor markers (VIP, PP) are consistently elevated pre-operatively.
3. For unresectable/metastatic disease, debulk; some recommend hepatic artery embolization.
   a. Steroids may provide temporary symptomatic relief in 50%, but relapse is the rule.
   b. > 90% remission rate with streptozotocin, many lasting for years; DTIC and 5-FU have also been used successfully.
   c. Several series have shown symptomatic relief using somatostatin analog (**Sandostatin®**), with a suggestion of tumor mass regression.

VII. SOMATOSTATINOMA

A. Very rare tumor of pancreatic islet; duodenal tumors also reported.

B. Termed "inhibitory syndrome"; classic triad of gallstones, diabetes, and steatorrhea are vague; duodenal tumors are usually asymptomatic. Thus, most tumors are discovered late in course with metastases already present.

C. In general, these are malignant, solitary, and virulent.

D. Symptoms are due to inhibition of exocrine and endocrine pancreas, gallbladder contraction, and gastric emptying (resulting in bloating, indigestion, nausea, and vomiting).

E. Diagnosis—usually discovered *incidentally* at cholecystectomy; plasma somatostatin can be measured and is markedly elevated.

F. Localization—most discovered incidentally, but CT and angiography are useful.

G. Treatment—resection should be attempted if possible; debulking recommended otherwise.

1. Duodenal somatostatinomas should be treated like carcinomas.
2. Tumor is rare; no information on chemotherapy is available.

H. Prognosis—in cases described is poor, with most patients surviving several months; early diagnosis and resection may be curative.

VIII. MULTIPLE ENDOCRINE NEOPLASIA (*MEN*) SYNDROMES

A. All are *autosomal dominant.*

MEN-I	MEN-IIa	MEN-IIb
Pituitary adenoma	Medullary thyroid carcinoma	Medullary thyroid carcinoma
Parathyroid hyperplasia	Pheochromocytoma	Pheochromocytoma
Pancreatic islet cell tumor	Parathyroid hyperplasia	Multiple mucosal neuromas

B. MEN-I (Wermer's syndrome, "3 Ps": pituitary, parathyroid, pancreas).

1. Peak incidence in 20s for women, 30s for men; most commonly present with peptic ulcer disease symptoms/complications; next most common is hypoglycemia (insulinoma); less common are headaches, visual field deficits, amenorrhea (pituitary adenoma).
2. ***Pituitary***—60-70% have adenoma, usually chromophobe with hypofunction; occasionally have functional tumor (e.g., acromegaly).
3. ***Parathyroid***—most consistent lesion; > 90% with generalized hyperplasia and hypercalcemia; may have renal stones, peptic ulcer disease.
4. ***Pancreas***—80% with pancreatic lesion; most common in gastrinoma, followed by insulinoma; *any* islet cell tumor is possible, including simple islet cell hyperplasia; tumors usually multicentric, often malignant, but slow-growing.
5. Diagnosis.
   a. Screen all patients with pancreatic tumor for hyperparathyroidism (Ca^{++}, PTH).
   b. Screen all family members of patients with gastrinoma or any other MEN-I associated lesions (pituitary, parathyroid).
   c. Pancreatic polypeptide may be good marker; seems to be elevated in nearly *all* cases.
6. ***Treatment.***
   a. Hyperparathyroidism—*treat first,* with subtotal parathyroidectomy; if peptic ulcer disease is present and persists with normal Ca^{++}, do work-up for gastrinoma.
   b. Since gastrinoma and other pancreatic lesions in MEN-I are often multiple and/or malignant, surgery may not be curative (see above sections for approach).
   c. Pituitary lesions—addressed surgically as indicated.

C. MEN-IIa (Sipple's syndrome) and IIb.

1. Both MEN-IIa and IIb are **autosomal dominant,** but sporadic cases have been reported.
2. ***Medullary thyroid carcinoma,*** preceded by thyroid C-cell hyperplasia, is present in 100% of these patients; multicentric and bilateral, unlike sporadic cases; **much more aggres-**

sive tumor in IIb syndrome, making early total thyroidectomy critical for successful treatment.

3. ***Pheochromocytoma***—present in 40-50%; 80% bilateral, almost always benign; peak incidence in teens, 20s.
4. ***Parathyroid hyperplasia*** is present in approximately 60% of MEN-IIa patients.
5. MEN-IIb patients have characteristic physical appearance with multiple **cutaneous neuromas.**
6. ***Diagnosis***—elevated plasma calcitonin level.
   a. Measurement of plasma calcitonin after **pentagastrin stimulation** (0.5 μg/kg IVP, measure calcitonin at 1-3 min, 30 min) detects medullary thyroid carcinoma in clinically normal patients who will have microscopic disease when thyroid is removed.
   b. Symptoms of pheochromocytoma (see "Adrenal Gland" section VI for work-up).
   c. Blood Ca^{++}, PTH levels for hyperparathyroidism.
7. ***Treatment.***
   a. Look for and treat **pheochromocytoma** first–abdominal, bilateral exploration due to frequency of bilateral lesions.
   b. Total thyroidectomy, with resection of nodes between the jugular veins from thyroid cartilage to sternal notch; neck dissection for more extensive lymphatic involvement; follow pentagastrin stimulation test to check for adequacy of resection, recurrence.
   c. Subtotal parathyroidectomy for patients with hyperparathyroidism, or total parathyroidectomy with reimplantation.
8. ***Prognosis.***
   a. Related to the extent of thyroid tumor.
   b. Extremely variable, even in same family. Overall, 10-year survival of patients with medullary thyroid carcinoma is 50%.

31

The Esophagus

J. Kevin Bailey, M.D.

I. ANATOMY

A. A hollow muscular tube approximately 25 cm long that begins 15 cm from incisors, at the cricopharyngeus muscle, and ends at the gastro-esophageal (GE) junction. It is narrowed at the level of the cricopharyngeal muscle (narrowest point), at the aortic arch and left main stem bronchus, and the diaphragmatic hiatus.

B. The esophagus enters the abdomen via the esophageal hiatus at the level of T11 and is accompanied by the vagal trunks. The distal 2-4 cm are intra-abdominal.

C. Blood supply.

1. Arterial supply is segmental from superior and inferior thyroid, aortic and esophageal branches, inferior phrenic, and left gastric arteries.
2. Venous drainage to hypopharyngeal, azygous, hemizygous, intercostal, and gastric veins. May become varices with portal hypertension.
3. Nervous supply from both parasympathetic and sympathetic systems. Right and left vagal trunks lie posteriorly and anteriorly, respectively, on the distal esophagus.

D. Histology.

1. Mucosa is squamous, changing to columnar epithelium at or near GE junction.
2. Submucosa contains glands, arteries, Meissner's neural plexus, lymphatics, and veins.
3. Muscularis composed of two layers, an outer longitudinal and inner circular layer. Nerves and blood vessels run between layers. Upper one-third composed of striated muscle, lower two-thirds smooth muscle.
4. Serosa–none. Contributes to increased potential for anastomotic leaks and early mediastinal invasion by cancer.

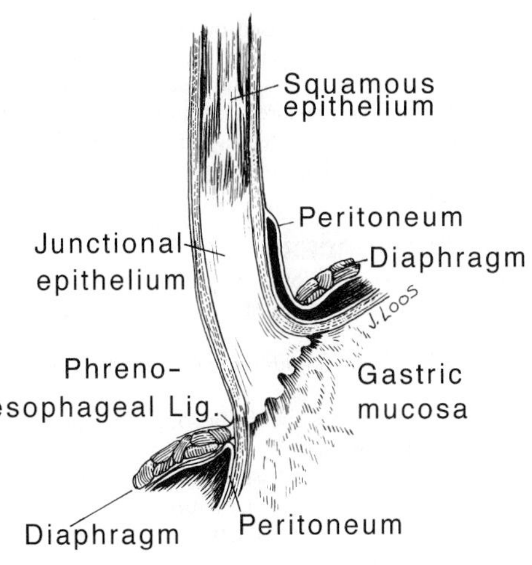

FIG. 1

II. PHYSIOLOGY

A. Function—transports swallowed material from pharynx to stomach, involving voluntary and involuntary actions.

B. Peristalsis.

1. Primary peristalsis initiated by relaxing upper esophageal sphincter (UES), which propels swallowed material from pharynx to stomach in a progressive and sequential manner.
2. Secondary peristalsis is involuntary waves caused by local distention in an attempt to clear the esophagus. Initiated in the smooth muscle of the lower esophagus.
3. Tertiary peristalsis is repetitive, non-progressive, and uncoordinated smooth muscle contractions.

C. Sphincters.

1. Upper esophageal sphincter (UES) is ~ 3 cm long. Resting pressure is 20-60 mm Hg.
2. Lower esophageal sphincter (LES).
   a. Not an anatomically defined sphincter in man; more appropriately called a zone of high pressure. Serves to reduce gastric regurgitation and reflux. It is located in distal 3-5 cm of esophagus and defined by "pull back" manometric studies. Its normal resting pressure is 10-20 mm Hg.
   b. Varies with respiration, increases with inspiration and drug/hormone levels.
      (1) Pressure increased by gastrin, caffeine, α-adrenergic drugs, bethanechol, and metoclopramide.

(2) Pressure decreased by secretin, cholecystokinin, glucagon, progesterone, alcohol, nitroglycerin, nicotine, anticholinergics, and β-adrenergic drugs.

c. Abdominal pressure transmitted to distal esophagus important for competence. Intra-abdominal position of segment of esophagus maintained by phreno-esophageal ligament.

III. MOTILITY DISORDERS

A. Definition—Conditions interfering with swallowing, not caused by intraluminal obstruction or external compression.

B. History.

1. Dysphagia with liquids more than solids suggest motility disorder.
2. Dysphagia progressive from solids to liquids suggests mechanical obstruction.
3. Odynophagia suggests spasm or esophagitis. Increased pain with cold liquids suggests spasm.
4. Difficulty with swallowing or nasopharyngeal reflux suggests neurologic or muscular disorder.
5. Symptoms of reflux.
6. Duration of symptoms.
7. Gurgling with swallowing, regurgitation of undigested food suggests a Zenker's diverticulum.
8. Hematemesis, weight loss, alcohol/tobacco use should be questioned.

C. UES dysfunction—cricopharyngeal achalasia.

1. Caused by abnormalities in central and peripheral nervous systems, metabolic, inflammatory myopathy, gastroesophageal reflux, and others.
2. Patients complain of "lump in throat", excessive expectoration of saliva, weight loss, and intermittent hoarseness.
3. Diagnosis by barium swallow and manometric studies; however, these may be normal.
4. Treatment depends on the cause–antireflux procedure, bougienage, or cervical esophagotomy.

D. Body of esophagus.

1. Achalasia–failure of relaxation.
   a. Abnormal peristalsis secondary to absence or destruction of Auerbach's (myenteric) plexus and failure of LES to relax. Affects body and distal esophagus.
   b. Etiology unknown, multiple associations.
   c. Patients complain of dysphagia, regurgitation, weight loss, retrosternal chest pain, and recurrent pulmonary infections.
   d. Barium swallow demonstrates "bird's beak" narrowing of distal esophagus with proximal dilation.
   e. Manometric studies show failure of LES to relax and lack

of progressive peristalsis. Tertiary waves are seen proximally. Methacholine increases LES pressure.

f. One to 10% of patients develop squamous cell carcinoma after 15-25 years of disease.

g. Treatment is palliative.

(1) Non-surgical treatment includes sublingual nitroglycerin, calcium channel blockers, and repeated dilation. Sixty-five percent improve with pneumatic or hydrostatic dilation.

(2) Surgical treatment involves a longitudinal (Heller) esophagotomy. Eighty-five percent of patients improve with a 3% rate of reflux following this procedure.

2. Diffuse esophageal spasm.
   a. Repetitive, simultaneous, high-amplitude contractions.
   b. Pain greater than dysphagia. Symptoms increased by emotional stress.
   c. Diagnosis by motility studies. Barium swallow may show "coiled spring."
   d. Treatment includes small, soft meals; calcium channel blockers, and extended esophagomyotomy.
3. Scleroderma.
   a. Fibrous replacement of esophageal smooth muscle and atrophy.
   b. LES loses tone and normal response to swallowing; results in gastroesophageal reflux.
   c. Medical/surgical treatment directed at antireflux measures to decrease esophagitis.

IV. DIVERTICULA

A. Epithelial-lined mucosal pouches that protrude from the esophageal lumen.

B. Pharyngoesophageal (Zenker's).

1. Located between oblique fibers of the thyropharyngeus muscle and the horizontal fibers of the cricopharyngeus.
2. Most common esophageal diverticula. "False" type contains only mucosa and submucosa.
3. Pulsion type created by elevated intraluminal pressure.
4. Patients usually 30-50 years of age. Complain of cervical dysphagia, effortless regurgitation of undigested food, choking, gurgling in throat, and recurrent aspiration.
5. Treatment includes diverticulectomy with myotomy of the cricopharyngeus muscle. Low mortality and recurrence rate; 2% and 4%, respectively.

C. Peribronchial.

1. Located near tracheal bifurcation.
2. Traction diverticulum resulting from inflammatory reaction, typically mediastinal granulomatous disease of adjacent

lymph nodes which adhere to esophagus and pull on wall during healing.
3. Rarely symptomatic, tend to be very small, and are discovered incidentally.

D. Epiphrenic.

1. Located in distal 10 cm of esophagus.
2. Pulsion type, arising from distal obstruction or motor dysfunction.
3. Patients complain of regurgitation, dysphagia, and retrosternal chest pain.
4. Treatment–usually none. If large, a long extramucosal thoracic myotomy and diverticulectomy.

V. HIATAL HERNIA AND GASTRO-ESOPHAGEAL REFLUX

A. Anatomy.

1. Normally, the distal 2-3 cm of esophagus are intra-abdominal.
2. Endo-abdominal fascia (continuous with transversalis fascia) inserts into esophageal wall at the esophageal hiatus.
3. No discrete LES in humans.

B. Etiology of reflux.

1. Decreased LES tone.
2. Delayed gastric emptying.
3. Increased intra-abdominal pressure due to obesity, tight garments, or large meal.
4. Motor failure of esophagus with loss of peristalsis.
5. Iatrogenic injury to LES.

C. Acid-protecting mechanisms.

1. Distal esophagus prevents reflux through influence of intra-abdominal pressure.
2. Peristalsis rapidly clears gastric acid.
3. Bicarbonate-rich saliva (1000-1500 ml/day.)

D. Reflux esophagitis.

1. Gastric acid and pepsin corrosive to mucosa.
2. Complications.
   a. Pain and spasm.
   b. Stricture.
   c. Hemorrhage.
   d. Shortening of esophagus.
   e. Ulceration.
   f. Barrett's esophagus.
      (1) Mucosal metaplasia of distal esophagus, squamous to columnar.
      (2) Associated with an increased risk of developing adenocarcinoma (10-15%).
      (3) Correction of reflux does not prevent malignant transformation. Requires serial endoscopic biopsy. Esophageal resection indicated for severe dysplasia.

g. Dysmotility.
h. Schatzki's ring–constrictive band at squamocolumnar junction composed of mucosa and submucosa, not esophageal muscle.
i. Aspiration pneumonia.

3. Symptoms.
   a. Heartburn, retrosternal pyrosis.
   b. Regurgitation of sour or bitter liquids, aggravated by postural changes.
   c. Nocturnal aspiration with recurrent pneumonia, lung abscesses, or bronchiectasis.
   d. Dysphagia secondary to obstruction or motility disorder.
4. Diagnosis.
   a. Upper GI series.
      (1) Spontaneous reflux in 40% of patients with true GE reflux.
      (2) Able to document stricture or ulcer.
   b. Esophagoscopy combined with mucosal brushings and biopsy are essential to diagnosis.
   c. Esophageal pH probe.
      (1) Accurate for determining magnitude and duration of reflux.
      (2) 24-h test most precise and quantitative method.
      (3) Acid reflux test–HCl is placed into the stomach. Monitor esophageal pH proximal to LES as intragastric pressure is increased. A pH less than 4 is a positive result.
   d. Bernstein test.
      (1) Reproduction of pain during instillation of acid into mid-esophagus. Acid is alternated with saline.
      (2) Normal individual able to clear acid.
   e. Manometry.
      (1) Does not test reflux; however, reflux more common with low LES pressure (less than 6 mm Hg).
      (2) May identify motility disorder.
5. Treatment.
   a. Medical.
      (1) Dietary.
         a) Avoid substances that decrease LES tone.
         b) Do not eat 2 h prior to sleep.
         c) Avoid excessive eating; eat small meals.
      (2) Avoid anticholinergics, tranquilizers, and muscle relaxants.
      (3) Reduce weight, if obese.
      (4) Elevate head of bed 6 inches on blocks.
      (5) Increase LES pressure.
         a) Metoclopramide 10 mg q 8 h.
         b) Bethanechol 10-50 tid or qid.
      (6) Decrease gastric acid.

a) Antacids.
b) H_2 blockers
c) Omeprazole.

b. Surgical-antireflux procedures.
(1) Goals.
a) Restore segment of intra-abdominal esophagus.
b) Maintain distal esophagus as small diameter tube.
c) Narrow the hiatus.
d) Avoid increasing resistance of relaxed sphincter to level that exceeds peristaltic force of esophagus.
(2) Indications.
a) Failure of medical therapy.
b) Esophagitis with frank ulceration or stricture.
c) Complications of reflux esophagitis.
(3) Procedures.

Procedure	Approach	Wrap	Features
Hill	Abdominal	180°	Phrenoesophageal ligament anchored to median arcuate ligament of diaphragm.
Belsey	Thoracic	270°	Exaggerated gastroesophageal angle, stomach anchored below diaphragm.
Nissen	Either	360°	Fundus is wrapped completely around the esophagus.
Angelchik	Abdominal	—	Silicone ring placed around esophagus below the diaphragm.
Collis	Abdominal	—	Lengthens the foreshortened esophagus by creating a "tube" of gastric mucosa.

(4) Complications.
a) Morbidity/mortality.
(1) Hill–8%/4%.
(2) Belsey–14%/0.5%.
(3) Nissen–24%/1%.
b) Excessively tight wrap–dysphagia.
c) Excessively loose or short wrap–reflux.
d) "Slipped-Nissen" occurs when wrap slides down, GE junction retracts into the chest, and the stomach is partitioned.
e) "Gas-bloat" syndrome"–difficulty with eructation due to a restored LES in a patient who swallows air.
f) The Angelchik ring has an excessive incidence of complications secondary to migration and erosion and is now generally avoided.
g) Incidence of splenectomy 7-15%.

E. Hiatal hernia.

1. ***Type I (sliding or axial)*** [Figure 2].
a. GE junction migrates above the diaphragm. Phrenoesophageal membrane is intact. No true peritoneal sac.

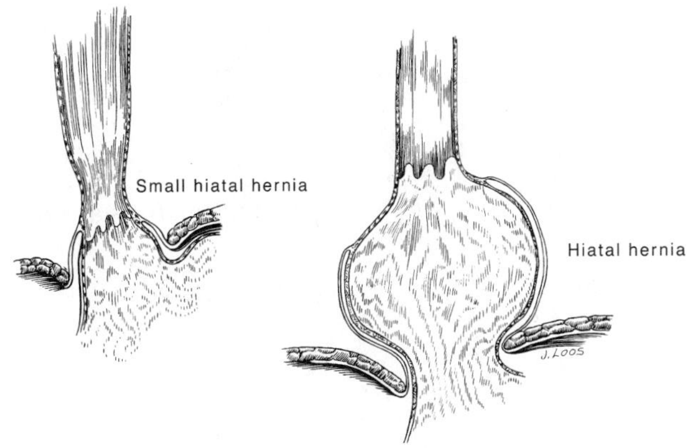

FIG. 2 Type I Hiatal Hernia

b. Most common hiatal hernia, 90%.
c. Significant only if reflux symptoms.
d. Etiology.
   (1) Chronically increased intra-abdominal pressure, including obesity.
   (2) Weakness of supporting structures at esophageal hiatus.

2. ***Type II (paraesophageal)*** [Figure 3].
   a. Gastric fundus herniates alongside esophagus; GE junction maintains its normal position.
   b. Peritoneal sac.
   c. Reflux rare.
   d. Uncommon type of hernia.
   e. Can result in gastric volvulus or strangulation.
   f. All type II hernias should be repaired.
3. ***Type III***—a combination of Types I and II.

VI. BENIGN TUMORS OF THE ESOPHAGUS

A. Incidence—rare, less than 1% of esophageal tumors.

B. Leiomyoma.

1. Most common benign tumor of esophagus (75%).
2. Less common in esophagus than stomach or small bowel.
3. Usually located in distal two-thirds.
4. Lesions smaller than 5 cm are usually asymptomatic.
5. Multiple in 3-10% of patients.
6. 97% are intramural in the circular muscle layer. Histologically, interlacing smooth muscle bundles.
7. Symptoms.
   a. Progressive intermittent dysphagia.

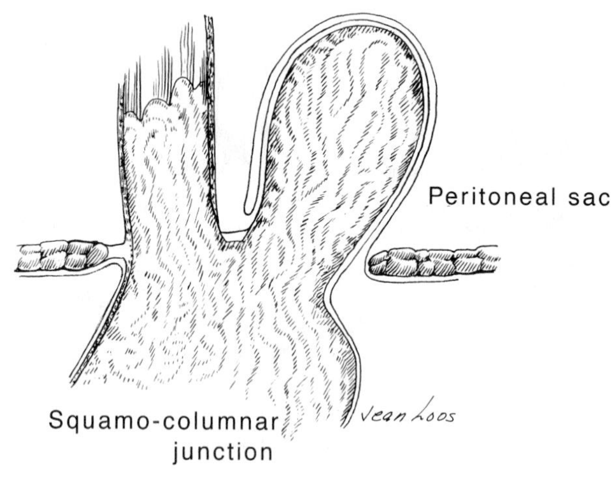

FIG. 3 Type II Hiatal Hernia

b. Vague retrosternal ache.
c. Heartburn.

8. Diagnosis by chest radiograph, barium swallow, and endoscopy (avoid biopsy if suspected).
9. Treatment.
   a. Excision of leiomyoma via thoracotomy, mortality less than 2%.
   b. Tumors not amenable to enucleation (10%) may require esophageal resection (mortality 10%).

C. Others include cysts, polyps, lipomas, and hemangiomas.

VII. ESOPHAGEAL CARCINOMA

A. Incidence.

1. Male:female 3:1.
2. Black:white 4:1.
3. Peak incidence 50-70 years of age.

B. Risk factors.

1. Alcohol and tobacco use.
2. Diet.
   a. Nitrosamines.
   b. Betel nuts.
   c. Chronic ingestion of hot foods and beverages.
3. Lower socioeconomic level.
4. Caustic ingestion (1-5% incidence with mean delay of 40 years).
5. Achalasia (2-8% incidence of squamous cell carcinoma).

6. Plummer-Vinson syndrome–esophageal webs, anemia, brittle nails, glossitis.
7. Vitamin and mineral deficiencies.
8. Barrett's esophagus–10% incidence of adenocarcinoma.

C. Pathology.

1. Seventy percent are squamous cell carcinomas (SCC).
   a. Cervical–8%.
   b. Upper or middle half–55%.
   c. Distal esophagus–37%.
2. Adenocarcinomas arise from gastric cardia or Barrett's esophagus.
3. Incidence increasing in United States.
4. Three growth patterns.
   a. Fungating–60%.
   b. Ulcerative–25%.
   c. Infiltrative–15%.
5. Tumors spread circumferentially and longitudinally via lymphatics, vascular invasion, and direct extension.
6. Seventy-five percent of patients with lymph node metastasis at diagnosis. Common distant metastatic sites are liver, lung, and bone.

D. Staging.

1. Tumor (T).
   a. T0–no tumor identified.
   b. Tis–carcinoma *in situ.*
   c. T1–tumor invading lamina propria or submucosa.
   d. T2–tumor invades muscularis propria.
   e. T3–tumor invading adventitia.
   f. T4–invasion of adjacent structures.
2. Lymph nodes.
   a. N0–no lymph node involvement.
   b. N1–regional node involvement.
3. Distant metastases.
   a. M0–none.
   b. M1–metastases present.
4. Stages.
   a. 0–TisN0M0.
   b. I–T1N0M0.
   c. IIA–T2N0M0, T3N0M0; IIB–T1N1M0, T2N1M0.
   d. III–T3N1M0, T4 any N M0.
   e. IV–Any T or N M1.

E. Clinical presentation.

1. Insidious onset, beginning as indigestion or retrosternal discomfort. Dysphagia, progressing from solids to liquids, is present in > 80% of patients. Pain is a late symptom and indicates extra-esophageal involvement.
2. Weight loss.
3. Odynophagia.
4. Regurgitation.

5. Anemia.
6. Hematemesis.
7. Vocal cord paralysis, left > right.
8. Aspiration pneumonia.
9. Tracheoesophageal or bronchoesophageal fistula.

F. Diagnosis.

1. Barium swallow has 92% accuracy. Able to identify abnormal peristalsis, mucosal irregularity, and annular constructions.
2. Fiberoptic endoscopy with biopsy or brushing is confirmatory in 95% of cases.
3. Bronchoscopy with biopsy to rule out involvement of the bronchus in upper two-third tumors and a synchronous lung primary.
4. Nasopharyngoscopy and direct laryngoscopy to rule out synchronous head and neck lesions and vocal cord involvement.
5. CT scan of chest with extension to liver and adrenals to assess tumor spread.

G. Therapy.

1. Principles.
   a. Vast majority of patients have advanced disease at presentation and are incurable.
   b. Fifty percent are resectable at presentation. Pre-operative chemotherapy increases operability rates.
   c. Palliation is the goal in most patients.
2. Surgical.
   a. Curative in early lesion, part of multimodal therapy in advanced cases.
   b. Esophagectomy techniques.
      (1) Ivor-Lewis involves esophagectomy, gastric mobilization, and gastroesophageal anastomosis in chest or neck. Done via midline abdominal incision and right thoracotomy.
      (2) Transhiatal via neck and abdominal incisions. Involves blunt esophagectomy, gastric mobilization, and gastroesophageal anastomosis in neck.
      (3) Esophageal reconstruction can also be completed with colon or jejunal interposition, or as free graft.
      (4) Mortality rates range from 5-30%.
      (5) Survival not improved with radical *en bloc* resections.
3. Radiation.
   a. Dosages to mediastinum range from 4,000 to 6,000 cGy.
   b. Primary treatment for poor-risk patients and palliation for unreactable lesions with obstructive symptoms.
   c. No increased survival with pre-operative treatment. May have value in post-operative therapy for residual mediastinal disease.

   d. Five-year survival for patients treated with radiation alone only slightly worse than surgery alone.
4. Chemotherapy.
   a. Current regimen–5-FU, cisplatinum, and vinblastine.
   b. Increased disease-free and long-term survival when given pre- and post-operatively to responding tumors.
   c. May decrease tumor mass pre-operatively.
5. Multimodal.
   a. Pre-operative chemotherapy, esophagectomy, and post-operative chemotherapy for responding tumors and radiation to residual mediastinal disease is treatment of choice.
   b. Seventy percent survival at 12 months in non-randomized trials.
6. Palliation.
   a. Resection or bypass best long-term palliation.
   b. Laser fulguration for relief of obstruction.
   c. Repeated dilation and pulsion placement of endoprosthesis is reserved for poor-risk, short-term patient. Fourteen percent mortality and 25% complication rate.
7. Prognosis.
   a. Eighty percent mortality at 1 year. Overall 5-year survival less than 10%.
   b. Radiotherapy 6-10%.
   c. Surgery 2-24%, average 10% 5-year survival.
   d. Multimodal therapy 5-year survival rates pending.

VIII. ESOPHAGEAL RUPTURE AND PERFORATION

A. Etiology.

1. Iatrogenic–most common.
   a. Endoscopic injury more common with rigid *vs.* flexible endoscope. Occurs most commonly at pharyngo-esophageal junction. Results from direct injury or foreign body removal.
   b. Dilation.
   c. Biopsy.
   d. Intubation (esophageal or endotracheal).
   e. Operative–devascularization or perforation with pulmonary resection, vagotomy, or anti-reflux procedure.
   f. Placement of nasoenteric tubes.
2. Non-iatrogenic.
   a. Barogenic trauma.
      (1) Postemetic (Boerhaave syndrome)–transmural tear following forceful or repeated vomiting. Usually associated with gluttony, bulimia, or alcoholic binge. Esophageal and gastric contents forced into chest under pressure.
      (2) Blunt chest or abdominal trauma.
      (3) Other–labor, convulsions, defecation.

b. Penetrating neck, chest, or abdominal trauma.
c. Foreign body.
d. Post-operative–anastomotic disruption.
e. Corrosive injury.
f. Erosion by adjacent inflammation.
g. Carcinoma.

B. Clinical presentation—can be dramatic and catastrophic with tachycardia, hypotension, and respiratory compromise. Other presentations include dyspnea, neck or chest pain, fever, subcutaneous emphysema, and pneumothorax.

C. Diagnosis.

1. Chest radiograph may reveal pneumothorax, pneumomediastinum, pleural effusion, or subdiaphragmatic air.
2. Contrast swallow. Controversy whether water soluble or barium is best. Most perform water-soluble study first because its effects on mediastinum are less than barium if perforation is present; however, this material is worse if aspirated. Barium study can be obtained if initial study is negative and suspicion remains high.

D. Treatment.

1. Early recognition and treatment are essential to survival. Must rule out myocardial infarction, perforated viscus, dissecting aortic aneurysms, and pulmonary embolus.
2. Basics.
   a. Drainage.
   b. NPO.
   c. Fluid resuscitation.
   e. Broad-spectrum antibiotics.
   f. Nutritional support in recovery period. Parenteral nutrition preferred.
3. Non-operative.
   a. Controversial; only applicable in patient with small perforation, cervical perforation, contained leak, no evidence of sepsis, and wide drainage back into esophagus.
   b. Nasogastric suction, antibiotics, close observation.
   c. Cervical.
      (1) Limited extravasation and extrathoracic perforation may initially be managed non-operatively.
      (2) Patient with crepitus or increased extravasation–operative drainage, antibiotics, closure of rupture if possible, and, potentially, a cervical esophagostomy.
   d. Thoracic.
      (1) Mortality is 10-15% in patients treated within 24 h of injury. Increases to greater than 50% if diagnosis delayed greater than 24 h.
      (2) Early–suture closure, wide drainage, and antibiotics. Bolstering repair with patch is of controversial benefit.

(3) Late–operative drainage and antibiotics. Suture closure is unlikely to hold. Some perform esophagectomy, oversew the cardia, and create a cervical esophagostomy.

4. Complications of esophageal perforation include sepsis, abscess, fistula, empyema, mediastinitis, and death.

IX. CAUSTIC INJURY

A. Etiology.

1. Usually results from ingestion of alkalis, acids, bleach, or detergents.
2. Patient usually younger than 5 years old or adolescent/adult attempting suicide.
3. Alkalis cause liquefactive necrosis, which results in greater depth of injury.

B. Clinical presentation.

1. Oral and oropharyngeal burns (pseudomembranes).
2. Signs and symptoms of laryngotracheal edema (hoarseness, stridor, aphonia, and dyspnea).
3. Signs and symptoms of esophageal or gastric perforation.
4. In absence of perforation, acute manifestations resolve in a few days. Clinical improvement may continue for several weeks until course complicated by stricture.

C. Diagnosis.

1. Esophagogastroscopy to establish severity of injury.
2. Contrast exam of esophagus can demonstrate injury as well as suspected perforation.

D. Treatment.

1. Initial therapy.
   a. Induction of emesis should be avoided as well as attempts to dilute the caustic agent (damage is nearly instantaneous, and intake of large volumes of fluid may only cause distention and emesis).
   b. NPO.
   c. IV hydration
   d. Broad-spectrum antibiotics after diagnosis confirmed.
   e. Use of corticosteroids to attempt to limit stricture debatable.
2. Operative intervention.
   a. Patients with evidence of esophageal or gastric perforation require immediate operation.
      (1) Best explored through an abdominal incision, but prepped from mandible to pubis to allow for possibility of cervical incision.
      (2) Restoration or alimentary continuity should await resolution of acute insult.
   b. Stricture formation tends to be the rule.
      (1) Dilatation is traditional therapy.

(2) Stricture that cannot be dilated or remains refractory to dilatation after 1 year requires esophageal substitution.
   a) Stomach is preferred substitute but often unusable secondary to scarring from original injury.
   b) Esophagus should be excised.

32

Gastric Tumors

TIMOTHY D. KANE, M.D.

I. ADENOCARCINOMA OF THE STOMACH

A. 90-95% of all gastric tumors.

B. Epidemiology.

1. 8th most common cause of cancer mortality in U.S.
2. Declining incidence (10 per 100,000).
3. Male:Female 2:1.
4. 70% of patients > 50 years old; peaks 7th decade.
5. Incidence highest in Asia (Japan, 80 x that in US).

C. Risk factors—genetic and environmental.

1. Environment.
   a. Diet–smoked foods, nitrosamine compounds, polycyclic hydrocarbons, and low consumption of fruits and vegetables.
   b. Occupational–heavy metals, rubber, asbestos.
   c. Cigarette smoking, alcohol consumption.
   d. Low socioeconomic status.
2. Genetic.
   a. Associated with blood type A (only 1.2 relative risk).
   b. Hereditary nonpolyposis colon cancer syndrome–Lynch syndrome II.
   c. Black race.
   d. Family history gastric cancer (1st degree relatives, 2-3 fold >risk).

D. Precursor conditions.

1. Pernicious anemia.
   a. Association with achlorhydria and atrophic gastritis.
   b. Increased risk of gastric cancer (2-10%), controversial.
2. Partial gastrectomy for benign disease.
   a. Most cases occur following Billroth II, 5% risk.
   b. Usually > 15 years after primary surgery (relative risk 1.5-3).
   c. Chronic exposure to biliary, pancreatic, and intestinal secretions with resultant gastritis is possibly the cause.

3. Gastric polyps.
   a. Inflammatory (75-90%) or adenomatous (10-20%).
   b. Adenomatous polyps associated with gastric cancer.
      (1) $>$ 2 cm–40% risk of malignant change.
      (2) $<$ 2 cm–1.5% risk.
4. Hypertrophic gastritis (Ménétrier's disease).
   a. Inflammatory disease of gastric epithelium.
   b. Up to 10% risk of malignant change.
5. Chronic atrophic gastritis with intestinal metaplasia.
6. Peptic ulcer disease–$<$ 1% risk of malignant change.
7. *Helicobacter pylori.*
   a. Gram-negative microaerophilic bacterium, possible promoter agent of gastric carcinoma.
   b. Patients with *H. pylori* infection have 3-6 times increased risk gastric cancer; also increased infection rate in patients with cancer.
   c. Increased incidence *H. pylori* infection in China, where rate of gastric cancer is high.
8. Barrett's esophagus–0.8% risk per year.

D. Pathology.

1. Location of primary tumor.
   a. Pyloric canal or antrum–30%.
   b. Body–20%.
   c. Cardia–37%.
   d. Entire stomach–12%.
2. Borrmann's classification.
   a. Type I (3%)–nonulcerated, polypoid, growing intraluminally.
   b. Type II (18%)–ulcerated, circumscribed with sharp margins.
   c. Type III (16%)–ulcerated, margin *not* sharply circumscribed.
   d. Type IV (63%)–diffuse, infiltrating, may be ulcerated; may involve entire stomach–"*Linitis plastica*".
3. Evidence of metastatic disease.
   a. Direct extension to adjacent organs.
   b. Lymphatic.
      (1) Regional nodes–greater/lesser curve, celiac axis.
      (2) Supraclavicular (**Virchow's node**).
      (3) Umbilical (**Sister Mary Joseph's node**).
   c. Hematogenous via portal or systemic circulation–ascites, jaundice, liver mass, pelvic mass.
   d. Peritoneal seeding to omentum, parietal peritoneum, ovaries (**Krukenberg's tumor**), or cul-de-sac (**Blumer's shelf**).

E. Clinical features—rarely present with early gastric carcinoma.

1. Weight loss (62%).
2. Pain/dyspepsia (52%).
3. Anemia (40-50%).
4. Palpable abdominal mass (30-50%).
5. Nausea/emesis (34%).

6. Dysphagia (26%).
7. Hematemesis is rare; melena (20%).
8. Early satiety (18%).
9. Ascites, pleural effusion, or lymphadenopathy from metastasis.

F. Diagnosis.

1. Radiology.
   a. Barium upper GI series with air contrast–90% accurate.
      (1) Evaluate for ulcer, mass, or infiltrating lesions.
      (2) Sensitivity poor if previous gastric surgery.
   b. Abdominal CT.
      (1) Delineates extent of primary tumor and presence of metastatic disease.
      (2) Accuracy 70% for regional node metastases.
2. Endoscopy.
   a. 90-95% accurate in diagnosing advanced cancers.
   b. Multiple biopsies, brush and lavage cytology improves accuracy.
   c. Less than 3% gastric ulcers evaluated by endoscopy/biopsy are malignant.
3. Endoscopic ultrasound.
   a. More accurate than CT for determining depth of tumor invasion, regional nodes, and invasion of adjacent structures.
   b. Used together with CT; ultrasound is unable to identify distant metastases.

G. T-N-M Classification.

Primary Tumor (T)

T1: Tumor limited to mucosa or submucosa.
T2: Tumor extends to serosa.
T3: Tumor penetrates serosa.
T4: Tumor invades adjacent structures.

Nodal Involvement (N)

N0: No metastases to regional lymph nodes.
N1: Metastases in perigastric nodes within 3 cm from tumor.
N2: Metastases in perigastric nodes > 3 cm from tumor.

Distant Metastasis (M)

M0: No known distant metastasis.
M1: Distant metastasis present.

Surgical Results (R)

R0: No residual tumor.
R1: Microscopic residual tumor.
R2: Macroscopic residual tumor.

H. Treatment.

1. Lymphadenectomy.
   a. Value of extended procedure controversial.
   b. Of benefit in Japan in patients with local or regional disease.
   c. R1–resection of stomach, omentum, and perigastric lymph nodes.

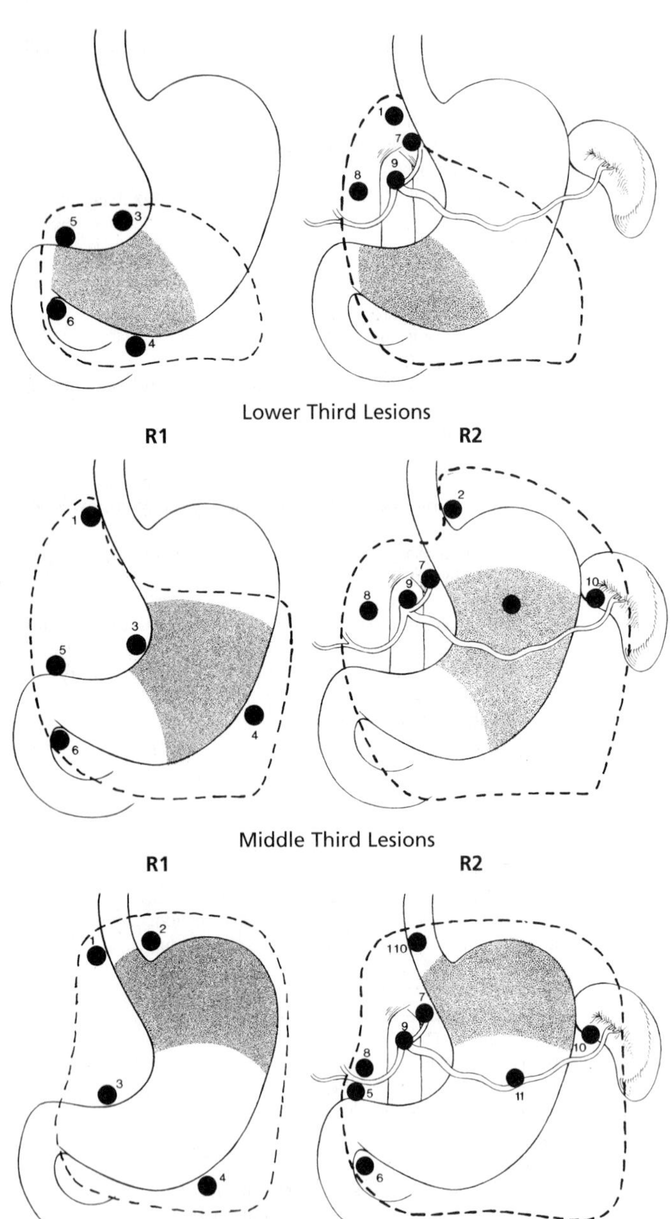
1
2
3
4
5
6
7
8
9
10
11
110
Lower Third Lesions
R1
R2
Middle Third Lesions
R1
R2
Upper Third Lesions (Includes Cardia)
R1
R2

d. R2—as in R1, with *en bloc* resection of superior leaf of transverse mesocolon pancreatic capsule, and lymph nodes along branches of celiac artery, and infraduodenal and supraduodenal areas.

e. R3—resection of above structures and lymph nodes along aorta and esophagus, along with the spleen and tail of the pancreas.

2. Surgical resection.
   a. Indicated for both curative intent and palliation.
   b. Curative resection.
      (1) **Cardia, fundus**—total gastrectomy including regional lymphadenectomy; reconstruction by Roux-en-Y esophagojejunostomy. In lesions confined to the cardia, proximal subtotal gastrectomy with lymphadenectomy is an alternative. Esophagogastrectomy is usually performed for tumors of the gastroesophageal junction.
      (2) **Body**—carcinomas can involve all regional nodal areas draining stomach. Options include radical subtotal or total gastrectomy. Total gastrectomy is associated with improved survival in patients with early gastric cancer.
      (3) **Antrum and pylorus**—subtotal gastrectomy with regional lymphadenectomy; optimal reconstruction by antecolic gastrojejunostomy. Need at least 1 cm margin in first part of duodenum and 5-7 cm margin in proximal stomach. Obtain frozen section evaluation of margins prior to anastomosis.
      (4) **Splenectomy** increases morbidity and has no survival benefit.
   c. Palliative surgery.
      (1) 65% have advanced disease such that curative resection is not possible; performed to relieve obstruction, bleeding, or pain.
      (2) Subtotal gastrectomy better than gastro-enterostomy bypass; good control of symptoms in 50%.
      (3) Endoscopic laser ablation or intubation.
3. Chemotherapy.
   a. FAM—5-fluorouracil, adriamycin, and mitomycin C.

FIG. 1 Lymphadenectomy (Redrawn from Smith JW, Shiu MH, Kelsey L, and Brennan MF: Morbidity of radical lympadenectomy in the curative resection of gastric carcinoma, *Arch Surg* 126:1469, 1991. Copyright by American Medical Association) [see facing page].

1, Right cardiac
2, Left cardiac
3, Lesser curvature
4, Greater curvature and short gastric
5, Suprapyloric (optional)
6, Infrapyloric (optional)
7, Left gastric artery
8, Hepatic artery
9, Celiac
10, Splenic hilar
11, Splenic artery
110, Para-esophageal (cardia lesions)

b. 30-40% partial remission rate; median response about 9 months.
c. No evidence of improved survival or palliation of symptoms beyond that associated with curative resection.

4. Radiation therapy.
   a. Radioresistant tumors marginal response to external beam irradiation.
   b. Used to palliate symptoms of cardia obstruction or chronic blood loss.

I. Prognosis (5-year survival, Western series).

1. Overall 5-year survival–10-21%.
2. Resection with curative intent–20-25%.
3. Early gastric cancer (T1)–90%.
4. Cancer of the cardia–< 10%.
5. Linitis plastica–< 5%.

II. GASTRIC LYMPHOMA

A. 5% of primary gastric malignancies; two-thirds of GI lymphomas.

B. 2% of all non-Hodgkin's lymphoma; most common extranodal lymphoma.

C. Clinical presentation.

1. Indistinguishable from those of gastric adenocarcinoma.
2. Up to 42% present as emergencies (bleeding, perforation, obstruction).

D. Predominant histology is histiocytic.

E. Diagnosis.

1. Endoscopy with biopsy and brush cytology: 80% accuracy.
2. Staging–chest radiograph, chest and abdominal CT scan, bone marrow biopsy, pedal lymphangiography, and biopsy of enlarged peripheral node.

F. Treatment.

1. Subtotal gastrectomy followed by chemotherapy; radiation reserved for residual bulky disease. Some centers use neoadjuvant chemotherapy (doxorubicin & cytoxan), reserving surgery and/or radiation therapy for incomplete responses or recurrent disease.
2. 75% resectable at exploration.
3. Microscopic positive margins do not affect survival.
4. Regional lymphadenectomy not necessary unless grossly involved.

G. Prognosis better than adenocarcinoma; 5-year survival 25-50%.

III. GASTRIC LEIOMYOSARCOMA

A. 1-3% of primary gastric malignancies.

B. Presentation—Usually present as bulky intraluminal mass with central area of necrosis. Tumor develops submucosally. Usually present with hemorrhage, pain, and/or weight loss.

C. Diagnosis—by endoscopy with biopsy and brush cytology.

D. Treatment of choice—total excision; not radiosensitive, chemotherapy of little benefit.
E. Hematogenous spread common; liver frequently involved.
F. 5-year survival—30-50%.

IV. BENIGN TUMORS OF THE STOMACH

A. 7% incidence overall.
B. Most common in the antrum and body.
C. Classification.

1. Hyperplastic polyp (40%).
2. Leiomyoma (40%).
3. Gastric adenoma (10%).
4. Heterotopic pancreas (7%).

D. Presentation—depends on tumor size, location, and histologic nature.
E. Diagnosis—by endoscopy with biopsy and brush cytology.
F. Treatment—depends on tumor size and type.

1. Remove symptomatic polyps endoscopically.
2. Open surgical excision is indicated for lesions > 2 cm, incomplete endoscopic excision, or if malignant neoplasm is identified.

33

Peptic Ulcer Disease

Betty J. Tsuei, M.D.

I. DUODENAL ULCER

A. Pathogenesis.

1. Higher rates of basal and stimulated acid secretion (noted in 40% of patients with duodenal ulcers).
2. Increased number of parietal cells and enhanced gastrin sensitivity.
3. Disturbances in gastric motility (accelerated gastric emptying).
4. *Helicobacter pylori*–Gram-negative organism associated with peptic ulcer disease.
   a. Although 70-90% of patients with duodenal ulcer and 50-70% of patients with gastric ulcer have concomitant *H. pylori* infection, not all patients with *H. pylori* have peptic ulcer disease.
   b. Pathogenesis is unclear, but infection may disrupt protective mucosal layers and predispose to peptic ulcer disease.
   c. Diagnosis is established with antral biopsy and CLO (*Campylobacter*-like organism) test, or serology.
   d. Treatment (see below) accelerates healing and decreases rate of ulcer recurrence.

B. Pathology.

1. Usually located 1-2 cm distal to the pylorus, commonly on the posterior wall, but can occur anteriorly and in the pyloric channel.
2. Duodenal ulcers are rarely malignant.
3. Multiple ulcers or those that occur in the second and third portions of the duodenum should raise suspicions of gastrinoma (Zollinger-Ellison syndrome–see "Miscellaneous Endocrine Disorders").

C. Clinical presentation.

1. Duodenal ulcers are most common in the younger population (25-35 years old); there is a male predominance.
2. Increased familial incidence.
3. Risk factors–alcohol, tobacco, aspirin, coffee, and steroids.

4. Pain typically presents as a burning sensation when the stomach is empty (i.e., several hours after eating) and is relieved by ingestion of food or antacids, which act to buffer acid secretion.
5. Epigastric tenderness may be present on physical exam.

D. Diagnostic studies.

1. ***Endoscopy*** is 95% accurate for diagnosis and may detect other lesions of esophagus, stomach and duodenum.
2. ***Upper GI series*** is 75-80% accurate and may reveal duodenal lesion.

E. Medical management should include discontinuation of risk factors and ulcerogenic medications when possible. Therapy is aimed at reducing acid output, increasing mucosal protection, and eliminating infectious agents.

1. Acid-reducing medications.
   a. **Antacids** should be given 1 h before and 3 h after each meal. Those containing magnesium can produce diarrhea; those with aluminum can produce constipation. Antacids are associated with healing rates of 80% at 4 weeks.
   b. **H_2 receptor antagonists** (cimetidine, ranitidine, famotidine) have ulcer healing rates exceeding 80% at 4 weeks. Approximately 5-10% of duodenal ulcers are refractory to H_2 receptor therapy, with recurrence rates up to 30% with long-term maintenance therapy.
   c. **Omeprazole** (Prilosec®)–blocks the proton pump and reduces acid secretion by 99%. Accelerates ulcer healing compared to other medications now available. Useful in ulcers refractory to H_2 blockers.
2. Cytoprotective agents.
   a. **Sucralfate** (Carafate®)–a basic aluminum sucrose sulfate that dissociates in an acidic medium.
      (1) The negatively charged polymerized molecule adheres to proteinaceous deposits found in the ulcer base. Binding lasts about 6 h with little systemic absorption.
      (2) Sucralfate requires an acidic medium and should be taken on an empty stomach. The standard dose is 1 g 1 h before each meal and at bedtime. Concomitant antacid use should be avoided.
      (3) Healing action may result from the physical barrier that prevents acid and pepsin from acting further on the ulcer. Healing rates (95% at 12 weeks) are similar to H_2 blockers.
      (4) Most common side-effect is constipation (7.5%).
   b. **Misoprostol** (Cytotec®)–a prostaglandin E_2 analog; is the only treatment with demonstrated effectiveness in prophylaxis of NSAID-induced ulcer disease.
3. Treatment of infectious agents.
   a. Treatment of *H. pylori* has been shown to increase the rate of ulcer healing and decrease the rate of recurrence.

b. Treatment regimens have consisted of bismuth, metronidazole, and tetracycline (or amoxicillin) for 2 weeks, but there are often side-effects of nausea, vomiting, or diarrhea.
c. With increased incidence of resistance to metronidazole, omeprazole and antibiotics (amoxicillin, tetracycline) may be useful.

4. Following diagnosis, a course of medical therapy (most often H_2 antagonist and/or antacids) should be tried. After 6-8 weeks, repeat diagnostic tests are indicated to document healing. Ulcers that do not heal after 8-12 weeks of medical management may require surgical intervention.

F. **Indications for operation**—only 10-20% of patients with peptic ulcer disease will require surgical intervention.
1. ***Bleeding***—most cases will stop spontaneously. Typically seen with posterior ulcers that erode into the gastroduodenal artery. Surgery is indicated for acute bleeds that require transfusion of 6 or more units of blood.
2. ***Perforation.***
   a. Typically seen in anterior wall duodenal ulcers.
   b. Indication for surgery in up to 30% of patients.
   c. Classic presentation is sudden onset of severe generalized abdominal pain associated with a rigid abdomen.
   d. Free air under diaphragm on upright chest radiograph seen in 75% of cases.
3. ***Gastric outlet obstruction.***
   a. Usually seen with prepyloric or duodenal ulcers; results from edema during acute phase or scarring of the duodenal bulb.
   b. History of emesis of undigested food shortly after eating; usually long history of peptic ulcer disease.
   c. Characteristic electrolyte abnormalities (hypokalemia, hypochloremia, and metabolic alkalosis).
   d. Saline load test for diagnosis. Empty stomach with nasogastric tube and instill 750 cc of normal saline. Place patient in sitting position for 30 min, then aspirate. Test is positive if aspirate > 400 cc.
4. ***Intractable pain*** despite maximal medical therapy.
5. ***Failure of medical management.***

G. **Surgical treatment.**
1. Resections.
   a. **Subtotal gastrectomy**—operative mortality 2-4%, recurrence rate 4%. Rarely performed today owing to increased incidence of post-gastrectomy syndromes.
   b. **Vagotomy and antrectomy**—mortality 1-3%, has the lowest recurrence (< 2% at 5 years) but a high incidence of post-operative diarrhea and dumping (10-20%).
   c. Most common reconstructions used after gastric resection procedure.
      (1) **Billroth I**—gastroduodenostomy (Figure 1).

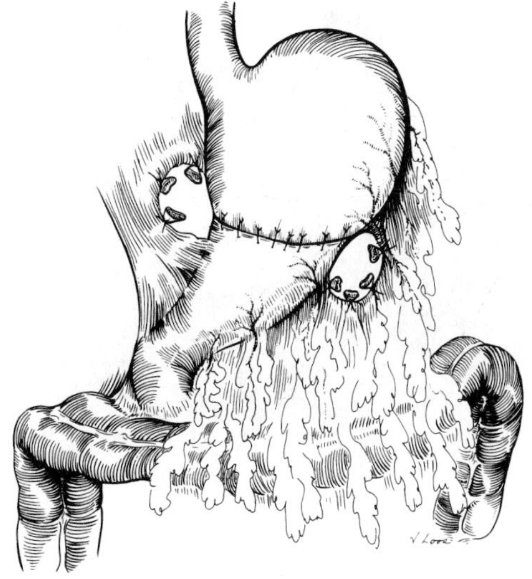

FIG. 1 Billroth I Reconstruction

(2) **Billroth II**—gastrojejunostomy with closure of the duodenal stump (Figure 2).

(3) Roux-en-Y gastrojejunostomy (Figure 3).

2. ***Vagotomy and drainage*** (pyloroplasty or gastrojejunostomy)—a mortality of 1% with recurrence rate of 5-10%. Useful in cases of active bleeding in conjunction with oversewing of the bleeding ulcer.
3. ***Selective vagotomy***—the entire stomach is denervated with preservation of the celiac and hepatic branches of the vagal nerves. A drainage procedure is often required, as gastric emptying is delayed.
4. ***Highly selective vagotomy***/parietal cell vagotomy.
   a. Only the parietal cell mass is denervated.
   b. As the motor function of the antrum and pylorus remains intact, no drainage procedure is needed. Very low incidence of post-gastrectomy syndromes.
   c. Results are highly dependent on operator experience. Mortality of 0.1-0.3% with long-term recurrence rate of at least 15%.
   d. *Contraindicated* for prepyloric or pyloric channel ulcers—higher recurrence rate.
5. ***Omental (Graham) patch*** for perforated ulcer may be an adequate procedure in patients without prior history of chronic

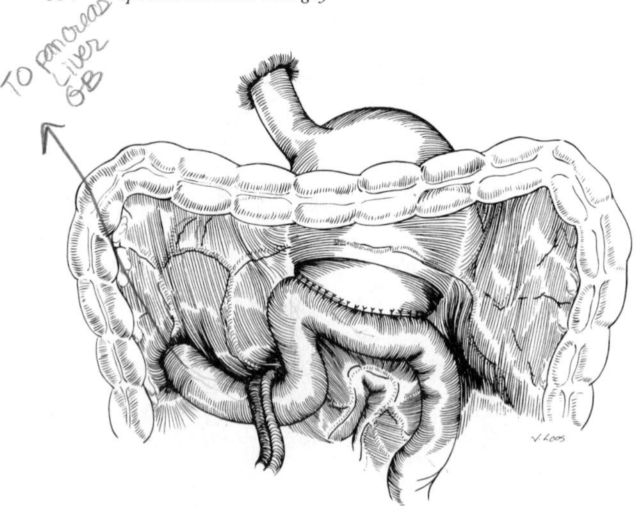

FIG. 2 Retrocolic Billroth II Reconstruction

ulcer disease, since 30% will have no further manifestation of their disease.

H. Post-operative complications.

1. ***Recurrent ulcers.***
   a. More common with duodenal ulcers.
   b. Usually occur at the anastomotic site (intestinal side) within the first 2 years after surgery ("marginal ulcer").
   c. Most commonly caused by incomplete vagotomy.
   d. Can be treated with medical management, but should be re-explored if these measures fail.
2. ***Early postprandial dumping***—most common postgastrectomy complication.
   a. Rapid emptying of hyperosmolar chyme causes intravascular fluid shifts, resulting in gastrointestinal and vasomotor symptoms.
   b. Symptoms of abdominal pain and fullness, vomiting, diarrhea, flushing, palpitations and dizziness occur within 30 minutes of a meal.
   c. Symptoms are relieved with supine position and prevented by frequent small high-protein and low-carbohydrate meals.
   d. If surgical intervention is required, an antiperistaltic jejunal loop between the gastric remnant and the small intestine or a Roux-en-Y loop may be successful.
3. ***Late postprandial dumping***/reactive hypoglycemia.

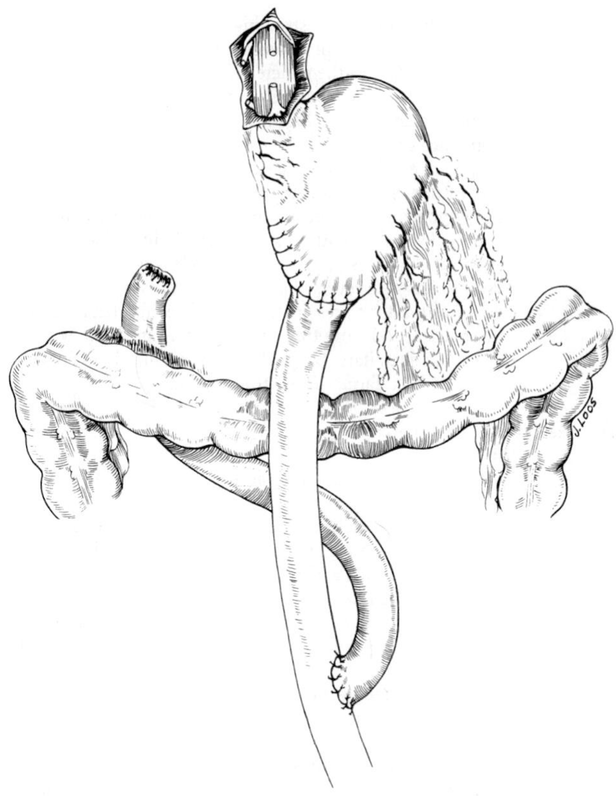

FIG. 3 Roux-en-Y Gastrojejunostomy

a. Large amounts of carbohydrates stimulate insulin release, which produces hypoglycemia several hours after eating.
b. Symptoms include tachycardia, dizziness, and diaphoresis 1.5-2 h after a meal.
c. Treatment consists of low-carbohydrate meals, with ingestion of carbohydrates once symptoms begin.
d. Surgical intervention consists of an antiperistaltic jejunal loop to delay gastric emptying.

4. ***Afferent loop syndrome.***
   a. Post-prandial distention, nausea, and RUQ pain relieved by bilious emesis.
   b. Acute form may be related to post-operative edema at the

gastrojejunostomy obstructing the afferent loop. Hyperamylasemia is common secondary to reflux of the duodenal contents into the pancreatic duct.
   c. Chronic form is caused by intermittent obstruction of a long afferent limb and results in bilious emesis without the presence of food.
   d. Operative correction of chronic form involves conversion to a Roux-en-Y gastrojejunostomy.
5. ***Post-vagotomy diarrhea*** is typically episodic and may occur in up to 30% of patients. First-line therapy includes constipating agents or cholestyramine to bind bile acids. Operative intervention using a reversed jejunal segment is rarely necessary.
6. ***Bile reflux gastritis*** presents as epigastric pain often associated with nausea and vomiting. Treatment is initiated with H_2 blockers or sucralfate. Surgical options include conversion to a Roux-en-Y or Tanner-19 gastrojejunostomy.

II. GASTRIC ULCERS

A. Pathogenesis.

1. ***Type I***—most common, and present as a solitary ulcer on the lesser curve.
   a. Caused by the reflux of duodenal contents through an incompetent pylorus, resulting in atrophic gastritis.
   b. Ulceration occurs at the junction of acid secreting and non-acid secreting mucosa.
   c. Most clearly related to defects in mucosal resistance. Nearly 1/3 of gastric ulcers are related to aspirin or non-steroidal agents.
2. ***Type II***—associated with concomitant duodenal ulcer.
3. ***Type III***—prepyloric ulcers (located within 2 cm of the pylorus) are similar in etiology to duodenal ulcers.

B. Presentation and diagnosis.

1. Gastric ulcers are less common than duodenal ulcers and occur in older patients.
2. Pain is the most common complaint, but there is less correlation to meals. The pain may actually be exacerbated by food. Completely asymptomatic lesions are also common.
3. 5-10% of gastric ulcers are malignant; those > 2 cm have a higher rate of malignancy.
4. Endoscopy and radiographic studies are used to confirm the diagnosis. Endoscopy is preferred, as biopsies can be taken at the time of diagnosis to **distinguish benign from malignant ulcers.** All gastric ulcers should be biopsied to rule out malignancy.

C. Medical treatment is similar to that of duodenal ulcers, except antacids are less effective. Failure to heal suggests malignancy. Complications of gastric ulcer are more frequent than duodenal ulcer; relapse rates are as high as 60% within 2 years.

D. Indications for surgery.

1. Failure to heal after 3 months of conservative therapy.

2. Dysplasia or carcinoma.
3. Recurrence.
4. Poor medical compliance.
5. Complications–bleeding (> 6 units acutely or recurrent), perforation.

E. Surgical intervention.

1. Type I ulcers are treated with distal gastrectomy (antrectomy) to include the ulcer without concomitant vagal section. Cure rate is about 95%.
2. Type II and type III ulcers should be treated as duodenal ulcers.
3. Proximal ulcer may be treated with local excision and closure; consider antrectomy or drainage if gastric stasis contributing factor.

III. STRESS GASTRITIS

A. Pathology.

1. Occurs in the setting of severe and prolonged physiologic stress, such as critically ill patients with severe trauma, burns, ARDS, renal failure, and sepsis.
2. Multiple superficial punctate lesions arise acutely in the proximal stomach. In 20% of patients, these can progress and coalesce to form multiple hemorrhagic ulcerations (acute hemorrhagic gastritis).
3. The cause appears to be a defect in mucosal membrane protection, since stress gastritis is not associated with acid hypersecretion.

B. Diagnosis is established with endoscopy.

C. Treatment.

1. The most effective form of treatment is prevention. Maintain intraluminal pH > 4.5 with H_2 blockers or antacids. Sucralfate is also an effective prophylactic agent.
2. In severe hemorrhage, endoscopy with coagulation, intra-arterial vasopressin or embolization can be used (see "GI Bleeding").
3. Surgical procedures are used only if non-operative management fails; associated with high rebleeding rates (25-50%) and mortality (30-40%).
   a. Oversewing of bleeding points and a vagotomy and drainage.
   b. Vagotomy and drainage for bleeding from the distal stomach is preferred to prevent rebleeding.
   c. Hemorrhage not controlled by (a) or (b) may require near-total gastrectomy.

IV. ZOLLINGER-ELLISON SYNDROME (see "Miscellaneous Endocrine Disorders")

34

Crohn's Disease

Christopher S. Meyer, M.D.

I. INFLAMMATORY BOWEL DISEASE (IBD)

Usually refers to two diseases that may be difficult to differentiate clinically.

- **A. Ulcerative colitis—**a diffuse inflammatory disease limited to the mucosa of the colon and rectum. Surgical resection is almost always curative.
- **B. Crohn's disease** (regional enteritis, granulomatous colitis)–a chronic, relapsing, transmural, usually segmental, and often granulomatous inflammatory disorder that can involve any portion of the GI tract. Operative therapy is usually reserved for the treatment of complications or intractable disease.

II. CROHN'S DISEASE

- **A. Etiology—**not known, but may be similar to that of ulcerative colitis. Others:
  1. Infectious–possibly atypical mycobacteria.
  2. Genetic–15-20% of patients have family history of IBD.
  3. Environmental–temperate climates, smoking.
- **B. Epidemiology.**
  1. Peak incidence between 2nd and 4th decades; late peak ages 50-60.
  2. Equal sex distribution.
  3. Incidence–6-7/100,000.
- **C. Clinical manifestations/evaluation.**
  1. *Signs and symptoms.*
     - a. Diarrhea–90% of patients, usually non-bloody.
     - b. Recurrent **abdominal pain**–mild colicky pain, often initiated by meals and relieved by defecation.
     - c. Abdominal symptoms (distention, flatulence).
     - d. Fever, malaise.
     - e. Anorectal lesions–chronic recurrent or non-healing anal fissures, ulcers, complex anal fistulas, perirectal abscesses (may precede bowel involvement).

f. Malnutrition–protein-losing enteropathy, steatorrhea, mineral and vitamin deficiencies, growth retardation.
g. Acute onset–an acute appendicitis-like presentation due to acute inflammation of the distal ileum; only 15% of these patients (with isolated terminal ileitis) develop chronic Crohn's disease. May be due to a different pathogen (i.e., *Yersinia*).
h. Extraintestinal manifestations in 30% (see II.E.1 above).

2. ***Disease distribution.***
   a. May involve entire GI tract (from lips to anus); distal ileum is most frequently involved; skip areas found in 12-35% of cases.
   b. Small bowel alone–30%.
   c. Distal ileum and colon–55%.
   d. Colon alone–15%.
   e. Duodenum–0.5-7%.
   f. Anorectum alone–5%.
3. ***Laboratory findings—*** nonspecific and varied.
   a. Anemia–iron or B_{12}/folate deficiency.
   b. Hypoalbuminemia and steatorrhea are common.
   c. Tests of small bowel function (D-xylose absorption, bile acid breath test) are abnormal with extensive disease.
4. ***Radiographic findings.***
   a. Upper GI with small bowel follow-through or enteroclysis if small bowel disease is suspected.
   b. Barium enema–thickened bowel wall, longitudinal ulcers, transverse fissures, cobblestone formation, and rectal sparing. Terminal ileum demonstrated by reflux from barium enema, may see stricture ("string sign").
   c. Abdominal CT scan is useful in complicated cases with intra-abdominal abscess.
5. ***Endoscopy.***
   a. Proctosigmoidoscopy reveals a normal rectum in 40-50% of patients with colonic disease. Biopsy from a grossly normal-appearing rectum may reveal histologic disease, however.
   b. Characteristic lesions (aphthous ulcers, mucosal ulcerations and fissures, cobblestoning) may be seen in colon and distal ileum.
   c. Involvement is typically patchy.
6. ***Intra-operative findings.***
   a. Creeping of mesenteric fat toward antimesenteric border.
   b. Serosal and mesenteric inflammation.
   c. Bowel wall thickening, strictures; foreshortening of bowel and mesentery.
   d. Enlargement of mesenteric lymph nodes; nodes adjacent to bowel indicate mucosal disease.
   e. Inflammatory masses, abscesses, adherent bowel loops.

D. Differential diagnosis.

1. Ulcerative colitis.
2. Acute ileitis (e.g., *Campylobacter, Yersinia*).
3. Acute appendicitis.

4. Tuberculosis.
5. Lymphoma.
6. Miscellaneous–carcinoma, amebiasis, ischemia, diverticulitis.

E. Complications.

1. Intestinal obstruction.
2. Abscess formation.
3. Fistula–internal and external.
4. Anorectal lesions–abscess, fistula, fissures.
5. Free perforation and hemorrhage are rare.
6. Carcinoma–much less common than in ulcerative colitis; usually occurs in surgically bypassed segments.
7. Toxic megacolon–occurs in 5% of patients with colonic disease; responds better to medical therapy than ulcerative colitis.
8. Extraintestinal (see II.E.1 above).
   a. More common with colonic involvement.
   b. Urinary–cystitis, calculi (oxalate), ureteral obstruction.

F. Medical management.

1. Drug therapy.
   a. **Steroids and sulfasalazine** for acute attack. Sulfasalazine is primarily indicated for colonic involvement.
   b. Immunosuppressants–indicated for steroid-sparing, refractory disease, or perianal disease, healing of some fistulas and possibly maintenance of remission.
      (1) Azathioprine (2.5 mg/kg/day).
      (2) **6-mercaptopurine** (50-100 mg/day).
      (3) May take 3-6 months to see beneficial effect.
   c. **Metronidazole** (Flagyl®) is often helpful, especially for anal complications; it requires long-term use. Some flare-ups may be due to presence of *Clostridium difficile,* which is treated with metronidazole as well.
2. Supportive measures.
   a. NPO, intravenous fluids, nasogastric suction as needed.
   b. TPN for fistulas and malnutrition.
   c. Low-residue/high-protein diet for mild relapses.

G. Surgical management—intervention is eventually necessary in 70-75% of cases over the lifetime of the disease. Reserved for treatment of complications of Crohn's disease.

1. ***Indications for surgery.***
   a. Small bowel obstruction–indication in 50% of surgical cases.
   b. Fistula.
   c. Abscess.
   d. Perianal disease (when unresponsive to medical therapy).
   e. Disease intractable to medical management.
   f. Failure to thrive (e.g., chronic malnutrition, growth retardation).
   g. Toxic megacolon.
2. ***Surgical procedures*** (not curative).

a. **Conservative resection** of diseased/symptomatic bowel segment, primary end-to-end anastomosis.
   (1) Only resect grossly diseased area with small "normal" margins. Unnecessary to get histologically free margins for anastomosis.
   (2) Distal ileum and cecal resection with ileocolostomy is common procedure.
   (3) 60% recurrence in long-term follow-up.

b. **Stricturoplasty**–relieves obstruction in chronically scarred bowel without resection. Especially useful for multiple symptomatic strictures.

c. Exclusion bypass–higher incidence of recurrence and carcinoma; may be indicated:
   (1) To bypass unresectable inflammatory mass.
   (2) Gastroduodenal Crohn's disease.
   (3) Multiple, extensive skip lesions.

d. Continent (Kock) ileostomy and mucosal proctectomy procedures are contraindicated.

H. Prognosis—Crohn's is a chronic disease; none of the available modes of therapy are curative.

1. Medical therapy–does not avoid surgery.
2. Recurrence rate 10 years after initial operation:
   a. Ileocolic disease–50%.
   b. Small bowel disease–50%.
   c. Colonic disease–40-50%.
3. Re-operation rates at 5 years:
   a. Primary resection–20%.
   b. Bypass–50%.
4. 80-85% of patients who require surgery lead normal lives.
5. Mortality rate: 15% at 30–disease tends to "burn out".

Inflammatory Bowel Disease

	Crohn's	Ulcerative Colitis
Epidemiology	15-30 years old 50-70 years old Male = Female White > Black	20-30 years old Jews > non-Jews Female > Male White > Black
Gross Pathology	bowel wall thickened longitudinal fissure cobblestones skip areas focal strictures	friable mucosa granular irregularity pseudopolyps continuous disease stove pipe narrowing
Microscopic Pathology	transmural granulomas mesenteric adenopathy	mucosal loss of goblet cells crypt abscess plasma cell infiltrate

Inflammatory Bowel Disease (cont.)

	Crohn's	Ulcerative Colitis
Anatomic Distribution	30% small bowel only 55% small bowel/colon 15% colon only 30% rectal disease 20% skip lesions 50% perianal disease	continuous from anus < 5% rectal sparing no skip lesions 10% terminal ileitis (backwash ileitis)
Clinical Features	diarrhea abdominal pain weight loss	bloody diarrhea abdominal pain weight loss
Complications	fistulas abscess obstruction arthritis uveitis/iridocyclidis pyoderma gangrenosum	anemia toxic megacolon perforation sclerosing cholangitis colon cancer
Mortality	3-6% elective surgery	2-3% elective surgery

35

Ulcerative Colitis

CHRISTOPHER S. MEYER, M.D.

I. INFLAMMATORY BOWEL DISEASE (IBD) usually refers to two diseases that may be difficult to differentiate clinically.

- **A. Ulcerative colitis—**a diffuse inflammatory disease limited to the mucosa of the colon and rectum. Surgical resection is almost always curative.
- **B. Crohn's disease** (regional enteritis, granulomatous colitis)–a chronic, relapsing, transmural, usually segmental, and often granulomatous inflammatory disorder that can involve any portion of the GI tract. Operative therapy is usually reserved for the treatment of complications or intractable disease.

II. ULCERATIVE COLITIS

- **A. Etiology** is unknown. Multiple theories include the following.
  1. Infectious–viral, bacterial, mycobacterial.
  2. Immunologic–possible defect in regulation of mucosal immunity with poorly regulated inflammatory response to exogenous antigens.
  3. Genetic–increased in whites, females, and Jews (2-4 x); familial predisposition; association with certain HLA phenotypes.
  4. Environmental–increased prevalence in urban dwellers.
- **B. Epidemiology.**
  1. Bimodal distribution of onset age–15-30, 50-70.
  2. Females affected slightly more frequently than males (1.3:1).
  3. Family history of ulcerative colitis present in 10-20% of cases.
  4. Incidence–5-12/100,000; prevalence 60/100,000.
- **C. Clinical manifestations/evaluation.**
  1. Signs and symptoms.
     - a. **Diarrhea** (79%), **abdominal pain** (71%), **rectal bleeding** (55%), pus and mucus in stool, weight loss (20%), tenesmus (15%), vomiting (14%), fever (11%).
     - b. Onset may be insidious, or acute and fulminant (15%).
     - c. Abdominal tenderness present with severe disease.
     - d. Extraintestinal manifestations–(see II.E.1 below).

2. Disease distribution.
   a. Confined to colon and rectum; no skip areas.
   b. **"Backwash" ileitis** in 10%; resolves after colonic resection.
   c. Almost always involves rectum (95%); ulcerative proctitis if only rectum involved.
3. Laboratory findings.
   a. Anemia, leukocytosis, elevated sedimentation rate.
   b. Negative stool cultures for ova and parasites.
   c. Severe disease–hypoalbuminemia; water/electrolyte/vitamin depletion; steatorrhea.
4. ***Radiographic findings.***
   a. Plain abdominal films–follow colonic size during acute phase to exclude toxic megacolon.
   b. Barium enema–mucosal irregularity, "collar-button" ulcers, and pseudopolyps. Chronic disease characterized by loss of haustrations, colonic narrowing and shortening; ileum typically spared; strictures are late manifestation and should raise suspicion of malignancy.
5. ***Sigmoidoscopy.***
   a. Essential to diagnosis and determination of disease extent.
   b. Rectal mucosa–granular, friable, dull, hyperemic, edematous.
   c. Uniform disease pattern.
   d. Biopsy findings.
      (1) Mucous depletion in goblet cells.
      (2) Inflammatory polyps in healing stage.
      (3) Crypt abscesses.
6. ***Colonoscopy***—valuable for specific investigations (stricture, rule out malignancy) and for cancer surveillance in chronic disease.

D. Differential diagnosis.

1. Crohn's disease–10% of IBD cases are indeterminate.
2. Diverticulitis.
3. Neoplasm.
4. Infectious enteritis–bacillary dysenteries (*Salmonella, Shigella, Campylobacter*), amebiasis, gonococcal proctitis, *Chlamydia trachomatis.*
5. Pseudomembranous (antibiotic-associated) colitis.
6. Ischemic colitis, spastic colitis.

E. Complications.

1. ***Extraintestinal*** (1/3 of cases).
   a. Skin–erythema nodosum, pyoderma gangrenosum, erythema multiforme, aphthous ulcers/stomatitis.
   b. Eyes–conjunctivitis, iritis (uveitis), episcleritis.
   c. Joints–arthritis, sacroileitis, ankylosing spondylitis (association of the HLA-B27 antigen with ankylosing spondylitis in patients who have ankylosing spondylitis and inflammatory bowel disease).

   d. Hepatobiliary–fatty liver, pericholangitis, hepatitis, bile duct carcinoma; ulcerative colitis probably leading cause of sclerosing cholangitis.
2. Anorectal–hemorrhoids, anal fissure, rectal strictures are common.
3. ***Toxic megacolon***—leading cause of death in ulcerative colitis; 40% of cases are fatal.
   a. Affects 3-5% of patients.
   b. Highest risk of perforation with initial attack of toxic megacolon.
   c. Pathology–inflammation extends into muscular layers of bowel wall; perforation can lead to localized abscess or generalized peritonitis.
   d. Clinical findings–systemic toxicity, transverse colon 8-10 cm in diameter on plain films.
   e. Treatment.
      (1) Intravenous fluid and electrolyte resuscitation.
      (2) NPO, nasogastric tube.
      (3) Parenteral antibiotics, consider TPN.
      (4) Positional maneuvers–redistributes intracolonic gas.
      (5) If no significant improvement within 2-5 days with conservative therapy, then surgery is indicated. Total abdominal colectomy, Brooke ileostomy, and Hartmann closure of the rectum is standard procedure.
4. ***Massive hemorrhage***—can occur in acute fulminant ulcerative colitis. Treatment is emergency total abdominal colectomy, Brooke ileostomy, and Hartmann closure of rectum; allows future sphincter-saving procedure.
5. ***Carcinoma of colon/rectum.***
   a. Begins to appear after 5-10 years of active disease. More common in patients whose colitis presented before age 25.
   b. Incidence–controversial.
      (1) 10 years–2-5%.
      (2) 20 years–20%.
      (3) 1-2% per year if disease present over 10 years.
   c. Predictors–**dysplasia** (if severe, then 10% chance of invasive carcinoma at distant site), extent of colitis, persistent disease.
   d. Vigilant surveillance with **colonoscopy** and **biopsies** mandatory.
   f. Strictures–rule out neoplasm.
   g. Short-term prognosis is worse than with idiopathic colon cancer, long-term (5-year) survival is equivalent.
6. Malnutrition–with acute, severe episodes. Growth retardation in children.

F. Medical management.

1. ***Sulfasalazine*** (Azulfidine®)–used in treatment of mild to moderate ulcerative colitis and to maintain disease remission.

a. Dose.
   (1) 2-8 g/day orally during acute attacks.
   (2) 2 g/day chronically to decrease relapse rate.
b. Metabolized by bacteria to 5-aminosalicylic acid (5-ASA), the active component, and sulfapyridine, which is responsible for the majority of side-effects.
c. Side-effects.
   (1) Oligospermia.
   (2) Inhibits folate absorption.
   (3) Hemolytic anemia.
   (4) Nausea, vomiting, headache, abdominal discomfort.
   (5) Allergic hypersensitivity (10-15%).
d. **5-ASA enemas** may be more effective in distal colitis and proctitis.

2. ***Corticosteroids.***
   a. IV steroids (hydrocortisone 100-300 mg/day; prednisolone 20-80 mg/day; ACTH 20-40 U/day as continuous infusion) for severe or fulminant disease.
   b. Oral steroids (prednisone 20-60 mg/day) for less severe or improving disease.
   c. Does not prevent relapse in inactive disease.
   d. Topical retention enemas for rectal disease.
3. ***Azathioprine*** (Imuran®)–recent studies suggest steroid-sparing effect and prevention of relapse.
4. Supportive measures.
   a. Acute exacerbation–NPO; nasogastric drainage; TPN may improve overall nutritional state and may reverse growth retardation in children.
   b. During remission–diet of choice, avoid milk products, opiates; loperamide, diphenoxylate, or psyllium may control diarrhea.

G. Surgical management.

1. ***Indications for surgery.***
   a. Severe, acute attack unresponsive to intense medical therapy.
   b. Colonic complications–perforation, toxic megacolon, massive hemorrhage, obstruction.
   c. Chronic, debilitating disease.
   d. Carcinoma or high risk for carcinoma.
   e. Growth failure in children.
   f. Severe extraintestinal complications.
2. ***Surgical procedures*** (total proctocolectomy is curative).
   a. **Total abdominal colectomy, mucosal proctectomy, ileal reservoir, and ileoanal anastomosis (Figure 1).**
      (1) Eliminates all diseased mucosa; preserves rectal continence and normal defecation in most patients.
      (2) In experienced centers has become the procedure of choice.

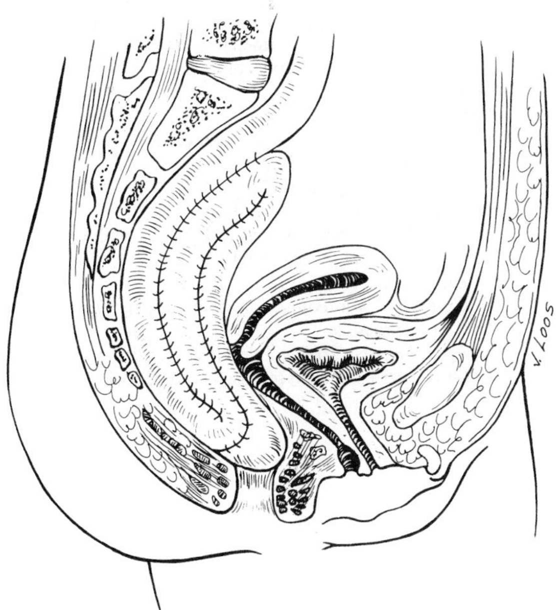

FIG. 1

(3) Disadvantages include frequent stooling, nighttime incontinence, pouchitis, and risk of intestinal obstruction.

b. **Total proctocolectomy with standard (Brooke) ileostomy.**
   (1) Until recently was "gold standard" operation; replaced by sphincter-saving operations to preserve continence.
   (2) 1-3% elective operative mortality.
   (3) 10-15% develop impotence.

c. **Total proctocolectomy with continent (Kock) ileostomy.**
   (1) Avoids need for conventional ileostomy/appliances.
   (2) Major problem is stability of continent nipple valve within ileal reservoir (40-50% may require re-operation).
   (3) Use is now limited to patients who strongly desire continence-restoring procedure following total proctocolectomy.

d. **Total abdominal colectomy with ileostomy, rectal preservation.**
   (1) Reserved for emergency procedures (hemorrhage, toxic megacolon) to decrease operative morbidity and mortality (3-10%).

(2) Mucosal proctectomy and ileoanal anastomosis can be subsequently performed to control proctitis, reduce cancer risk, and preserve continence.

H. Prognosis.

1. Mortality.
   a. 5% death rate over 10 years (pancolitis).
   b. Elective surgery (2%).
   c. Emergency surgery (8-15%).
2. Left-sided colitis and pancolitis.
   a. Acute intermittent (60%); most relapses within first year.
   b. Chronic, unremitting (20%).
   c. Fulminant (10%).
   d. Up to 50% will require colectomy in first 10 years.
3. Ulcerative proctitis.
   a. Approximately 20% will develop left-sided colitis.
   b. Only 2-15% reported to progress to pancolitis.

36

Appendicitis

Tory A. Meyer, M.D.

I. EPIDEMIOLOGY

A. **Frequency—**Appendicitis is the most common cause of acute abdomen requiring surgery; there are nearly 300,000 cases/year in the U.S.; it affects 7% of the population.

B. **Incidence—**decreasing in western societies, most likely secondary to an increase in dietary fiber.

C. **Peak incidence—**in adolescents and young adults, with a slight male predominance in that age group.

D. **Overall mortality—**0.3% for non-perforated cases; 1% for perforated cases.

E. **Infants and elderly** have a much higher morbidity and mortality owing to an increase in the perforation rate from 21% to nearly 85% for infants and 65-75% for elderly adults.

II. PATHOPHYSIOLOGY

A. **Obstruction** of the appendiceal lumen is felt to be the initiating event, most commonly secondary to a fecalith in adults and lymphoid hyperplasia in children.

B. **With continued mucosal secretion,** luminal pressure rises and eventually exceeds capillary venous and lymphatic pressures, causing venous infarction in watershed areas (middle and proximal antimesenteric regions).

C. **Bacterial overgrowth** occurs in the inspissated mucus.

1. Polymicrobial infection with anaerobes > aerobes, 3:1.
2. *E. coli, Bacteroides fragilis, Psuedomonas* present in 80%, 70%, and 40% respectively.

D. **Worsening edema, high luminal pressure, and bacterial proliferation** lead to occlusion of arterial blood flow and gangrenous appendicitis.

E. **Transmural necrosis and bacterial penetration** into the appendiceal wall is associated with perforation, which may be either walled off by omentum or spread throughout the abdomen, inducing diffuse peritonitis.

III. PRESENTATION

A. History.

1. Classical presentation occurs in only 50% of patients.
2. Pain usually begins in peri-umbilical or epigastric region (dermatome = T10), due to appendiceal distension and referred pain along lesser splanchnics.
3. Anorexia and nausea occur almost uniformly *after* the pain. Almost all adults have anorexia, whereas children with appendicitis may remain hungry.
4. Pain localizes to the RLQ as the parietal peritoneum in that area becomes irritated.
   a. If the appendix lies in the pelvis or retrocecal area, the location of the pain (and tenderness) will change accordingly with peritoneal irritation.
   b. If perforation occurs, diffuse peritonitis ensues, with pain throughout the abdomen.
5. Patients may have constipation, diarrhea, or no change in bowel habits.

B. Physical examination.

1. Fever may be present, but the temperature is rarely greater than 38°C unless perforation and/or abscess formation have occurred.
2. Patients usually prefer to lie on their side, with legs drawn up.
3. When appendix lies anteriorly, tenderness is present at McBurney's point; 1/3 of the distance between the anterior superior iliac spine and the umbilicus (Figure 1).
4. With peritoneal irritation, guarding, rebound, and indirect rebound tenderness may occur.
5. Rovsing's sign is pain in RLQ with palpation of the LLQ.
6. Cutaneous hyperesthesia may be present in distribution of T10-T12 and is tested by rolling the skin between the thumb and forefinger, which normally does not cause pain.
7. Rectal exam will elicit suprapubic pain if the inflamed appendix tip lies in the pelvis.
8. The psoas sign is pain occurring with extension of the right thigh and indicates an irritative focus overlying that muscle.
9. The obturator sign is pain with passive internal rotation of the flexed right thigh and similarly indicates inflamation overlying that muscle.

C. Laboratory and radiologic findings.

1. The diagnosis of appendicitis is largely a clinical one, however, some objective data may be useful.
2. WBC elevation from 10,000 to 18,000/mm^3 is expected, with a left shift on differential.
3. Urinalysis may be normal or reveal few RBCs or WBCs only.
4. Abdominal radiograph may show a fecalith in the RLQ, loss of the right psoas shadow, or fat pad, paucity of RLQ gas, and/or a few dilated loops of bowel.
5. Although not specific, barium enema may rule out appendi-

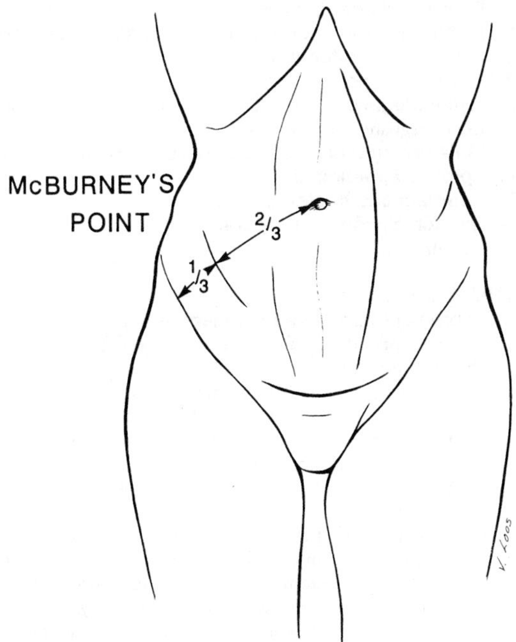

FIG. 1

citis if normal filling of the appendix occurs. May be useful for children or difficult adult patients.

a. Mass effect on the cecum or terminal ileum is seen with appendicitis.
b. 10% false-negative rate.

6. Ultrasound has been shown to be 86% sensitive and is useful for ruling out ovarian pathology or mesenteric adentitis; these conditions may not require operative therapy.
7. Technetium 99m albumin colloid WBC scan (TAC-WBC) is uniformly accurate if positive; however, 24% of scans are "indeterminate".

IV. DIFFERENTIAL DIAGNOSES

A. **Gastroenteritis.**
B. **Diverticulitis** (adults).
C. **Acute mesenteric adenitis** (children).
D. **Meckel's diverticulitis.**
E. **Intussusception** (infants and children).
F. **Regional enteritis.**

G. **Perforated peptic ulcer.**
H. **Perforating carcinoma of cecum or sigmoid colon.**
I. **Urinary tract infection.**
J. **Ureteral stone.**
K. **Gynecologic disease** (e.g., pelvic inflammatory disease, ectopic pregnancy, ovarian cyst).
L. **Male urologic disease** (e.g., testicular torsion, epididymitis).
M. **Epiploic appendicitis.**
N. **Spontaneous bacterial peritonitis.**
O. **Henoch-Schönlein purpura.**
P. **Yersinosis.**

V. TREATMENT

A. **Immediate operative management** is indicated in all cases of acute appendicitis unless there has been a perforation with abscess formation.
   1. Most surgeons use a McBurney (or Rockey-Davis) incision over McBurney's point with a muscle-splitting technique.
   2. If there is reasonable doubt over the diagnosis, some surgeons prefer a paramedian or midline incision.
   3. After resection of the appendix, the ligated stump is usually inverted.
   4. In the case of a perforated appendix with phlegmon formation (or significant cecal inflammation), an "interval" (or delayed) appendectomy is usually performed. Drains are brought out to drain discrete collections only, and the fascia is closed while the skin and subcutaneous tissue is left open.
   5. Patients with a walled-off abscess may be managed by ultrasound- or CT-guided percutaneous drainage followed by interval appendectomy.
   6. Peri-operative antibiotics have been shown to be beneficial in lowering the infectious complications, and many authors recommend 3-5 days of antibiotics in patients with confirmed appendicitis.
   7. If no appendiceal inflammation is present, a careful search for other causes of the symptom should be undertaken.
      a. Examination of pelvic organs.
      b. Gallbladder and gastroduodenal area are inspected.
      c. Gram stain of any peritoneal exudate.
      d. Inspection of the mesentery for lymph nodes.
      e. Thorough examination of the small bowel to rule out regional enteritis and Meckel's diverticulum.
      f. Palpation of the colon and kidneys.

VI. SPECIAL CIRCUMSTANCES

A. **Elderly patients.**
   1. Account for more than 50% of the deaths from appendicitis.
   2. Higher mortality is due to delay of definitive treatment, uncontrolled infection, and a high incidence of coexistent disease.

3. Constellation of symptoms is usually much more subtle.
   a. Abdominal pain may be minimized.
   b. Fever and leukocyte count are less reliable signs.
4. Morbidity and mortality are much higher due to the delay in accurate diagnosis.

B. Infants.

1. Similarly high rate of rupture and secondary complications due to delayed or atypical presentation.
2. Accurate diagnosis is made more difficult by the fact that infants are unable to give a history, the index of suspicion is usually lower, and progression of disease is usually faster.
3. The more inefficient ability of the infant to wall off perforated appendicitis enables rapid diffuse peritonitis and distant abscesses.

C. Pregnant women.

1. Although appendicitis is the most common extrauterine surgical emergency in pregnant patients, it occurs with the same frequency in pregnant women as it does in non-pregnant women.
2. It occurs more frequently in the first two trimesters.
3. Diagnosis is obfuscated by the lateral and superior displacement of the appendix by the gravid uterus with an accompanying change in the point of maximum tenderness.
4. Diagnosis is also made more difficult by the fact that abdominal pain, nausea, vomiting, and an elevated WBC are "normal" findings during pregnancy.
5. Although maternal mortality is very low, early operative intervention is essential, as perforation and peritonitis results in fetal mortality rates as high as 35%.

VII. LAPAROSCOPIC APPENDECTOMY (see also "Laparoscopic Appendectomy")

A. Advantages—Laparoscopy offers the potential advantage of both diagnostic and therapeutic interventions for patients with suspected appendicitis.

B. Technique—The procedure is carried out in a nearly identical manner as the open procedure.

C. Studies in adults have demonstrated shorter hospital stays but generally at some increased cost versus open appendectomy.

D. The advantages of shorter hospital stay and decreased morbidity from laparoscopic appendectomy are not as well supported in pediatric patients.

(MANTRELS) — ≥7 suggestive appendicitis; ≥5 nearly all pts have
Movemt. pain RLQ
Anorexia / Acetone urine
Nausea c̄ vomiting
Tenderness in (R) lower quad. (2) McBurney
Rebound tenderness
Elev. Temp >100.4°F
Leukocytosis
Shift of WBC >75% neutrophils

37

Colorectal Cancer

Keith M. Heaton, M.D.

I. INCIDENCE

A. **Colorectal cancer accounts for 14% of all cases of cancer,** excluding skin malignancies.
B. **Second in incidence only to breast cancer in females** and third in incidence in males behind prostate cancer and lung cancer.
C. **Accounts for 14% of all yearly cancer deaths.**
D. **Peak incidence** is in the 7th decade of life. Colon cancer has a slight female predominance, whereas rectal cancer has a male predominance.

II. ETIOLOGY

A. **Environmental factors—**Western countries have higher incidence of colorectal cancer than countries in Asia and Africa. Immigrants from Asia and Africa have higher incidence of colorectal cancer than their countrymen, suggesting an environmental etiology such as the low-fiber, high-fat diet common in the West.
B. **Genetic predisposition—**well-described polyposis syndromes include the following.
   1. Familial polyposis–adenomatous polyposis of the colon with a 100% risk of malignancy; may also occur in the proximal GI tract. Autosomal dominant inheritance.
   2. Gardner's syndrome–polyposis associated with exostoses, soft tissue tumors, and osteomas; also has a 100% incidence of malignant degeneration.
   3. Turcot's syndrome–polyposis of the colon associated with CNS tumors. Autosomal recessive inheritance.
   4. Cronkhite-Canada syndrome–GI polyposis with alopecia, nail dystrophy, hyperpigmentation. Minimal malignant potential. No inheritance pattern.
   5. Peutz-Jeghers syndrome–hamartomatous polyps of the entire GI tract with mucocutaneous deposition of melanin in lips,

oral cavity, and digits. Slightly increased malignant potential. Autosomal dominant inheritance.

C. Inflammatory bowel disease.

1. Ulcerative colitis and, to a lesser extent, Crohn's disease are associated with increased rates of colon cancer.
2. After 10 years, the risk of cancer in ulcerative colitis is 1-2%/year.

D. Adenomatous polyps—probably premalignant lesions. Thought to represent transformation of normal mucosa to cancer, although the majority of polyps will not progress to carcinoma. Increasing size and increased number of polyps are associated with an increased risk of developing cancer.

1. Tubular adenomas–65% of adenomas; 15% have carcinoma *in situ* or frank invasive cancer.
2. Tubulovillous adenomas–25% of adenomas; 19% have carcinoma *in situ* or invasive cancer.
3. Villous adenomas–10% of adenomas; 25% have carcinoma *in situ* or invasive cancer.

E. Summary of major risk factors.

1. Hereditary polyposis syndromes.
2. Adenomatous polyps.
3. Previous colorectal cancer.
4. Inflammatory bowel disease.
5. Family history of colorectal cancer.
6. Age > 50 years.

III. DIAGNOSIS

A. Presentation—Colorectal cancer may present with different symptoms and manifestations related to the region of the bowel from which it arises.

1. Right-sided lesions are typically bulky, fungating, ulcerative lesions that project into the lumen.
   a. Anemia–microcytic, chronic intermittent occult blood loss in the stools.
   b. Systemic complaints–anorexia, fatigue, weight loss, or dull persistent abdominal pain; abdominal mass with more advanced tumors.
   c. Obstruction is rare secondary to the liquid consistency of the stool and the large diameter of the bowel.
   d. Triad–anemia, weakness, RLQ mass.
2. Left-sided lesions–annular, "napkin-ring" lesions that often obstruct the bowel.
   a. Change in bowel habits–obstipation, alternating constipation and diarrhea, small-caliber "pencil" stools.
   b. Obstructive symptoms are more prominent as a result of growth pattern of tumor, small caliber of bowel, and solid stool.
3. Rectal cancer–blood streaking in stools, tenesmus. This finding must *not* be attributed to hemorrhoids without fur-

ther investigation. Obstruction is uncommon, but is a poor prognostic sign when present.
4. Abdominal pain is the most common presenting symptom for lesions in all locations.

B. Signs of local extension or metastasis.
1. Abnormal liver function tests, jaundice, or hepatomegaly.
2. Fistula formation.
3. Mass fixed to sacrum on rectal exam.

C. Diagnostic studies.
1. Rectal exam–all patients undergo rectal exams. Up to 10% of lesions are *palpable* on rectal exam.
2. Stool guaiac–up to 50% of positive results are due to colorectal cancer. The test should be repeated yearly on at least 3 separate occasions in patients > 40.
3. Barium enema or flexible sigmoidoscopy for routine screening every 3-5 years in patients over 50; may substitute with colonoscopy if index of suspicion is high. Flexible sigmoidoscopy should detect almost 50% of colorectal cancers.
4. Work-up for metastatic disease in biopsy-proven cases.
   a. Must evaluate the entire colon; 6% incidence of synchronous lesions.
   b. Chest radiograph.
   c. Liver function tests.
   d. Abdominal CT for intra-abdominal metastasis and extracolonic spread.
   e. Carcinoembryonic antigen (CEA) pre-operatively.
   f. IVP–optional in patients with low-lying lesions or urinary symptoms.

IV. PATHOLOGY

A. Location—The majority are located in the distal colon, however, there is an increasing incidence of right-sided lesions.

B. Gross description.
1. Polypoid–bulky polypoid lesions are more common in the right colon.
2. Scirrhous–annular ("apple-core") lesions. More common in the left colon.
3. Ulcerated.
4. Nodular.

C. Routes of spread.
1. Intramural–along bowel wall.
2. Direct extension into surrounding tissues (e.g., ovary, small bowel).
3. Intraluminal.
4. Peritoneal.
5. Lymphatic.
6. Hematogenous.

D. Histologic staging.
1. Duke's classifications–there have been several modifications to the original classification.

a. Astler-Coller (1959) modification is most commonly used.
   (1) Stage A–limited to mucosa (above lymphatic channels).
   (2) Stage B_1–into the muscularis propria.
   (3) Stage B_2–through the muscularis propria.
   (4) Stage C_1–into the muscularis propria, with (+) nodes.
   (5) Stage C_2–through the muscularis propria, with (+) nodes.
b. Stage D (not part of original classification) metastases or unresectable.
c. American Joint Committee for Cancer Staging and End Results (TNM).
   (1) Primary Tumor (T)
      Tx Primary tumor cannot be assessed
      T0 No evidence of primary tumor
      Tis Intraepithelial, carcinoma *in situ*
      T1 Tumor invades the submucosa
      T2 Tumor invades the muscularis propria
      T3 Tumor invades into the subserosa or nonperitonealized pericolic structures
      T4 Tumor directly invades other organs or perforates
   (2) Regional Lymph Nodes (N)
      Nx Regional lymph nodes cannot be assessed
      N0 No regional lymph node metastasis
      N1 Metastasis in 1-3 pericolic lymph nodes
      N2 Metastasis in 4 or more pericolic lymph nodes
      N3 Other distant lymph node metastasis
   (3) Distant Metastasis (M)
      Mx Presence of metastases cannot be assessed
      M0 No distant metastases
      M1 Distant metastases
d. Prognosis is related to the stage of disease, not size of the tumor.
   (1) Five-year survival using the Astler-Coller modification:
      a) Stage A–> 90%.
      b) Stage B_1–70-85%.
      c) Stage B_2–55-65%.
      d) Stage C_1–45-55%.
      e) Stage C_2–20-30%.
      f) Stage D–< 1%.
      g) Patients with isolated hepatic metastases that are resected for cure have a 5-year survival rate of 15-25%.
   (2) Rectal cancer has an increased local recurrence rate and decreased 5-year survival compared with colonic tumors.
   (3) Only 70% of colorectal cancer patients are resectable for cure at presentation.

a) Ten percent of primary lesions are unresectable.
b) Twenty percent of patients have distant metastases at presentation.

(4) Forty-five percent of patients are cured by primary resection.
(5) Of the 25% of patients who develop a recurrence, 20% will be cured by further resection.
(6) Overall 5-year disease-free survival is about 50% for colon cancer and about 40% for rectal cancer resected for cure.

V. TREATMENT

A. An adequate cancer operation requires resection of tumor-containing bowel with 3- to 5-cm margins and resection of the mesentery at the origin of the arterial supply, including the primary lymphatic drainage of the tumor. Recent studies suggest that 90% of tumors can be adequately handled by 2-cm margins. This is especially important for lesions of the lower 1/3 of the rectum, which may be managed with a low anterior resection and primary anastomosis.

B. Pre-operative preparation.

1. Mechanical bowel preparation and pre-operative oral antibiotics have been shown to reduce wound and intra-abdominal infections.
2. Peri-operative systemic antibiotics may decrease incidence of infectious complications.
3. CEA level must be obtained prior to operation.

C. Choice of operation (Figure 1).

1. Lesions of the **cecum** and **ascending colon**—treated by resection of the distal ileum to the mid-transverse colon, including the ileocolic, right colic, and middle colic vessels with accompanying mesentery.
2. Tumors in the **left transverse colon** and **splenic flexure**—require resection of the transverse and proximal descending colon. The middle and left colic arteries are removed.
3. Tumors in the **descending** and **sigmoid colon**—require removal from the splenic flexure to the rectosigmoid. The left colic and sigmoidal arteries are removed.
4. Tumors in the **upper 1/3** of the **rectum**—treated by an anterior resection.
5. Lesions **between 5 and 10 cm** from the anal verge—treated by a low anterior resection or an abdominal-sacral resection (Kraske, York-Mason).
6. Lesions in the **lower 1/3** of the **rectum** (0-5 cm)—usually require an abdominoperineal resection (Miles procedure) with a permanent end-sigmoid colostomy; may be amenable to a low anterior resection with anastomosis using a stapler (EEA). At least 4 cm of rectal stump is necessary for fecal continence.

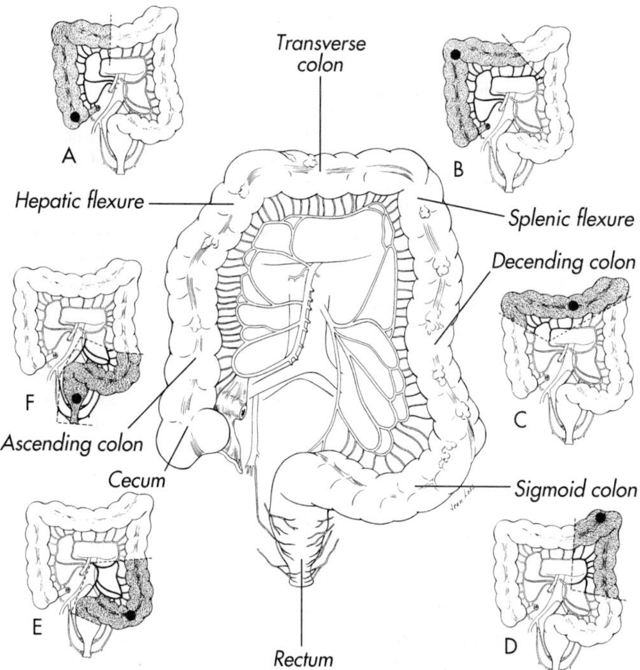

FIG. 1 Anatomic resection commonly employed for cancer at different sites within the large bowel: A, right hemicolectomy; **B**, extended right hemicolectomy; **C**, transverse colectomy; **D**, left hemicolectomy; **E**, sigmoid colectomy; **F**, abdominal perineal resection.

7. Pre-operative multimodality therapy using both chemotherapy and radiation–may aid in "down-staging" locally advanced rectal carcinoma so that otherwise unresectable lesions may be resected.
8. Selected patients with rectal cancer have equal survival following wide local excision via a transanal approach. Criteria for local excision:
   a. Mobile tumor in the lower 1/3 of the rectum.
   b. Size < 3 cm.
   c. Stage A or B_1 by endorectal ultrasound.
   d. Well- or moderately-differentiated histology.
   e. No detectable pararectal lymph node involvement clinically or by endorectal ultrasound.

9. Bilateral oophorectomy may be reasonable at the time of initial resection, since about 6% of patients will have microscopic involvement of the ovaries.
10. Direct adherence of the tumor to adjacent structures may result from inflammation rather than from tumor extension. A cure in the presence of local invasion may still be possible with resection of the involved structures or, if local invasion is more extensive, by total pelvic exenteration.

D. Adjuvant therapy.

1. For patients with Dukes' **C colon** adenocarcinoma, postoperative therapy with 5-FU and levamisole or leucovorin has been shown to be effective in improving both disease-free and overall survival. Radiation therapy has not been shown to be an effective adjuvant treatment for colon adenocarcinoma.
2. For patients with Dukes' B_2 or C **rectal** carcinoma, postoperative combined modality therapy with radiation and chemotherapy improves both disease-free and overall survival and also improves local tumor control and should be considered standard therapy after either abdominal-perineal or low anterior resection. Some recent data suggest chemotherapy alone may be just as beneficial, however. The use of preoperative radiation is controversial, but may be helpful, especially with large, bulky tumors.

VII. POST-OPERATIVE FOLLOW-UP

A. Recurrence—Approximately 80% of recurrences occur within 2 years of resection, most often in the form of hepatic metastases or local recurrence.

B. Detection and treatment of recurrent disease remains problematic. Careful history, physical exam, liver function tests, carcinoembryonic antigen (CEA) screening, and stool guaiacs will detect greater than 90% of recurrent disease.

1. Follow-up protocol.
   a. Routine physical exam, stool guaiac, CBC, liver function tests–every 3 months for 2 years, then every 6 months for 2 years, then annually.
   b. CEA–every 3 months for 2 years, then every 6 months for 2 years, then annually.
   c. Colonoscopy–baseline at 3-6 months, then annually for 4 years, then every 2-3 years. Barium enema should be performed if complete visualization is not achieved by colonoscopy.
2. CEA helpful only if initially elevated and returns to normal postresection.
3. An increase in CEA (> 5 ng/ml) requires prompt investigation, including abdominal CT, chest radiograph, and colonoscopy or barium enema. If no abnormalities are found, some advocate a second-look laparotomy. Whether this results in

increased 5-year survival is controversial; however, recurrences detected by frequent CEA screening alone are more frequently resectable than recurrences detected by the appearance of symptoms.

4. Other screening tests–tissue peptide antigen (TPA) and CA 19-9 are not as sensitive or specific as CEA.

C. Treatment of recurrent disease.

1. Local recurrence.
   a. Should attempt a cure by resection in selected patients or to palliate symptoms whenever possible.
   b. Resectability can only be determined by re-exploration. Debulking procedures (tumor resections with gross disease left behind) are rarely indicated.
   c. Recurrence following low anterior resection usually requires an abdominal-perineal resection.
   d. Pelvic recurrences following abdominal-perineal resection are usually unresectable, but occasionally pelvic exenteration is possible.
2. Distant metastases.
   a. Involves the liver, lung, bone, brain (in order of frequency).
   b. Approximately 35-50% of all colorectal carcinoma patients develop hepatic metastases during the course of their disease.
   c. 10-20% of patients with hepatic metastases may benefit from resection, with 5-year survival of 25% in some studies. Relative contraindications to resection:
      (1) Positive hepatic nodes.
      (2) Extrahepatic metastases.
      (3) More than 4 hepatic metastases.
   d. When synchronous hepatic metastasis is found during operation for primary colorectal malignancy, the hepatic lesion may be removed simultaneously or at second operation 2-3 months later.
   e. No difference in survival has been demonstrated for lobectomy *vs.* wedge resection (when possible).
   f. For unresectable hepatic metastases, an implantable pump for intra-arterial (hepatic artery) infusion of 5-FU or FUDR has shown tumor response rates of 40-60%; however, toxicity remains a significant problem.
   g. Pulmonary metastases most often present as disseminated disease. For metastatic nodules, up to 38% 5-year survival has been demonstrated with surgical resection (usually wedge). Patients with solitary nodules and nodules < 3 cm in size may have better survival.
   h. For unresectable systemic disease, chemotherapy (5-FU and leucovorin) is used, but results continue to be disappointing.

38

Diverticular Disease of the Colon

David L. Brown, M.D.

DIVERTICULOSIS

I. DEFINITION

Saccular outpouchings of the colon.

A. Acquired (false/pseudo) diverticuli.

1. Most common type of diverticulum.
2. Contains only the mucosal and submucosal layers.
3. These diverticuli occur at weak points in the bowel wall where arterioles penetrate the circular muscle layer, primarily on the mesenteric side of the antimesenteric tenia (Figure 1). They do not occur below the peritoneal reflection.
4. Diverticuli may occur throughout the GI tract, but are most common in the large bowel, especially the sigmoid colon.

B. Congenital (true) diverticuli.

1. Rare. Usually single.
2. Contain all layers of the bowel wall.
3. Predominantly located in the right colon, in or near the cecum.

II. INCIDENCE

A. M = F.

B. Age—10% by age 40; 75% in those greater than 80 years old.

C. Region—Higher in industrialized nations (see III.E.2. below).

III. PATHOPHYSIOLOGY

A. 80% are asymptomatic.

B. Symptoms (secondary to hypermotility, not to the diverticula themselves)–pain, diarrhea, constipation.

C. 95% of cases involve the sigmoid colon.

D. 65% of cases are limited to the sigmoid colon.

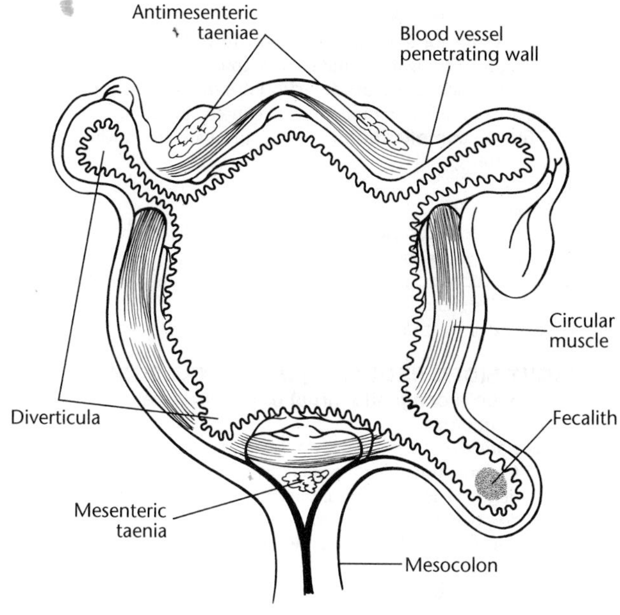

FIG. 1

E. The etiology of this disease is still unproven. Two extremes in pathophysiology are recognized:

1. The first occurs in people with essentially normal colonic musculature, likely as a result of weakness in the wall due to aging or a connective tissue disorder. This form is usually asymptomatic and tends to involve the entire colon.
2. The second is associated with hypermotility and thickening of the musculature. An increased incidence has been seen in industrialized nations since the introduction of flour milling in the late 1800s. The resulting decrease in the consumption of fiber translates to less stool bulk, and therefore higher intraluminal pressures in the colon (presumably causing both muscular hypertrophy and diverticuli at points of weakness). This can be explained by Laplace's Law: $P=T/R$, which states that pressure (P) within a tube varies inversely with the radius (R) of the lumen. (T = wall tension.) Laplace's Law also explains the increased incidence of diverticuli in the sigmoid, the narrowest region of the colon.

IV. COMPLICATIONS

A. **Complications** include infection (diverticulitis), perforation, bleeding, fistulization, and obstruction.

B. **10-20% will develop diverticulitis or hemorrhage,** and 30% of these will require operative intervention.

C. **75% of complications** occur in patients without prior symptoms.

V. TREATMENT

A. **Asymptomatic patients—**a high-fiber diet with avoidance of peanuts and popcorn is recommended.

B. **Symptomatic patients—**constipation is improved by a high-fiber diet; pain is not.

C. **Surgery** for complications.

VI. RIGHT-SIDED (ISOLATED) DIVERTICULOSIS

A. **May be a congenital (true) or acquired (false) diverticulum.**

B. **Location.**

1. Cecum–usually congenital with approximately 1-2% incidence. The majority are asymptomatic. The most common complication is inflammation.
2. Ascending colon–most are acquired. Most common complication is bleeding.

C. **Presentation.**

1. Usually occur in younger (30-40) age group.
2. Inflammation can mimic appendicitis.
3. Symptoms may be prolonged and persistent.

D. **Diagnosis.**

1. CT scan–for atypical presentation of appendicitis, particularly in older patients.
2. Barium enema or flexible colonoscopy if no perforation.
3. Must rule out malignancy.
4. The diagnosis usually is not made pre-operatively.

E. **Therapy.**

1. Isolated ileo-right colectomy is usually necessary.
2. Has a lower morbidity and mortality rate than does diverticulectomy.

DIVERTICULITIS

I. PATHOPHYSIOLOGY

A. **Age—**Occurs in 20% of patients > age 40 with diverticulosis.

B. **Inspissated stool** lodges in the diverticulum, producing increased intraluminal pressure with impairment of venous return. Venous hypertension with impaired capillary filling results in ischemia and mucosal injury with subsequent inflammation.

C. **Ischemia** usually leads to "peridiverticulitis," a contained perforation into the mesentery or pericolic fat, causing focal inflammation and localized peritonitis.

D. **10-15% of patients with diverticulitis** have free perforation producing generalized peritonitis. This is more common in immunosuppressed, debilitated and steroid-dependent patients.

II. PRESENTATION

A. Symptoms.

1. Pain–most common–usually in left lower quadrant, but may be anywhere in lower abdomen due to the redundancy of the sigmoid colon. The pain is typically dull and achy, but may be crampy and associated with tenesmus.
2. Fever, malaise, anorexia, nausea with/without emesis.
3. Change in bowel habits–diarrhea, constipation, alternating diarrhea and constipation, change in stool caliber, obstipation, tenesmus.
4. Urinary symptoms–frequency, nocturia and/or dysuria due to pericystic inflammation. Pneumaturia (presenting symptom in 3-5%) and/or polymicrobial urinary tract infections in noncatheterized patients are seen with colovesical fistulas.

B. Signs.

1. Tenderness and guarding.
2. Distention due to ileus or mechanical bowel obstruction.
3. Palpable tender mass, especially on pelvic or rectal exam.
4. Hypoactive or absent bowel sounds with peritonitis.
5. Hyperactive, high-pitched bowel sounds with obstruction.
6. Guaiac positive stools.

C. Laboratory exam.

1. Mild to moderate leukocytosis, often with left shift.
2. Urinalysis–leukocytes may be present as a result of inflammation around ureters and bladder.

III. DIAGNOSTIC TESTS

Initial diagnosis is made on clinical assessment–diagnostic studies are performed for confirmation of clinical suspicion. The diagnosis must be confirmed objectively at some point to rule out the possibility of colon cancer.

A. **CT scan—**study of choice.

1. Has therapeutic advantage of option of abscess drainage.
2. Superior to contrast enemas for defining pericolic inflammation and evaluating complications of diverticulitis.

B. Contrast enema.

1. Deferred until peritoneal signs subside (usually 2-4 weeks). If used in acute setting, use water-soluble contrast.
2. Barium and stool combined cause a more severe peritonitis than either alone.

C. **Flexible sigmoidoscopy** (with minimal insufflation) used to rule out a perforated colon cancer.

D. Colonoscopy—mandatory once acute process has resolved in the case of bleeding or the possibility of cancer radiographically.

IV. TREATMENT

A. Initial management—non-operative.

1. ***Outpatient management*** with oral antibiotics is appropriate for mild tenderness and low-grade fever. Admission criteria include high fever, increasing abdominal pain, and failure to improve on oral antibiotics.
2. ***NPO, IV hydration,*** and nasogastric suction (if ileus or small bowel obstruction is present).
3. ***Parenteral antibiotics***—gram-negative and anaerobic coverage (e.g., an aminoglycoside and clindamycin or metronidazole). Continue for 7-10 days, or until afebrile with normal WBC and non-tender exam.
4. ***Pain control*** with meperidine.
5. ***Serial exams*** to detect worsening or complicated disease.
6. ***Oral antibiotics*** (e.g., trimethoprim-sulfamethoxazole plus metronidazole; or ciprofloxacin) may be used for 7-10 days for mild attacks, or for 1-2 weeks after discontinuation of parenteral antibiotics for more severe attacks.
7. ***Diet***—clear liquids followed by a low-residue diet for 2-4 weeks after an acute attack. Patients are then placed on a high-fiber diet including psyllium. This may decrease the rate of further symptoms, but probably does not decrease the incidence of complications.

B. Surgical management.

1. 50% of all patients admitted to the hospital resolve their diverticulitis with conservative therapy. Only 25% return with a subsequent attack.
2. Of the 50% who do not respond during initial hospitalization:
   a. 60% do not resolve (or recur) after discontinuation of antibiotics.
   b. 30% have free perforation, requiring immediate surgery.
   c. 9% have urinary fistulas.
   d. 1% have a solitary right-sided diverticulum.
3. 10-20% of patients diagnosed with diverticulitis on clinical grounds are subsequently found to have carcinoma of the colon; therefore, it is necessary to rule out carcinoma following resolution of the acute attack.
4. ***Indications for operation.***
   a. Repeated attacks (two or more).
      (1) The rate of complications is less than 20% with the first occurrence, but increases to 60% with subsequent attacks.
      (2) 30-40% of patients will have subsequent attacks.
   b. Complications–abscess, obstruction, fistula, stricture.
   c. Failure to improve with conservative management after 3-4 days.

d. First episode in young patient (<50 years old).
e. Inability to exclude carcinoma.
f. Right-sided diverticulitis.

5. ***Operative procedures.***
   a. **Single-stage**—resect all diverticulum-bearing colon with a primary anastomosis; usually an elective operation on prepared bowel.
   b. **Two-stage.**
      (1) The safe creation of an anastomosis is not possible in the presence of edematous bowel or gross contamination because of the high incidence of resultant leaks.
      (2) First stage—primary resection of diseased colon with end colostomy and mucous fistula or Hartmann pouch.
      (3) Alternative first stage—primary resection and anastomosis with a proximal diverting colostomy.
      (4) Second stage—reanastomosis after 2-6 months.
   c. **Three-stage** (rarely used).
      (1) Employed for severe peritonitis with localized abscess cavity, on any unstable patient, or for a prohibitively difficult resection.
      (2) Disadvantage—leaves diseased colon holding column of stool in place.
      (3) First stage—drainage of abscess and proximal diverting colostomy.
      (4) Second stage—resection of involved colon with anastomosis.
      (5) Third stage—closure of diverting colostomy.

VI. COMPLICATIONS

A. Abscess.

1. CT-guided drainage:
   a. Effective drainage of an abscess can allow the performance of an elective procedure when the acute process has subsided, with lower morbidity and mortality than an emergent one, and can avoid the need for a colostomy.
   b. A one-stage operation is then possible in 50-90% of patients after effective percutaneous drainage.
2. Hartmann's operation is usually indicated during a celiotomy in the face of an undrained abscess.

B. Fistula.

1. ***Colovesical fistula.***
   a. Occurs in 2-4% of cases of diverticulitis.
   b. Accounts for 50% of fistulas secondary to diverticulitis.
   c. Cancer is the second most common cause of colovesical fistulas (after diverticulitis) and therefore must be ruled out.
   d. 3:1 male to female preponderance owing to absence of interposed uterus and adnexa.
   e. Ascending infections (i.e. pyelonephritis) are rare, except in the face of distal obstruction.

f. Presentation–typically fecaluria, pneumaturia or recurrent UTIs. Major abdominal symptomatology is the exception, not the rule.

g. Diagnosis.
   (1) CT with intraluminal contrast is the most sensitive. Air will be seen in the bladder in 90% of patients.
   (2) Barium enema is <50% sensitive.
   (3) Cystoscopy–usually only induration and edema are seen.

h. Treatment.
   (1) 50% will close spontaneously.
   (2) If the fistula was caused by colon cancer, the resection must include a disc of bladder; otherwise, the colon may be dissected free, leaving the bladder intact.
   (3) Methylene blue distention of the rectum or bladder may help delineate the hard-to-find fistula tract.

2. ***Colovaginal fistula.***
   a. Almost all patients are s/p hysterectomy.
   b. Barium enema is <50% sensitive.
   c. Speculum exam–fistula is visible in 85%.
3. ***Coloenteric fistula***—usual treatment is single-stage *en bloc* resection and primary anastomosis of both colon and small bowel.

HEMORRHAGE (*see also "GI Bleeding"*)

I. GENERAL

A. **The close anatomic relationship** between the diverticulum and the penetrating artery provides the opportunity for bleeding.
B. **70% of lower GI bleeding** is caused by diverticulosis.
C. **70% of bleeds secondary to diverticulosis** stop spontaneously.
D. **75% of those that stop spontaneously** don't recur. (see III.I.B. below)

II. DIFFERENTIAL DIAGNOSIS

A. **Angiodysplasia**—the most important distinction, because 50% of those with bleeds secondary to angiodysplasia also have diverticulosis.
B. **Upper GI bleed** (rapid).
C. **Hemorrhoids.**
D. **Carcinoma/polyps.**
E. **Colitis** (ischemic, inflammatory).

III. TREATMENT

A. **Acute stabilization**—(see "GI Bleeding").
B. **Initial bleed**—Seventy percent of diverticular bleeds stop spontaneously. Continued bleeding despite transfusing 6 or more

units of blood in 24 h is the main indication for emergent surgical intervention. A segmental colon resection with primary anastomosis can be performed if the bleeding source has been localized. If attempts at localization are unsuccessful, total abdominal colectomy with ileoproctostomy should be performed because of the high incidence of rebleeding if segmental resection is performed without adequate localization.

C. Subsequent episodes—Resection should be performed in any patient who stops bleeding spontaneously on the initial episode but subsequently rebleeds. Primary resection should be performed even in light of spontaneous cessation of hemorrhage for the second episode, due to the high rate of further rebleeding and the associated morbidity and mortality.

39

Colitis and Enteric Infections

DAVID L. BROWN, M.D.

I. MICROBIOLOGY

A. **The colon is sterile at birth.**

B. **Approximately 400 bacterial species** comprise normal fecal flora.

C. **99% of these species** are anaerobic (*B. fragilis* is most prevalent at 10^{10}/g).

D. **1% aerobic—**coliforms (*E. coli*–10^7/g, *Klebsiella, Proteus, Enterobacter*) and enterococcus (*Strep. faecalis*).

II. DIARRHEA

A. **Definition** (imprecise)–increased number of stools and increased fluid loss.

B. **Normal stool—**$\leq$ 200 g/day. Diarrhea–$>$ 250 g/day.

C. **Mechanisms—**increased motility, presence of osmotically active substances, inflammatory exudate, increased secretion by mucosa.

D. **Bacterial toxins—**cause increased mucosal secretion.

1. Cytotonic (i.e., cholera, enterotoxigenic *E. coli*)–do not damage mucosal epithelium. Increase mucosal secretion by increasing cAMP via activation of adenylate cyclase.
2. Cytotoxic (i.e., shigella, enterohemorrhagic *E. coli*)–cause direct damage to epithelium. Increase secretion via a different pathway.

E. **Diagnosis.**

1. Stool smear.
   a. WBCs–likely an exudative process (IBD or infectious enteritis).
   b. RBCs, no WBCs–ischemia, cancer, amebic colitis, pseudomembranous colitis.

2. High stool fat content–malabsorption due to IBD, short gut, pancreatic insufficiency, infection, or interruption of enterohepatic bile circulation.
3. Osmolarity–mucosa is permeable to water; therefore, stool and serum osmolarity should be approximately equal. If stool osmolarity is greater than serum osmolarity by 50 mOsm or more, then an osmotically active cation is likely present.

III. PSEUDOMEMBRANOUS COLITIS

A. Pathogenesis.

1. Almost always due to *Clostridium difficile,* a gram-positive obligate anaerobe.
   a. 3-5% of the population are carriers.
   b. Can be found in 15-20% of asymptomatic patients treated with antibiotics.
2. Nosocomial transmission.
   a. Opportunity for epidemic outbreaks, particularly on surgical wards and ICUs.
   b. *Hand washing* is the primary means of controlling spread of the disease.
3. Antibiotic use causes alterations in the normal flora of the colon, allowing for overgrowth of *C. difficile.* Almost all antibiotics have been implicated (although clindamycin, ampicillin, and the cephalosporins are most common).
4. Damage to the mucosal integrity is caused by toxins produced by the bacterium. These toxins also have additional specific actions.
   a. Toxin A (enteropathic)–disrupts protein synthesis.
   b. Toxin B (cytopathic)–enhances chemotaxis of granulocytes.
5. Pseudomembranes–dead mucosal cells and WBCs, along with mucous and fibrin, which give a characteristic appearance.
6. Usually most severe in the sigmoid and rectum, but 10% of cases are located solely on the right side.

B. Signs and symptoms.

1. Severity–may vary from mild to severe. Complications include perforation and megacolon.
2. Copious watery diarrhea (rarely grossly bloody), crampy pain, fever, and leukocytosis.
3. Typically occurs 5-10 days after starting the offending antibiotic, but up to 20% of cases are seen as long as 6 weeks after discontinuation.

C. Diagnosis.

1. WBCs will be present in less than 50% of patients' stools. Therefore, a positive test rules out benign etiologies, but a negative one is not necessarily helpful.
2. Endoscopy, stool culture and stool for *C. difficile* toxin titres.

D. Treatment.

1. Stop offending antibiotic, if possible.
2. In toxic, elderly, and immunocompromised patients, start therapy empirically while waiting for culture and toxin titres to return.
3. Do not use an antiperistaltic agent.
4. Vancomycin–100% of cases are sensitive. The drug is poorly absorbed from the GI tract. 125 mg PO q 6 h has been shown to be equivalent to 500 q 6 h.
5. Metronidazole–approximately 90% of cases are sensitive. It is significantly cheaper than vancomycin, but cannot be used in infants and pregnant patients. Dosage: 500-750 mg PO TID, or 250 QID.
6. There is a 20% recurrence rate, despite drug choice.

IV. ULCERATIVE COLITIS (see "Inflammatory Bowel Disease.")

V. CROHN'S COLITIS (see "Inflammatory Bowel Disease.")

VI. ISCHEMIC COLITIS (see "Mesenteric Ischemia.")

VII. NEUTROPENIC COLITIS

A. Occurs with AML (25%), aplastic anemia, and chemotherapy.

B. Primarily affects the cecum and ascending colon.

C. Pathogenesis—unknown, but hypothesized to be secondary to necrosis of intramural leukemic cells, which then cause mucosal ulceration.

D. Symptoms/signs—diarrhea, abdominal pain, fever, distention, RLQ tenderness.

E. Treatment—hydration, NG decompression, antibiotics. Operative intervention is reserved for complications (perforation, hemorrhage, obstruction) or unresponsive sepsis.

VIII. ENTERIC INFECTIONS

A. Amebic colitis (*Entamoeba histolytica*).

1. Typically a tropical disease, although 5% of U.S. citizens are carriers.
2. The most common complication is a hepatic abscess.
3. Fecal-oral transmission.
4. trophozoite–invasive, motile form–causes ulcerations in the colon, primarily the cecum.
5. Cyst–infective form.
6. Most infected people are carriers.
7. Symptoms/signs–mild dysentery to severe colitis.
8. Diagnosis–trophozoites can be seen microscopically in the stool in 90% of cases. Differentiation from ulcerative colitis is critical, as steroids can cause colonic perforation and lead to dissemination.

9. Ameboma–an inflammatory mass in the wall of the colon that can cause obstruction and may mimic a colon cancer diagnostically.
10. Treatment–metronidazole–kills the invasive trophozoite. Iodoquinol–kills the organisms within the lumen of the bowel. Operative therapy is indicated for an ameboma that is unresponsive to antibiotics.

B. Giardia (*Giardia lamblia*).

1. A protozoan infection obtained from drinking contaminated water.
2. Primarily inhabits the duodenum and jejunum.
3. Symptoms/signs–cramps, anorexia, steatorrhea.
4. Diagnosis–50% detection in the stool; duodenal biopsy is most sensitive.
5. Treatment–metronidazole.

C. Cytomegalovirus colitis.

1. 90% of AIDS patients are infected (in various organs) with CMV.
2. 10% of AIDS patients get CMV colitis.
3. The most frequent cause for emergent exploration in AIDS patients.
4. Symptoms/signs–diarrhea, hematochezia, fever.
5. Diagnosis–CMV inclusions are demonstrated on biopsy.
6. Treatment–gancyclovir.
7. Survival–50% at 6 months.

D. Chagas' disease (*Trypanosoma cruzi*).

1. A protozoan endemic to South America.
2. Destroys the myenteric plexus of Auerbach, primarily in the rectum, creating a functional obstruction, which can cause proximal megacolon.
3. Treatment–resection.

E. Bacteria.

1. *E. coli*–"traveller's diarrhea."
   a. Present in all stool.
   b. Most treated with TMP-SMX, but resistance is emerging.
   c. 5 pathogenic strains–entero-toxigenic, pathogenic, hemorrhagic, invasive, and adherent.
2. *Shigella*–noted for adherence to and penetration of mucosa. Treat with TMP-SMX or tetracycline.
3. *Salmonella*–typhoid fever.
   a. Penetration of mucosa ⇒ lymphatic invasion ⇒ access to bloodstream ⇒ R.E.S. ⇒ recurrent bacteremia.
   b. Hyperplasia of Peyer patches can cause ulceration and/or perforation.
   c. Treatment–ampicillin or TMP-SMX.
4. *Campylobacter*–number one cause of bacterial diarrhea.
5. *Yersinia*–suspect at negative appendectomy with findings of mesenteric adenitis and inflammation of the terminal ileum.

F. Actinomycosis (*Actinomyces israelii*).

1. Gram-positive anaerobic bacteria.
2. Normal oral flora.
3. Typically a head and neck infection–20% primarily involve the chest; 20% the abdomen. Abdominal involvement most commonly occurs as a cecal infection following an appendectomy.
4. Causes chronic inflammation and sinus formation.
5. Treatment–drainage and antibiotics (tetracycline or PCN).

G. Food poisoning.

1. Results from bacterial toxins produced in the food prior to ingestion. Inadequate cooking heat to kill the bacteria allows for multiplication while cooling, prior to eating.
2. Causes.
   a. *Clostridium perfringens*–a 12-h, self-limited illness involving severe crampy pain without vomiting.
   b. *Staphylococcus aureus* (coagulase +)–24-48 h primarily of vomiting, but also involving cramps and diarrhea.
   c. *Bacillus cereus*–both diarrheal and vomiting forms.

IX. INFECTIONS OF THE ANORECTUM (see "Anorectal Disorders.")

40

Anorectal Disorders

Scott C. Hobler, M.D.

I. ANATOMY

A. Rectum.

1. The rectum is 12-15 cm in length extending from the sacral promontory to the levator ani muscles.
2. The three teniae spread and fuse into a continuous smooth muscle layer with obliteration of the haustral markings.
3. Three horizontal rectal folds are visible internally as the *valves of Houston.*
4. The peritoneum covers the upper 2/3 of the rectum anteriorly, but only the inner 1/3 laterally and posteriorly.

B. Anal canal.

1. Anatomic canal–extends from the dentate line to the anal verge.
2. Surgical canal–extends from the top of the anorectal ring to the anal verge.
3. The rectum is lined by colonic columnar epithelium. Transitional epithelium lines the anal canal from the columns of Morgagni to the dentate line (commonly termed the transition zone), and below the dentate line the anal canal is lined by squamous epithelium.
4. ***Internal sphincter***—thickened continuation of the circular smooth muscle of the rectum under control of the autonomic nervous system (involuntary).
5. ***External sphincter***—three rings of striated muscle with somatic innervation (voluntary).
   a. Deep external sphincter–the *puborectalis.*
   b. Superficial external sphincter–attached by the anococcygeal ligament to the coccyx.
   c. Subcutaneous external sphincter.

C. Levator ani muscle—composed of *iliococcygeus* and *pubococcygeus,* it constitutes the pelvic floor and is innervated by the fourth sacral nerve.

D. Blood supply and lymphatic drainage.

1. Arterial supply–segmental but with rich anastomoses.
   a. Superior hemorrhoidal–last branch of the IMA.
   b. Middle hemorrhoidal–branch of the internal iliac artery.
   c. Inferior hemorrhoidal–branch of the internal pudendal artery.
2. Venous drainage–parallels the arterial supply.
   a. Superior hemorrhoidal–drains the rectum and upper part of anal canal into the portal system.
   b. Middle hemorrhoidal–drains rectum and upper anal canal into internal iliac vein (systemic circulation).
   c. Inferior hemorrhoidal vein–drains rectum and lower anal canal into the systemic venous return.
   d. The superior, middle, and inferior hemorrhoidal veins converge to form the inferior hemorrhoidal plexus in the submucosa of the columns of Morgagni.
3. Lymphatic drainage.
   a. Superior and middle rectum–drains into the IMA nodes.
   b. Lower rectum and upper anal canal–drains into the superior rectal lymphatic (leading to the IMA) and to the internal iliac nodes.
   c. Anal canal distal to the dentate line–has dual drainage to the inguinal nodes and the internal iliac nodes.

II. HEMORRHOIDS

A. Types.

1. Internal hemorrhoids–dilated submucosal veins of the superior rectal plexus that lie proximal to the dentate line. Typically seen in three locations.
   a. Left lateral (3 o'clock).
   b. Right posterior lateral (7 o'clock).
   c. Right anterolateral (11 o'clock).
   d. Classification.
      (1) First degree–bleed but do not descend through the anal orifice.
      (2) Second degree–protrude during defecation and return spontaneously.
      (3) Third degree–protrude during defecation and must be replaced manually.
      (4) Forth degree–are permanently prolapsed.
2. External hemorrhoids–dilated veins arising from the inferior hemorrhoidal plexus below the dentate line and covered with squamous epithelium. Generally asymptomatic, unless thrombosed.

B. Signs and symptoms.

1. Pain, pruritus, rectal bleeding (usually bright red with spotting of the toilet paper), perianal moistness or drainage.
2. Symptoms are most commonly due to prolapsing internal hemorrhoids. Perianal moisture is caused by columnar mucous prolapsing beyond the anal verge.

3. Severe pain is not typically associated with internal hemorrhoids and is commonly seen with thrombosis of external hemorrhoids.

C. Treatment.

1. Initial treatment is nonoperative, except with symptomatic thrombosed hemorrhoids. Sitz baths provide symptomatic relief and improve hygiene. Stool softeners and bulk agents (psyllium) will minimize constipation and straining. Anusol HC® suppositories and Tuck's® pads help resolve inflammation.
2. ***Non-operative treatment*** (usually used for 1st- and 2nd-degree hemorrhoids).
   a. Rubber band ligation–used in the treatment of internal hemorrhoids, rubber bands must be placed above the dentate line, where mucous does not have somatic pain innervation.
   b. Sclerotherapy–submucosal injection of hemorrhoid with sclerosing agent, which obliterates the hemorrhoid by fibrosis.
   c. Other therapies–include cryotherapy, bipolar diathermy, infrared coagulation, and direct current therapy.
3. ***Hemorrhoidectomy*** indicated for prolapse, pain, or persistent bleeding.
   a. Dissection should be carried out in no more than 3 quadrants of the anal canal to avoid stricture formation (Whitehead deformity).
   b. The hemorrhoidal vein is ligated and then dissected free. The mucous is closed for homeostasis, but left open distally for drainage.
   c. Injection of long-acting local anesthetic is helpful.
   d. Rectal packs may aid homeostasis but can be very uncomfortable.
   e. Sitz baths are started the next day as well as stool softeners or bulk laxatives.
4. Thrombosed external hemorrhoids–these can be extremely painful and should be excised if seen within 48 h. Beyond this time, conservative therapy with analgesics and Sitz baths is appropriate.

III. ANAL FISSURE

One of the most frequent causes of severe anal pain.

A. Represents an acute or chronic tear in the anal squamous epithelium in the anterior or posterior midline. The fissure extends from the dentate line to the anal verge. Lateral or multiple fissures should raise suspicion of trauma, inflammatory bowel disease, lymphoma, neoplasm, or infection.

B. Equal frequency among males and females; most common in young adults.

C. Posterior location is more common.

D. Typically associated with spasm of the internal sphincter.

E. Signs and symptoms—sharp, shearing, or burning pain associated with defecation. Blood may streak the toilet paper. Pain is thought to be caused by spasm of the internal anal sphincter.

F. Treatment.

1. Non-operative–typically used in acute fissures and chronic fissures with mild or moderate symptoms.
   a. Stool softeners and bulk laxatives relieve straining.
   b. Sitz baths offer symptomatic relief and improve hygiene.
   c. Anesthetic suppositories may be helpful.
2. Operative therapy indicated for failure of conservative therapy. The goal of surgery is to modify the function of the internal sphincter, thereby breaking the cycle of spasm and pain.
   a. Anal dilation–disrupts the internal sphincter in a nonpredictable way. May lead to incontinence.
   b. Lateral-internal sphincterotomy–predictable and effective. The lateral-internal sphincter is divided to relieve the spasm. Pain is alleviated, and most fissures will heal with continued conservative care. Fissurectomy is rarely, if ever, needed.
   c. Fissurectomy and midline sphincterotomy–effective but often has a 6-8 week healing period. Up to 10% of patients will have a "keyhole" deformity with chronic soiling.

IV. ANORECTAL ABSCESS

Originate from an infection arising from the anal crypts. The abscess typically forms in the inter-sphincter space. Subsequent spread can occur along various paths (Figure 1). The distinction between an anorectal abscess and fistula is typically based on its time course. Abscesses typically represent an acute episode, whereas a fistula represents a more chronic process. The exact etiology of anorectal abscess is not known. Factors implicated in the development of abscess include constipation, diarrhea, trauma, Crohn's disease, tuberculosis, actinomysis, anorectal malignancy, leukemia, and lymphoma. The most common associated medical problems include hypertension, diabetes, heart disease, and inflammatory bowel disease. More common in males (3:1). Typically polymicrobial (*E. coli, Proteus, Streptococcus,* and *Bacteroides* common).

A. Classification.

1. Perianal abscess–a superficial abscess that lies beneath the skin of the anal canal but does not traverse the external sphincters.
2. Ischiorectal abscess–occupy the ischiorectal fossa below the levators and lateral to the sphincters. The abscess can cross the midline to form a bilateral ("horseshoe") abscess.
3. Intersphincteric abscess–located between the external and

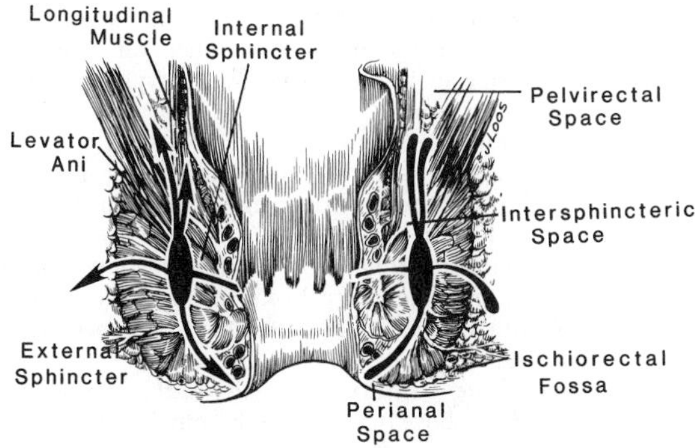

FIG. 1 **Pathways of Infection in Perianal Spaces**

internal sphincter muscle. Most common in the posterior quadrant. Typically without evidence of perianal swelling or induration.

4. Supralevator abscess–occurring above the levators, these are more difficult to diagnose and drain. Can mimic intra-abdominal condition.

B. Signs and symptoms—usually presents with extreme perianal pain. A mass is commonly felt on rectal exam. Cellulitis and fluctuance are often seen. Vague pain and high, ill-defined mass may be evidence for a supralevator abscess.

C. Treatment—surgical drainage is always indicated, and drainage alone is usually sufficient therapy.

1. Most small, superficial perianal abscesses can be drained in the E.R. Packing is left in overnight and removed, and Sitz baths or showers are instituted. Exploration of the fistula tract is not necessary.
2. Antibiotics are indicated for significant cellulitis or with immunosuppressed patients.
3. Perirectal abscesses and all abscesses in diabetics or immunocompromised patients should be drained in the operating room. A fistula is identified in 30% of cases. Necrotizing fasciitis and Fournier's gangrene are feared complications if left undrained.
4. Proximal fecal diversion may be necessary in complex cases, particularly with supralevator abscesses.

V. FISTULA *IN ANO*

An abnormal communication between the anal canal (internal opening) at about the level of the dentate line and the perianal skin (external opening). Typically represents the incomplete healing of a drained anorectal abscess and commonly occurs secondary to a pyogenic process and, less frequently, a granulomatous disease. Those fistula arising above the dentate line are typically secondary to diverticulitis or trauma.

A. Classification.

1. Intersphincteric fistula (70%)–located in the intersphincteric space with external opening typically on the perianal skin near the anal verge.
2. Transsphincteric fistula (23%)–starts in the intersphincteric space, traverses the external sphincter into the ischiorectal fossa, with external opening lateral to the perianal skin. Horseshoe fistula falls into this category.
3. Suprasphincteric fistula (5%)–starts in the intersphincteric space, passes above the puborectalis muscle, and tracts laterally between the levator and the puborectalis muscle.
4. Extrasphincteric fistula (2%)–complicated fistula. Passes from the perianal skin through the ischiorectal fossa and levator ani muscles and subsequently through the rectal wall.

B. Goodsall's Rule (Figure 2)–relates the position of the internal opening of a fistula to the external opening. Fistulas with external openings anterior to a transverse line through the anal opening have a fistula tract that extends directly to the anal canal anteriorly. Those fistulas with external openings posterior or greater than 3 cm from the verge have a tract that curves and has its internal opening in the posterior midline. Fistulas defying this rule should raise the suspicion of inflammatory bowel disease. Anterior midline is the 12 o'clock position by convention.

C. Signs and symptoms—chief complaint is typically intermittent or constant drainage. Typically a history of recurrent

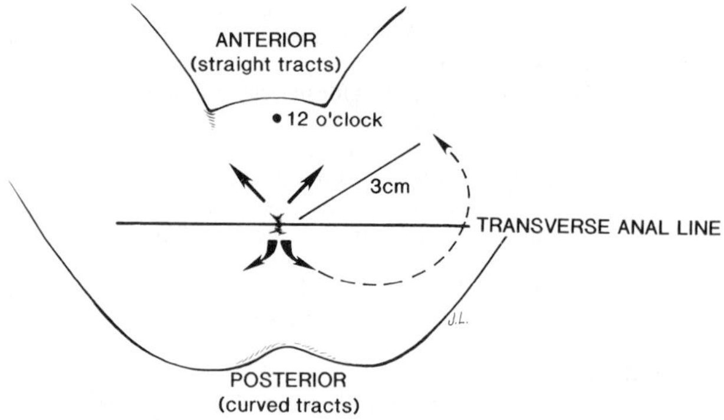

FIG. 2 Goodsall's Rule

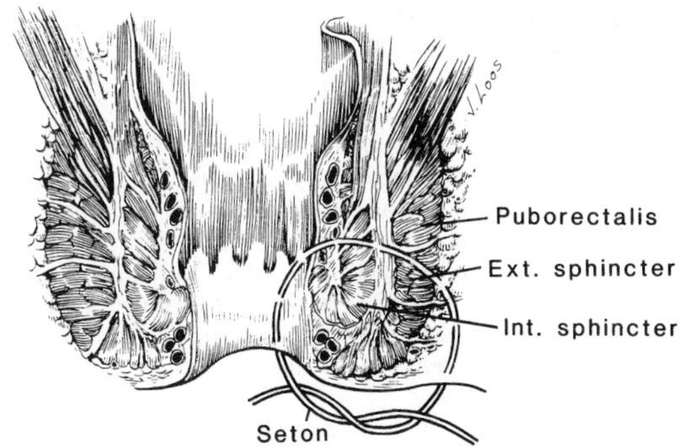

FIG. 3 Use of a Seton in High Fistula

perianal abscess is found, but not always. External opening is typically represented by a red cluster of granulation tissue. A cord-like tract may be palpated on rectal exam.

D. Treatment.

1. Delineation of the fistula tract is most important but is only possible in 2/3 of cases. This must be performed under appropriate anesthesia.
2. The entire tract must be unroofed for drainage. The wound will heal secondarily. Actual excision of the tract (fistulectomy) is rarely necessary.
3. Since unroofing may require the division of one or both sphincters, setons may be indicated for any fistula crossing both sphincters (Figure 3). A heavy suture is passed through the tract to improve drainage and stimulate fibrosis of the tract. The seton may be sequentially tightened, and after significant fibrosis the tract is ultimately opened with a greatly reduced risk of incontinence.
4. Horseshoe fistulas involve infection of the deep postanal space with extension into the ischiorectal spaces on both sides. These can be treated by opening the postanal space and placing appropriate counter-incisions laterally for drainage.

VI. PILONIDAL DISEASE

A common skin lesion of the sacrococcygeal area.

A. Affected population—Most frequently seen in young men.

B. Etiology—It is believed to be an acquired disease that develops secondary to obstruction of the hair follicle in this area. This obstruction can subsequently lead to formation of cysts, sinuses or abscesses.

C. Sinuses or cysts are typically seen in the midline.

D. Presentation—Most patients present with pain and swelling secondary to the development of infection.

E. Treatment.

1. Acute abscess–incision and drainage with curettage of the cavity and removal of present hair. Incision is made lateral to the midline to improve healing. Wound is packed open. Following incision and drainage, up to 40% will develop chronic pilonidal sinuses, which will require further therapy.
2. Chronic pilonidal sinus–many treatment options are available for the treatment of this problem, and their use depends on the severity of the disease. The surgical options include the following.
   a. Simple pilonidal cystectomy.
   b. Excision and marsupialization.
   c. Excision with Z-plasty or flap advancement.

VI. ANAL AND PERIANAL INFECTIONS

A. Condyloma acuminata (venereal warts)–caused by the human papilloma virus. May occur on perianal skin, anal or rectal mucous, vulva, vaginal wall, or penis. Incubation period is 1 to 6 months. Presenting symptoms include lump in the perianal region, pruritus ani, bleeding, or pain. Examination reveals coliform-like masses that are typically pink or white and tend to grow in rows.

B. Treatment—combination of local ablation and improved hygiene with concomitant treatment of sexual contacts. Genital lesions should be treated concurrently.

1. Podophyllin resin–25% solution in mineral oil or tincture of benzoin for small, scattered lesions.
2. Fulguration under anesthesia for extensive involvement.
3. Surgical excision of large masses may be necessary.

B. Anorectal herpes—usually presents with severe pain. Characteristic herpetic lesions are seen on exam and are confirmed by viral culture. Treatment is generally symptomatic, although acyclovir decreases the time to healing and the frequency of recurrence.

C. Gonococcal proctitis—confirmed by culture, the treatment is the same as with genital involvement. Symptoms include pain and discharge. Anoscopy reveals mucosal erythema and purulence of the anal crypts.

VII. PRURITUS ANI

Common symptom of perianal itching that affects up to 1-5% of the population.

A. Etiology—There is a long list of causes, but in general, any condition that leads to moisture, drainage, or soiling increases its prevalence.

B. Up to 50% will ultimately be classified as "idiopathic."

C. Hygiene is the mainstay of treatment, even when surgically correctable problems such as hemorrhoids exist. Improved hygiene may solve pruritus and improve other symptomatology, obviating surgery.

D. Surgically correct hemorrhoids, fissures, fistula, etc.

E. Other causes include fungi, pinworms, other infectious agents.

F. Underlying disease—diabetes, jaundice, Crohn's disease.

G. Topical or dietary sensitivities.

H. Neoplasm—carcinoma, melanoma, Paget's, Bowen's disease.

VII. ANAL NEOPLASM

Malignancies of the anal canal are relatively uncommon and represent only 2-3% of all large bowel carcinomas. Position of the tumor in the anal canal relative to the dentate line is important to the biological behavior of the tumor. This is based on the lymphatic drainage in these two areas. Most tumors spread by direct extension and via the lymphatic system. Hematologic spread is much less common. Anal tumors are classified into two groups based on location: (1) anal canal tumor and (2) anal margin tumors.

A. Tumors of the anal canal.

1. Epidermoid carcinoma (1-2% of all colorectal carcinomas).
   a. Typically seen in patients between 50-70 years.
   b. More frequent in women
   c. Two cell types–squamous cell (keratinizing) and transitional cell (non-keratinizing).
   d. Rectal pain, bleeding, or mass are common presenting symptoms.
   e. 40-50% have pelvic lymph node involvement at diagnosis, 15-36% have inguinal nodes, and 10% have distant metastasis at the time of diagnosis.
   f. 5-year survival is dependent on grade but averages about 50%.
   g. Chemotherapy with mitomycin-C and 5-FU combined with radiation is treatment of choice. This may be followed by surgical resection. Abdomino-perineal resection is indicated for residual disease or recurrence.
2. Malignant melanoma (0.5-1.0% of malignant anal tumors).
   a. Anal canal is the third most common site after skin and eyes.
   b. Typically occurs adjacent to the dentate line.
   c. Rectal bleeding is the most frequent complaint.
   d. Most are not highly pigmented, and diagnosis is difficult.
   e. Tumor is aggressive and often widely metastatic. Abdominal-perineal resection is only appropriate in selected patients.

f. Tumors often radio-resistant and unresponsive to chemotherapy.
g. 5-year survival is less than 15%.

B. Tumors of the anal margin.

1. These tumors are similar to skin tumors elsewhere and are treated in the same manner.
2. Include squamous cell and basal cell carcinomas, Bowen's disease, and Paget's disease.

VIII. RECTAL PROLAPSE

A. Classification (Figure 4).

1. Type I (false prolapse or mucosal prolapse)–redundant rectal mucous prolapsed with radial furrows.
2. Type II (incomplete prolapse)–rectal intussusception without a sliding hernia.
3. Type III (true prolapse or complete prolapse)–protrusion of the entire rectal wall through the anal orifice with herniation of the pelvic peritoneum or cul de sac. Circular furrows present. This is the most common type.

B. Clinical features.

1. 85% of patients are female; maximal incidence is in the 5th and subsequent decades. Also seen in children under 5 years old.
2. Many patients have had prior gynecological surgery.
3. In men, the incidence is more evenly distributed throughout the age range.
4. High incidence of associated chronic neurological or psychiatric disorders (5-50%).
5. Possible pathogenesis include either sliding-type hernia, in which the rectum herniates through a defect in the pelvic fascia, or intussusception of the rectum.
6. Presenting complaints may be related to the prolapse itself or to the disturbance of anal continence that frequently coexists and include the following.
   a. Extrusion of a mass with defecation, exertion, coughing, sneezing, etc.
   b. Difficulty in bowel regulation–tenesmus, constipation, fecal incontinence.
   c. Permanently extruded rectum with excoriation, ulceration, and constant soiling.
   d. Associated urinary incontinence or uterine prolapse.
7. Physical findings.
   a. Demonstrated prolapse during Valsalva.
   b. Compromised sphincter tone.
   c. Excoriation or circumferential inflammation of midrectum on proctosigmoidoscopy.

C. Evaluation.

1. Replace the prolapsed area, if possible, and perform sigmoidoscopy to determine the condition of the bowel and the presence of any associated lesion or carcinoma.

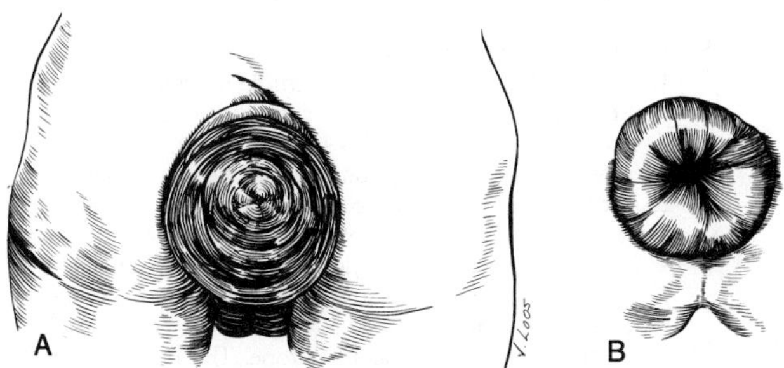

FIG. 4 **Differential Diagnosis of True Rectal Prolapse, A *vs.* Type I Mucosal Prolapse, B**

2. Assess sphincter tone and the degree of fecal continence by exam. Many patients with prolapse have poor sphincter tone.
3. Barium enema or colonoscopy.
4. Intravenous pyelogram–the ureters may be pulled with the rectum into the sliding hernia.
5. Radiographs of the lumbar spine and pelvis–look for neurologic disease.
6. Cinedefacography–useful in the evaluation of occult prolapse (Type II).
7. Transit time studies will document functionally delayed transit as a cause of chronic constipation and straining.

D. Treatment options.

1. False prolapse.
   a. Common in very young children. Conservative therapy is often successful. Gently replace the prolapsed area after each defecation or straining. Excision of redundant mucous is rarely necessary.
   b. In adults, hemorrhoidectomy with excision of redundant mucous is effective.
2. True prolapse–typically a progressive disorder that is not responsive to non-surgical therapy. Many procedures have been described that indicate the difficulty and chronicity of the problem. Basic features of the repairs include correction of the following anatomical characteristics.
   a. Abnormally deep or wide cul-de-sac.
   b. Weak pelvic floor with diastasis of the levators.
   c. Patulous anal sphincter.
   d. Redundant rectosigmoid.
   e. Lack of fixation of the rectum to the sacral hollow with abnormal mobility and loss of the normal horizontal position of the lower rectum.

f. Associated incontinence is not treated initially since it may resolve after treatment of the prolapse.

E. Abdominal approaches.

1. ***Abdominal proctopexy with sigmoid resection.*** The lateral rectal stalks are used to anchor the rectum to the presacral fascia and periosteum. This is amenable to a laparoscopic approach. Treatment option in young healthy patients.
2. ***Rectal sling*** (Ripstein procedure)–the rectum is fixed to the sacrum using a sling of synthetic mesh. This must be loose enough to prevent obstruction. Foreign material makes concomitant sigmoid resection more hazardous and provides an increased risk of pelvic sepsis.
3. ***Ivalon sponge***—popular in Europe. The rectum is mobilized posteriorly and attached to the sacrum with a polyvinyl alcohol sponge.

F. Perineal approach—very useful in debilitated patients who would not tolerate an abdominal incision.

1. ***Perineal rectosigmoidectomy*** (Altemeier procedure)–involves resection of the redundant prolapsing bowel with primary anastomosis, high ligation of the hernia sac, and approximation of the levator ani muscles. This is well tolerated even in high-risk patients and may be performed under regional anesthesia.
2. ***Thiersch procedure***—this is of historical interest only and is rarely (if ever) done. This technique was used in those too ill to tolerate even a perineal resection. The sphincters are encircled with a wire or band of synthetic material.

G. Transsacral approach—resection of the coccyx and lower sacrum with subsequent resection of the redundant prolapsing bowel with primary anastomosis. This technique has not gained popularity.

IX. ANOSCOPY

A. Indications—examination of the lower rectum and anal canal.

B. Patient preparation—none necessary. Enema is desirable, depending on the clinical situation.

C. Technique.

1. Position patient in right or left lateral decubitus position with hips and knees flexed.
2. Inspection–note presence of fissures, hemorrhoids, skin tags, blood, or pus.
3. Palpation–digital exam must be done prior to anoscopy.
   a. Note masses, induration, spasm, tenderness, or discharge.
   b. Palpate normal structures including prostate.
   c. Inspect examining finger for blood, pus, stool, or mucus.
4. Anoscopy.
   a. Lubricate generously and insert obturator.
   b. Introduce anoscope into anus and point in direction of

umbilicus. Once upper end of the anal canal is reached, direct anoscope posteriorly toward sacral hollow.

c. Note character of mucus, presence of lesions, masses, or foreign body.
d. Slowly withdraw scope, observing the mucus as it passes the scope.

X. RIGID SIGMOIDOSCOPY

A. Reach—Rigid sigmoidoscopy will reach to 25-30 cm.

B. Patient preparation—Milk of Magnesia®, magnesium citrate, or castor oil the evening before procedure. Clear liquids after midnight. The patient is given an enema that morning or prior to the procedure.

C. Technique.

1. Position the patient in the lateral decubitus position or in elbow-to-chest position over a sigmoidoscopy table.
2. Inspect the perianal area and perform a digital exam as in anoscopy.
3. Insert the scope into the anus, direct toward the umbilicus.
4. As soon as the rectum is entered, remove the obturator and close the window. The scope should only be advanced further under direct visualization of the lumen. Insufflation is used as needed.
5. Slowly advance the scope though the lumen of the bowel. Movements are initially posterior into the sacral hollow, then anterior and left into the sigmoid colon.
6. Once the scope is fully inserted, it is slowly withdrawn in a circular fashion to carefully examine all of the mucous.
7. Biopsy should be performed last so that blood does not obscure the rest of the exam.
8. Before removing the scope, insufflated air should be allowed out for the patient's comfort.

41

Gynecological Oncology

Alexander A. Parikh, M.D.

I. CERVICAL CANCER

Incidence of *invasive cancer* has steadily declined secondary to the Pap smear, but the frequency of diagnosis of *carcinoma in situ* has increased, and it is now the third most common gynecological malignancy. More prevalent in women with early age at first intercourse, multiple sexual partners, lower socioeconomic status, early childbearing, HPV infection, and those who smoke cigarettes. Pre-invasive intraepithelial carcinoma occurs primarily in women of age 20-30, whereas invasive carcinoma usually presents between ages 40-60. Predominantly squamous cell carcinoma (85-90%) or adenocarcinoma (10-15%). Other types include adenosquamous carcinoma, small cell variants, and cervical lymphoma. Adenocarcinoma appears to be more aggressive and appears at a more advanced stage than squamous.

A. Clinical presentation.

1. Most commonly presents with vaginal bleeding or brownish discharge (especially after intercourse or douching and between periods) that is usually light, but can be profuse.
2. Advanced lesions may present with pain (pelvic, lower back and/or lower extremity), dysuria, hematuria and weight loss. The lesions may be exophytic, ulcerative, or endophytic.

B. Diagnostic workup.

1. Yearly routine Pap smears recommended at age 18 or at initiation of sexual activity.
2. Colposcopic evaluation with biopsies and endocervical curettage (ECC) for high-grade and sometimes low-grade squamous intraepithelial lesions, and any other suspicious lesions.
3. Cone biopsy under the following conditions.
   a. ECC shows intraepithelial or microinvasive carcinoma.
   b. Cytologic abnormality (Pap) not consistent with tissue diagnosis.
   c. The entire transformation zone is not visible.

d. Microinvasive carcinoma is diagnosed by direct biopsy.
e. Premalignant or malignant glandular epithelium detected.

4. Staging provides the basis for therapeutic decisions and prognosis and requires tissue and histological diagnosis, a thorough history and physical exam (including bimanual pelvic and rectal exams), and radiological and laboratory studies as appropriate.

C. Staging.

Stage 0: Carcinoma *in situ,* intraepithelial carcinoma.

Stage I: Confined to the cervix; pre-clinical, with minimal microscopic stromal invasion **(IA1),** or with a maximum invasion of 5 mm in depth from the base of the epithelium, and a maximum of 7 mm horizontal spread **(IA2).** All tumors larger than IA2 are **IB.** *Overall 5-year survival 65-90%.*

Stage II: Extends beyond cervix, involves upper two-thirds of vagina, does not extend to the pelvic wall; no obvious parametrial involvement **(IIA or IIB);** *overall 5-year survival 45-80%, 30-40% if adenocarcinoma.*

Stage III: Either extends to pelvic wall or invades the lower third of the vagina. **IIIA** does not extend to the pelvic wall, while **IIIB** either extends to the wall and/or is associated with hydronephrosis or a nonfunctioning kidney. *5-year survival as high as 61%; 20-30% if adenocarcinoma.*

Stage IV: Extension beyond the true pelvis or has clinically involved the mucosa of the bladder or rectum; spread to adjacent organs **(IVA),** or spread to distant organs **(IVB).** *Overall 5-year survival <15%.* Other prognostic factors include age, tumor volume, histologic grade, lymphatic and vascular invasion, performance status, Her-2/neu and c-myc oncogene overexpression, and tumor aneuploidy.

D. Management.

Stage IA: Conservative surgery (Conization, simple hysterectomy) for lesions with ≤3 mm stromal invasion, no invasion of blood or lymphatic channels, no areas of confluence, and negative margins. Conization especially helpful in patients who wish to preserve fertility. Other lesions should be treated like Stage IB lesions, and poor surgical candidates can be treated with intra-cavitary radiation.

Stage IB: 15% of patients have metastases to pelvic lymph nodes, and therefore options include radical hysterectomy and pelvic lymphadenectomy, or external pelvic combined with intracavitary irradiation.

Stage IIA: Most recommend combination radiotherapy, although radical hysterectomy with lymphadenectomy may be appropriate for small-volume lesions.

Stages IIB, III, IVA: Primarily with external and intracavitary irradiation, combined with radio-sensitizing agents (hydroxyurea, 5-FU, cisplatin). External field irradiation for para-aortic lymph nodes has shown to be of some benefit in long-term survival. Stage IVA, barring evidence of distant or unresectable disease, can occasionally be cured with pelvic exenteration.

Stage IVB: Treated with chemotherapy (primarily cisplatin); radiation given for palliation.

E. Recurrence.

1. Approximately 35% have recurrent or persistent disease that generally develops within 2-3 years.
2. The pelvis is the most common site of recurrence, followed by the uterus and distant organs.
3. Signs and symptoms include unexplained weight loss, lower extremity edema, pelvic and lower extremity pain, serosanguinous vaginal discharge, progressive ureteral obstruction, and lymphadenopathy.
4. *For locally recurrent cervical cancer,* after previous irradiation, treatment includes pelvic exenteration or rarely hysterectomy. If previously treated with surgery, irradiation therapy is appropriate.
5. *For metastatic cervical cancer,* systemic chemotherapy (cisplatin) is the treatment of choice.
6. Overall poor prognosis, with a 10-15% 1-year survival for all patients with recurrent disease.

F. Surveillance.

1. Physical and pelvic exam and Pap smear every 3 months for the first year, every 4 months for the second year, every 6 months for years 3-5, and annually thereafter.
2. Radiologic and laboratory studies include annual chest radiograph (may not be necessary in stages I-IIA), IVP annually, or at any time for patients with hydronephrosis (also may not be necessary for stages I-IIA), and CBC, BUN, creatinine every 6 months to yearly.

II. ENDOMETRIAL CANCER

Most common gynecologic malignancy in the U.S., and the fourth most common malignancy in women. Mean age of onset is 63 years, but about 25% of cases occur in pre-menopausal women. Chronic, unopposed exposure to estrogen is the principal predisposing factor; other risk factors include early menarche, late menopause, obesity, chronic anovulation, nulliparity, estrogen-secreting tumors, complex atypical hyperplasia, and ingestion of unopposed estrogen (progestins can nullify this risk). Other associations include pelvic radiation, hypertension, diabetes mellitus, and a history of breast or ovarian malignancy. The use of oral contraceptives is *negatively* correlated with the incidence of endometrial cancer. Histologically, about 75% are adenocarcinomas, followed by adenosquamous (15-20%), papillary serous, and clear cell. Other types include mucinous carcinoma, squamous, undifferentiated, and mixed type.

A. Clinical presentation and diagnosis.

1. Presenting signs and symptoms include any bleeding or abnormal vaginal discharge in post-menopausal women; or abnor-

mal menstruation or intermenstrual bleeding in peri- and premenopausal women.

2. Diagnostic workup in suspected patients includes a careful inspection of the vulva, anus, vagina, and cervix; a Pap smear from the endo- and ectocervix; an endometrial biopsy and endocervical curettage or aspiration; biopsies of any suspicious genital lesions; testing for occult blood in the stool; and a chest radiograph, CBC, UA, renal and hepatic profiles.

B. Staging.

Once cancer is proven by biopsy, a total abdominal hysterectomy and bilateral adnexectomy, peritoneal cytology, careful inspection of the abdominal and pelvic organs, and biopsy of pelvic and aortic nodes are required for proper staging.

Stage I: Confined to the body of the uterus with tumor limited to the endometrium (*IA*), or invasion to less than (*IB*) or more than (*IC*) of the myometrium; *75-100% overall 5-year survival.*

Stage II: Involves the body and cervix, but not outside the uterus with endocervical glandular involvement only (*IIA*) or cervical stromal invasion (*IIB*); *5-year survival is about 60%.*

Stage III: Extends outside the uterus, but confined to the true pelvis or involves para-aortic nodes; IIIA invades uterine serosa and/or adnexa and/or has positive peritoneal cytology, IIIB has vaginal metastasis and IIIC involves pelvic and/or para-aortic lymph nodes. *5-year survival 30-50%.*

Stage IV: Involves adjacent organs (*IVA*) or distant metastases (*IVB*); *10-20% 5-year survival.*

HISTOPATHOLOGIC GRADING:

G1: 5% or less of a nonsquamous or nonmorular solid growth pattern.

G2: 6-50% of a nonsquamous or nonmorular solid growth pattern.

G3: More than 50% of a nonsquamous or nonmorular solid growth pattern.

NOTE: Although staging and grade usually correlate, the clinical stage is more influential in the prognosis.

C. Management.

1. ***Low-risk patients*** (grade 1 or 2 tumors confined to the fundus with ≤ 33% myometrial invasion)—*require no further therapy.*
2. ***Intermediate-risk patients*** (grade 1 or 2 tumors with middle third invasion and no extrauterine spread)—*post-operative radiation (whole-pelvis or intracavitary) improves local/regional control.*
3. ***High-risk patients***—with adnexal spread, pelvic node metastasis, outer third myometrial invasion, cervical invasion, or grade 3 tumors with any invasion—may benefit from adjuvant whole-pelvis radiotherapy. If positive aortic nodes are found, external field radiation is recommended.
4. ***Patients with intra-abdominal metastatic disease***—may benefit from debulking surgery and adjuvant whole-abdomen radiotherapy, chemotherapy (doxorubicin, cisplatin or multiagent), or progestin therapy combined with radiation.

5. ***Patients with distant metastatic disease***—usually treated with single agent or combination chemotherapy.

D. Recurrent disease is managed with radiotherapy for patients originally treated with radiation alone, or chemotherapy or progestin therapy for patients having received radiation.

III. OVARIAN CANCER

Accounts for about 25% of all gynecological malignancies, but for about 50% of gynecological cancer-related deaths because of the usual advanced stage at presentation. Risk of developing ovarian cancer is 1 in 70 and increases with age until 70 years. Other risk factors include family history (first-degree relatives), low parity, decreased fertility, and delayed childbearing if not using oral contraceptives. The use of oral contraceptives has been shown to decrease the risk of epithelial ovarian cancer in patients aged 40-59 years. Most (85-90%) are epithelial in origin; the other types (germ cell and sex cord-stromal tumors) are rarer.

A. Screening.

1. Unfortunately, no effective screening program exists; therefore most patients present clinically with advanced-stage carcinoma, with only 30% of the cases confined to the ovaries.
2. Careful pelvic examination remains the only effective screening method to date.
3. Pelvic ultrasound, especially vaginal, offers some promise; however, tumor markers such as CA 125 are not sensitive or specific enough to be helpful as a *screening tool.*

B. Clinical presentation and diagnosis.

1. Most presenting symptoms are those associated with increasing tumor mass, spread of tumor along the surfaces of other organs, and disseminated disease. These include abdominal discomfort, upper abdominal fullness, early satiety, constipation, dysuria, and polyuria as well as constitutional symptoms.
2. Physical findings include pelvic pain and ascites associated with a pelvic mass. An adnexal mass that is bilateral, irregular, solid, or fixed is suggestive of malignancy, although not diagnostic.
3. Pelvic ultrasound, especially transvaginal, may detect the presence of mural nodularity, septations, and internal echoes, which are more suggestive of malignancy, if a mass is noted.
4. When ovarian cancer is suspected, the work-up is aimed at excluding other causes of an adnexal mass. This includes a thorough history and physical exam, including pelvic and rectal examination and Pap smear; pelvic ultrasound (as discussed above), CT or MRI to detect extraovarian disease and lymphadenopathy; colonoscopy, proctoscopy, or barium enema to exclude colonic involvement, colon cancer, or inflammatory bowel disease; EGD/UGI if upper abdominal symptoms are present to exclude gastric malignancy with metastases to the ovaries; mammogram to rule out metastases to the ovaries; IVP

or cystoscopy to rule out ureteral or bladder involvement, if indicated; chest radiograph to rule out metastatic disease or pleural effusion; and blood tests, including CA-125 (elevated in 80-85%). Other tumor markers such as CA 19-9 (mucinous epithelial ovarian carcinomas), AFP and HCG (germ cell tumors), LDH (dysgerminoma), and CEA (epithelial ovarian carcinoma) may also be useful.

C. **Staging**—Ovarian cancer is a staged by laparotomy, noting any ascites, and performing cytologic washes upon entering the abdomen. The abdominal cavity should then be explored systematically and biopsies taken as indicated.

Stage I: Growth limited to one ovary (*IA*) or both ovaries (*IB*) with no tumor on external surface(s), capsule(s) intact and no ascites; or involving the surface of one or both ovaries, capsule(s) ruptured or with ascites or peritoneal washings containing malignant cells (*IC*); *60-90% 5-year survival.*

Stage II: Growth involving one or both ovaries with extension and/or metastases to the uterus and/or tubes (*IIA*), extension to other pelvic tissues (*IIB*), or stage IIA or IIB, but involving the surface of one or both ovaries, capsule(s) ruptured, or with ascites or peritoneal washings containing malignant cells (*IC*); *40-70% 5-year survival.*

Stage III: Tumor involving one or both ovaries grossly limited to the true pelvis with negative nodes but with histologically confirmed microscopic seeding of abdominal peritoneal surfaces, including small bowel, omentum, and liver surfaces (*IIIA*); histologically confirmed implants of abdominal peritoneal surfaces, none exceeding 2 cm in diameter and negative lymph nodes (IIIB) or abdominal implants greater than 2 cm in diameter and/or positive retroperitoneal or inguinal lymph nodes (*IIIC*); *4-15% overall 5-year survival.*

Stage IV: Involves one or both ovaries with distant metastasis, positive pleural effusion cytology, or parenchymal liver metastasis. *5-year survival 0-5%.* Factors affecting survival include stage of disease, cell type, grade of the tumor, residual tumor at the end of initial surgery, response to adjuvant therapy, and functional level of the patient.

D. Management.

1. ***Surgical*** management is aimed at resection of as much tumor as is safely possible. If a malignant tumor is identified, a thorough abdominal exploration, total abdominal hysterectomy, bilateral salpingo-oophorectomy, node biopsy, omentectomy, and removal of all gross cancer comprise standard surgical therapy. If there is no extra-ovarian spread, care should be taken not to rupture the capsule when removing the adnexa, as this may seed the peritoneal cavity and increase the stage of the cancer. All roughened or suspicious surfaces in the peritoneal cavity should be biopsied. Cytoreductive surgery and debulking procedures in which residual disease is minimized, ideally to less than 2 cm of residual disease, have shown improved

long-term survival in stage II and III cancers, may provide palliation in stage IV, and therefore should be performed.

2. ***Adjunctive therapy.***
   a. Stage I lesions that are poorly differentiated, associated with dense adhesions to adjacent structures, or IC disease warrant further therapy. Multi-agent chemotherapy including cisplatin or intraperitoneal chromium phosphate has been shown to be equally effective.
   b. Stage II lesions can be managed with intraperitoneal ^{32}P, total abdominal irradiation, or systemic chemotherapy followed in 1 year by a second-look surgery with similar survival statistics.
   c. Stage III lesions are treated with removal of as much tumor as possible, followed by combination chemotherapy (cisplatin, paraplatin, and cytoxan).
   d. Stage IV lesions are treated similar to stage III, but the overall results are disappointing.

E. Recurrent disease.

1. Platinum-based chemotherapeutic agents, if not used in the past or used over 6 months prior to recurrence, are the standard regimen.
2. Second-line agents, including taxol (about a 30% response rate), are used for patients not meeting this criterion.
3. Cytoreductive surgery is only used in those who have had a long disease-free survival and if the recurrent disease is amenable to surgery.

F. Special considerations.

1. ***Borderline epithelial tumors*** account for about 15% of epithelial tumors, are of low malignant potential, and usually occur in pre-menopausal women. Stage I can even be treated with unilateral salpingo-oophorectomy if preservation of fertility is desired; more advanced tumors are treated similar to the usual epithelial ovarian cancers.
2. ***Germ cell tumors*** account for 2-3% of ovarian cancers and usually occur in younger women. The majority are unilateral, and unilateral salpingo-oophorectomy can be performed for stage IA lesions if the contralateral ovary appears normal (biopsies are often taken). Chemotherapeutic agents such as BEP (bleomycin, etoposide, and cisplatin) are often used, even for IA lesions, since such lesions tend to be sensitive.
3. ***Sex cord-stromal tumors*** account for about 2% of ovarian cancers, and include granulosa cell and Sertoli-Leydig cell tumors. Majority are unilateral and can be managed similar to the germ cell tumors.

G. Evaluation of the incidental ovarian mass.

1. ***Pre-menopausal:*** Masses < 5 cm diameter can be carefully followed with physical exam and/or ultrasound. Masses > 5 cm diameter that are cystic require cystectomy (any cyst in patients taking oral contraceptives), and solid masses require oo-

phorectomy, both with frozen section. If the mass is clinically suspicious or the pathology equivocal, a formal staging laparotomy should be performed.

2. ***Post-menopausal:*** A bilateral oophorectomy should be done with a complete staging laparotomy if clinically suspicious or pathology equivocal.

IV. VULVAR CANCER

Accounts for only 5% of gynecological malignancies; 90% of them are of squamous cell origin. Risk factors include advanced age, low socioeconomic status, smoking, hypertension, obesity, diabetes, previous neoplasm of the cervix or vagina, and immunosuppression. HPV infection has been associated with vulvar cancer, but the relationship is not as clear as in cervical cancer. Clinical signs and symptoms include a mass or a lump on the vulva and vulvar itching and/ or irritation. Bleeding, discharge, and dysuria are less common. On physical examination, the lesion is usually raised and may appear fleshy, ulcerated, leukoplakic or wartlike. Diagnosis is based on biopsy; evaluation should include a thorough pelvic and rectal examination with colposcopy, since vulvar cancer is associated with other malignancies of the lower genital tract. Vulvar cancer spreads by 1) direct extension to adjacent structures, 2) lymphatic embolization to regional lymph nodes, and 3) hematogenous spread to distant organs, including the liver, lungs, and bone.

A. Staging.

Stage 0: Carcinoma *in situ;* intraepithelial carcinoma

Stage I: Confined to the vulva and/or perineum; 2 cm or less in greatest diameter; no nodal metastasis; *5-year survival about 90%.*

Stage II: Confined to the vulva and/or perineum; more than 2 cm in greatest diameter; no nodal metastases; *5-year survival 75-80%.*

Stage III: Tumor of any size with 1) adjacent spread to the lower urethra and/ or the vagina, or the anus, and/or 2) unilateral regional lymph node metastasis; *overall 5-year survival about 50%.*

Stage IV: Tumor invades upper urethra, bladder mucosa, rectal mucosa, pelvic, bone, and/or bilateral regional node metastasis (*IVA*), or involves distant metastasis, including pelvic lymph nodes (*IVB*). *Overall 5-year survival 20-70%, depending on extent of metastasis.*

B. Management.

1. Radical vulvectomy with bilateral inguinal lymphadenectomies through separate incisions and occasional bilateral pelvic lymphadenectomy comprises the preferred treatment for most vulvar cancers, but is associated with a high morbidity rate.
2. Pre-operative radiation is used in patients with advanced disease to reduce the need for exenteration, and post-operative radiation is often used to decrease the incidence of inguinal node recurrence in patients with 2 or more positive inguinal lymph nodes.
3. Cancers that are not poorly differentiated, less than 2 cm in

diameter, and no more than 1 mm thick can often be treated with deep wide excision alone, without lymph node dissection. Locally advanced lesions can be treated with external beam radiation with radiosensitizing agents followed by excision.

C. Follow-up—A pelvic exam and Pap smear should be done every 3 months for 2 years, every 6 months for 5 years, and then yearly.

D. Other vulvar carcinomas.

1. ***Melanoma*** is the second most common vulvar malignancy and presents similar to squamous cell carcinoma. Diagnosis is confirmed by biopsy, and the primary lesion should be excised with at least a 2 cm margin. Tumors with invasion of more than 0.75 mm should be removed *en bloc* with removal of the regional nodes. Prognosis is related to the thickness, with overall 5-year survival about 30-35%.
2. ***Bartholin gland carcinoma*** accounts for 5% of vulvar cancers, but is often misdiagnosed. Any persistent mass in the region of the gland, especially in patients over 40, should be biopsied. Radical vulvectomy with bilateral inguinal node dissection is the traditional treatment, but less radical surgery such as hemivulvectomy or radical local excision may be as effective. Postoperative radiation may reduce the incidence of local recurrence.
3. ***Paget's disease*** of the vulva predominantly affects postmenopausal Caucasian women. It presents with pruritus and local soreness and an erythematous, scaly lesion. Second primary lesions occur in about 30% and usually involve the GU or GI tract or the breasts. Treatment requires wide local excision. If an underlying adenocarcinoma or underlying stromal invasion is present, a more radical local excision or radical vulvectomy is needed in combination with a regional lymphadenectomy.
4. ***Verrucous carcinoma*** requires an adequate biopsy to distinguish it from a benign condyloma or a squamous cell carcinoma. These tumors are slow growing, locally destructive and usually occur in post-menopausal women. Treatment should be by radical local excision.

V. VAGINAL CANCER

Accounts for only 1-2% of all gynecological malignancies, with mean age 60-65; 80-90% are squamous cell and are usually located in the upper posterior wall of the vagina. The next most common is malignant melanoma, which usually involves the lower third of the vagina. Clear cell adenocarcinoma is usually a rare vaginal carcinoma, but is much more common in women who have been exposed to DES. Patients usually present with abnormal vaginal bleeding or discharge; pelvic pain and dysuria are late symptoms. Physical examination requires careful inspection and palpation of the vagina, and colposcopy and/or biopsies are performed as appropriate.

A. Staging.

Stage 0: Carcinoma in situ; *5-year survival 95%.*
Stage I: Confined to the vaginal mucosa; *5-year survival 80%.*
Stage IIA: Subvaginal infiltration, but not into parametrium; *50% 5-year survival.*
Stage IIB: Parametrial infiltration, but not to pelvic side wall; *40% 5-year survival.*
Stage III: Extending to the pelvic side wall; *5-year survival 35%.*
Stage IV: Extending to bladder or rectum or metastasis outside true pelvis; *5-year survival 10%.*

B. Management.

1. Carcinoma *in situ* is usually managed by surgical excision or laser ablation; topical 5-FU has also been used.
2. For stage I lesions that do not involve the upper vaginal fornices, radiotherapy (usually intracavitary) is the standard form of treatment.
3. Lesions involving the upper fornices can be treated with a radical hysterectomy, pelvic lymphadenopathy, and partial vaginectomy.
4. Stage IIA lesions are usually treated with external radiation +/- intracavitary radiation. More advanced tumors are also treated with external beam and intracavitary radiation.
5. Recurrent disease is usually treated with surgery, from wide local excision to pelvic exenteration.
6. Chemotherapy has also been tried, with varying degrees of success.
7. Clear cell adenocarcinoma usually requires radical hysterectomy, pelvic lymphadenectomy, and removal of most of the vagina with reconstruction.
8. Advanced lesions are treated with radiation, similar to squamous cell neoplasms.

VI. CANCER OF THE FALLOPIAN TUBE

A. Frequency—The rarest of gynecological malignancies, accounting for only 0.3 to 1.0% (metastatic disease to the fallopian tube is ten times more common than primary tumors). Primarily affects older women.

B. Diagnosis—Although the combination of abnormal vaginal bleeding and discharge, lower abdominal pain, and an adnexal mass in a post-menopausal woman is considered pathognomonic, these symptoms are not very common. Usually, the diagnosis is made on surgical exploration, and most are adenocarcinoma. There are no official staging criteria for fallopian tube carcinoma, but the prognosis is related to the "spread" of the disease to adjacent organs, the peritoneum and to regional and para-aortic lymph nodes.

C. Management includes a total abdominal hysterectomy, bilateral salpingo-oophorectomy, peritoneal cytology, and lymph node dissection. Post-operative intra-peritoneal ^{32}P or whole-abdominal radiation is indicated for positive peritoneal cytology, and abdomino-perineal radiation, including to the para-aortic lymph nodes, is used when spread involves adjacent organs. Combination chemotherapy is also often used for intra-peritoneal spread or recurrent disease.

D. *Overall 5-year survival is about 40%.*

42

Jaundice

Gregory M. Tiao, M.D.

There are numerous etiologies of jaundice. A thorough history and physical examination and appropriate laboratory and diagnostic studies can identify the causes of jaundice that are surgically correctable.

I. GENERAL CONSIDERATIONS

A. Bilirubin metabolism.

1. Hemoglobin (Hgb), myoglobin ⇒ biliverdin ⇒ bilirubin.
2. 70-90% from Hgb, RBC breakdown.
3. 10-30% from myoglobin breakdown, liver enzymes, non-Hgb heme, and non-Hgb porphyrin.
4. Indirect–bilirubin complexed with albumin; water insoluble (unconjugated).
5. Direct–bilirubin conjugated with glucuronide; water soluble (conjugated).
   a. Conjugation occurs in the liver.
   b. Diglucuronide–normal.
   c. Monoglucuronide–present in hepatocyte injury; may react as "direct".

B. Enterohepatic circulation—conjugated bilirubin excreted by liver ⇒ biliary system ⇒ duodenum. Bilirubin reduced to urobilinogen by small intestine bacteria. Terminal ileum: 10-20% absorbed and re-excreted by the liver and kidneys.

C. Clinical jaundice—evident when total bilirubin > 2 mg/dl.

II. HISTORY AND PHYSICAL

A. History.

1. Abdominal pain, fever, nausea, vomiting.
2. Dark urine, light stools.
3. Itching.
4. Diarrhea, malabsorption.
5. Alcohol, IV drug abuse.

B. Physical exam.

1. Clinical jaundice–skin, sclera, oral mucosa under tongue.
2. Abdominal tenderness.

3. Abdominal masses.
   a. Hepatomegaly, splenomegaly.
   b. Palpable gallbladder.
4. Stigmata of chronic liver disease.
   a. Spider angiomata, palmar erythema, caput medusa.
   b. Ascites, muscle wasting.
   c. Asterixis, encephalopathy.

III. LABORATORY TESTS

A. Bilirubin—in jaundice of hemolysis and hepatocellular disease, indirect bilirubin makes up 90-95% of total. In obstructive jaundice, direct bilirubin makes up > *50%* of total bilirubin.

	Normals (mg/dl)	Hemolysis	Hepatocellular disease	Bile duct obstruction
Serum bilirubin:				
Indirect	0.2-1.3	Increased	Increased	Normal
Direct	0-0.3	Normal	Increased	Increased
Urine:				
Urobilinogen	2-4	Increased	Increased	Absent
Bilirubin	Negative	Negative	Positive	Positive
Fecal:				
Urobilinogen	40-280	Increased	Decreased	Absent

B. CBC.
1. Microcytic anemia with an increased reticulocyte count suggests hemolysis. Peripheral smear will reveal sickle cells, spherocytes, target cells.
2. Increased WBC is consistent with infectious etiology, but is non-specific.

C. Transaminases—increased with hepatocellular injury (viral, alcoholic, or drug-induced hepatitis).
1. Serum glutamic-pyruvic transaminase (SGPT) or alanine serum transaminase (ALT)–more specific for liver than SGOT.
2. Serum glutamic-oxaloacetic transaminase (SGOT) or aspartate serum transaminase (AST)–found in liver, heart, skeletal muscle, kidney, pancreas.

D. Alkaline phosphatase—increased production by proliferating terminal biliary ductules in response to intrahepatic or extrahepatic obstruction.
1. Sources–liver, bone, placenta, kidney, WBCs, intestine.
2. Increased level may also be due to hepatic infiltrative diseases (tuberculosis, sarcoid, lymphoma), space-occupying lesions (abscess, neoplasm), bone disease, pregnancy.

E. 5′-Nucleotidase—comparable sensitivity to alkaline phosphatase, but with increased specificity. Sources–liver (bile canaliculi and sinusoidal membranes), intestine, heart, brain, blood vessels, endocrine pancreas (also increase during third trimester of pregnancy).

F. **Gamma glutamyl transferase (GGT)**—sensitivity and specificity greater than alkaline phosphatase.

G. **Prothrombin time (PT).**
   1. Dependent upon hepatic synthesis of factors V, VII, and X, prothrombin and fibrinogen, and intestinal absorption of vitamin K.
   2. Helpful in assessment of hepatic reserve.
   3. If PT > 3 sec above control, treat with vitamin K 10 mg SQ or IV.
      a. Corrects within 48 h if due to cholestasis or deficiency.
      b. Remains prolonged if due to hepatocellular insufficiency.

H. **Albumin.**
   1. Reflection of hepatic synthetic function and nutritional status.
   2. Half-life of approximately 15-20 days; not as valuable in detecting acute liver injury; short-turnover proteins (retinol binding protein, etc.) are more indicative of current synthetic status.

I. **Urobilinogen**—total absence from urine and feces indicates complete biliary obstruction.

J. **Hepatitis serology** (Table 1).
   1. Hepatitis A.
      a. IgM–acute and transient.
      b. IgG–appears during recovery and persists.
   2. Hepatitis B (Figure 1).
      a. HBsAg–surface antigen; first marker to appear; absent by 3 months.
      b. HBcAg–core antigen.
      c. HBeAg–internal component of the nucleocapsid gene of

TABLE 1
Serologic Features of Viral Hepatitis

Form of Infection	Serologic Markers	Interpretation
Hepatitis A	IgM anti-HAV	Acute disease
	IgG anti-HAV	Remote infection and immunity
Hepatitis B	HBsAg	Acute or chronic disease
	HBeAg	Active replication
	IgM anti-HBc (high titer)	Acute disease
	IgG anti-HBc	
	IgG anti-Hbc positive	Past infection and immunity
	IgG anti-HBc negative	Immune response from vaccination
Hepatitis C	Anti-HCV	Acute, chronic, or resolved disease
Hepatitis D	HBsAg and anti-HDV	Acute disease
	IgM anti-HBc positive	Co-infection
	IgG anti-HBc negative	Superinfection
Hepatitis E	None	

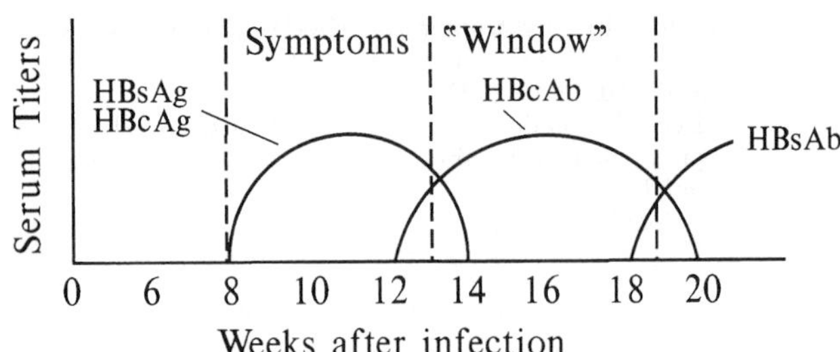

FIG. 1

hepatitis B virus (HBV). Indicates ongoing viral replication. HBV is most infectious when this is detected in the serum.

d. HBsAb–surface antibody; appearance variable, but usually persists for life.

e. HBcAb–core antibody; present during "window" period when HBsAG and HBsAB are too low to measure.

f. Important risk factor for hepatocellular carcinoma.

3. Hepatitis C.
   a. Responsible for > 90% of post-transfusion hepatitis.
   b. Chronic hepatitis develops in 50% of patients.
   c. Anti-HCV (hepatitis virus C) is not detectable in 10-20% of chronic hepatitis C patients.
4. Hepatitis D.
   a. Can develop in patients with HBsAg in serum.
   b. IV drug abusers and hemophiliacs at particular risk.
5. Hepatitis E.
   a. Enterically transmitted non-A non-B hepatitis.
   b. Transmitted by contaminated water.
   c. Does not lead to chronic infection.

IV. DIAGNOSTIC STUDIES

A. Abdominal flat plate.

1. Gallstones–15% are radiopaque.
2. Gas in biliary tree–seen in gallstone ileus and surgical anastomoses with intestinal tract, cholangitis with gas-producing organism.
3. Emphysematous cholecystitis–gas in gallbladder wall, extremely rare, is usually seen in diabetics.

B. Ultrasonography.

1. Accuracy > 90% for cholelithiasis.
2. Can identify dilated intra- and extrahepatic ducts, common duct stones, hepatic and pancreatic masses.
3. Accuracy affected by obesity, ascites, bowel gas, skill of technician and radiologist.

C. Nuclear biliary scan (HIDA, etc.).

1. Unreliable if bilirubin > 20 mg/dl (hepatic secretion of agent decreases as serum bilirubin exceeds 5 mg/dl).
2. Visualization of bile ducts but not gallbladder suggests cystic duct obstruction; 95% sensitive for acute cholecystitis.
3. Visualization of the duodenum rules out *complete* common duct obstruction.

D. Liver scan—reveals liver and spleen size, masses (> 2 cm), and parenchymal disease better than HIDA scan.

E. Computed tomography—most effective in identifying liver and pancreatic masses and level of extrahepatic biliary obstruction.

F. Percutaneous transhepatic cholangiography (PTC).

1. Identifies cause, site, extent of obstruction prior to surgery.
2. Obtainable in 95% of patients with dilated ducts secondary to extrahepatic biliary obstruction.
3. Contraindications.
   a. Coagulopathy–prolonged PT, PTT; platelets < 40,000.
   b. Ascites–unable to tamponade liver puncture.
   c. Peri- or intrahepatic sepsis.
   d. Disease of right lower lung or pleura.
4. Complications–bile peritonitis, bilothorax, pneumothorax, sepsis, hemobilia, bleeding.

G. Endoscopic retrograde cholangiopancreatography (ERCP) (see "Surgical Endoscopy").

1. Visualization of upper GI tract, ampullary region, biliary and pancreatic ducts.
2. Allows collection of cytology and biopsy specimens.
3. Complications–traumatic pancreatitis (1-2%), pancreatic or biliary sepsis (pre-procedure coverage with broad-spectrum antibiotic is recommended).

I. Percutaneous liver biopsy.

1. Histologic evaluation of liver parenchyma.
2. Contraindications–see PTC above.

V. DIFFERENTIAL DIAGNOSIS OF JAUNDICE

A. Pre-hepatic jaundice.

1. *Hemolysis.*
   a. Increased indirect bilirubin; unconjugated bilirubin is bound with albumin and cannot be excreted in urine.
   b. Production of bile pigments can raise total bilirubin by only 3 mg/dl (total bilirubin > 5 mg/dl indicates associated liver disease or biliary obstruction).
2. *Gilbert's disease*—defect in hepatocyte uptake of indirect bilirubin.
3. *Crigler-Najjar* (type I & II)–decreased conjugation secondary to impaired enzyme production or function.

B. Hepatic jaundice.

1. Viral hepatitis.

a. Insidious onset of symptoms: anorexia, malaise, fever, nausea, arthralgias, myalgias, headache, photophobia, pharyngitis, cough, coryza, and low-grade fever–usually precede abdominal pain.
b. Tender enlarged liver.
c. Serologic markers (see section III.J above)–cytomegalovirus (CMV) titers.

2. Alcoholic hepatitis–long history of alcohol abuse.
3. Drug-induced hepatitis–acetaminophen, halothane, erythromycin, isoniazid, chlorpromazine, valproic acid, phenytoin, oral contraceptives, 17,α-alkyl, substituted anabolic steroids, chlorpropamide, methimazole.
4. Cirrhosis (see "Cirrhosis").
5. ***Dubin-Johnson syndrome***–impaired hepatic excretion of conjugated bilirubin.

C. Post-hepatic/obstructive jaundice.

1. General considerations.
   a. Increased total bilirubin, bilirubin present in urine (dark-colored, "Coca-Cola™ urine), clay-colored stool.
   b. When total bilirubin > 3 mg/dl, both direct and indirect fractions are increased.
   c. Abdominal pain usually precedes symptoms of systemic disease.
   d. Painless jaundice with palpable gallbladder suggests cancer distal to the cystic duct (Courvoisier's Law).
   e. **Charcot's triad**–fever, RUQ pain, jaundice; suggests extrahepatic obstruction with ascending cholangitis; a surgical emergency.
   f. **Reynolds' pentad**–Charcot's triad, shock, mental obtundation.
2. Choledocholithiasis (see "Gallbladder and Biliary Tree").
3. Cholangitis (see "Gallbladder and Biliary Tree").
4. ***Sclerosing cholangitis.***
   a. Non-bacterial inflammatory narrowing of bile ducts–predominantly affects men ages 20-50; etiology unknown.
   b. Present with fatigue, weight loss, anorexia, insidious development of jaundice and pruritus, intermittent RUQ pain.
   c. Estimated that 50% of patients with sclerosing cholangitis have or will develop ulcerative colitis.
   d. ERCP and biopsy used for diagnosis–rule out malignancy.
   e. Treatment.
      (1) Medical–corticosteroids, long-term antibiotics to prevent cholangitis, immunosuppression, bile-acid binding agents, penicillamine.
      (2) Surgical–T-tube, transhepatic stent, other decompressive procedure.
   f. May progress to secondary biliary cirrhosis with ascites, varices, and hepatic failure requiring transplantation.

5. ***Benign biliary stricture.***
   a. 95% caused by surgical trauma, 5% caused by abdominal trauma, chronic pancreatitis, or impacted stone.
   b. Presents with intermittent cholangitis, jaundice.
   c. Diagnosis with PTC or ERCP–stricture usually within 2 cm of bifurcation.
   d. Treatment.
      (1) Antibiotics for cholangitis.
      (2) Surgical repair requires tension-free anastomosis and mucosal apposition: choledochoduodenostomy, choledochojejunostomy, or end-to-end bile duct anastomosis.
   e. Complications (if untreated):
      (1) Infection–cholangitis, abscess, sepsis.
      (2) Liver/biliary disease–cirrhosis, portal hypertension.
6. ***Carcinoma of the bile ducts (Klatskin's tumor).***
   a. Diagnosis usually made in 7th decade–commonly metastatic at presentation.
   b. Associated conditions–ulcerative colitis (incidence unaffected by colectomy), *Clonorchis sinensis* infection (oriental liver fluke), chronic typhoid carrier state, choledochal cyst, sclerosing cholangitis.
   c. Presentation includes insidious onset of jaundice, pruritus, anorexia, pain, and possible cholangitis.
   d. Diagnosis–PTC or ERCP with abdominal CT scan.
   e. Therapy.
      (1) Curative resection (rarely possible)–wide resection and reconstruction of biliary tree.
      (2) Palliative resection–cholecystojejunostomy, choledochojejunostomy, U-tube or other stent.
      (3) Both post-operative and palliative radiation may prolong life.
   f. Prognosis–5-year survival 10-15%.
7. Carcinoma of the head of pancreas (see "The Pancreas").
8. ***Carcinoma of the Ampulla of Vater.***
   a. 10% of obstructing tumors of common duct.
   b. Presentation–early jaundice, occult blood in stool.
   c. Diagnosis with CT and biopsy during ERCP.
   d. Spread locally with slow rate of metastasis.
   e. Therapy–pancreaticoduodenectomy.
      (1) 5-10% operative mortality.
      (2) Prognosis–5-year survival 39%.
9. ***Choledochal cyst***–congenital cyst of the extrahepatic biliary tree.
   a. Classic triad consists of RUQ mass, jaundice, pain.
   b. Four times more common in females.
   c. One-third diagnosed before age 10.
   d. Natural history–if left untreated, may progress to complete

biliary obstruction, cholangitis, secondary biliary cirrhosis, spontaneous rupture (frequently occurs during pregnancy), or carcinoma.

e. Five subtypes—all treated surgically.
   (1) Type I—cystic dilation of entire common hepatic and common bile duct. Excision of cyst with Roux-en-Y hepaticodochojejunostomy is the procedure of choice.
   (2) Type II—diverticulum of common bile duct. Excise diverticulum.
   (3) Type III—cystic dilation of the distal common bile duct (choledochocele). Marsupialize the diverticulum with a long sphincteroplasty or divide the common bile duct with Roux-en-Y choledochojejunostomy.
   (4) Type IV—extrahepatic and intrahepatic biliary cystic dilatation (Caroli's disease).
   (5) Type V—fusiform extrahepatic and intrahepatic dilatation. Both type IV and type V are treated by Roux-en-Y hepaticojejunostomy with transhepatic stent placement.

43

Cirrhosis

Gregory M. Tiao, M.D.

Cirrhosis means the formation of scar tissue and is the end result of parenchymal liver damage and regeneration. With scar formation there is a change in liver architecture such that resistance to blood flow, especially that of portal blood flow, increases. The result is the formation of spontaneous portasystemic shunts.

I. ETIOLOGY

There is a long list of possible causes of cirrhosis.

A. Ethanol abuse—responsible for up to 70% of cirrhosis in U.S.

B. Post-hepatitic—viral hepatitis B and C.

C. Hereditary—hemolytic anemia, α_1-antitrypsin deficiency.

D. Occupational exposure—carbon tetrachloride, beryllium, vinyl chloride.

E. Schistosomiasis.

F. Nutritional—long-term total parenteral nutrition (TPN).

G. Congestive heart failure—chronic.

II. DIAGNOSIS

A. History—Cirrhosis is a chronic disease process. Patients are often aware of their diagnosis and have a history of exposure to one of the etiologic agents listed above.

B. Physical exam—jaundice, dark urine, muscle wasting, ascites, peripheral edema, purpura, encephalopathy, splenomegaly, spider angiomata, caput medusa, asterixis, gynecomastia, testicular atrophy, palmar erythema, loss of body hair, Dupuytren's contractures. Liver size is variable.

C. Liver function tests.

1. Bilirubin.
   a. Direct hyperbilirubinemia is seen when the liver is unable to excrete conjugated bilirubin.
   b. Indirect hyperbilirubinemia is seen when the liver cannot clear the pigment it receives.
   c. Clinical jaundice is apparent when total bilirubin > 2 mg/dl.
   d. Conjugated bilirubin is spilled into urine.

2. Serum enzymes.
   a. Alkaline phosphatase.
      (1) Produced in bone, placenta and liver.
      (2) Excreted in bile.
      (3) Elevated alkaline phosphatase can signal obstruction of bile ducts (in the absence of bone disease and pregnancy).
   b. Transaminases.
      (1) Aspartate aminotransferase (AST, SGOT).
      (2) Alanine aminotransferase (ALT, SGPT).
      (3) ALT > AST in viral hepatitis.
      (4) AST > ALT in alcoholic hepatitis.
      (5) Transaminase may be normal in long-standing disease despite acute exacerbation.
3. Serum proteins.
   a. Albumin–is low when hepatic function is impaired.
   b. Coagulation factors.
      (1) Prothrombin time (PT) reflects adequacy of fibrinogen, prothrombin, coagulation factors V, VII, IX, X.
      (2) PT is prolonged when fat absorption, and subsequent vitamin K absorption, is impaired due to biliary obstruction as well as synthetic abnormalities.

D. Radiologic procedures.

1. Scintillation scans–reflect hepatic functional capacity; "cold spot" is seen when hepatocyte function is decreased or absent.
2. CT scan–assesses liver size, ascites, and presence of varices.
3. Ultrasound.
4. Angiography–can directly measure hepatic pressures, as well as define portal vein flow during the venous phase (see below).

E. Percutaneous liver biopsy.

1. Allows histologic diagnosis.
2. Contraindications–coagulopathy, thrombocytopenia, cholangitis, tense ascites.
3. Complications–bile leak or peritonitis, pneumothorax, bleeding, pain.

F. Paracentesis.

1. Relieves dyspnea and anorexia due to increased intra-abdominal pressure.
2. Cytologic exam of ascitic fluid can distinguish cause–cancer *vs.* cirrhosis–and diagnose spontaneous bacterial peritonitis.
3. Complications–infection, bleeding, perforation of viscus.

III. CIRRHOSIS and LIVER FUNCTION

To appreciate the impact of cirrhosis, it is important to understand that the liver is the "metabolic clearing house" and regulates almost every aspect of metabolism. Although cirrhosis implies nothing about the state of hepatic function, a cirrhotic liver is usually dysfunctional, which affects body-wide metabolism.

A. Carbohydrate metabolism.

1. Glycogenesis <-> glycogenolysis.
2. Glycolysis <-> gluconeogenesis.
3. Derangements result in hyperglycemia (early cirrhosis) and hypoglycemia (advanced failure).

B. Protein metabolism

1. Amino acids and bacterially produced ammonia from the gut are metabolized to urea by the liver. (Increased serum ammonia may be cause of encephalopathy, but 10% of encephalopathic patients have a normal serum ammonia level.)
2. Proteins synthesized in the liver include blood clotting factors, albumin, transferrin, immunologic proteins. Decreased production results in ascites, edema, and coagulopathy.

C. Fatty acid metabolism.

1. Fatty infiltration of the liver may be seen when fatty acids cannot be metabolized.
2. Serum cholesterol levels may be lowered in liver disease states.

D. Hormone metabolism—both activation and inactivation of various hormones are carried out in the liver.

1. Estrogen, testosterone, thyroxine, corticosteroids, aldosterone.
2. Altered hormonal metabolism may result in gynecomastia, testicular atrophy, loss of axillary and pubic hair, palmar erythema, and increased total body water.

E. Drug metabolism.

1. Uptake, detoxification, and excretion of drugs occurs in the healthy liver.
2. Dosage requirements in cirrhotics may be different for drugs such as antibiotics, anti-inflammatory agents, antiarrhythmics, and anticonvulsants.

IV. PATHOPHYSIOLOGY

Alterations in liver function and the development of portasystemic shunts results in the pathophysiologic diseases processes that characterize a patient with cirrhosis.

A. Portal hypertension.

1. Defined as portal venous pressure $\geq$ 18 mm Hg by direct measurement, or a wedged hepatic vein pressure (WHVP) $>$ 4 mm Hg above inferior vena cava (IVC) pressure; usually becomes clinically significant when WHVP $>$ 12 mm Hg above IVC pressure.
2. Portal hypertension is commonly classified by the level of venous obstruction.
   a. Pre-hepatic (or pre-sinusoidal)–portal vein thrombosis, tumor encasement, primary biliary cirrhosis.
   b. Intra-hepatic (sinusoidal)–alcoholic and post-necrotic viral cirrhosis.
   c. Post-hepatic (or post-sinusoidal)–hepatic vein occlusion (Budd-Chiari syndrome), vena caval web.

d. In the absence of obstruction, portal hypertension can occur with increased portal flow (i.e., splenic arteriovenous (A-V) fistula or hepatic artery/portal vein A-V fistula).

3. Portal vein pressure is decompressed through portosystemic collateral veins (varices–Figure 1).
   a. Esophageal.
   b. Gastric.
   c. Abdominal wall.
   d. Hemorrhoidal.
4. Diagnosis.
   a. Portal venography–obtained by venous phase imaging during mesenteric arteriography.
      (1) Defines size and location of dilated veins, and provides qualitative estimate of hepatic portal perfusion.
      (2) Hepatopedal flow (away from liver) *vs.* hepatofugal flow (towards liver).
   b. Hepatic vein wedge injection.
      (1) Visualize portal vein if hepatopedal flow present.
      (2) Used to determine adequacy of portal perfusion.
   c. Measurement of portal pressure.
      (1) Direct–measured during operation or venography.
      (2) Indirect–WHVP; compare to IVC pressure (see III.A.1 above).

B. Ascites.

1. Local causes.
   a. Portal hypertension–increased hydrostatic pressure.
   b. Lymphatic outflow obstruction–ascitic fluid can be seen weeping from surface of liver at surgery.
2. Systemic causes.
   a. Hypoalbuminemia–results in low intravascular oncotic pressure, with water loss into the extravascular space.
   b. Secondary hyperaldosteronism.
      (1) Caused by increased secretion and/or decreased inactivation of aldosterone by the impaired liver.
      (2) Results in increased total body water and sodium as a result of augmented sodium resorption in the distal tubule.
   c. Increased antidiuretic hormone (ADH) secretion.
      (1) Caused by relative hypovolemia, as detected by the carotid body and central nervous system.
      (2) Results in decreased free water clearance.

C. Cardiovascular changes.

1. High cardiac output and low systemic vascular resistance (SVR) are seen; may cause cardiac failure.
2. Low SVR is not completely understood, but several contributing factors are hypothesized:
   a. Peripheral shunting (splanchnic, muscle, skin).
   b. Increased vasoactive intestinal polypeptide (VIP) release.
   c. Decreased estrogen metabolism.

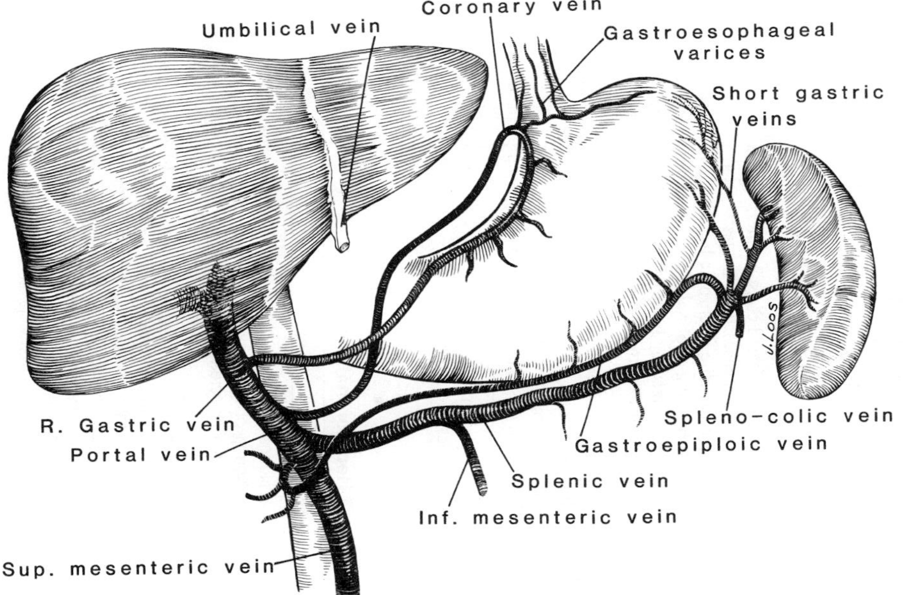

FIG. 1 Portal Venous Anatomy

d. Accumulation of "false" or "weak" neurochemical transmitters (phenylethylamine, tyramine, octopamine), displacing sympathetic adrenergic transmitters (norepinephrine).

D. Renal dysfunction—hepatorenal syndrome may result (Table 1). Oliguria with elevated BUN and creatinine.

1. Type 1–resolved by relief of ascites and improved volume status/renal perfusion.
2. Type 2–resolved by improved hepatic function and increased SVR.
3. Urine sodium ≤ 10 mEq/L.

E. Encephalopathy.

1. Characterized by altered consciousness, asterixis ("liver flap"), rigidity, hyper-reflexia, EEG changes.
2. May be seen in acute or chronic hepatic dysfunction.
3. Etiology–shunting of portal blood, containing toxins and nutrients metabolized by healthy hepatocytes, around the liver. Factors implicated include ammonia, mercaptans, aromatic amino acids, etc.
4. Precipitating factors.
   a. GI hemorrhage.
   b. Portosystemic shunting procedure.
   c. Infection, especially spontaneous bacterial peritonitis.
   d. Excessive dietary protein.
   e. Constipation.
   f. Narcotics and sedatives.

TABLE 1
Classification of Hepatorenal Syndrome

Characteristic	Type I	Type II
Blood pressure	Normal or low	Increased
Cardiac index	Normal of decreased	Increased
Peripheral resistance	Normal or increased	Decreased
Intravascular volume	Low	Normal
Urinary sodium	< 10 mEq/L	< 10 mEq/L
Pathophysiology	Effective hypovolemia Portorenal reflex	Maldistribution of blood flow
Associated findings	Intractable ascites Pressure gradient between IVC and right atrium High hepatic vein wedge pressure	Hepatic encephalopathy Acute hepatic insult
Therapy	Volume infusion Ascites reinfusion Peritoneal-atrial shunt "Side-to-side" portal decompression	α-Adrenergic agents Levodopa (Neither of these results in survival unless hepatic function improves)

V. CHILD'S CLASSIFICATION

Patients with cirrhosis are at increased risk for any kind of surgery. When elective surgery is being considered, prophylactic treatment for the complications of cirrhosis should be considered (see below). Child's classification was initially described as a prognostic guide to the outcome of portal decompressive surgery. It is an indicator of the severity of liver dysfunction and has been used as a guide to the risk for any kind of surgery on patients with liver disease. With proper pre-operative intervention (i.e., nutritional support, bowel preparation with antibiotics), liver function can be improved (as indicated by improved Child's class) and the risk of surgery reduced.

Child's Classification

	A	B	C
Ascites	none	controlled	uncontrolled
Bilirubin	<2.0	2.0-2.5	>3.0
Encephalopathy	none	minimal	advanced
Nutritional status	excellent	good	poor
Albumin	>3.5	3.0-3.5	<3.0
Operative mortality (portacaval shunt)	2%	10%	50%

VI. TREATMENT OF COMPLICATIONS OF CIRRHOSIS

A. Prophylaxis.

1. Fluid and electrolyte management.
   a. Sodium and water restriction.
   b. Cautious diuresis–over-diuresing can result in hepatorenal syndrome.
2. Maintain or improve nutritional status.
   a. Patients are hypermetabolic and require as much as 1.1 g protein/kg/day to maintain nitrogen balance.
   b. Hepatamine® is a specifically defined TPN solution high in branched-chain amino acids, low in aromatic amino acids that can be used in patients with liver dysfunction.
3. Prevent GI bleeding, which increases intraluminal protein load.
   a. H_2 blockers.
   b. Neutralize gastric pH.
4. Reduce intestinal flora to decrease bacterial production of ammonia.
   a. Oral neomycin (500 mg po q 6 h) to decrease intraluminal bacterial counts.
   b. Lactulose (15-30 cc po bid) is metabolized to organic acids in the colon; NH_3 (easily absorbed and delivered to the liver via the portal circulation) is readily converted to NH_4^+, which is poorly absorbed owing to the change in colonic pH.

B. Gastrointestinal bleeding

1. Diagnosis.
   a. Endoscopy (EGD).
   b. In cirrhotics, 50-90% of upper GI bleeds are due to variceal hemorrhage.
   c. Remaining percentage due to Mallory-Weiss tears, portal hypertensive gastropathy, peptic ulceration, gastric or esophageal neoplasm.
2. Natural history.
   a. 15-30% of cirrhotics have varices; less than 50% bleed from them.
   b. 20-50% mortality from first variceal hemorrhage; of those who live, more than 70% will rebleed within 1 year.
   c. Bleeding is rare unless WHVP exceeds IVC pressure by 12 mm Hg.
3. Treatment.
   a. Large-bore nasogastric tube; saline lavage; Foley catheter.
   b. Volume resuscitation.
      (1) Blood and blood products.
      (2) Maintain hematocrit above 27-30%.
   c. Correct coagulopathy.
      (1) Fresh frozen plasma, cryoprecipitate, platelets as appropriate.
      (2) Vitamin K, 10 mg IV (does not work immediately).
   d. Intravenous vasopressin—will control bleeding in 75% of patients.
      (1) Initial bolus of 20 U over 20 min.
      (2) Continuous drip at 0.2-0.8 U/min.
      (3) After bleeding stops, wean off by 0.1 U increments over 48 h; watch closely because rebleeding is common.
      (4) Vasopressin is a potent splanchnic vasoconstrictor that should be combined with nitroglycerine 50 μg/min IV to protect against cardiac ischemia.
   e. Esophageal balloon tamponade (Sengstaken-Blakemore, Minnesota tubes).
      (1) Initial success rate is high, but rebleeding occurs in 40-70%.
      (2) Gastric erosion, gastric and esophageal perforation, aspiration pneumonia are complications.
      (3) Consider prophylactic endotracheal intubation to prevent aspiration.
   f. Endoscopic sclerotherapy.
      (1) Acute control of bleeding accomplished in up to 90% of patients, with 20-30% mortality.
      (2) Sclerosing agents are administered into the varix directly, around the varix, or both, with similar results.
      (3) Sclerosing agents include ethanolamine oleate, sodium morrhuate, and sodium tetradecyl sulfate.

g. Portal decompression.
   (1) *Nonselective* shunt (e.g., portacaval); eliminates portal venous flow; most effective at controlling bleeding, but followed by a high rate of encephalopathy and hepatic failure.
   (2) *Selective* shunt (e.g., distal splenorenal); preserves portal venous flow to the liver.
   (3) Operative mortality may reach 40-50% in Child's class "C" patients.

4. Therapeutic options in prevention of recurrent variceal hemorrhage.
   a. Pharmacologic therapy–beta blockers, nitrates, and calcium channel blockers have been studied; most have not been demonstrated to be beneficial especially over the long term.
   b. Endoscopic sclerotherapy.
      (1) Decreases the frequency of recurrent variceal hemorrhage (48-58%) when compared to conventional medical management. Five-year survival not significantly different from that in those patients who undergo portosystemic shunt procedures.
      (2) Injection sclerotherapy should be performed until all varices are eradicated. Despite complete eradication, varices have been shown to recur at a mean interval of 1 to 2 years. Rebleeding rate is about 15% per year after obliteration of varices is achieved.
      (3) Patients with gastric varices, or whose varices are difficult to eradicate or have recurrent bleeding during therapy, should have early consideration for portosystemic shunt.
   c. Non-selective (total) portosystemic shunts.
      (1) Portacaval shunt–end-to-side (Eck fistula) and side-to-side portacaval shunts are the "gold standard" by which other shunts are evaluated.
         a) Prospective, randomized trials have failed to show any survival benefit compared to conventional medical therapy. When data from these trials are combined, however, some survival benefit is probable.
         b) Very effective in preventing recurrent variceal hemorrhage (> 90%). Hepatic encephalopathy occurs in about 15-30% of cases, whereas hepatic failure is a major cause of post-shunt mortality (13-18%).
         c) The failure to show significant survival benefit has significantly decreased use of total portosystemic shunts. At present, the most common indications include the use of an end-to-side shunt in acute variceal hemorrhage and a side-to-side shunt in the treatment of refractory ascites.

(2) Interposition H-graft shunts–mesocaval, portacaval, and mesorenal.
   a) Grafts > 10 mm in diameter are generally considered total shunts.
   b) Increased frequency of late thrombosis compared to conventional portacaval shunts.
   c) Useful in patients who are transplant candidates.

(3) Central splenorenal shunt (Linton shunt).
   a) Includes splenectomy with anastomosis of portal side of splenic vein to the left renal vein.
   b) Physiologically and hemodynamically similar to a side-to-side portacaval shunt.
   c) Results similar to portacaval shunts, but probably has a higher thrombosis rate.

(4) TIPS–transjugular intrahepatic portosystemic shunt. Radiologically guided, percutaneously placed shunt. Obviates the need for surgery, useful in high-risk or pretransplant patients. Long-term data not yet available.

d. Selective portosystemic shunts.

(1) Distal splenorenal (Warren-Zeppa) shunt.
   a) Most commonly employed selective shunt used in U.S. Splenic vein is divided, and splenic side is anastomosed end-to-side to left renal vein. Spleen remains *in situ,* and the coronary vein is ligated.
   b) Varices are decompressed via the short gastric veins. Decompresses the varices while maintaining portal perfusion in about 90% of patients.
   c) Operative mortality (7-10%) and long-term survival are similar to non-selective shunts in patients with alcoholic cirrhosis. Survival seems to be improved in patients with non-alcoholic cirrhosis.
   d) Possibly lower incidence of late hepatic failure and encephalopathy compared to non-selective shunts (in 3 of 6 studies).
   e) Long-term survival (60% 5-year survival) following distal splenorenal shunt is similar to that of endoscopic sclerotherapy. Rate of rebleeding is higher in sclerotherapy, but shunting may lead to progression of liver dysfunction.
   f) Splenic vein must be ≥ 7 mm in diameter and ascites must be absent or medically controlled.

(2) Small-bore (8-10 mm) portacaval H-grafts–may be effective in controlling rebleeding with less post-shunt encephalopathy.

(3) Left gastric-venacaval shunt–not used much in U.S.

e. Esophageal transection (including stripping of coronary veins–*Sugiura procedure*)–has met with limited success in the U.S. when compared to Japan.

f. Orthotopic liver transplantation.

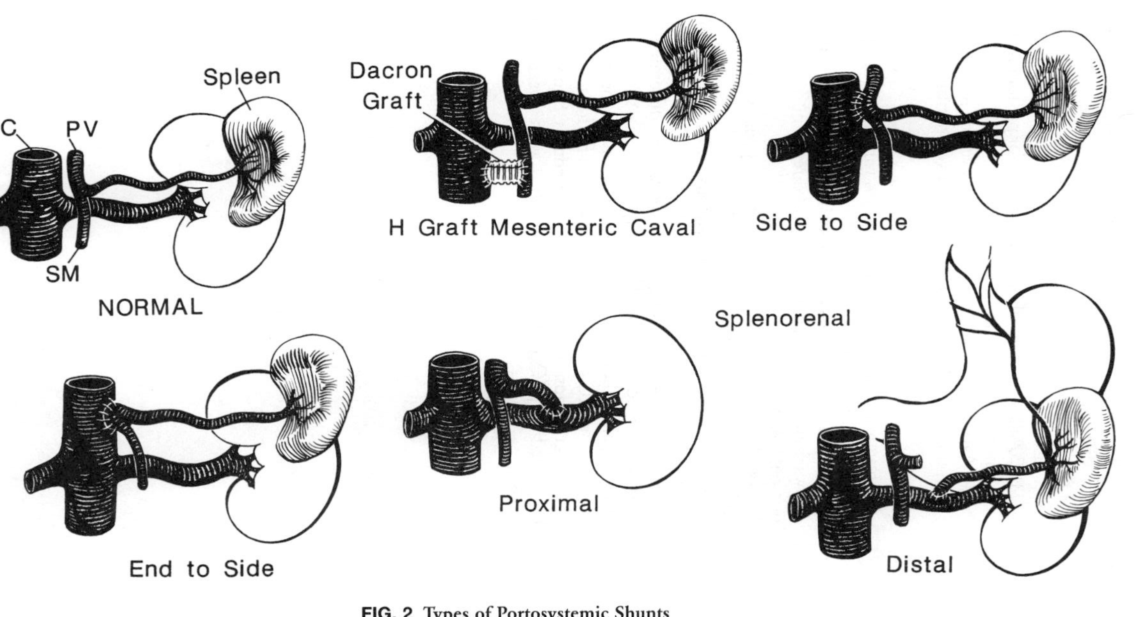

FIG. 2 Types of Portosystemic Shunts

(1) Treats both portal hypertension and underlying liver disease.
(2) Limited availability of donor organs prevents routine use.
(3) 70% 5-year survival in major centers for predominantly non-alcoholic cirrhotics.
(4) Avoid portacaval shunt in patients awaiting transplant–use sclerotherapy, TIPS, or selective shunting where possible.

g. Splenopneumopexy–anastomosis of spleen to lung through the diaphragm to decompress varices through pulmonary circulation.

C. Surgical treatment of ascites—peritoneovenous shunt.

1. Allows drainage of intraperitoneal fluid directly into the superior vena cava.
2. *LeVeen* shunt has a one-way valve that opens when intra-abdominal pressure exceeds 3 cm H_2O.
3. *Denver* shunt incorporates a subcutaneous pump that prevents clogging by active pumping.
4. Complications–sepsis, congestive heart failure, disseminated intravascular coagulation (DIC), hypokalemia, shunt malfunction, air embolism, and superior vena cava thrombosis.
5. Monitor for DIC post-operatively with serial fibrinogen levels, fibrin degradation products, and platelet counts. Shunt must be ligated if DIC cannot be controlled with coagulation factors.

44

Gallbladder and Biliary Tree

Scott R. Johnson, M.D.

I. CHOLELITHIASIS AND CHRONIC CALCULOUS CHOLECYSTITIS

A. Incidence.

1. Gallstones are found in 8% of male and 17% of female adults.
2. Predisposing conditions include obesity, multiparity, diabetes mellitus, cirrhosis, pancreatitis, chronic hemolytic states, malabsorption, inflammatory bowel disease, and certain racial/genetic factors (Blacks, Pima Indians).

B. Etiology—most important factor is composition of bile, which has three major constituents.

1. Bile salts (primary: cholic and chenodeoxycholic acids; secondary: deoxycholic and lithocholic acids).
2. Phospholipids (90% lecithin).
3. Cholesterol–although insoluble, both lecithin and cholesterol are incorporated along with bile salts into more soluble mixed micelles.
   a. Conditions that affect the relative concentrations of these components give rise to lithogenic bile.
   b. Bile containing excess cholesterol relative to bile salts and lecithin is predisposed to gallstone formation.

C. Types of gallstones.

1. ***Mixed*** (80%).
   a. Most common, usually multiple.
   b. Cholesterol usually predominates (approximately 70% of content).
   c. 15-20% may ultimately calcify and therefore become radiopaque.
2. ***Pure cholesterol*** (10%).
   a. Often solitary with large (> 2.5 cm), round configuration.
   b. Usually not calcified.

3. ***Pigment*** (10%).
   a. Composed of unconjugated bilirubin, calcium, and variable amounts of organic material.
   b. 50% are radiopaque.
   c. Black pigment stones are associated with cirrhosis and chronic hemolytic states. Bile is usually sterile, and choledocholithiasis is unusual.
   d. Earthy calcium bilirubinate stones are found more frequently in common bile duct. Associated with states that predispose to bile stasis (i.e., biliary strictures).

D. Natural history.
1. 80% of gallstones are asymptomatic. Each year, approximately 2% of patients with asymptomatic stones develop symptoms, most commonly (75%) biliary colic.
2. Incidence of development of symptoms in patients with asymptomatic stones is approximately 15-30% over 15 years.
3. Elective cholecystectomy is recommended for patients with cholelithiasis who develop symptoms.

E. Biliary colic—pain arising from gallbladder without established infection. Often difficult to differentiate between colic and intermittent chronic cholecystitis.
1. ***Etiology***—thought to be due to transient gallstone obstruction of the cystic duct.
2. ***History***—generally presents with moderate intermittent RUQ and epigastric pain.
   a. Pain may radiate to back or below right scapula.
   b. Pain usually begins abruptly and subsides gradually, lasting from minutes to hours.
   c. Pain of biliary colic is usually steady, not undulating like that of renal colic.
3. ***Physical exam.***
   a. No associated fever.
   b. May have some mild epigastric or RUQ tenderness, or palpable gallbladder.
4. ***Differential diagnosis***—pancreatitis, peptic ulcer disease, hiatal hernia with reflux, gastritis, hepatic flexure carcinoma, hepatobiliary carcinoma, cardiopulmonary disease.
5. ***Complications.***
   a. Prolonged cystic duct obstruction may allow bacterial growth and progress to acute cholecystitis.
   b. Stones may pass into common bile duct with consequent obstruction or pancreatitis.

F. Diagnosis.
1. ***Lab findings.***
   a. None are diagnostic.
   b. Liver function tests, amylase, and WBC count should be obtained.
   c. Elevation of alkaline phosphatase is common in biliary disease, but nonspecific.

2. 10-15% of gallstones are radiopaque and may be detected on plain films of the abdomen.
3. Oral cholecystogram (Graham-Cole test)–evaluates presence of gallstones as well as gallbladder function. Rarely used today because of use of ultrasound. Unreliable in the presence of jaundice (bilirubin ≥ 3.0) or hepatic dysfunction; variable GI absorption of contrast.
4. ***Ultrasound.***
   a. Has become the diagnostic procedure of choice. Identifies stones, determines wall thickness, presence of masses, ductal dilatation, and fluid collections; the pancreatic head may also be examined.
   b. Technical difficulties include obese patients, large amount of bowel gas, and skill of technician and interpretation.
   c. Sensitivity 95%, with overall specificity approximately 90%.
5. ***Radionuclide scan (HIDA).***
   a. Diagnoses acute cholecystitis (up to 95% accuracy) if gallbladder does not visualize within 4 h of injection and the radioisotope is excreted in the common bile duct.
   b. Reliable with a bilirubin up to 20.
   c. CCK-HIDA.

G. Treatment—cholecystectomy should be performed in most patients with symptoms and demonstrable stones if symptoms cannot be attributed to other disease states.

H. Management of asymptomatic stones.

1. Truly asymptomatic patients do not require cholecystectomy unless it can be performed safely during laparotomy for another condition ("secondary cholecystectomy"). Postoperative cholecystitis has been reported in up to 20% of patients with cholelithiasis undergoing a second major abdominal procedure.
2. Prophylactic cholecystectomy should be considered in asymptomatic patients in the following situations.
   a. Diabetics may have an increased frequency of serious complications (empyema, emphysematous cholecystitis) and increased morbidity/mortality, although some reports challenge the need for prophylactic cholecystectomy.
   b. Patient with a non-functioning gallbladder on oral cholecystogram (OCG).
   c. The patient with a calcified "porcelain" gallbladder (15-20% associated with carcinoma).
   d. Any patient with a history of biliary pancreatitis.

II. ACUTE CALCULOUS CHOLECYSTITIS

A. General considerations—95% of cases of acute cholecystitis are associated with obstruction of the cystic duct by a gallstone. Approximately 30% of patients with biliary colic will develop acute cholecystitis within 2 years.

B. Symptoms—constant severe RUQ or epigastric pain that may radiate to the infrascapular region. Anorexia, nausea, and vomiting are common.

C. Physical exam.

1. RUQ tenderness on palpation, and signs of focal peritoneal irritation may be present.
2. ***Murphy's sign***—the examiner palpates the RUQ and asks the patient to inhale deeply. The diaphragm descends and pushes the inflamed gallbladder against the examiner's fingertips, causing enough pain that the patient arrests his/her inspiration.
3. Low-grade fever.
4. Palpable gallbladder–uncommon.

D. Lab findings.

1. Moderate leukocytosis (10-20,000).
2. Frequent mild elevation of bilirubin (elevation > 4 mg/dl is unusual in simple cholecystitis and suggests the presence of choledocholithiasis).
3. Frequent elevation of alkaline phosphatase; transaminases and amylase may be elevated.

E. Differential diagnosis—acute peptic ulcer disease with or without perforation, pancreatitis, acute appendicitis, cecal volvulus, right lower lobe pneumonia, myocardial infarction, passive hepatic congestion, acute gonorrheal perihepatitis (Fitz-Hugh-Curtis syndrome), viral or alcoholic hepatitis.

F. Complications.

1. ***Hydrops***—cystic duct obstruction leads to a tense gallbladder filled with mucus ("lime bile"). May lead to gallbladder wall necrosis if pressure exceeds capillary blood pressure.
2. ***Gangrene and perforation***—may be localized, leading to abscess that is confined by the omentum, or free perforation may occur, leading to generalized peritonitis and sepsis. Emergency laparotomy indicated.
3. ***Empyema of the gallbladder*** (suppurative cholecystitis)–a condition in which the gallbladder contains frank pus. The patient is often toxic, and urgent surgery is indicated.
4. ***Cholecystenteric fistula.***
   a. Results from repeated attacks of cholecystitis.
   b. Duodenum, colon, and stomach involved, in decreasing order.
   c. Air is present in the biliary tree in 40% of cases (visible on plain films of the abdomen).
   d. May not cause symptoms unless the gallbladder is partially obstructed by stones or scarring.
   e. Symptomatic cholecystenteric fistulas should be treated with cholecystectomy and fistula closure.
5. ***Gallstone ileus***—gallstones causing the cholecystenteric fistula pass into the enteric lumen and cause intermittent bouts of small bowel obstruction ("tumbling ileus").

a. Symptoms of acute cholecystitis immediately preceding onset of bowel obstruction are uncommon (25-30%).
b. Stones < 2-3 cm usually pass spontaneously and do not cause bowel obstruction.
c. Terminal ileum is most common site of obstruction.
d. Overall responsible for 1-2% of bowel obstructions.
e. Mortality 10-15% (reflects elderly patients, in whom this is more common).
f. Small bowel enterotomy proximal to point of obstruction is usually required to remove the stone; fistula usually does not require immediate cholecystectomy or repair.

G. Treatment of acute cholecystitis.

1. Preferred treatment is cholecystectomy (open procedure or laparoscopic) within 3 days of the onset of symptoms. Conservative management with IV fluids and antibiotics (1st- or 2nd-generation cephalosporin) may be justified in some high-risk patients to convert an emergency procedure into an elective procedure. In some high-risk patients (chronic steroid use, diabetes mellitus), immediate operative treatment is recommended. Lack of noticeable improvement within 1 to 2 days of initiation of conservative treatment suggests possible complicated acute cholecystitis, necessitating more urgent operative intervention. In extremely high-risk patients, cholecystostomy and drainage may be indicated to decompress the gallbladder, saving formal cholecystectomy until the patient is more stable. This can be done percutaneously with interventional radiology.
2. The risk of gangrene and perforation is relatively low during the first 3 days after the onset of symptoms. After this period, the incidence increases to approximately 10%.
3. ***Microbiology and antibiotics.***
   a. *E. coli, Klebsiella, enterococcus,* and *Enterobacter* account for > 80% of infections.
   b. 1st- or 2nd-generation cephalosporins are first choice of antibiotic coverage, although they do not cover *enterococcus.*
   c. Broader-spectrum antibiotics are used depending on the severity of the infection and the patient's response to treatment. Ampicillin, aminoglycoside, and metronidazole (or clindamycin) may be indicated in overtly septic patients.

H. Acute acalculous cholecystitis—5% of cholecystitis occurs in the absence of cholelithiasis; 50-80% present in an advanced state (gangrene, perforation, abscess).

1. Acalculous cholecystitis is primarily seen as a complication of prolonged fasting after an unrelated operation or trauma (e.g., acute burns, multiple organ failure, multiple fractures). Etiologies are believed to include the following.
   a. Bile stasis results from a lack of cholecystokinin-stimulated gallbladder contraction.

b. Dehydration leads to formation of an extremely viscous bile, which may obstruct or irritate the gallbladder.
c. Bacteremia may result in seeding of the stagnant bile.
d. Sepsis with resultant mucosal hypoperfusion may promote gallbladder wall invasion of organisms.
e. Ischemia of the gallbladder during episodes of relative hypoperfusion.
f. May be associated with large amounts of parenterally administered narcotics with resultant spasm of the sphincter of Oddi.

2. Acalculous cholecystitis may also be due to cystic duct obstruction by another process, such as tumor or nodal enlargement.
3. The diagnosis may be difficult and is often delayed, because patients often are in the ICU setting with multiple medical problems; requires high degree of suspicion.
4. Diagnosis is obtained by HIDA scan or ultrasound; treatment is emergent cholecystectomy.

III. CHOLEDOCHOLITHIASIS

A. General considerations.

1. Approximately 8-16% of patients with cholelithiasis will be found to have stones in the common bile duct (CBD).
2. Most CBD stones arise from the gallbladder and pass into the CBD (secondary stones).
3. Stones forming *de novo* within the CBD are referred to as primary common duct stones; almost always associated with partial duct obstruction.
4. Complications include biliary colic, cholangitis, pancreatitis, late benign biliary stricture, and biliary cirrhosis.

B. Diagnosis.

1. Elevations of serum bilirubin, alkaline phosphatase, and 5′-nucleotidase are characteristic; amylase is elevated with concomitant biliary pancreatitis. WBC elevated if cholangitis present, normal otherwise.
2. Ultrasound is not useful in detecting common duct stones but is very sensitive in detecting associated intra-hepatic and extra-hepatic ductal dilatation.
3. Endoscopic retrograde cholangiopancreatography (ERCP) is procedure of choice after ultrasound. Can define biliary anatomy as well as upper GI anatomy and can be therapeutic as well as diagnostic (e.g., sphincterotomy or placement of stents as necessary).
4. Intra-operative cystic duct cholangiography.

C. Treatment—surgical treatment of stones within the biliary tree requires opening the CBD with removal of all stones and debris and establishment of free flow of bile into the GI tract. A T-tube is placed to drain bile externally.

1. Indications for mandatory operative cholangiography include obstructive jaundice, history of biliary pancreatitis, small stones in the gallbladder with a wide cystic duct, and a single faceted stone in the gallbladder.
2. Absolute indications for CBD exploration.
   a. Palpable stones in the CBD (90% reliable).
   b. Jaundice with acute suppurative cholangitis.
   c. Proven presence of CBD stones on cholangiogram.
3. Relative indications for CBD exploration.
   a. Dilated CBD over 15 mm (35% reliable).
   b. Bilirubin > 8 mg/dl.
4. Choledochoenteric bypass (choledochoduodenostomy or choledochojejunostomy) should be performed for the presence of > 5 CBD stones, marked CBD dilatation, impacted stones that cannot be removed safely, history of previous choledocholithotomy, primary common duct stones.
5. Management of T-tube.
   a. T-tube cholangiogram on post-operative days 5-7.
   b. If no evidence of leakage or retained CBD stones, may clamp tube.
   c. Remove tube in 2-3 weeks as outpatient.

D. Retained common duct stones—found in up to 5% of patients undergoing CBD exploration.

1. Options for the patient with a T-tube in place.
   a. Remove stones with a basket passed through a mature T-tube tract using fluoroscopic control (> 90% success rate).
   b. Dissolve stones using a litholytic agent (monooctanoin) administered via the T-tube.
      (1) Of radiolucent stones, 25% will dissolve, 25% will decrease in size, and 50% will show no response.
      (2) Radiopaque stones do not dissolve.
2. Patients without a T-tube:
   a. Endoscopic papillotomy and "basket" removal of stones transduodenally.
   b. Percutaneous transhepatic biliary catheter placement with stone dissolution.
   c. Re-operation.
   d. Extracorporeal shock wave lithotripsy (ESWL).

IV. CHOLANGITIS

A. General considerations.

1. A life-threatening disease that requires prompt recognition and treatment.
2. Caused by obstruction of the biliary tract and biliary stasis, leading to bacterial overgrowth, suppuration, and subsequent biliary sepsis under pressure.

B. Etiology.

1. Choledocholithiasis (60%).

2. Benign post-operative strictures.
3. Pancreatic or biliary neoplasms.
4. Miscellaneous–invasive procedures, biliary-enteric anastomoses, foreign bodies, parasitic infections.

C. Clinical findings.

1. ***Charcot's triad***–RUQ pain, jaundice, fever and chills; the classic Charcot's triad is seen in only 50-70% of cases.
2. ***Reynold's pentad*** may be seen–Charcot's triad, shock, and mental obtundation.

D. Diagnosis.

1. Leukocytosis, hyperbilirubinemia, elevated liver function tests.
2. Initial study should be RUQ ultrasound; presence of ductal dilatation and gallstones is suggestive. Thickening of bile duct walls, liver abscess, or gas in the biliary tree are strong supportive evidence.

E. Management—the immediate goal is to decompress the biliary tree. The method by which this is accomplished depends upon the particular clinical situation.

1. Initially, provide supportive care with hydration, electrolyte correction, and broad-spectrum antibiotics.
2. The toxic patient is prepared for immediate surgical decompression by CBD exploration.
3. Patients with a protracted course usually have more complicated obstruction and may require percutaneous cholangiography or ERCP. PTC may be therapeutic in the acute situation by decompressing the biliary tree.
4. ERCP may be effective in decompressing the biliary tree by papillotomy or by the endoscopic placement of biliary stents or nasobiliary tube.

V. GALLBLADDER CARCINOMA

A. General considerations.

1. Associated with gallstones in >90% of cases.
2. Increased incidence in patients with diffuse gallbladder wall calcification ("porcelain gallbladder"), cholecystenteric fistula, and adenoma.
3. Male:female ratio 1:2.
4. Adenocarcinoma most common cell type (82%).

B. Presentation.

1. Most commonly found incidentally at the time of elective cholecystectomy. A loss of clear dissection planes in the gallbladder bed or near the hilum is common.
2. Symptoms include RUQ pain, jaundice, and symptoms secondary to metastases.

C. Treatment.

1. *In situ* lesions require cholecystectomy only.
2. For advanced lesions, cholecystectomy with wedge resection

of adjacent liver and regional lymphadenectomy; radical hepatic resections do not influence survival.

3. Relieve ductal obstruction if present.
4. Adjuvant chemotherapy or radiation therapy are largely ineffective.

D. Prognosis: poor–> 90% mortality at 1 year.

45

Liver Tumors

KEITH M. HEATON, M.D.

I. DIFFERENTIAL DIAGNOSIS

A. Benign.

1. Neoplastic.
   a. Adenoma.
   b. Focal nodular hyperplasia.
   c. Cavernous hemangioma.
   d. Hemangioendothelioma.
2. Non-neoplastic.
   a. Simple cysts.
   b. Polycystic liver disease.
   c. Choledochal cyst.
   d. Echinococcal cyst.

B. Malignant.

1. Primary.
   a. Hepatocellular carcinoma–about 90% of primary malignant lesions.
   b. Cholangiocarcinoma–about 7% of primary malignant lesions.
   c. Hepatoblastoma.
   d. Sarcoma–angiosarcoma, leiomyosarcoma, others.
   e. Epithelioid hemangioendothelioma.
2. Metastatic.

II. BENIGN LIVER TUMORS

A. Adenoma.

1. Occurs primarily in young women in association with the use of oral contraceptives.
2. Usually solitary, often present with abdominal pain and palpable mass.
3. Should be resected, since approximately 1/3 present with either rupture or bleeding.
4. Malignant potential.

B. Focal nodular hyperplasia.

1. Usually found in young women.
2. Etiology thought to be due to local ischemia and tissue regeneration.
3. Rarely produces symptoms, and rupture is exceedingly rare.
4. On CT scan, a central stellate scar may be apparent, although often difficult to distinguish from adenomas.
5. Usually $<$ 5 cm in diameter.
6. Resection not necessary if diagnosis is secure.

C. Cavernous hemangioma.

1. The most frequent benign liver tumor.
2. Most are small and do not cause symptoms; however, larger lesions can produce significant pain.
3. Rarely, may cause congestive heart failure secondary to a large arteriovenous shunt.
4. Inappropriate use of percutaneous biopsy may lead to massive hemorrhage and therefore should *not* be attempted if hemangioma is suspected.
5. Accurate pre-operative diagnosis can usually be made by a delayed-phase CT angiogram that demonstrates pooling of dye in the lesion.
6. In general, it is not necessary to resect asymptomatic lesions.

D. Hemangioendothelioma.

1. Rare, usually appear during the first 2 years of life.
2. May be accompanied by similar lesions in the skin and other parts of the body.
3. May respond to prednisone; if not, resection may be necessary.

III. MALIGNANT TUMORS OF THE LIVER

A. Hepatocellular carcinoma (HCC).

1. Epidemiology.
   a. Relatively uncommon in U.S.; 1-7 per 100,000 annually. Up to 160 per 100,000 in parts of Asia and Africa.
   b. Four to five times more frequent in males.
2. Etiology.
   a. Viral hepatitis–HBsAG carriers have 220 x increased risk.
   b. Alcohol consumption–promotes cirrhosis, 15% of HCC in the U.S. may be attributable to alcohol.
   c. Exogenous steroid hormones–3.2 x increased risk for women who have used oral contraceptives.
   d. Inheritable liver diseases that progress to cirrhosis–α_1-antitrypsin deficiency, hemochromatosis, etc.
   e. Cigarette smoking–2.4 x increased risk.
   f. Chemical carcinogens–aflatoxin, vinyl chloride, Thorotrast®.
3. Pathology–two distinct histologic subtypes.
   a. Nonfibrolamellar–most frequent, often associated with hepatitis B and cirrhosis. Resectability rate is low; median survival of 22 months.

   b. Fibrolamellar–marked perihepatocyte fibrosis. Often no association with hepatitis B or cirrhosis. Usually well differentiated, more often resectable, and associated with a median survival of 50 months.
4. Signs and symptoms.
   a. Weakness, malaise, upper abdominal or shoulder pain, and weight loss.
   b. Most common sign is hepatomegaly. Other signs–jaundice, ascites, splenomegaly.
   c. A minority of patients present with an acute abdominal event secondary to rupture of the tumor or hemorrhage.
   d. In patients with stable cirrhosis, a sudden clinical worsening or sudden appearance of portal hypertension and variceal bleeding may herald the rapid growth of a HCC.
   e. Paraneoplastic syndromes may be present–parathyroid hormone, erythropoietin, carcinoid syndrome, or hypertrophic pulmonary osteodystrophy.
5. Diagnosis.
   a. Tumor markers.
      (1) Alpha-fetoprotein (AFP).
         a) Useful as a screening tool in patients at risk (alcoholics, chronic liver disease, cirrhosis).
         b) > 70% of patients with hepatoma larger than 3 cm have increased AFP.
         c) A significant number of patients with acute or chronic hepatitis and cirrhosis, as well as some pregnant women, have elevated AFP without HCC.
      (2) Carcinoembryonic antigen (CEA)–mild elevation in the majority of patients.
      (3) New markers.
         a) Alpha-1-fucosidase (elevated in 75%).
         b) DES-gamma-carboxyprothrombin (elevated in 46%).
   b. Radiologic evaluation.
      (1) Ultrasound important in early diagnosis in combination with AFP. Can detect lesions < 1 cm (better than CT).
      (2) Angiography provides information about anatomic features of the tumor and its possible involvement in vascular structures.
      (3) Contrast CT detects > 90% of lesions larger than 2-3 cm.
      (4) MRI, with greater sensitivity than CT.
6. Treatment.
   a. Surgery.
      (1) Although liver resection is the only therapy that substantially increases survival, its overall role is limited because of the usual background of cirrhosis, poor condition of the patient, and advanced tumor.
      (2) Only 10% of patients have resectable tumors.

(3) Five-year survival in resected patients is 11-40% and 5-year survival in all patients is only 5%.
(4) Pre-operative assessment.
a) Physical exam, chest radiograph, CT of abdomen to rule out extra-hepatic sites of disease.
b) Contrast CT/MRI/angiography to evaluate factors that determine extent of resection–proximity to major vessels, tumor thrombus in major veins or biliary tree.
c) Document adequate functional reserve capacity of the liver–albumin, SGOT, total bilirubin, prothrombin time, and MEG-X. Galactose elimination capacity is used in some centers.
d) Evidence of cirrhosis with portal hypertension is a major surgical risk factor, and Child's classification should be determined.
(5) Resection should attain at least a 2-cm tumor-free margin to minimize recurrence.
(6) Transplantation has been performed in selected subgroups (incidental tumors found at the time of transplant, small localized fibrolamellar tumors in patients with severe cirrhosis that precludes liver resection).

b. Nonsurgical treatment.
(1) Chemotherapy–recent trials with adriamycin have shown some promise.
(2) Radiation–poor response overall.
(3) Others–hepatic artery ligation, arterial embolization.

B. Intra-hepatic cholangiocarcinoma.

1. Epidemiology/etiology.
   a. Accounts for 7% of primary hepatic malignancies.
   b. Much less common than their extra-hepatic counterpart.
   c. Associated with chronic cholestasis, congenital cystic diseases of the liver, and infestation with *Clonorchis sinensis* (liver fluke).
2. Signs/symptoms.
   a. Pruritus, vague abdominal pain, mild cholangitis, and jaundice are the usual presenting symptoms.
   b. Signs–slight hepatomegaly possible, jaundice.
3. Treatment of choice remains surgical resection, but long-term survival rates remain poor.

C. Hepatoblastoma.

1. Arises in infants and children (> 60% younger than 2 years old).
2. Usually relatively low grade.
3. Up to 60% 5-year survival with resection.
4. Newer protocols show promise using pre-operative combination therapy with chemotherapy and radiation.

D. Sarcomas.

1. Angiosarcoma–associated with Thorotrast® and vinyl chloride. Usually occurs as multiple nodules. No cure.

2. Leiomyosarcoma, fibrosarcoma, and rhabdomyosarcoma rarely occur.

E. Epithelioid hemangioendothelioma.

1. Characteristic diffuse involvement of liver.
2. High metastasis rate.
3. Clinical course extremely variable.

F. Metastasis.

1. By far the most common malignancy found in the liver.
2. Bronchogenic carcinoma is the most common primary cause of hepatic metastasis. Next most common are colorectal, pancreas, breast, stomach.
3. Symptoms–pain, ascites, jaundice, palpable mass, weight loss, anorexia.
4. Most lesions favorable for resection have been found by early laboratory detection before the onset of symptoms or signs. For this reason, liver function tests and CEA are part of the recommended follow-up protocol for colorectal cancer.
5. Colorectal adenocarcinoma–liver is the most common site of metastasis. (see "Colorectal Cancer.")
6. Carcinoma of the stomach, pancreas, gallbladder, ovary, breast, and head and neck have not responded favorably following resection of hepatic metastasis.
7. Major hepatic resections for palliation of symptoms from carcinoid tumors or insulinomas have been performed.
8. Need at least 2-cm tumor-free margins in resection to decrease the incidence of recurrence.
9. Chemotherapy may be effective in the treatment of certain hepatic metastasis; hepatic artery infusion via implantable pump may be used in colorectal carcinoma metastasis.

46

The Pancreas

Stephen P. Povoski, M.D.

I. ANATOMY

A. General considerations.

1. Occupies a retroperitoneal position, lying posterior to the stomach and lesser omentum at the level of the 1st and 2nd lumbar vertebrae.
2. Anterior surface covered by peritoneum; posteriorly lies in proximity to inferior vena cava, aorta, superior mesenteric vessels, inferior mesenteric and splenic veins.
3. Adult pancreas weighs 75-125 g and is 15-20 cm in length.
4. Divided into five portions.
   a. **Head**–lies within confines of duodenal C-loop to right of the superior mesenteric vessels.
   b. **Uncinate process**–inferior projection of the head that passes behind superior mesenteric vessels and portal vein and anterior to inferior vena cava and aorta.
   c. **Neck**–narrowed portion overlying superior mesenteric vessels and portal vein.
   d. **Body**–lies left of the neck and is superior and adjacent to 4th portion of duodenum, ligament of Treitz, and proximal jejunum; forms posterior floor of lesser sac.
   e. **Tail**–lies left of the body and extends into the splenic hilum.

B. Ductal system.

1. **Main pancreatic duct (Duct of Wirsung).**
   a. Begins at the tail and extends to right through the midportion of the gland, lies slightly closer to the posterior surface of the pancreas.
   b. Turns inferiorly in the head and joins the intrapancreatic portion of the common bile duct (CBD) at the papilla of Vater.
   c. Diameter: 3.0-4.8 mm in head, 2.0-3.5 mm in body, 0.9-2.4 mm in tail.

2. ***Accessory pancreatic duct (Duct of Santorini).***
    a. Lies in the head in a more ventral plane, beginning at its junction with the main duct in the neck and terminates at the minor papilla at a point about 2 cm proximal to the papilla of Vater.
    b. Drains the anterior portion of pancreatic head.
3. ***Ampulla of Vater.***
    a. Dilatation at entrance of CBD and main pancreatic duct into 2nd portion of duodenum on its posteromedial wall.
    b. Associated with a series of adjacent muscular coats at the pancreaticobiliary duct junction called the sphincter of Oddi.

C. Vasculature.

1. Arterial supply.
    a. Gastroduodenal artery–branch of the hepatic artery that gives rise to the **superior anterior** and **posterior pancreaticoduodenal arteries,** which form marginal arcades with branches of the SMA to supply the head of the pancreas.
    b. Superior mesenteric artery (SMA)–gives rise to **inferior anterior** and **posterior pancreaticoduodenal arteries,** which join the above arcades.
    c. Blood supply to the neck, body, and tail is more variable and consists of the **superior dorsal pancreatic artery, inferior transverse pancreatic artery,** and multiple **short branches** of the **splenic** and **left gastroepiploic arteries.**
2. Venous drainage–parallels arterial supply quite closely, but lies superficial to its arterial counterpart; drains into the portal system via the superior mesenteric and splenic veins.
3. Lymphatic drainage–drains into the pancreaticoduodenal and pre-aortic lymph nodes, which are in close proximity to the SMA and celiac trunk, respectively. Tail of pancreas drains into splenic hilum nodes.

II. ACUTE PANCREATITIS

A. General considerations.

1. Acute pancreatitis presents as a broad spectrum of pathological changes in the pancreas that range in severity from mild parenchymal edema to fulminant hemorrhagic necrosis.
2. The majority (80-95%) of patients will experience only mild to moderate symptoms with a self-limiting course and will recover fully with only supportive care.
3. 10-15% of patients, however, will develop acute hemorrhagic or necrotizing pancreatitis, with considerable associated morbidity and mortality despite maximal intensive supportive care.
4. Over the past several decades, mortality from acute pancreatitis has decreased from 25% to 5%. This change most likely reflects improved supportive care as well as better awareness

and earlier recognition of potentially life-threatening complications.

B. Etiology—gallstones and alcohol are by far the most common causes, accounting for over 90% of cases of acute pancreatitis.

1. ***Gallstones.***
   a. May be related to obstruction of the anatomic common channel between CBD and pancreatic duct.
   b. Two-thirds of private hospital cases of pancreatitis; one-third of charity hospital cases.
2. ***Alcohol.***
   a. Exact mechanism of alcohol-related injury unknown; most recent evidence suggests that ethanol increases ductal permeability by both a toxic metabolic mechanism and by causing a small increase in ductal pressure.
   b. Two-thirds of charity hospital cases; one-third of private hospital cases.
3. ***Hyperlipidemia***—types I, IV, and V have been implicated.
4. ***Hypercalcemia*** (e.g., hyperparathyroidism, multiple myeloma).
5. ***Trauma.***
   a. External (penetrating or blunt).
   b. Post-operative.
      (1) Following surgery on the biliary tract, upper gastrointestinal tract, pancreas, colon, and spleen.
      (2) Occasionally after operations remote from the pancreas (i.e., cardiopulmonary bypass).
   c. Retrograde pancreatography (ERCP).
6. ***Pancreatic duct obstruction***—ampullary stenosis, tumor, pancreatic divisum, duodenal diverticulum, ascaris infestation.
7. ***Ischemia***—circulatory shock, emboli, vasculitis, polyarteritis nodosum, aortic graft, hypothermia.
8. ***Drugs***—azathioprine, estrogens, thiazides, furosemide, ethacrynic acid, sulfonamides, tetracycline, steroids, procainamide, valproic acid, clonidine, pentamidine, phenformin, L-asparaginase.
9. ***Infection***—viral (mumps, CMV, hepatitis B), mycoplasmal.
10. ***Others***—scorpion venom, posterior penetrating peptic ulcer, post-renal transplant.
11. ***Familial.***
12. ***Idiopathic.***

C. Clinical presentation.

1. Generally, the first episode of acute pancreatitis is the most severe.
2. ***Symptoms.***
   a. **Abdominal pain** (> 90% of patients), usually constant midepigastric pain with maximal intensity within several hours of onset. Usually occurs several hours after a heavy

meal or within 12-24 h of an alcoholic binge, 50% with pain radiating to back. Alleviated by sitting up and aggravated by motion.

b. **Nausea** and **vomiting** usually accompany pain.

c. **Anorexia.**

3. *Signs.*

a. **Epigastric tenderness** or less commonly diffuse abdominal tenderness with peritoneal signs. RLQ tenderness may be present owing to fluid/inflammation tracking down right paracolic gutter.

b. **Abdominal distension** with diminished or absent bowel sounds due to paralytic ileus.

c. **Fever, tachycardia.**

d. Palpable epigastric mass–may be secondary to pancreatic phlegmon.

e. Left flank ecchymosis **(Grey-Turner's sign)** and periumbilical ecchymosis **(Cullen's sign)** occur in 1-3% of cases and suggest severe hemorrhagic pancreatitis. They are the result of blood-stained retroperitoneal fluid tracking through tissue planes of the abdominal wall to the flank or along the falciform ligament to the umbilical area, respectively.

f. Jaundice–uncommon.

D. Diagnosis.

1. Usually based on clinical impression supported by appropriate laboratory and radiologic evaluation.

2. *Laboratory tests.*

a. CBC with differential, platelets, PT, PTT, electrolytes, Ca^{++}, Mg^{++}, glucose, BUN, creatinine, amylase, lipase, alkaline phosphatase, bilirubin, SGOT, SGPT, LDH, GGT, triglycerides, arterial blood gas, urinalysis.

b. EKG–exclude myocardial infarction.

c. **Serum amylase.**

(1) Elevated in 90% of cases.

(2) Increase occurs within 24 h of onset of symptoms and gradually returns to normal range within 5-7 days.

(3) Degree of initial elevation does not correlate with severity of attack, nor does it predict clinical outcome. High values are suggestive of gallstone pancreatitis.

(4) Hyperamylasemia is not specific for pancreatitis. Other causes include the following.

a) Pancreatic–trauma, carcinoma, pseudocyst, ascites, abscess.

b) Intra-abdominal–biliary tract disease, intestinal obstruction, mesenteric ischemia or infarction, ruptured aortic aneurysm, perforated peptic ulcer, peritonitis, acute appendicitis, afferent loop syndrome, ruptured ectopic pregnancy, ruptured graafian follicle, salpingitis.

c) Salivary gland disorders–mumps, parotitis, trauma

(amylase isoenzymes may help differentiate), impacted calculi, irradiation sialadenitis.
d) Impaired amylase excretion–renal failure, macroamylasemia.
e) Miscellaneous–severe burns, diabetic ketoacidosis, pregnancy, head trauma, pneumonia, liver disease, drugs.

e. **Amylase isoenzymes**–may be useful to determine if hyperamylasemia is of non-pancreatic origin; not widely used.
f. **Serum lipase.**
   (1) Remains elevated longer than serum amylase.
   (2) More specific but less sensitive than serum amylase.
   (3) May be elevated in intestinal ischemia, perforated peptic ulcer or acute cholecystitis.
g. **Diagnostic paracentesis**–elevated peritoneal fluid amylase and lipase; invasive test; not frequently used.

3. ***Radiologic procedures.***
   a. **Chest radiograph.**
      (1) Findings suggestive of but not specific for acute pancreatitis include left pleural effusion, elevated left hemidiaphragm, or basilar atelectasis.
      (2) As baseline in the event of respiratory deterioration.
      (3) To rule out pneumoperitoneum or pneumonia.
   b. **Abdominal radiograph** (nonspecific findings).
      (1) Air in duodenal loop.
      (2) "Sentinel loop sign"–dilated proximal jejunal loop.
      (3) "Colon cut-off sign"–distended colon to midtransverse colon with no air distally.
      (4) Nonspecific ileus pattern.
      (5) Others–cholelithiasis, loss of psoas margins, pancreatic calcifications.
   c. **Ultrasound**–useful in initial evaluation of pancreas to rule out cholelithiasis and pseudocyst.
   d. **CT scan**–more sensitive and specific than ultrasound for demonstration of pancreatic abnormalities, but not for cholelithiasis. Dynamic CT scan (contrast-enhanced) is preferred because it can identify pancreatic necrosis.
   e. **ERCP** (endoscopic retrograde cholangiopancreatography)–contraindicated for diagnosis of acute pancreatitis; indicated after resolution for recurrent disease, or if anatomic abnormality is suspected.

E. Prognosis.

1. Approximately 10-15% of patients with acute pancreatitis develop severe prolonged illness with significant morbidity and mortality.
2. ***Ranson's criteria***–11 prognostic signs for identifying high-risk patients.
   a. At admission.
      (1) Age > 55 years.

(2) WBC > 16,000 cells/mm^3.
(3) Glucose > 200 mg/dL.
(4) LDH > 350 IU/L.
(5) SGOT > 250 IU/dL.

b. **During initial 48 h.**
(1) Hematocrit decrease > 10 percentage points.
(2) BUN increase > 5 mg/dL.
(3) Serum Ca^{++} < 8 mg/dL.
(4) Arterial Po_2 < 60 mm Hg.
(5) Base deficit > 4 mEq/L.
(6) Fluid sequestration > 6 L.

c. **Mortality**–correlates with incidence of pancreatic sepsis.
(1) < 3 signs = 1%.
(2) 3-4 signs = 15%.
(3) 5-6 signs = 50%.
(4) ≥ 7 signs = approximately 100%.

F. Therapy.

1. ***Intravenous fluids*** and **electrolyte replacement**–cornerstone of therapy; use of lactated Ringer's solution or normal saline to maintain urine output of 0.5-1.0 cc/kg/h.
2. ***Foley catheter***—facilitates accurate measurement of intake and output; indirect assessment of tissue perfusion.
3. ***Nasogastric suction***—indicated if vomiting present or persists. Has not been shown to alter clinical course in mild cases by randomized prospective trials.
4. NPO until abdominal pain, tenderness, and ileus have resolved and amylase is normal or near normal.
5. Parenteral nutrition–indicated in severe, complicated cases of pancreatitis or when the patient is expected to be NPO > 7 days. Incidence of severe complications and overall mortality are not affected. Administration of lipid preparations is safe.
6. ***Analgesia***—meperidine preferred to morphine because it is thought to have less potential for sphincter of Oddi spasm.
7. ***Respiratory monitoring***—respiratory complications occur in 15-55% of cases. May require careful monitoring of ABGs or pulse oximetry.
8. ***Antibiotics***—not beneficial in uncomplicated cases, but may be indicated in presence of pancreatic necrosis.
9. ***Serial labs***—close monitoring of CBC, electrolytes (including Ca^{++} and Mg^{++}), and amylase.
10. ***Alcohol withdrawal prophylaxis*** for selected patients with alcohol-induced pancreatitis. Scheduled dose of a benzodiazepine; thiamine 100 mg qd x 3 days; folate 1 mg qd x 3 days; multivitamins qd.
11. ***Histamine (H_2) blockers***—no proven benefit in acute pancreatitis; may be indicated in critically ill patients as ulcer prophylaxis or in treatment of associated upper GI disease.
12. ***ICU monitoring***—indicated in moderate to severe cases or

in patients at high risk as determined by Ranson's criteria. Endotracheal intubation and PEEP ventilation may be indicated in face of progressive respiratory insufficiency unresponsive to other treatment.

13. ***Peritoneal dialysis***—may decrease early systemic complications of severe pancreatitis, but no influence on overall outcome.
14. No evidence to support use of agents that either suppress pancreatic exocrine secretion or inhibit activation of pancreatic enzymes.
15. ***Surgical management: Specific indications.***
    a. **Uncertainty of diagnosis** is such that life-threatening intra-abdominal processes cannot be ruled out.
    b. **Progressive deterioration** despite optimal supportive care.
    c. **Complications** of pancreatitis (abscess, pseudocyst).
    d. Treatment of **gallstone pancreatitis.**
        (1) Current recommendations: either surgery (cholecystectomy with intra-operative cholangiogram) after the acute attack has subsided but during the same hospitalization period (5-7 days) or early operation within 48 to 72 h of onset of symptoms.
        (2) 30% recurrence rate if surgery delayed 4 to 6 weeks.

G. Complications.

1. ***Pancreatic necrosis.***
    a. Diagnosed by dynamic CT or elevated serum acute-phase reactants (e.g., C-reactive protein).
    b. Approximately 40% of patients operated on for pancreatic necrosis will have positive bacterial tissue cultures at laparotomy.
    c. Decreased rate of pancreatic and non-pancreatic sepsis has been demonstrated by prophylactic use of imipenem/cilastatin in sterile pancreatic necrosis.
    d. Surgical debridement and serial open packing indicated for clinical deterioration or evidence of pancreatic sepsis.
2. ***Pancreatic sepsis / abscess.***
    a. A serious and life-threatening complication of acute pancreatitis.
    b. Occurs in 2-5% of patients and in over 50% of those with 6 or more Ranson's prognostic signs.
    c. Characterized by extensive necrosis of retroperitoneal fat, mesentery, and mesocolon, while the pancreas remains relatively intact but inflamed.
    d. **Pathogens**—most commonly enteric organisms; includes *Klebsiella, E. coli, Proteus, Enterobacter, Enterococcus, Serratia, Pseudomonas,* anaerobic species, *Staphylococcus, Streptococcus,* and *Candida;* 50% are polymicrobial.
    e. **Diagnosis**—usually occurs 1-4 weeks after onset of pancreatitis.

(1) Fever, abdominal pain, tenderness/distension, paralytic ileus, and leukocytosis.
(2) Persistent hyperamylasemia and nonspecific liver function tests in 50% of cases.
(3) **CT scan**—most accurate mode for diagnosis; finding of air bubbles in a peripancreatic fluid collection or areas of liquefactive necrosis; CT-guided percutaneous needle aspiration is helpful to differentiate infected *vs.* sterile fluid collection.

f. **Treatment.**
(1) Broad-spectrum antibiotics.
(2) Surgical drainage consisting of either laparotomy with debridement and wide-sump drainage or laparotomy with debridement and serial open packing.

3. ***Pseudocyst.***
a. Definition—collection of pancreatic secretions within a cyst lacking a true epithelium; consists of surrounding tissues walling off a pancreatic duct disruption.
b. Most common complication of pancreatitis (2-10% of patients), appears 2-3 weeks after initial attack.
c. **Signs and symptoms**—early satiety, abdominal pain, nausea, vomiting, epigastric tenderness, abdominal mass, and persistent hyperamylasemia.
d. **Diagnosis**—CT and ultrasound each have 90% accuracy; ERCP may demonstrate site of duct disruption, multiple cysts, and/or ductal anatomy.
e. **Complication rate**—if untreated, 20% by 6 weeks and 67% if cyst persists for 12 weeks; includes secondary infection, hemorrhage, or rupture.
f. **Treatment.**
(1) 50% resolve spontaneously by 4-6 weeks.
(2) Expectant, supportive management for 6-8 weeks until a thick, fibrous, reactive wall has formed and the cyst remains unchanged. Then **internal drainage** via a **cystogastrostomy, cystojejunostomy,** or **cystoduodenostomy.** *Always biopsy* a pseudocyst wall to rule out malignant cystic neoplasm.
(3) **External drainage** for infected pseudocysts or immature walls.
(4) Pseudocysts restricted to the pancreatic tail may be resected by distal pancreatectomy.

4. ***Pancreatic ascites.***
a. Secondary to pseudocyst disruption (more common) or direct pancreatic duct disruption.
b. Painless massive ascites may be associated with a left pleural effusion.
c. **Diagnosis**—made by paracentesis; high amylase (> 1000 U/L) and high protein (> 3.0 g/dL).
d. **Treatment**—NPO, TPN for 4-6 weeks. Somatostatin has been shown to lead to resolution of pancreatic ascites. If

does not resolve, ERCP to delineate ductal anatomy and then surgical internal drainage or distal resection.

5. ***Pancreatic fistulas.***
   a. Secondary to complicated acute pancreatitis, pancreatic surgery, or abdominal trauma.
   b. **Treatment**–NPO, TPN for 4-6 weeks. Somatostatin has been shown to be effective in accelerating the closure rate of pancreatic fistulas. If does not resolve, ERCP to delineate ductal anatomy and then surgical internal drainage or distal resection.
6. ***Hemorrhage.***
   a. Usually due to erosion of arterial pseudoaneurysm secondary to pseudocyst, abscess, or necrotizing pancreatitis. Hemorrhage may be gastrointestinal, intraperitoneal, or retroperitoneal. Incidence up to 10% with pseudocysts.
   b. **Signs and symptoms–abdominal pain, increasing size of abdominal mass, hypotension, falling hematocrit.**
   c. **Diagnosis**–angiography to localize if patient stable.
   d. **Treatment**–immediate surgery if patient is unstable or bleeding is uncontrolled; surgery is necessary in most cases; if secondary to pseudocyst, resection of entire cyst is preferable if possible.

III. CHRONIC PANCREATITIS

A. Characteristics—Chronic pancreatitis is characterized by recurrent or persistent abdominal pain that is generally associated with evidence of exocrine and endocrine pancreatic insufficiency as a result of irreversible destruction and fibrosis of pancreatic parenchyma.

B. Etiology—most commonly associated with history of alcohol abuse; also seen with hyperparathyroidism, pancreatic trauma, and pancreas divisum.

C. Clinical manifestations.

1. Recurrent or chronic abdominal pain–typically epigastric and radiates to back.
2. Anorexia and weight loss are common.
3. Steatorrhea and malabsorption.
4. IDDM (insulin dependent diabetes mellitus) occurs in up to 30%.
5. History of narcotic analgesic abuse frequently seen.

D. Diagnosis.

1. Suspected based on clinical findings. Routine laboratory tests not generally helpful; amylase may be normal or only mildly elevated.
2. ***Radiologic evaluation.***
   a. **Abdominal radiograph**–pancreatic calcifications (95% specific for chronic pancreatitis).
   b. **CT scan**–useful for evaluation of both parenchymal and ductal disease.
   c. **ERCP**–vitally important role for planning surgical man-

agement since it provides a "road-map" of pancreatic ductal system.
(1) Early changes–dilated duct with filling of secondary and tertiary branches.
(2) Later changes–ductal strictures and calculi; pseudocyst may be present; characteristic "chain of lakes" due to areas of alternating ductal dilatation and stricture (less frequently observed than uniform ductal dilatation).

d. CT and ERCP are mandatory prior to consideration of surgical management.

E. Non-operative management.

1. Control of abdominal pain.
   a. Abstinence from alcohol.
   b. Frequent, small-volume, low-fat meals.
2. Treatment of IDDM.
3. Exogenous pancreatic enzyme supplementation to treat steatorrhea and malabsorption.

F. Indications for surgery.

1. Debilitating abdominal pain.
2. Common bile duct obstruction.
3. Duodenal obstruction.
4. Persistent pseudocyst.
5. Pancreatic fistula and/or pancreatic ascites.
6. Variceal hemorrhage secondary to splenic vein obstruction–treated by splenectomy.
7. Rule out pancreatic carcinoma.

G. Surgical management.

1. Goal–to relieve incapacitating abdominal pain while attempting to preserve pancreatic exocrine and endocrine function.
2. Pancreatic duct drainage.
   a. **Duval procedure**–distal pancreatectomy with end-to-end pancreaticojejunostomy.
      (1) Originally used to relieve proximal duct obstruction by allowing simple retrograde drainage of the pancreas via its tail.
      (2) Does not adequately decompress the ductal system in cases of widespread ductal disease.
      (3) Currently, applicable to the rare case of isolated proximal ductal stenosis not involving the ampulla.
   b. **Puestow procedure**–lateral side-to-side pancreaticojejunostomy.
      (1) Most widely used and preferred surgical treatment.
      (2) Involves unroofing and incising the pancreatic duct along its entire length from a point adjacent to the duodenum to the distal portion of the pancreatic tail (with or without removal of the spleen or mobilization of the pancreas) and side-to-side anastomosis to an overlying Roux-en-Y limb of jejunum.

(3) Allows for decompression of the entire pancreatic duct.
(4) The presence of a pancreatic duct > 10 mm in diameter, an anastomosis > 6 cm in length, and pancreatic calcifications are determinants of a successful Puestow procedure.
(5) Provides substantial pain relief in about 65-85% of patients.

3. Pancreatic resection.
   a. Major drawback–development of pancreatic endocrine and exocrine insufficiency.
   b. **Limited distal pancreatectomy**–resection of 40-80% of gland extending no further than to pancreatic neck; only applicable for true focal disease in distal pancreas.
   c. **Subtotal distal pancreatectomy**–resection of 80-95% of gland including inferior portion of head and uncinate process, but leaving intrapancreatic portion of CBD in continuity. Higher incidence of late deaths, diabetes, and steatorrhea than limited resection.
   d. **Pancreaticoduodenectomy (Whipple procedure).**
      (1) Involves resection of head of pancreas to the level of the superior mesenteric vein, as well as duodenum, pylorus, distal stomach, gallbladder, and distal CBD.
      (2) Restoration of gastrointestinal continuity involves bringing up the proximal jejunum through the transverse mesocolon and creating a pancreaticojejunostomy, choledochojejunostomy, and gastrojejunostomy.
      (3) Considered in patients with chronic pancreatitis who have parenchymal disease primarily restricted to pancreatic head.
      (4) Also useful in cases associated with biliary or duodenal obstruction.
      (5) Preserves endocrine function of pancreas.
      (6) With proper patient selection, up to 80% of patients can obtain satisfactory pain relief.
   e. **Pyloric-preserving pancreaticoduodenectomy (modified Whipple procedure).**
      (1) Same as standard Whipple except for preservation of entire stomach, pylorus, and first portion of duodenum.
      (2) Re-establishment of GI continuity involves a duodenojejunostomy as well as pancreaticojejunostomy and choledochojejunostomy.
      (3) Leaves motor, secretory, and reservoir functions of stomach intact and thus reduces the risk of dumping syndrome.
   f. Duodenum-preserving resections of the pancreatic head.
      (1) **Beger procedure**–proposed as alternative to standard Whipple for patients with disease localized to head and

uncinate process. Involves duodenum-preserving subtotal resection of pancreatic head combined with Roux-en-Y drainage of the retained proximal and distal portions of the pancreatic duct.

(2) **Frey procedure**—consists of a non-anatomical resection ("coring-out") of the pancreatic head, leaving the posterior pancreatic capsule and a rim of pancreatic tissue intact along the duodenal C-loop. Proximal pancreatic duct is ligated and distal duct is opened widely. Drainage is via a Roux-en-Y side-to-side pancreaticojejunostomy.

g. **Total pancreatectomy**—last-resort option for patients with continued pain despite previous lesser resections; 100% risk of developing IDDM, steatorrhea, and malabsorption.

4. ***Pancreatic denervation***—lumbodorsal sympathectomy and splanchnicectomy; high failure rate with only short-term relief seen.
5. ***Islet and segmental pancreatic autotransplantation***—adjuvant treatment to subtotal or total pancreatectomy in face of brittle IDDM; limited indication and utility.

H. Endoscopic management—involves endoscopic pancreatic duct stone removal, sphincterotomy, and placement of ductal endoprosthesis; very recent technology; performed at only a few centers.

IV. PANCREATIC CANCER

A. Epidemiology.

1. Fifth most common cause of cancer death in the United States, accounting for over 26,000 cancer deaths annually.
2. Nearly incurable, with cancer death rate closely paralleling cancer incidence.
3. Overall survival rate 10% at 1 year and $< 2\%$ at 5 years.
4. Mean survival for unresectable disease is 3 months.
5. Incidence increases steadily with increasing age; median age of presentation is 69 years with nearly three-fourths of all patients 60 years or older.
6. Male to female ratio 1.7:1.
7. Incidence in black males is 30-40% higher than white males.

B. Etiology.

1. ***Cigarette smoking***—most clearly established risk factor (two- to five-fold increased relative risk with heavy smoking).
2. Other suggested (but not proven) risk factors.
   a. Specific occupations–chemists, metal workers, coke and gas plant workers.
   b. Long-term exposure to benzidine and beta-naphthylamine.
   c. Heavy alcohol consumption.
   d. High-fat diet.
   e. Diabetes mellitus.

f. Chronic pancreatitis.
g. Familial pancreatitis.

C. Histopathologic classification.

1. Ductal adenocarcinoma–most common type (75-80%).
2. Giant cell carcinoma (4%).
3. Adenosquamous carcinoma (3%).
4. Mucinous carcinoma (2%).
5. Mucinous cystadenocarcinoma (1%).
6. Acinar cell adenocarcinoma (1%).
7. Unclassified (10%).

D. Anatomic distribution.

1. Pancreatic head–70%.
2. Pancreatic body–20%.
3. Pancreatic tail–5-10%.

E. Clinical staging.

1. Staging system for pancreatic carcinoma is based on the extent of primary tumor (defined by extension through the pancreatic capsule), the status of regional lymph nodes, and the presence of metastatic disease.
2. *TNM classification.*
   a. Primary tumor (T).
      T_x–Primary tumor cannot be assessed.
      T_0–No evidence of primary tumor.
      T_{1a}–Tumor limited to pancreas, ≤ 2 cm in diameter.
      T_{1b}–Tumor limited to pancreas, > 2 cm in diameter.
      T_2–Tumor extends to duodenum, bile duct, or peripancreatic tissues.
      T_3–Tumor extends directly to stomach, spleen, colon, or adjacent large vessels.
   b. **Nodal involvement (N).**
      N_x–Regional lymph nodes cannot be assessed.
      N_0–Regional lymph nodes not involved.
      N_1–Regional lymph nodes involved.
   c. **Distant metastasis (M).**
      M_x–Presence of distant metastasis cannot be assessed.
      M_0–No distant metastasis.
      M_1–Distant metastasis present.
3. *TNM staging system.*
   a. **Stage I–T_1,** T_2, N_0,M_0; no direct extension beyond duodenum, bile duct, or peri-pancreatic tissues without regional nodal involvement.
   b. Stage II–T_3, N_0, M_0; direct extension into adjacent tissues without regional nodal involvement.
   c. **Stage III**–Any T, N_1, M_0; regional lymph node involvement with or without direct tumor extension.
   d. **Stage IV**–Any T, Any N, M_1; distant metastatic disease present.
4. *R classification*–to indicate presence or absence of residual tumor following surgical intervention.

a. **R_0**–No residual tumor.
b. **R_1**–Microscopic residual tumor.
c. **R_2**–Macroscopic residual tumor.
d. **R_0** corresponds to curative resection; **R_1** and **R_2** to non-curative resection.

F. **Clinical presentation**—The early signs and symptoms of pancreatic cancer are vague and nonspecific; thus, the majority of patients present with disease advanced beyond the scope of potentially curative treatment.

1. ***Abdominal pain.***
   a. Occurs in 80-90% of patients and is the presenting symptom in 65% of cases.
   b. Typically located in the midepigastrium and is characterized as a deep-seated dull ache or boring pain that is progressive and often worse at night; pain may radiate to the low thoracic or upper lumbar back.
   c. Severe pain is slightly more common with carcinoma of body and tail.
2. ***Weight loss*** (60%).
3. ***Anorexia*** (60%)–a feature of anorexia associated with pancreatic cancer is that patients may feel hungry until they begin to eat, at which time they rapidly lose appetite.
4. ***Jaundice.***
   a. Only presenting symptom in 30% of cases.
   b. Much more commonly associated with carcinoma of head (80%) compared to carcinoma of body and tail.
   c. Signifies fairly advanced disease with obstruction of intrapancreatic common bile duct.
   d. *Painless* jaundice is *not* common in pancreatic cancer, but occurs more often with ampullary or primary bile duct tumors.
   e. **Courvoisier's sign**–a palpable, dilated gallbladder in the face of painless jaundice; seen in less than 20% of patients.
5. Other signs and symptoms.
   a. **Weakness, fatigue** (30%).
   b. **Diarrhea** (25%) or **constipation** (10%).
   c. **Steatorrhea** (10%).
   d. **Fever** and **chills** (10%)–may indicate associated ascending cholangitis.
   e. Recent onset of **diabetes mellitus** (5-15%).
   f. **Hematemesis** and/or **melena** (8%)–may be caused by direct invasion of the stomach or duodenum.
   g. **Trousseau's sign** (6%)–migratory thrombophlebitis.
6. Surgical Dictum: *Vague abdominal pain with weight loss,* with or without jaundice, in an older patient (> 50 years old) *is pancreatic cancer until proven otherwise.*

G. **Diagnostic studies.**

1. ***Ultrasound.***
   a. Useful as screening method and for evaluating biliary ducts.

b. Nondiagnostic in up to 25% of cases.
c. Will miss more than 25% of all pancreatic carcinomas and over 50% of small (< 3 cm) lesions.
d. Potential role for endoscopic ultrasound.

2. ***Abdominal CT scan.***
   a. Mainstay of both diagnosis and evaluation of disease spread.
   b. Sensitivity 82-90%; specificity > 90%.
   c. CT-guided percutaneous needle aspirate of mass may be helpful in tissue diagnosis.
3. ***ERCP.***
   a. Most sensitive imaging technique to diagnose pancreatic cancer. Sensitivity 92%; specificity > 95%.
   b. Can be combined with cytologic analysis of pancreatic or duodenal secretions or brush cytology.
   c. Findings suggestive of pancreatic cancer include:
      (1) Pancreatic duct obstruction.
      (2) Ductal stenosis (localized or multiple) or displacement of duct, with or without proximal duct dilatation.
      (3) Necrotic cavity formation secondary to diffuse or focal disease.
   d. Associated with a small but significant risk of serious complications (e.g., pancreatitis, hemorrhage).
4. ***PTHC (percutaneous transhepatic cholangiography).***
   a. Largely replaced by ERCP because of lower complication rate.
   b. Useful in evaluation of patient suspected of pancreatic cancer when there is no visualization of common bile duct by ERCP.
5. ***Selective angiography.***
   a. Sensitivity 70-94%.
   b. Largely replaced as primary diagnostic study by less invasive imaging techniques.
   c. Used to determine presence of abnormal vasculature, such as right hepatic artery arising from SMA, and to determine unresectability based on encasement of the SMA, SMV, hepatic artery, or portal vein.
6. ***Laparoscopy.***
   a. Invasive.
   b. May be helpful tool in staging pancreatic cancer since it can detect hepatic and peritoneal metastases missed on CT.
7. ***Serum chemistries***—generally nonspecific and of little use in diagnosis.
   a. Hepatic profile–elevated bilirubin, alkaline phosphatase; sometimes slight increase in transaminases.
   b. Glucose intolerance.
   c. Occasional elevation of amylase, lipase, or elastase.
8. ***Serological tumor markers.***
   a. CA 19-9 (sensitivity 83%; specificity 82%).

b. CEA (sensitivity 56%; specificity 75%).
c. Not useful as screening test but may be useful for follow-up to monitor for recurrent disease after resection or response to adjuvant therapy.

H. Treatment.

1. A number of patients presenting with pancreatic cancer are candidates for resectional or palliative surgical treatment, although most patients present with advanced disease.
2. ***Non-operative management.***
   a. Potential option for documented distal metastases, unresectable local disease, and in those with associated acute or chronic debilitating illnesses.
   b. Attempt tissue diagnosis by percutaneous needle biopsy of primary tumor, cytologic determination at ERCP or PTHC, or biopsy of distant metastases.
   c. Palliation of pain–analgesics or percutaneous celiac ganglion block.
   d. Palliation of biliary obstruction–percutaneous transhepatic drainage catheter or endoprosthesis; marginal success.
   e. Palliation of duodenal obstruction–external beam radiation (minimal success); percutaneous endoscopic gastrostomy.
3. ***Resectional surgical therapy.***
   a. At operation, the abdomen and pelvis are thoroughly explored for extra-pancreatic disease (e.g., liver, omentum, serosal implants, mesentery, and lymph node metastases outside the potential resection margins) before proceeding with pancreatic dissection. The next step is determination of resectability. Encasement of the hepatic artery, superior mesenteric vessels, or portal vein by tumor is indicative of nonresectability.
   b. For all patients explored with curative intent, only 10-20% are candidates for resection.
   c. **Pancreaticoduodenectomy (Whipple procedure).**
      (1) The traditional resection procedure for pancreatic cancer.
      (2) See section III.G.3.d. for details.
      (3) Overall operative mortality is about 5% in experienced centers.
      (4) Most common post-operative complication is pancreatic fistula in 5-20% of patients.
      (5) Recent support for aggressive curative resection procedures involving extended regional lymph node dissection. Resection of arterial and portal vein segments as well as involved neighboring organs may be indicated in some cases.
   d. **Pyloric-preserving pancreaticoduodenectomy (modified Whipple procedure).**

(1) See section III.G.3.e. for details.
(2) No compromise in survival compared to standard Whipple procedure.

e. **Total pancreatectomy.**
(1) No advantage over pancreaticoduodenectomy, but higher morbidity, including very brittle diabetes mellitus.
(2) May be indicated when invasive carcinoma present at resection line or when the friable texture of the pancreatic remnant prohibits creating a safe pancreaticojejunal anastomosis.

f. **Distal pancreatectomy and *en bloc*** splenectomy.
(1) For rare patient with potentially resectable pancreatic cancer of body and tail.
(2) Prognosis still poor, but serves as good palliation of tumor-associated pain.

4. ***Palliative surgery.***
a. Performed on patients with unresectable disease discovered at time of laparotomy.
b. Goal is to alleviate biliary obstruction, duodenal obstruction, and tumor-associated pain.
c. Biliary obstruction–treated by choledochojejunostomy or cholecystojejunostomy.
d. Duodenal obstruction–treated by gastrojejunostomy.
e. Pain–treated by intra-operative chemical splanchnicectomy (injection of 50 cc of either 50% alcohol or 6% phenol along both sides of celiac axis). May be done percutaneously.
f. Some surgeons advocate resectional palliation.

5. ***Adjuvant therapy.***
a. **Chemotherapy.**
(1) Most commonly used agents are 5-FU, mitomycin C, streptozocin, doxorubicin, and methyl-CCNU.
(2) Currently, chemotherapy alone has little or no role after curative or palliative surgery.
(3) 5-FU has potentiating effect on radiation therapy.

b. **Radiation therapy.**
(1) Modalities–external-beam radiotherapy (EBRT), intraoperative radiotherapy (IORT), and interstitial implants (brachytherapy).
(2) Positive responses reported with radiation therapy for both resectable and unresectable disease.
(3) Beneficial in relieving pain from pancreatic cancer.

c. **Multimodality therapy (chemoradiotherapy).**
(1) Combination chemoradiotherapy with EBRT and 5-FU following surgical resection can significantly improve median survival.
(2) Pre-operative chemoradiotherapy presently undergoing

prospective analysis to determine whether this may be better tolerated and possibly "downstage" previously unresectable tumors.

V. PRIMARY CYSTIC NEOPLASMS OF THE PANCREAS

A. General considerations.

1. Important to distinguish these neoplasms from the more routine and mundane inflammatory pancreatic pseudocysts because their respective management differs so radically.
2. Patients with primary cystic neoplasms tend to be older (>50 years), are more commonly female (approximately 80%), have no history of pancreatic abnormalities, and are seen at diagnosis with signs and symptoms related to the mass effect of the lesion, but are truly asymptomatic in up to 40% of patients with discovery of the cystic mass at the time of evaluation for an unrelated disorder.
3. CT scan generally show multiple cysts without other pancreatic or peripancreatic inflammatory changes, and ERCP generally shows a normal pancreatic duct without communication with the cystic mass.

B. Histopathologic classification.

1. *Serous cystadenoma.*
   a. Virtually always benign with little tendency for malignant transformation.
   b. Composed of a honeycomb of multiple (> 6) small-diameter, sometimes "microscopic cysts" (< 2 cm) lined by a glycogen-rich, low-cuboidal epithelium.
   c. Generally 6-10 cm in overall gross size, located in the head of the pancreas and contain clear cyst fluid.
   d. Resection generally advocated, but can be managed by close observation in frail/elderly patients or patients with high operative risks.
2. Mucinous cystadenoma/cystadenocarcinoma spectrum.
   a. Represent a diverse, heterogenous spectrum of related neoplasms, ranging from benign mucinous cystadenoma to overt malignant cystadenocarcinoma.
   b. Mucinous cystadenoma have tremendous latent malignant potential (> 80%).
   c. Composed of a tall columnar epithelium that expresses mucin that can have papillary invaginations with multiple areas of atypia, dysplasia, carcinoma *in situ*, and overtly invasive carcinoma.
   d. Generally appear as "macroscopic cysts" (> 2 cm) with less than 6 cysts, are 8-10 cm in overall gross size, and are more often located in the body and tail of the pancreas.
   e. All mucinous neoplasms should be considered malignant and managed by potential curative resection.
   f. Five-year survival is > 50% for mucinous cystadenocarcinoma resected for cure.

3. ***Unusual cystic neoplasms.***
   a. Acinar cell cystadenocarcinoma.
   b. Cystic choriocarcinoma.
   c. Cystic teratoma.
   d. Angiomatous cystic neoplasms.

47

Surgical Diseases of the Spleen

Robert J. Burnett, III, M.D.

I. ANATOMY AND FUNCTION

A. Adult anatomy.

1. Average adult spleen weighs 75-175 g.
2. Splenic pedicle–in the hilum contains the splenic artery, vein, lymphatics, and the tail of the pancreas.
3. Micro-anatomy–trabecular connective tissue framework from the inner capsular surface divides the spleen into compartments filled with pulp.
   a. Red pulp–sinusoids with intervening splenic cords.
   b. White pulp–lymphocytes, plasma cells, and macrophages that form nodules with germinal centers.
   c. Marginal zone–between white and red pulps, consists of ill-defined vascular space.

B. Function.

1. Hematopoiesis until 5th month of life, repair of red cell membrane abnormalities.
2. Destruction of bacteria (especially encapsulated) and foreign cells, aged and abnormal hematologic cells, and cellular components such as nuclear remnants (Howell-Jolly), denatured hemoglobin (Heinz), and iron granules (Pappenheimer). Also removes antibody coated or parasite infested cells.
3. IgM production-particulate antigens are transported by macrophages to the germinal centers, where humoral response is initiated.
4. Role of surveillance of malignancy–not well understood.

II. INDICATIONS FOR SPLENECTOMY

A. General—Indications for splenectomy have changed in recent years owing to improved treatment for underlying disorders.

Mortality rate of splenectomy for hematologic disease is < 1%, with a morbidity rate of 10%.

B. Trauma (see "Trauma").

C. Splenectomy as primary therapy.

1. Congenital hemolytic anemias.
   a. Hereditary spherocytosis.
      (1) Relatively common, autosomal dominant, RBC membrane disorder. Caused by a defect in spectrin, a membrane component responsible for shape and strength.
      (2) Patients are characterized by splenomegaly, fluctuating jaundice, cholelithiasis, spherocytosis, and reticulocytosis.
      (3) Splenectomy is indicated in all patients and is curative of the anemia. Pre-operative RUQ ultrasound used to look for concomitant gallbladder disease.
   b. Hereditary elliptocytosis–another congenital hemolytic anemia in which splenectomy is uniformly beneficial.
   c. Hereditary pyropoikilocytosis–rare congenital hemolytic anemia that may evolve into elliptocytosis. Splenectomy is beneficial.

D. Splenectomy as secondary therapy.

1. Immune thrombocytopenic purpura (ITP).
   a. Average age 36, usually female. ITP associated with AIDS is more common in males.
   b. Symptoms of bruising, petechiae, mucosal hemorrhage, menorrhagia, or prolonged bleeding are common.
   c. Propensity for hemorrhage directly related to the platelet count, with prolonged bleeding at 20,000-50,000 and spontaneous bleeding below 20,000.
   d. Diagnosis requires the exclusion of drug-dependent antibodies, collagen vascular disease, lymphoproliferative disorders, thyroid disease, recent viral illness, and spurious thrombocytopenia.
   e. Characterized by increased platelet production (4-5 x normal) and higher megakaryocyte mass on bone marrow biopsy.
   f. Thrombocytopenia due to IgG antibodies directed at a platelet antigen. The spleen is usually small or normal in size.
   g. Medical treatment–achieves remission in 15% of adult patients.
      (1) Platelet transfusions for active bleeding or severe risk of life-threatening hemorrhage.
      (2) Corticosteroids–shown to increase platelet production in 3-7 days; usually a 2-week course is given.
      (3) IV gamma-globulin.
      (4) In childhood, most cases follow a viral illness and are self-limited with resolution within 1 year.
   h. Splenectomy–indicated when medical management fails or for recurrence of disease.

(1) Pre-operative steroids or gamma-globulin to increase platelets to acceptable level may be used.
(2) Complete remission following splenectomy is 80% and is more likely in persons responsive to steroids pre-operatively.
(3) Thorough search should be performed intra-operatively for accessory splenic tissue.
(4) Patients who are thrombocytopenic after splenectomy require further therapy with danazol, cyclophosphamide, vinca alkaloids, or IV gamma-globulin.

2. Autoimmune hemolytic anemia (AIHA).
   a. Acquired hemolytic anemia from anti-red cell antibodies.
   b. Hemolysis, fluctuating jaundice, splenomegaly, and reticulocytosis.
   c. Positive direct Coombs' test–warm (IgG) or cold (IgM).
   d. IgG-coated cells are sequestered in the spleen.
   e. Disease can be associated with certain drugs (penicillin, cephalothin, streptomycin, methyldopa, quinidine, and sulfonamides).
   f. Blood transfusions and steroids are primary treatment, resulting in improvement in 80% of patients.
   g. Splenectomy indicated in warm reactive AIHA not responsive to medical management or requiring large steroid doses for maintenance.
3. Felty's syndrome.
   a. Triad of rheumatoid arthritis, granulocytopenia, and splenomegaly.
   b. Primary therapy is medical with antibiotics, gold, and lithium.
   c. Splenectomy is considered for patients with considerable transfusion requirements or serious neutropenia, recurrent infections, and chronic non-healing leg ulcers.

E. Splenectomy for symptoms.

1. ***Hypersplenism.***
   a. Refers to the effects of increased splenic function.
      (1) Anemia, leukopenia, or thrombocytopenia (any combination).
      (2) Splenomegaly (may or may not be present).
      (3) Improvement after splenectomy.
   b. Also divided into primary hypersplenis, in which underlying disease is unknown, and secondary hypersplenism, in which the primary disease accounts for the increased splenic function.
   c. Categories of hypersplenism by mechanism with examples of the underlying disease.
      (1) Work hypertrophy, immune response–subacute bacterial endocarditis, infectious mononucleosis, Felty's syndrome.
      (2) Work hypertrophy, red cell destruction–spherocytosis,

thalassemia, autoimmune hemolytic anemia, sickle cell anemia.
(3) Congestion–cirrhosis, splenic vein thrombosis.
(4) Myeloproliferative-chronic myelogenous leukemia, myeloid metaplasia.
(5) Infiltrative-sarcoid, amyloid, Gaucher's disease.
(6) Neoplastic-lymphoma, hairy-cell leukemia, chronic lymphocytic leukemia, metastasis.

2. Thalassemia and sickle cell disease.
   a. Both disorders characterized by abnormalities in hemoglobin structure.
   b. Splenectomy indicated for painful splenomegaly.
3. Splenic vein thrombosis.
   a. Fifty percent are caused by pancreatitis, but pancreatic carcinoma, pseudocyst, and penetrating gastric ulcer are other causes.
   b. Results in gastric varices that can be the cause of upper gastrointestinal hemorrhage.
   c. Splenectomy resolves both problems and should be done once other causes of portal hypertension are ruled out.
4. Infectious mononucleosis.
   a. Splenomegaly common in Epstein-Barr virus infection.
   b. "Spontaneous" rupture probably just susceptibility to injury with minor trauma.
   c. May require splenectomy.

F. Hematologic malignancies.

1. Hairy-cell leukemia.
   a. Most patients with hematologic malignancies are not considered for early splenectomy with the exception of hairy-cell leukemia.
   b. Splenectomy is first treatment.
   c. Secondary therapy consists of alpha-interferon and 2′-deoxycoformycin if splenectomy fails to improve the cytopenias.
   d. Chemotherapy is first therapy if bone marrow cellularity is > 85%.
2. ***Hodgkin's disease.***
   a. A malignant lymphoma characterized by "Reed-Sternberg" cells.
   b. Incidence peaks in late 20s and again begins increasing over the age of 45. More common in males.
   c. Commonly presents as asymptomatic lymphadenopathy, and constitutional symptoms (B symptoms) of fever, night sweats, weight loss usually indicate widespread disease and a less favorable prognosis.
   d. Treatment and ultimate survival depend on disease distribution, the presence or absence of B symptoms, and histologic subtype.
   e. Staging–Ann Arbor Staging Classification.

(1) Stage I–single node region involved.
(2) Stage II–2 or more node regions involved on same side of diaphragm.
(3) Stage III–2 or more node regions involved on opposite sides of diaphragm.
(4) Stage IV–diffuse disease.
(5) A or B depending on presence of symptoms.
(6) E for local extranodal disease.

f. The staging laparotomy.
(1) Consists of exploratory laparotomy with liver biopsy, splenectomy, para-aortic node sampling, and bone marrow biopsy.
(2) Indications are Stage I & II disease, in which treatment is usually radiation therapy alone. Stage III & IV patients, in whom chemotherapy or combined modality therapy will be used, are not candidates for staging laparotomy.
(3) A change in clinical stage occurs in 35-40% of patients:
a) 25-35% are upstaged (higher stage) after staging laparotomy.
b) 5-15% are downstaged.

g. Survival (5-year).
(1) Stage I-II–85%.
(2) Stage IIIA–70%.
(3) Stage IIIB–50%.
(4) Stage IV–40%.

G. Splenectomy not indicated—thrombotic thrombocytopenic purpura (TTP).

1. Condition of thrombocytopenia, microangiopathic hemolytic anemia, neurological abnormalities, fever, and renal failure secondary to platelet microthrombi.
2. 90% idiopathic, female > male, with peak in 3rd decade.
3. Poor prognosis, with 10% 1-year survival.
4. Treatment focuses on plasmapheresis, high-dose steroids, and anti-platelet drugs.
5. Splenectomy may be performed for poor response to above treatments, with few reports of improvement.

III. OTHER SPLENIC DISORDERS OF SURGICAL SIGNIFICANCE

A. Splenic artery aneurysm.

1. Rare, but occur more in women than in men.
2. Medial dysplasia is usual cause in women, atherosclerosis in men.
3. May cause vague abdominal pain.
4. Occasionally ruptures with early containment by lesser sac or exsanguinating hemorrhage into peritoneal cavity. Fewer than 10% rupture; of these, 20% are during pregnancy.

5. Elective aneurysm excision should be performed in patients who are good surgical risks or women of childbearing age.
6. Splenic function should be preserved.

B. Splenic abscess.

1. Rare and usually occurs with a primary focus, such as other abscesses or endocarditis.
2. Fever, chills, LUQ tenderness, and splenomegaly.
3. Diagnosed by CT or sonogram.
4. Splenectomy is preferred treatment unless abscess is unilocular and subcapsular, in which case percutaneous drainage may be effective.

C. Splenic cysts.

1. Pseudocysts–50-75%, related to previous injury.
2. Epithelial (non-parasitic)–10% of cysts, prone to rupture if > 10 cm in size. May be lymphangiomas, dermoid cysts, or cystic hemangiomas. Symptomatic cysts are treated with aspiration; splenectomy indicated if cysts are very large or diagnosis uncertain.
3. Parasitic–echinococcal most common, should not be aspirated.

D. Ectopic spleen.

1. Normal spleen found in the lower abdomen.
2. Young, multiparous women most commonly affected.
3. Elongated splenic pedicle predisposes to splenic torsion. If splenic torsion occurs, splenectomy is required.
4. When recurrent vague symptoms are present or found incidentally, splenopexy may be performed.

IV. COMPLICATIONS OF SPLENECTOMY

A. Immediately post-operatively.

1. Peripheral blood changes.
   a. Leukocytosis.
   b. Thrombocytosis.
   c. Presence of Howell-Jolly bodies.
2. Hemorrhage–from splenic pedicle or short gastric vessels. Many advocate nasogastric tube post-operatively to decompress the stomach and decrease chances of bleeding from the short gastrics.
3. Atelectasis (usually left lower lobe) is the most common complication.
4. Subphrenic abscess or hematoma–presents as fever and LUQ pain or left shoulder pain, usually about 5 days post-operatively. This may require re-exploration or percutaneous drainage.
5. Pancreatitis or pancreatic fistula from manipulation.

B. Post-splenectomy sepsis.

1. Overwhelming sepsis, usually with an encapsulated organism such as pneumococcus or haemophilus. Incidence in splenectomized patients is 40 x that of the general population.

2. Occurs in 4.25% of splenectomized patients, with a higher rate associated with hematologic disease. Rates for trauma splenectomies are less than 1%.
3. Fatal 50% of the time.
4. Vaccinations for *Streptococcus pneumoniae* and *Haemophilus influenza* should be given to all splenectomy patients. Vaccines are more effective if given 10-14 days pre-operatively.
5. Prophylactic penicillin is given to children under 18 and reduces the incidence significantly.

48

Abdominal Wall Hernias

Timothy D. Kane, M.D.

It has only been within the past century, when we have gained an improved understanding of inguinal anatomy, aseptic technique, and improvements in suture material, that significant improvements in hernia management have occurred.

I. TERMINOLOGY

A. **Hernia**—the protrusion of a part or structure through tissues normally containing it.

B. **Reducibility**—contents can be restored to their anatomic location.

C. **Incarceration**—an irreducible hernia; may be acute and painful or chronic and asymptomatic.

D. **Strangulation**—an incarcerated hernia with vascular compromise of the herniated contents. Usually indirect, femoral, and umbilical hernias.

E. **Sliding hernia** (Figure 1)–a portion of the hernial sac composed of a wall of a viscus (frequently cecum or sigmoid colon).

F. **Richter's hernia** (Figure 2)–only one wall of a viscus lies within the hernial sac (i.e., a "knuckle" of small bowel); may incarcerate or strangulate without obstructing.

II. INCIDENCE

A. **Male:female** = 7:1.

B. **Lifetime risk of developing a hernia**—males 5%, females 1%.

C. **Most common surgical disease of males.**

D. **Most common groin hernia in either sex** is indirect inguinal hernia; however, femoral hernias are more common in females.

III. ANATOMICAL CONSIDERATIONS

A. **Layers of the abdominal wall**—skin, subcutaneous fat, Scarpa's fascia, external oblique, internal oblique, transversus abdominus, transversalis fascia, peritoneum.

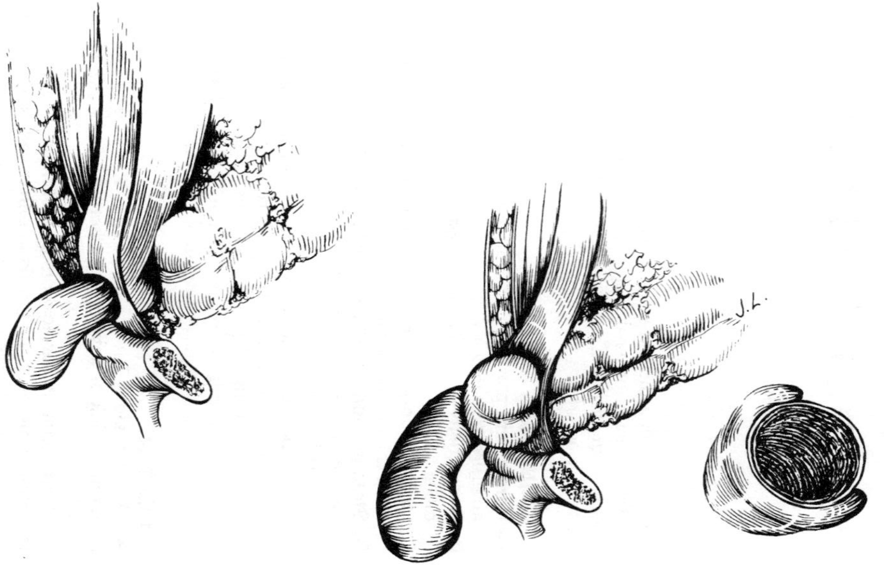

FIG. 1 Sliding Hernia

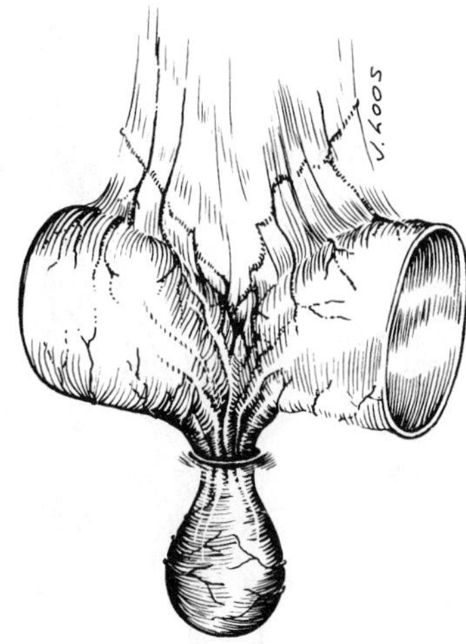

FIG. 2 Richter's Hernia

B. Hesselbach's triangle—bordered by lateral edge of rectus sheath, inferior epigastric vessels and inguinal ligament. *Note:* These tissues are not in the same plane.

C. Inguinal ligament—runs from anterior superior iliac spine to the pubic tubercle. Formed from external oblique aponeurosis.

D. Lacunar ligament—inguinal ligament reflected from the pubic tubercle onto the iliopectineal line of the pubic ramus.

E. Cooper's ligament—a strong, fibrous band on the iliopectineal line of the superior pubic ramus.

F. External ring—opening in external oblique aponeurosis through which the ilioinguinal nerve and spermatic cord or round ligament pass.

G. Internal ring—bordered superiorly by internal oblique muscle, and inferomedially by inferior epigastric vessels and transversalis fascia.

H. Processus vaginalis—a diverticulum of parietal peritoneum that descends from the abdomen along with the testicle and comes to lie adjacent to the spermatic cord. There is subsequent obliteration of its lumen in normal individuals.

I. Femoral canal—bordered by inguinal ligament, lacunar ligament, Cooper's ligament, and femoral sheath.

IV. CLASSIFICATION OF HERNIAS

A. Groin hernias (Figure 3).

1. ***Indirect inguinal hernia*** — sac lies anteromedial to cord, exit-

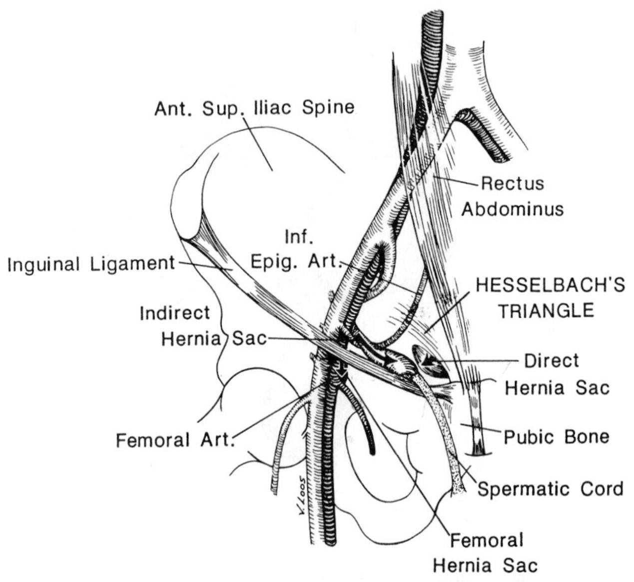

FIG. 3 Groin Hernias

ing through the internal ring; lateral to inferior epigastric artery.

2. ***Direct inguinal hernia*** — passes through Hesselbach's triangle (medial to inferior epigastric artery).
3. ***Pantaloon hernia*** — components of both direct and indirect inguinal hernias.
4. ***Femoral hernia*** — passes through femoral canal, medial to femoral vein.

B. Ventral hernias.

1. Umbilical hernia–congenital or acquired.
2. Incisional hernia–develops in previous fascial closure.
3. Epigastric hernia–defect in linea alba above the umbilicus.

C. Miscellaneous hernias.

1. ***Littre's hernia*** — inguinal hernia sac that contains a Meckel's diverticulum.
2. ***Spigelian hernia.***
   a. Ventral hernia occurring at the semilunar line (lateral edge of rectus).
   b. Usually occurs where semilunar line and semicircular line intersect and rectus sheath becomes completely anterior.

3. ***Petit's hernia***—through lumbar triangle.
4. ***Obturator hernia***—through obturator foramen.
5. ***Perineal hernia***—defect occurs in the muscular floor of the pelvis; anterior, posterior, or complete rectal prolapse.
6. ***Sciatic hernia***—rarest of all hernias; sac exits through the greater or lesser sacrosciatic foramen.

V. ETIOLOGY

A. Indirect inguinal hernia—congenital patency of processus vaginalis; herniation through internal ring facilitated by a weak inguinal floor.

B. Direct inguinal hernia—acquired weakness in the floor of Hesselbach's triangle.

C. Contributing factors—obesity, chronic cough, pregnancy, constipation, straining on urination, ascites, previous hernia repair.

VI. DIAGNOSIS

A. History of a palpable, soft mass that increases with straining; may reduce spontaneously or manually; there may be pain with straining.

B. Examination—palpable mass that increases in size while the patient strains. Examine patient when upright and supine.

1. Femoral hernia may reflect superiorly over the inguinal ligament, presenting in the inguinal region.
2. Obesity may make identification of small hernias difficult.
3. Obturator, lumbar, sciatic, and even femoral hernias may be easily missed by physical exam.
4. Abdominal radiograph or CT scan may demonstrate hernias not detectable by physical exam.

C. Small bowel obstruction–may be first manifestation of a hernia.

VII. REPAIR OF HERNIAS

A. Inguinal hernias—need to repair defect in transversalis fascia.

1. High ligation of sac–in children, where only defect is patent processus vaginalis, no further repair is needed.
2. Bassini–transversalis fascia and transversus abdominus arch (conjoined tendon) are approximated to the shelving edge of inguinal ligament. Can be done in 2 layers:
   a. Transversalis repair.
   b. Transversus abdominus arch to inguinal ligament.
3. McVay (Cooper's ligament repair)–transversus abdominus arch approximated to Cooper's ligament; must use relaxing incision in rectus sheath or mesh.
4. Halsted I–Bassini-type repair except the imbricated external oblique reinforces the repair beneath the spermatic cord, which lies in the subcutaneous tissue. Rarely used.

5. Ferguson–Bassini-type repair; however, spermatic cord lies beneath reconstructed inguinal floor.
6. Preperitoneal–expose hernial defect from beneath abdominal wall fascia in the preperitoneal space. Useful approach for repair of recurrent hernia.
7. Shouldice–2-layer running overlapping repair of transversalis fascia, reinforced by a 2-layer running overlapping approximation of transversus abdominus arch to inguinal ligament.
8. Lichtenstein repair–Marlex® mesh, tension-free repair. Lowest recurrence rate, but infection risk of foreign body.
9. Laparoscopic repair–preperitoneal or transperitoneal repair using synthetic material.

B. **Femoral hernias—**require a Cooper's ligament repair (McVay), shouldice repair or preperitoneal repair. Many large direct hernia are repaired in this manner.

C. **Ventral hernias—**wide mobilization, primary repair of fascial defect if possible; often requires synthetic material (polypropylene or PTFE).

VIII. POST-OPERATIVE COMPLICATIONS

A. **Scrotal hematoma—**from blunt dissection and inadequate hemostasis.

B. **Deep bleeding** will enter the retroperitoneal space and may not be apparent initially. Suspect this with hypotension, orthostasis, or tachycardia.

C. **Difficulty voiding—**more common in elderly males.

D. **Painful scrotal swelling** from compromised venous return of testes.

E. **Neuroma/neuritis—**entrapment or severance of nerves at the repair site. Usually resolve spontaneously.

IX. RECURRENCE

A. **2-3% with indirect inguinal hernias;** some "recurrences" are direct hernias that were missed at the initial operation. Lowest for shouldice or Lichtenstein.

B. **Higher with direct hernias** and when the underlying process (chronic cough, constipation, urinary obstruction) causing increased intra-abdominal pressure has not been corrected.

C. **Technical errors.**

1. Excessive tension on suture line.
2. Internal ring too loose.
3. Indirect hernia sac not identified at the time of operation.
4. Inadequate tissue strength despite adequate reconstruction (requires Marlex® or other reinforcement).
5. Failure to identify concomitant femoral hernia at time of repair of inguinal hernia.
6. Failure to repair "pre-hernia" laxity in floor.

X. MISCELLANEOUS

A. Marlex® (polypropylene) mesh placed over the fascial defect may be used if the defect cannot be closed because of inadequate tissue or excessive tension. Often used to reinforce repairs.

B. Repair of bilateral inguinal hernias is recommended in children.

C. Consider orchiectomy in elderly males with multiple recurrences.

D. Reduction of incarcerated hernia.

1. Trendelenburg position, sedation, and gentle continuous compression may allow reduction of a recently incarcerated hernia.
2. Significant tenderness, induration, erythema, or leukocytosis suggest possible strangulation and necessitate immediate surgical exploration. *(No reduction should be attempted!)*
3. Use of a truss can result in distortion of anatomy as a result of fibrosis of the inguinal canal, complicating and delaying the required surgery; a truss should be avoided in all but extremely high-risk patients.
4. Reduction *en masse*–reduction of hernia sac and contents from the extracavitary position with persistent entrapment of the contents within the sac. Patients should be observed post-reduction for signs and symptoms of strangulation.

49

Surgical Endoscopy

Karl J. Bertram, M.D.

I. INTRODUCTION

A. **Endoscopy provides a non-invasive view** of the GI tract.

B. **The advances in fiberoptics** have enhanced the capabilities of diagnosis and treatment of GI tract disorders.

II. INSTRUMENTATION AND TECHNIQUES

A. **The basic instrument** has a head with an eyepiece and controls, a variable-length shaft, and a maneuverable tip (Figure 1). Video monitors may be used instead of the standard eyepiece.

B. **Centrally located flexible fiberoptic light** and viewing bundles allow for maneuverability of instrument while providing a clear image.

C. **The fiberoptics** are arranged so that the scope may be either forward viewing or side viewing.

D. **The flexibility of the tip** allows for up and down and side-to-side deflection of $> 180°$.

E. **Shaft** is torque-stable, allowing rotary movements to be transmitted the length of the scope.

F. **Keeping the shaft of the instrument relatively straight** allows rotatory movements to be transmitted to the tip.

G. **The scope has 2 or more channels** for the passage of instruments and introduction of air and water (Figure 2).

H. **Light source** is attached to scope via an "umbilical cord." An air pump, water pump and suction are frequently built into the light source, and their channels pass through the umbilical cord.

I. **Maneuverability**—The instrument can be controlled with one hand.

J. **After introduction of the scope,** orientation is maintained by use of marker at the 12 o'clock position in the field of view, with upward deflection being toward the mark (Figure 3).

K. **Important rules for endoscopic examination.**

1. Prepare patient.
2. *Protect airway at all times.*

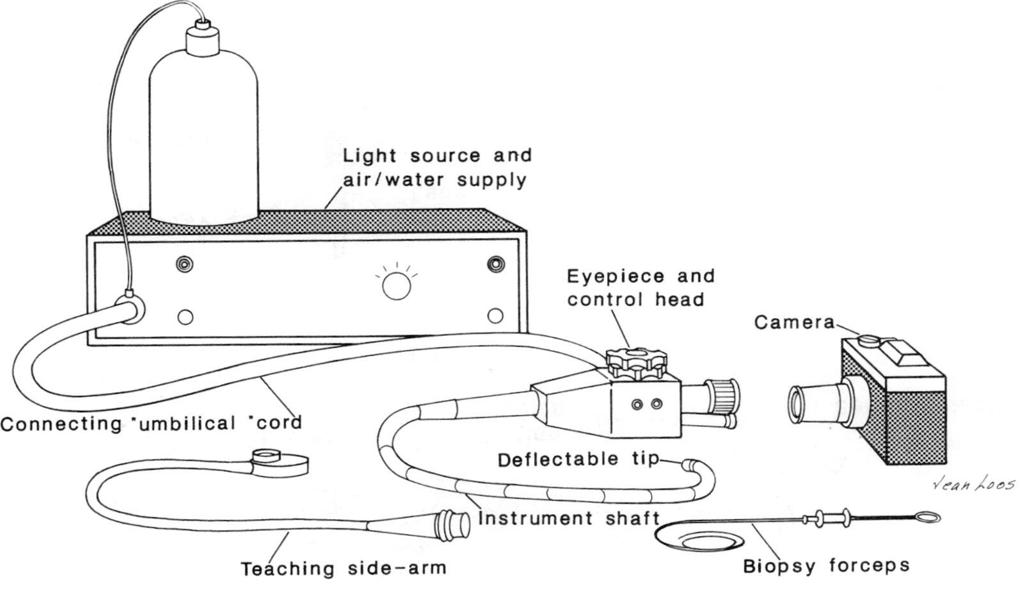
Light source and
air/water supply
Eyepiece and
control head
Camera
Connecting "umbilical" cord
Deflectable tip
Instrument shaft
Teaching side-arm
Biopsy forceps
Jean Loos

FIG. 1

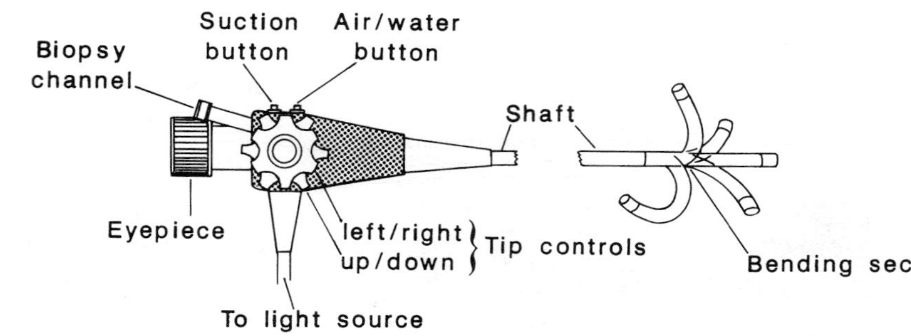
Suction button
Air/water button
Biopsy channel
Shaft
Eyepiece
left/right
up/down
Tip controls
Bending section
To light source

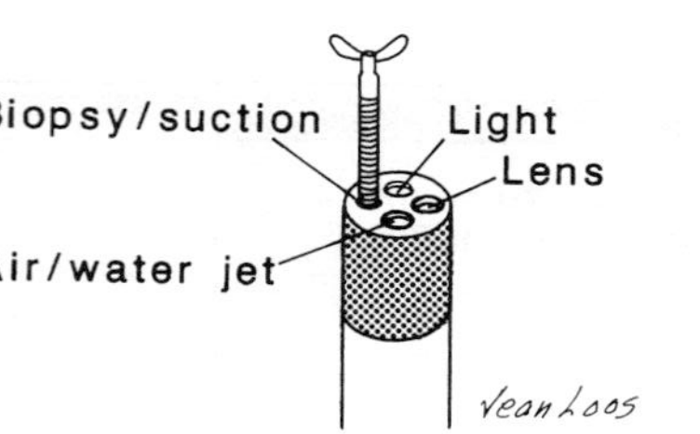
Biopsy/suction
Light
Lens
Air/water jet
Jean Loos

FIG. 2

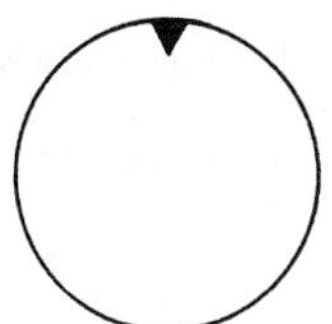

FIG. 3

3. ***Do not advance without vision.***
4. If in doubt, withdraw.
5. Tissue can be obtained for histologic and cytologic exam during most of the multiple endoscopic procedures.
6. Biopsies should be taken from multiple areas of suspected pathology (specimens placed in formalin).
7. Most common complications are perforation and bleeding.

III. ESOPHAGOGASTRODUODENOSCOPY (EGD)

Used for evaluation and selective treatment of diseases of the esophagus, stomach, and proximal duodenum.

A. Indications.

1. Upper abdominal pain unresponsive to medical therapy.
2. Upper abdominal pain with signs or symptoms suggestive of organic disease.
3. Foreign bodies.
4. Persistent esophageal reflux despite medical therapy.
5. Dysphagia or odynophagia.
6. Persistent vomiting of unknown cause.
7. Upper GI radiographs suggestive of carcinoma, gastric or esophageal ulcer, or evidence of stricture or obstruction.
8. Gastrointestinal bleeding.
   a. Surgery contemplated.
   b. Recurrent bleeding.
   c. Portal hypertension–esophageal and gastric varices, portal gastropathy.
   d. Rule out aorto-enteric fistula in patient with previous aortic surgery.
   e. Iron-deficiency anemia with negative colonoscopy.
9. Surveillance of Barrett's esophagus.

B. Preparation.

1. NPO for a minimum of 4-6 h prior to study.
2. Urgent EGD may require prior gastric lavage and decompression.
3. ***Ensure airway is protected.***
4. IV sedation is recommended (e.g., midazolam 1 mg IVP), titrate for desired effect.

5. Topical anesthesia for pharynx (e.g., Cetacaine® spray).

C. Technique.

1. A 120-cm forward-viewing scope is used.
2. The patient is placed in a left lateral decubitus position.
3. The instrument may be introduced manually or by having the patient swallow the scope.
4. The instrument is further safely advanced **under direct vision of the lumen** through the esophagus into the stomach and duodenum.
5. Important landmarks are the cricopharyngeal sphincter, lower esophageal sphincter, incisura, pylorus, and superior duodenal angle. The distance from the incisors for each landmark should be noted in the report.
6. Careful inspection of the upper GI tract, noting abnormal mucosal findings and gastrointestinal motility, is performed during insertion and withdrawal of the scope.
7. Retroflexion of the scope is performed to inspect the incisura, cardia, and the gastric side of the esophageal hiatus.
8. The "pinch line" (corresponds to the diaphragmatic crus) may be visualized by having the patient sniff with the scope in the lower esophagus. The "Z-line" (squamocolumnar junction) can be visually identified.
9. The vocal cords should be seen on withdrawal through the hypopharynx.

D. Contraindications.

1. Uncooperative or combative patient.
2. Acute corrosive or phlegmonous esophagitis.
3. Relative contraindications.
   a. Pulsion diverticulum.
   b. Bleeding diathesis.
   c. Aneurysm of ascending aorta.
   d. Large goiter.
   e. Large cervical osteophytes (increases risk of esophageal perforation).

E. Complications—risk of occurrence is approximately 2%.

1. Perforation–most common at level of pharynx, cervical esophagus, cardia, or superior duodenal angle.
2. Bleeding.
3. Aspiration.
4. Vasovagal response–associated bradycardia and hypotension.
5. Cardiac arrhythmias.
6. Transmission of infection (no documented instances).
7. Mortality 0.02%–cardiac dysrhythmias are the most common cause of EGD-associated deaths.

F. Therapeutic options.

1. Esophageal strictures and dilation therapy.
   a. Strictures amenable to dilation therapy.
      (1) Peptic stenosis–most common, usually secondary to reflux.

(2) Achalasia.
(3) Erosive stricture.
(4) Esophageal webs.
(5) Neoplastic stenosis.
(6) Post-surgical strictures.
(7) Schatzki rings.

b. Technique.
(1) Dilate to eliminate dysphagia.
(2) Do not use more than 3 dilators of successive size (6-9 French of dilation) per treatment.
(3) Continue till obtain diameter 14-15 mm (~45 French).
(4) 80-90% patients successfully treated–50% will require a second dilation.

c. Complications.
(1) Perforation (0.1-0.3%)–most common–increased risk with achalasia (1-5%) or malignancy (2-10%).
(2) Bleeding.
(3) Bacteremia.

2. Foreign bodies.
a. General information.
(1) Population.
a) Children ages 1-5.
b) Adult–obtunded, inebriated, psychotic disorder, prisoners.
(2) 60-90% pass spontaneously, 10-20% endoscopically removed, 1% require surgery.
(3) Removal necessary if no progression in 48 h.
(4) Objects wider than 2 cm or longer than 5 cm rarely pass and require removal.
(5) Signs of respiratory compromise or inability to handle secretions **require immediate removal.**

b. Technique.
(1) **Maintain airway.**
(2) Place patient in Trendelenburg position to prevent object from falling into trachea.
(3) May require overtube.

c. Types.
(1) Coins.
a) Usually pass if in stomach.
b) Those that remain in esophagus must be removed owing to risk of pressure necrosis or fistula formation.
(2) Meat.
a) Most common in adults.
b) Must remove if in esophagus > 12 h.
c) Must use endoscope even if passes, because obstructing lesion is found in 75-90% of patients.
(3) Sharp objects.
a) Remove with pointed end distally.
b) Risky endoscopic removal best managed by surgery.

c) Passage beyond endoscope.
   1) Conservative treatment and daily radiographs.
   2) Failure to progress > 2-3 days or signs of perforation require surgery.

3. Non-variceal upper GI bleeding.
   a. General.
      (1) Perform as soon as patient stabilized.
      (2) Endoscopy will reveal source in 80-90% of patients.
   b. Technique.
      (1) Lavage GI tract free of all blood and clots.
      (2) Look for active bleeding or stigmata of recent hemorrhage (clot, black spots, or a visible vessel).
      (3) 70-80% of bleeding will stop spontaneously. Hemostasis should be performed with active bleeding, ulcers with a non-bleeding visible vessel, or a sentinel clot (use as marker for artery below it; hemostatic attempts should not be performed on the clot itself).
      (4) Either injection therapy or thermal therapies may be used (80-95% successful, perforation rate 0.5-2%).
4. Variceal bleeding–technique.
   a. Volume and coagulation factor replacement.
   b. Metoclopramide (20 mg IV)–contracts the lower esophageal sphincter and decreases cephalad flow to esophageal varices.
   c. Massive bleeding may require use of Sengstaken-Blakemore tube for 12-24 h prior to sclerotherapy.
   d. Sclerotherapy–sclerosant is injected intraluminally beginning distally and moving proximally at 2-3 cm intervals until small-caliber vessels encountered. Should not exceed 20 ml of sclerosant per session.
   e. Repeat treatments should be performed 5 days after first treatment and then at 1- to 3-week intervals until the varices are ablated.
   f. Controls hemorrhage in 85% and lowers rate of rebleed.

IV. ENDOSCOPIC RETROGRADE CHOLANGIOPANCREATOGRAPHY (ERCP)

Used for evaluation and treatment of pancreaticobiliary disorders.

A. Preparation.

1. Same as for EGD.
2. Prophylactic antibiotic coverage for enteric organisms.
3. Correction of coagulopathy if present.

B. Technique.

1. The 120-cm side-viewing scope is used.
2. Introduction of the instrument is the same as for EGD, except scope is passed relatively blindly through the cricopharyngeus due to its side-viewing nature.
3. The instrument is passed into the second portion of the duodenum until the ampulla of Vater is identified.

4. Intestinal paralysis is obtained with glucagon (0.25 mg).
5. The ampulla is cannulated, and dye is injected under fluoroscopic control. Subsequently, radiographs of the biliary and pancreatic systems are obtained. Attention to radiographic detail is critical.
6. Sphincterotomy if indicated is performed by placing sphincterotome at 11-12 o'clock position and then applying electrical current to expose the bile duct mucosa.

C. Indications.

1. *Diagnostic ERCP.*
   a. Jaundice of undetermined etiology.
   b. Suspected bile duct pathology.
   c. Evaluation of chronic pancreatitis.
   d. Suspected pancreatic carcinoma.
   e. Suspected pancreatic divisum.
   f. Pancreatic ductal trauma.
2. *Endoscopic sphincterotomy.*
   a. Choledocholithiasis–retained or recurrent.
   b. Acute cholangitis.
   c. Papillary stenosis.
   d. Sphincter of Oddi dysfunction.
   e. Preparation of endoprosthesis insertion.
   f. Gallstone pancreatitis.
   g. Chronic pancreatitis with elevated pancreatic sphincter pressures.
   h. Palliation of ampullary tumor.
   i. Sump syndrome.
   j. Choledochocele.

D. Contraindications.

1. Same as for EGD.
2. Relative–acute pancreatitis. Recommended for severe biliary pancreatitis.

E. Complications—occur in 6-10% of cases; can usually be treated conservatively. Surgery is required for 20-30% of complications. Mortality rate is 1%.

1. Hemorrhage.
2. Cholangitis.
3. Pancreatitis.
4. Perforation.
5. Basket impaction.

F. Endoprosthesis insertion.

1. Indications.
   a. Malignant biliary obstruction–90% can be successfully stented; mortality 2%.
      (1) Pancreatic carcinoma.
      (2) Cholangiocarcinoma.
      (3) Gallbladder carcinoma.
      (4) Metastatic carcinoma.
   b. Benign biliary obstruction.

(1) Anastomotic stricture.
(2) Surgical trauma.
(3) Pancreatitis.
(4) Sclerosing cholangitis.

c. Choledocholithiasis.
d. Biliary fistula.

2. Complications.
   a. Clogging–most common, secondary to bacterial biofilm and deposition of biliary sludge. Average stent survival 6 months.
   b. Reflux.
   c. Obstruction.
   d. Migration of stent.
   e. Perforation.

V. ENDOSCOPIC ULTRASOUND (EUS)

Provides high-resolution images of the gut wall layers and surrounding organs.

A. Preparation.

1. Same as for EGD.
2. IV sedation and topical anesthesia.

B. Technique.

1. Fiberoptic endoscope with mechanically rotated transducer in tip of scope, providing 360 degree real-time sonographic image.
2. Biopsy channel and optical lens located proximal to transducer mounted at 45-degree angle provide optically but not ultrasonically directed biopsy.
3. Intraluminal instillation of water and the use of a water-filled balloon around the transducer reduce the problem of bowel gas interference.
4. Ultrasound resolves gut wall into at least five discrete layers.
   a. Perechoic first band–interface of lumen and superficial mucosa.
   b. Hypoechoic second band–interface between mucosa and submucosa.
   c. Hyperechoic third band–represents the submucosa layer.
   d. Hypoechoic fourth band–represents the muscularis propria.
   e. Hyperechoic fifth band–depicts adventitia or serosa.

C. Indications.

1. Staging of esophageal, gastric, ampullary, distal bile duct, and pancreatic carcinomas.
2. Determining the nature of subepithelial GI lesions.
3. Staging of gastric lymphoma.
4. Localization of pancreatic neuroendocrine tumors.
5. EUS-directed biopsy to differentiate benign and malignant lymph nodes.
6. Evaluate thickened gastric folds.

D. Contraindications—similar to EGD.
E. Complications—similar to EGD.

VI. COLONOSCOPY

Allows for diagnostic evaluation of the colon and terminal ileum. Most accurate diagnostic modality available for the lower GI tract. Allows for early detection of colorectal carcinoma.

A. Preparation.

1. Mechanical bowel prep prior to procedure (e.g., Golytely® 4 L over 4 h at least 12 h prior to study).
2. Clear liquids for 24-48 h prior to procedure.
3. NPO for 6 h preceding the procedure.
4. Normal coagulation profile.

B. Technique.

1. The 140-180 cm forward-viewing scope is used.
2. The patient is placed in left lateral decubitus position with knees flexed, and the instrument is introduced through the anus.
3. The instrument is passed **under direct visualization** until the cecum/terminal ileum is reached.
   a. Endoscopically, the lumen of the ascending colon is circular and the lumen of the transverse colon is triangular.
   b. Splenic and hepatic flexures may be identified by the extra-luminal bluish hue of the spleen and liver.
   c. The appendiceal orifice may be identified as the point of fusion of the tinea.
4. As with EGD, careful inspection is performed during insertion and withdrawal of the scope.
5. Adequate insufflation of the colon must be maintained to completely evaluate all mucosal surfaces.

C. Indications.

1. Lower GI bleeding.
2. Unexplained iron-deficiency anemia.
3. Diagnosis of persistent diarrhea.
4. Abnormalities on barium enema.
5. Chronic inflammatory bowel disease, if more precise diagnosis or determination of disease activity will influence immediate management.
6. Surveillance of colonic neoplasia (see "Colorectal Cancer.")

D. Contraindications.

1. Acute inflammatory disease of colon/rectum–relative.
2. Toxic megacolon.
3. Peritonitis.
4. Recent myocardial infarction.
5. First trimester of pregnancy.

E. Complications—complication rate is approximately 0.14%.

1. Perforation.
2. Cardiac dysrhythmias.
3. Vasovagal response.

4. Mesenteric hematoma.
5. Splenic injury.
6. Bleeding.

F. Therapeutic options.

1. Lower GI bleeding.
   a. Colonoscopy indicated.
      (1) Chronic bleeding with history of melena.
      (2) Hematochezia or blood-streaked stool.
      (3) Fecal occult blood.
      (4) Recent severe, but currently inactive bleed.
      (5) Active severe bleed–only for persistent bleeding with negative radionucleotide scan and/or angiogram.
   b. Technique.
      (1) Adequate resuscitation, correction of coagulation parameters.
      (2) Bowel prep with sodium sulfate-based solution.
      (3) Colonoscopy looking for stigmata of recent bleeding.
         a) Active bleeding.
         b) Adherent clot in a single diverticulum or ulcerative lesion.
         c) Non-bleeding visible vessel in an ulcer.
      (4) Hemostasis obtained by injection or thermal therapies.
2. Malignant colonic polyps.
   a. Removal.
      (1) Prep as for standard colonoscopic exam.
      (2) Correction of coagulation deficits.
      (3) Pedunculated polyps can usually be removed with a snare and electrocoagulation of the stalk. It is important to constantly move polyp during transection to avoid burning the opposite colonic wall.
      (4) Sessile polyps.
         a) Ulcerative and indurated polyps best removed surgically.
         b) Polyps less than 2 cm can usually be removed in one piece with a snare.
         c) Larger polyps may require piecemeal removal in 1-1.5 cm segments.
      (5) Once transected, it is critical to retrieve the polyp for histologic examination.
3. Colonic decompression.
   a. **Ogilvie's syndrome**–acute pseudo-obstruction of the colon, characterized by massive dilation of the cecum and colon without organic obstruction.
      (1) Colonoscopy is successful in 80-85% of patients.
      (2) Conservative treatment for patients with cecal diameters less than 9-10 cm (NPO, NG suction, correction of electrolytes, and cessation of narcotics).
      (3) Decompression indicated for cecal diameter greater

than 11-12 cm, or if there is no improvement in 48-72 h.

(4) Technique.

a) Air insufflation should be kept to a minimum.

b) Attempt to reach the cecum; however, successful decompression has been achieved with passage to the hepatic flexure.

c) Colonic lumen is collapsed by applying intermittent suction as the endoscope is withdrawn.

d) Care must be taken to center the colonoscope tip in the bowel lumen to permit decompression of gas and liquid without trapping mucosa.

e) A soft rectal tube may be placed endoscopically to prevent recurrence.

b. Volvulus.

(1) **Sigmoid volvulus.**

a) Frequent in elderly, institutionalized patients.

b) Decompression is temporizing measure and allows the patient and the colon to be prepared for an elective operation. Although colonoscopy is frequently successful, recurrence is frequent (50-70%) without operative treatment.

c) Allows assessment of bowel viability–important prognostic factor. Bloody colonic contents or dark blue or black mucosa suggests necrosis and mandates emergent operative treatment.

(2) **Cecal volvulus.**

a) Symptoms similar to small bowel obstruction.

b) Colonoscopic decompression of cecal volvulus is not indicated since it is frequently unsuccessful and delays operative treatment.

c) Surgical treatment–detorsion and cecopexy.

4. Dilation of colonic strictures.

a. Strictures amenable to dilation.

(1) Anastomotic–best results.

(2) Diverticular.

(3) Malignant.

(4) Inflammatory.

(5) Radiation.

(6) Ischemic.

b. Must determine cause of stricture. May require biopsies and/or mucosal brushing.

c. Performed same as with upper GI strictures.

VII. PROCTOSIGMOIDOSCOPY

Allows visualization of the anal canal, rectum, and proximal portion of sigmoid colon from 30-60 cm.

A. Preparation.

1. Two Fleet® enemas prior to the procedure.
2. Adequate rectal exam.

B. Technique.

1. A 30-cm rigid or 30- to 60-cm flexible scope can be used.
2. The longer flexible scope affords better visualization and a higher yield, as well as greater patient comfort.
3. The procedure can be performed with the patient in the lateral decubitus position with knees flexed, lithotomy, or knee-chest (genupectoral) position.
4. The instrument is passed per rectum under direct vision.

C. Indications.

1. Hematochezia.
2. Anorectal symptoms.
3. Change in bowel habits.
4. Routine exam for population > 40. American Cancer Society recommendations:
   a. Rectal exam every year > 40.
   b. Sigmoidoscopy every year > 50; if two successive exams are negative, then repeat every 3-5 years.
5. 30% of colorectal cancers can be detected by rigid sigmoidoscopy (50-60% by lower flexible sigmoidoscopy).
6. Good screening tool as 60% of all colorectal tumors occur within 30 cm of the anal verge.

D. Contraindications.

1. Fulminant colitis.
2. Active diverticulitis.
3. Uncooperative patient.
4. Toxic megacolon.
5. Peritonitis.

E. Complications—lowest risk of any endoscopic diagnostic procedure.

1. Perforation.
2. Bleeding.
3. Mesosigmoid hematoma.
4. Cardiac dysrhythmias.

50

Laparoscopic Cholecystectomy

John J. Bruns, Jr., M.D.

A. History.

1. Charles Filipi performed the first laparoscopic cholecystectomy in the early 1980s.
2. Phillipe Mouret performed the first laparoscopic cholecystectomy in humans in 1988.
3. First performed in the U.S. by McKernan and Saye.

B. Indications—same as for open cholecystectomy.

C. Contraindications.

1. Absolute.
   a. Sepsis and peritonitis or cholangitis.
   b. Inability to tolerate general anesthesia (spinal anesthesia cases are reported).
   c. Biliary fistula.
   d. Uncorrectable severe coagulopathy.
   e. Suspected carcinoma of the gallbladder.
   f. Pregnancy in later trimesters.
2. Relative.
   a. Acute cholecystitis with suspected empyema or perforation.
   b. Prior upper abdominal surgery.
   c. Cirrhosis or portal hypertension.
   d. Pregnancy.
   e. Morbid obesity.
   f. Common bile duct stones, especially if large or multiple.
   g. Surgeon inexperience.
   h. Severe COPD with hypercarbia.
   i. Acute gallstone pancreatitis.

D. Pre-operative evaluation(see "Cholecystitis").

E. OR setup.

1. Position supine on x-ray compatible OR table with appropriate straps and footboard for possible frequent repositioning.

2. Foley, nasogastric tube, anti-embolic bilateral LE compression boots.
3. Surgeon on patient's left, first assistant on patient's right, and camera manipulator next to surgeon.
4. Monitors at head of bed.

F. Technique.

1. Pneumoperitoneum–Veress or Hussan technique in infra-umbilical position.
2. Trocar insertion.
   a. 10-to 11-mm trocar in infra-umbilical position, camera port.
   b. Under direct vision, insert the surgeon's trocar (a 10- to 11-mm trocar) just to the right of the falciform ligament.
   c. Under direct vision, place assistant's trocars (two 5-mm trocars) below liver edge at the right anterior axillary line and right mid-clavicular line. It is helpful to grasp gallbladder (GB) via operative port and retract to RUQ to assess optimal position of assistant trocars.
3. Cholecystectomy.
   a. Grasp the fundus with the anterior axillary port access and retract the dome of the GB anterior and cephalad to expose the neck and cystic duct.
   b. Grasp Hartmann's pouch with the mid-clavicular line port and retract laterally to expose the cystic duct away from the CBD.
   c. Begin at the GB neck and dissect toward the cystic duct and CBD. (This junction must be identified during dissection.) During the dissection, the infindibulo-cystic vessels of glomus must be controlled. They are an invariable pair of vessels passing through the triangle of calot, perpendicular to the junction of the infindibulum and cystic duct.
   d. A cholangiogram can be attempted through a partially transected cystic duct after proximal clip application.
   e. If filling defects are present, the CBD can be cleared by the following procedures.
      (1) Simple irrigation.
      (2) Trans-cystic common duct exploration using Domier Lapkit or Fogarty embolectomy catheters.
      (3) Laparoscopic choledochoscopy.
      (4) Laparotomy with CBD exploration.
      (5) Post-operative endoscopic papillotomy.
   f. The cystic artery is then identified, isolated, and divided between clips.
   g. The GB is then carefully dissected from the liver starting at the neck and using the hook or spatula electrocautery with alternating medial and lateral traction, ensuring meticulous hemostasis with frequent irrigation.
   h. Remove the GB through one of the 10-mm ports.
   i. Irrigate and suction any residual intra-abdominal debris, bile, blood, or fluid.

   j. Re-inspect peritoneum, ensure hemostasis, then remove all trocars under direct vision.
   k. Close the fascia of the umbilical incision and the skin of all incisions.

G. Conversion to open procedure.

1. Required in 1-5% of cases.
2. Suspected injury to bile duct, viscus, or major blood vessel.
3. Unclear anatomy.
4. Unsuspected pathological findings–cancer, fistula.

H. Complications.

1. Complication rates of 1-5%.
2. Pneumoperitoneum.
   a. Gas embolism.
   b. Vagal reaction.
   c. Cardiac dysrhythmias.
   d. Hypercarbia with acidosis.
   e. Pulmonary compromise.
3. Trocar insertion.
   a. Bowel or bladder injury.
   b. Bleeding.
   c. Special considerations must be made for patients who have undergone previous abdominal surgery.
4. Cholecystectomy.
   a. Injury to bile ducts.
   b. Bleeding.
   c. Wound infection.

51

Laparoscopic Inguinal Hernia Repair

Gregory M. Tiao, M.D.

Over 500,000 inguinal hernias are repaired every year. To date, there exists no "perfect" inguinal hernia repair. Hernias repaired traditionally using autologous tissue to close the hernia have a recurrence rate between 5-10%. Hernias repaired using prosthetic mesh and tension-free suture lines appear to have a lower recurrence rate. Laparoscopic hernia repair is a recently developed alternative to traditional and mesh herniorrhaphy. Potential advantages of laparoscopic hernia repair include faster post-operative recovery rates and potentially lower recurrence rates. Disadvantages include the need for general anesthesia, the use of a posterior, buttressed repair with mesh, undefined recurrence rates, and potentially higher in-hospital costs.

A. Approach—There are three recognized laparoscopic approaches.

1. Trans-abdominal pre-peritoneal (TAPP).
2. Extra-peritoneal laparoscopic repair with laparoscopic mesh (ELM).
3. Intra-peritoneal laparoscopic onlay mesh (IPOM).

B. Anatomy of the pre-peritoneal space.

1. Laparoscopic approaches require understanding the inguinal anatomy in the pre-peritoneal space. In Figure 1, the key anatomical landmarks in the pre-peritoneal space are identified along with typical locations of a direct, indirect, and femoral hernia.
2. In both TAPP and ELM repairs, the herniated contents are reduced from within the abdomen and the defect in the abdominal wall is identified. The defect is closed with mesh stapled to the posterior surface of the abdominal wall, reinforcing the floor of all three hernia spaces. The mesh is tacked medially to the rectus sheath, inferiorly to the iliopubic tract beginning at Cooper's ligament, and superiorly and laterally to transversalis fascia, thus buttressing the myopectineal orifice. To avoid the femoral blood vessels medially and the genitofemoral and lateral femoral cutaneous nerves laterally, it is important not to staple below the iliopubic tract.

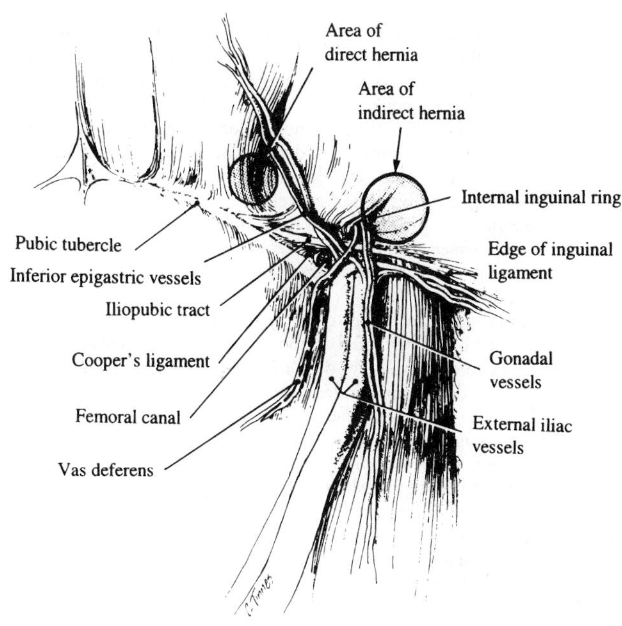

FIG. 1

C. Pre-operative preparation.

1. History and physical examination.
   a. In older patients with new hernia, consider etiology of straining (i.e., prostate cancer, colon cancer, pulmonary disease).
   b. Pre-operative antibiotic (i.e. 2nd-generation cephalosporin).
2. Relative contraindications to laparoscopic hernia repair.
   a. Previous lower abdominal operation.
   b. Known sliding or inguinal-scrotal hernia; reduction of these hernias can be difficult.
   c. Poor candidate for general anesthesia.

D. TAPP.

1. Operative procedure.
   a. Intra-abdominal laparoscopy using three ports, a 10-mm infraumbilical camera port, a 10-mm dissection port placed lateral to the rectus abdominis on the contralateral side to the hernia, and a 5-mm ipsilateral dissection port.
   b. Reduction of herniated abdominal contents and the peritoneum from the inguinal canal into the abdominal cavity.
   c. Incision of peritoneum high over hernia defect and entry into preperitoneal space.

d. Dissection within the preperitoneal space, exposing the abdominal wall defect. Cooper's ligament, the inferior epigastric vessels, the gonadal vessels, the vas deferens, and the internal inguinal ring should be identified.
e. Reinforcement of the posterior abdominal wall with mesh, thus closing the abdominal wall defect. The mesh is secured with staples medially to Cooper's ligament and the rectus sheath extending laterally to the transversalis fascia.
f. Reapproximation of the peritoneum, thus preventing direct contact between the abdominal viscera and the prosthetic mesh.
g. Closure of laparoscopy ports.

2. Advantages.
   a. Best established laparoscopic approach.
   b. Reduction of herniated abdominal contents is easier than with ELM, and the viability of the contents in a strangulated hernia may be determined under direct visualization.
   c. Easier to unroll and place mesh.
3. Disadvantages.
   a. If the peritoneum is not closed completely, there may be direct contact between mesh and abdominal contents, which may increase the risk for small bowel adhesions.
   b. This is an intra-abdominal procedure and has the attendant risks of perforation of intra-abdominal viscus and blood vessels on trocar placement.

E. ELM.

1. Operative procedure.
   a. Incision of the infra-umbilical anterior fascia, placement of a dissecting balloon below the rectus abdominis muscle, anterior to the posterior fascia. The dissecting balloon is advanced in this plane to the pubis and inflated developing the pre-peritoneal space. Low-pressure (10 mm Hg) CO_2 insufflation maintains the pre-peritoneal cavity.
   b. Placement of a 10-mm infraumbilical camera port, a 10-mm port between pubis and umbilicus, and a 5-mm port just above pubis; all ports placed in the midline.
   c. Reduction of herniated contents, including peritoneum from within the pre-peritoneal space.
   d. The dissection of the abdominal wall defect and its repair with mesh is similar to the TAPP procedure.
2. Advantages.
   a. Ideally, because the peritoneum is never violated, the risk of contact between intra-abdominal contents and mesh is minimized.
   b. Dissection of the abdominal wall defect can be easier than the TAPP.
   c. Avoids intra-abdominal cavity.
   d. Can be performed under regional anesthesia.
3. Disadvantages.
   a. Reduction of a large hernia sac can be more difficult than with the TAPP.

   b. If the peritoneum is accidentally entered, pneumoperitoneum can reduce the pre-peritoneal space, making the dissection difficult.

F. Results.

1. Retrospective studies.
   a. Results suggest that laparoscopic approach is viable with low complication rates and faster return to activity.
   b. Major limitation is short-term follow-up in all of the studies (maximum of 36 months). Studies of open repair have shown that a large percentage of hernia recurrences occur 5-10 years after surgery.
2. Prospective studies.
   a. Several small prospective randomized trials.
   b. Results indicate that patients repaired laparoscopically return to work faster with less post-operative pain. Medical cost may be higher, but the societal benefit of early return to work has not been measured.
   c. Follow-up is a limitation of all the studies.
3. Complications.
   a. Mortality 0.1%.
   b. Morbidity 0-6%.
   c. Recurrence 2-3%.

G. Conclusions.

Exact role of laparoscopic herniorrhaphy still remains to be determined. Laparoscopic hernia repair is a viable alternative to standard repairs. Patients with bilateral and recurrent hernias appear to be the best candidates for this type of approach. Large prospective randomized studies with long follow-up are needed to validate the use of laparoscopic herniorrhaphy.

52

Laparoscopic Appendectomy

MICHAEL J. GORETSKY, M.D.

I. HISTORY

A. First laparoscopic removal of an appendix was performed by Semm in 1983.

B. First laparoscopically resected inflamed appendix was performed by Schrieiber in 1987.

II. INDICATIONS—SAME AS FOR OPEN APPENDECTOMY

A. Proposed advantages.

1. Evaluation of the abdomen/pelvis when the diagnosis is in question.
   a. Women in childbearing years—can visualize pelvis, fallopian tubes, and ovaries.
   b. Elderly—can evaluate for perforated cecal cancer or diverticulitis.
2. Smaller incisions.
3. Better exposure in an obese patient.
4. Able to evaluate the entire abdomen.
5. Less post-operative pain.
6. Shorter hospital stay.
7. Earlier return to activities and work.
8. Reduction in the incidence of postop adhesions.
9. Reduced incidence of wound infections.

B. Results have been from a limited number of comparative prospective studies. The only significant difference between laparoscopic and open appendectomy has been a decrease in the incidence of wound infections for laparoscopy, which is believed to be secondary to removing the appendix through cannulas without touching the wound.

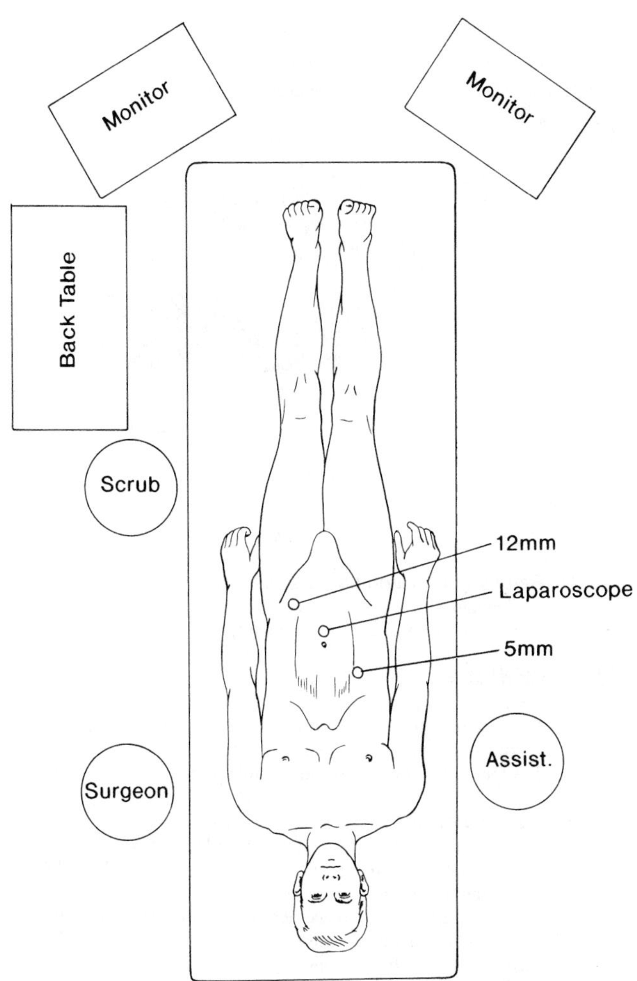

FIG. 1

III. CONTRAINDICATIONS

A. Absolute contraindications.

1. Patient cannot tolerate general anesthesia.
2. Coagulopathy.

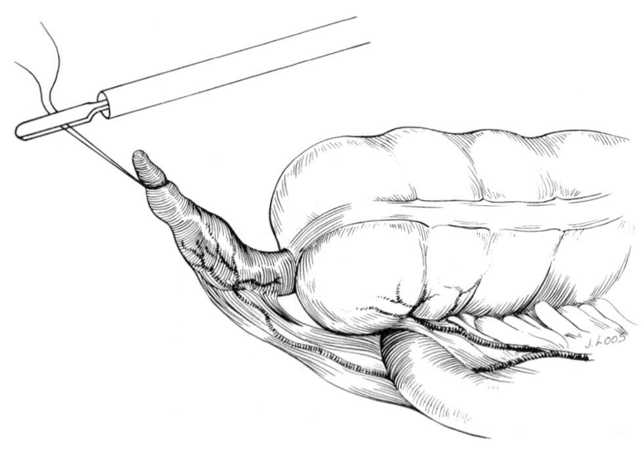

FIG. 2

B. Relative contraindications.

1. Pregnancy.
2. RLQ adhesions from previous surgery.

IV. TECHNIQUE

A. Setup.

1. Procedure performed under general anesthesia with bladder and stomach decompression.
2. Operating room setup and cannula placement is shown in Figure 1.

B. Cannula placement.

1. Infra-umbilical plament of a 10-mm laparoscope cannula.
2. LLQ (lateral to rectus muscle) placment of a 10- to 12-mm operative cannula.
3. RUQ/right midline placement of a 5-mm retractor cannula.

C. Procedure—many variations exist. In general, the technique used in Cincinnati is as follows.

1. The appendix is grasped with a forceps or an endoloop to expose its base through the RUQ cannula (Figure 2).
2. Using either a vascular stapler or clips to ligate vessels, the mesoappendix is taken down.
3. The appendix can either be amputated with a linear stapler or excised after an endoloop is placed at its base.
4. The appendix is removed through the 10- to 12-mm cannula after placing it in a bag. Care should be taken to avoid contact between the subcutaneous tissue and the inflamed appendix.

V. RESULTS

A. **No significant differences** have been found between laparoscopic and open appendectomies exist with regards to complications, length of hospital stay, and recovery time.

B. **When patients are subdivided by disease state,** patients with perforated appendicitis treated laparoscopically had a shorter hospital stay and received fewer days of antibiotics.

C. **Operative time costs are higher in laparoscopic appendectomies.**

53

Miscellaneous Laparoscopic Surgery

W. BRADLEY CRAFT, M.D.

I. LAPAROSCOPIC SURGERY

A. **First performed by Dr. George Kelling** in dogs in 1901.

B. **Only recently accepted into general surgical practice**—the first laparoscopic cholecystectomy was reported by Muehe in 1986.

C. **Current abdominal laparoscopic procedures** being performed include the following.

1. Abdomino-perineal resection.
2. Adhesiolysis.
3. Adrenalectomy.
4. Appendectomy.
5. Cyst aspiration.
6. Cholecystectomy and common bile duct exploration.
7. Colectomy.
8. Diagnostic–abdominal pain, abdominal trauma, malignancy.
9. Esophageal myotomy.
10. Gastric resection/gastroplasty.
11. Gynecological procedures.
12. Hernia repair–all types.
13. Ligamentum teres cardiopexy.
14. Meckel's diverticulectomy.
15. Nephrectomy.
16. Graham patch for perforated ulcer.
17. Splenectomy.
18. Staging of abdominal malignancy.
19. Ultrasonography.
20. Urologic procedures.
21. Vagotomy–highly selective, posterior truncal, anterior seromyotomy.

D. Proposed benefits.

1. Increased patient acceptance and satisfaction.
2. Decreased post-operative pain and narcotic use.
3. Shorter post-operative course and hospital stay.
4. Shorter convalescence.
5. Smaller wound with improved cosmesis.
6. Preserved abdominal wall strength.
7. Reduced costs.

E. Potential disadvantages.

1. Lack of controlled clinical trials.
2. Requires general anesthesia.
3. Requires training with a steep learning curve.
4. Anatomical limitations.
   a. Morbidly obese patients.
   b. Patients who have undergone previous surgeries.
5. Technical limitations.
   a. Two-dimensional operative field.
   b. Lack of tactile sense.
6. Longer operative times.
7. Increased costs.

II. LAPAROSCOPIC NISSEN FUNDOPLICATION

A. General.

1. All open abdominal surgical procedures for the treatment of gastroesophageal reflux have proved to be feasible laparoscopically. The Nissen repair is the most commonly used procedure.
2. Morbidity appears lower and mortality is similar to that obtained in open surgery.
3. Indications for operation are identical to the open technique.

B. Results.

1. Most series report good to excellent short-term symptomatic relief in > 90% of patients with gastroesophageal reflux disease (GERD) refractory to medical treatment.
2. Intra-operative complications occur in about 5% of cases; and there is an additional 5% post-operative morbidity. The most severe complication is mediastinal and peritoneal infection due to undetected esophageal injury. Mortality is less than 1%. These are similar to the results obtained with the open procedure.
3. Conversion to laparotomy is necessary in about 6% of cases, mostly as a result of difficult exposure or severe bleeding.
4. Post-operative feeding may be resumed the night of surgery, and hospital stay is typically 1-3 days.
5. Long-term results are not yet available for the laparoscopic treatment of GERD. As the procedures involved are the same as those used in open surgery, with equivalent short-term outcomes, the long-term results are expected to be similar.

III. LAPAROSCOPIC COLON RESECTION

A. General.

1. Laparoscopic approaches have been used for benign and malignant diseases and for resection of all areas of the colon.
2. The surgical techniques that are used are seldom purely laparoscopic. In most cases a mini-laparotomy is performed to remove the specimen or perform an anastomosis.
3. There currently are no prospective, randomized, controlled trials comparing open *vs* laparoscopic colectomy.
4. The laparoscopic approach has not been validated for the treatment of malignant tumors. Uncertainty persists regarding tumor recurrence at trocar sites. Several reports have documented early tumor recurrence in trocar and incision sites following laparoscopic colon resection for malignant disease.

B. Results.

1. Morbidity–studies report an average morbidity of 16.9% associated with laparoscopic colon resection. This compares favorably with the 21% morbidity associated with open procedures. Complications of laparoscopic colon resection have included enterotomy, splenic injury, hemorrhage, cerebrovascular accidents, bowel obstruction, abscess, anastomotic leak, UTI, ileus, wound infection, and upper GI hemorrhage.
2. Mortality ranges from 0 - 3.6%; for open colon resection mortality is 2 - 5%.
3. Conversions to open resection are high and vary from 7-41%. Reasons for conversion include unclear anatomy, adhesions, intra-abdominal abscess, bleeding, extensive malignant disease, and inability to locate the lesion laparoscopically.
4. Operative time has been reported to range from 40-310 min in most series, with an average of 158 minutes for colon resection by the most experienced surgeons.
5. Resumption of diet occurs on average at 2 days with discharge at 4.6 days, which is significantly shorter on average than following most open colon resections.

IV. LAPAROSCOPIC SPLENECTOMY

A. General.

1. Laparoscopic splenectomy was first reported in the literature in 1992 by Dr. A. DeLaitre from Paris.
2. Indications are identical to those for open splenectomy. Indications are idiopathic thrombocytopenic purpura (ITP), autoimmune anemia, hereditary spherocytosis, thrombotic thrombocytopenia purpura (TTP), and staging laparoscopy for Hodgkin's disease. Spleen size > 30 cm is a relative contraindication for laparoscopic splenectomy.
3. Several small series demonstrating the feasibility of laparoscopic splenectomy have been published; however, no prospective, randomized, controlled clinical trials are available to compare open *vs* laparoscopic splenectomy.

4. The spleen may be removed through a left lower quadrant muscle-splitting incision or through a trocar site if a tissue morcellator is used.
5. Operative time ranges from 2.5 to 7 h.
6. Procedure morbidity is in the 10-20% range; and mortality is 0-2%.

54

Non-Invasive Vascular Laboratory Studies

Kevin J. Ose, M.D.

The non-invasive vascular laboratory provides the clinician with an objective means of non-invasively and reproducibly assessing the hemodynamic effects of a variety of vascular lesions as well as following patients after medical or surgical intervention.

I. PERIPHERAL ARTERIAL STUDIES

A. Doppler arterial survey.

1. The presence of an audible signal in any vessel confirms its patency.
2. A normal multiphasic signal strongly suggests the absence of a significant proximal lesion.

B. Segmental limb pressures—measurement of multilevel, segmental, systolic pressures.

1. Most generally accepted and widely applied non-invasive technique for diagnosing extremity arterial occlusive disease.
2. Simple, reproducible, inexpensive, and well-tolerated.
3. Ankle/brachial index (ABI) [or the ankle pressure index (API)] is a simple ratio of ankle systolic pressure to arm systolic pressure that can establish the severity of the extremity ischemia. This can be performed at bedside with a blood-pressure cuff and a hand-held Doppler instrument.
   a. ABI 0.9-1.0–normal.
   b. ABI 0.5-0.8–claudication range.
   c. ABI < 0.3–rest pain range.
   d. Be sure to measure the systolic pressure of both brachial arteries and to use the highest value.
4. Disadvantages–localization of specific responsible lesions may be difficult.
   a. Aortoiliac disease in the presence of superficial femoral artery occlusion is particularly difficult to identify.

b. Segmental limb pressures in patients with calcified vessels that are not compressible (associated with diabetes mellitus or chronic renal failure) are meaningless.
c. Examiner must remember that distal pressures may represent the combined effects of more than one lesion.

C. Waveform analysis—segmental pulse volume waveforms.
1. Excellent assessment of segmental limb perfusion.
2. Less technician-dependent.
3. Not limited by vessel wall calcification.
4. Rapidly obtained using the same cuffs placed for segmental limb pressures.
5. Can be analyzed qualitatively with great accuracy.

D. Stress testing—allows quantitation of the physiologic impact of arterial lesions and the resulting functional disability.
1. Useful in studying patients who have exercise-related peripheral arterial complaints.
2. Treadmill exercise best reproduces exercise-induced reactive hyperemia in symptomatic patients.
3. In patients who cannot exercise, temporary pneumatic cuff occlusion is used to produce reactive hyperemia.

E. Upper extremity evaluation.
1. Atherosclerotic arterial occlusion is rare in the upper extremity; however, vasospasm, emboli, and trauma may result in ischemic symptoms, and non-invasive vascular studies may be helpful.
2. Useful in differentiating between vasospasm and collagen vascular disease of the upper extremity.
3. Evaluation of vascular complications of thoracic outlet syndrome.

F. Penile blood flow.
1. Detect impotence due to vascular insufficiency.
2. Penile-brachial index (PBI).
   a. PBI < 0.60 is compatible with vasculogenic impotence.
   b. PBI ≥ 0.75 is the lower limit of normal.

G. Color Flow Duplex Scanning (CFDS).
1. Pulse volume recording (PVR) tracings and segmental limb pressures are now often accompanied by CFDS. The CFDS is able to localize and quantify many of the lesions initially screened for by segmental limb pressures.
2. CFDS is also used to diagnose and size aneurysms and pseudo-aneurysms of the upper and lower extremities.
3. Bypass grafts of the upper or lower extremities are ideally scanned immediately post-operatively, 3 months, 6 months, and one year.

II. CEREBROVASCULAR STUDIES

A. A variety of tests are available. They are "indirect" if they evaluate hemodynamic alterations, and "direct" if they examine the anatomy at the carotid bifurcation.

B. Ocular plethysmography (OPG)—indirect measure of cerebrovascular occlusive disease. Two types are available: One device detects delay in pulse arrival in the eye (OPG-K), the second device measures ophthalmic systolic pressure (OPG-G). The second type, OPG-G, is most commonly used.

1. ***Advantages.***
   a. Sensitive and specific in recognizing hemodynamically significant lesions > 75% diameter reduction.
   b. More objective and less technician-dependent than other forms of indirect testing.
2. ***Disadvantages.***
   a. Small risk of minor eye irritation.
   b. Sensitive to only the most severe stenoses.
3. Criteria for significant stenosis (OPG-G).
   a. Right-to-left ophthalmic pressure difference ≥ 5 mm Hg.
   b. Right-to-left ophthalmic pressure difference of 1-4 mm Hg with ophthalmic-brachial pressure index < 0.66.
   c. No ophthalmic pressure difference, but an ophthalmic-brachial pressure index < 0.60. (Invalid if the patient is severely hypertensive.)
   d. Difference of ocular pulse amplitude ≥ 2 mm Hg.

C. Duplex scanners—combination of real-time B-mode image with pulse Doppler real-time frequency analysis. Velocity analysis also used as a diagnostic tool.

1. Color flow Doppler now available–more technician-dependent; however, can improve diagnostic accuracy.
2. Accurate but expensive diagnostic tool for assessing extracranial carotid and vertebral arteries.
3. Requires patient cooperation and skilled technologists for accurate reporting–> 90% positive predictive value with skilled technologist when compared to angiography.

III. NON-INVASIVE TESTING IN VENOUS DISEASE

A. Venous Doppler survey—inexpensive, simple means of assessing the presence of *proximal* venous obstruction.

1. Highly subjective and only used when other modalities unavailable.
2. Normal venous signals are phasic with respiratory variability and augment with compression of the extremity distal to the point of investigation.
3. A continuous venous flow signal lacking variation and unable to augment suggests either a proximal obstruction or external compression (i.e., tumor, pregnancy).
4. ***Advantages.***
   a. Applicability at the bedside.
   b. Ability to repeat the study frequently without patient discomfort.
   c. Low cost.

5. ***Disadvantages.***
   a. Accuracy is very technician-dependent.
   b. Limited to proximal (iliofemoral) venous obstruction.
   c. Accuracy decreases with isolated calf clot because of the presence of paired veins and extensive collaterals.

B. Plethysmography—the study of changes in limb volume.

1. Two principal types.
   a. Occlusive techniques–strain-gauge plethysmography, IPG.
   b. Non-occlusive techniques–phleborrheography.
2. IPG studies the changing resistance to passage of an electrical current (impedance) through the lower extremity relative to changes in its blood volume.
3. IPG measures resting limb volume and records the response to temporary venous occlusion and its subsequent relief.
   a. A pneumatic cuff is placed on the thigh and temporarily inflated to 50-60 cm of H_2O pressure, and changes in calf volume (as reflected in decreasing electrical impedance) are measured.
   b. When tracing plateaus, the cuff is released and the decrease in venous volume (as reflected in increased electrical impedance) is measured over 3 sec.
   c. During cuff inflation, a normal limb will exhibit a rapid increase in calf volume due to unobstructed arterial inflow.
   d. Upon release of the cuff, the veins will empty rapidly and cuff volume will return to baseline within 3 seconds.
   e. The obstructed venous system will frequently demonstrate reduced filling, since the obstruction has already engorged the veins, and venous emptying through collateral channels is inefficient and results in a marked slowing of venous outflow.
4. Numerous studies comparing IPG to venography document a sensitivity of 60-75% and specificity of 50%.
5. ***Disadvantages.***
   a. False-positive results may occur as a result of other causes of venous outflow obstruction (gravid uterus, tumor, edema, etc.) or hemodynamic impairment (congestive heart failure, severe arterial insufficiency, chronic lung disease).
   b. The patient who is cold, anxious, or uncooperative may present difficulties in interpretation owing to vasoconstriction or muscular contraction.

C. Venous photoplethysmography (PPG)—used to assess the degree of chronic venous insufficiency.

1. Measures changes of skin blood content after standard exercise.
2. Photo-electric cells placed on the skin over the malleolus, and venous refilling time is recorded after repeated dorsiflexion of the foot.

   a. Normal–venous refilling time is often > 25 sec.
   b. In venous valvular incompetency–refilling time is greatly shortened (< 20 sec) because of constant reflux from incompetent venous valves.
3. Tourniquet is then applied to thigh, calf and ankle at a pressure of 50 mm Hg to occlude the superficial venous system.
   a. Test is then repeated.
   b. Differentiates superficial from deep venous insufficiency.
4. Color flow Doppler now used to assess venous insufficiency–valve site imaged (i.e., common femoral vein or popliteal vein) and while imaging, patient uses Valsalva maneuver. The technologist records the presence or absence of reflux. *Disadvantage:* Not quantifiable and very technician-dependent.

D. Duplex venous imaging and color flow Doppler.

1. Most exams now performed use color flow Doppler information in conjunction with the B-mode image; portable studies are sometimes limited to conventional duplex scanning. These modalities provide both anatomic and hemodynamic information of vessels tested.
2. Criteria used to determine the presence of a thrombus.
   a. Compressibility–normal veins are under very low pressure and do not have the elastic walls of arteries. In the presence of a non-occlusive thrombosis the vein will partially compress, whereas normally the vein will compress wall to wall.
   b. Doppler and/or color Doppler exam–presence or absence of respiratory variation and augmentation.
   c. Dilation of veins–in acute, occlusive deep venous thrombosis, the veins are dilated 2-3 times the size of the adjacent artery.
   d. Echogenicity–normal vessels without thrombus appear different from acutely thrombosed vessels.
3. Duplex scanning may differentiate fresh from chronic thrombus and can even identify a new clot superimposed on preexisting chronic disease.
4. With experienced technicians, accuracy of the study approaches 100% and has all but replaced venography in the evaluation of lower extremity deep venous thrombosis.
5. ***Disadvantages.***
   a. Accessibility is limited to vessels of the upper and lower extremity and extrathoracic jugular system. Imaging of the iliac veins and intrathoracic veins are less accurate because of interference by intra-abdominal and intrathoracic structures.
   b. This is expensive, time-consuming, technician-dependent study.

E. Diagnosis of suspected acute deep venous thrombosis (algorithm).

1. Use of any one of the non-invasive venous tests is superior to the clinical diagnosis of deep venous thrombosis.

2. A combination of IPG and duplex scan theoretically takes advantage of the strength of each and minimizes the possibility of missing clinically important thrombosis, but results in a decrease in specificity.
   a. A negative IPG rules out the possibility of proximal venous obstruction.
   b. A scan is able to evaluate calf veins for thrombosis.
3. Visualization of thrombus on a scan is sufficient to warrant institution of therapy, as is an unequivocally positive IPG in a patient without a previous history of ipsilateral deep venous thrombosis.
4. Venography is reserved for confirmation of positive or equivocal Duplex scan when one of the clinical sources of a false-positive result (congestive heart failure, arterial insufficiency, etc.) is present.

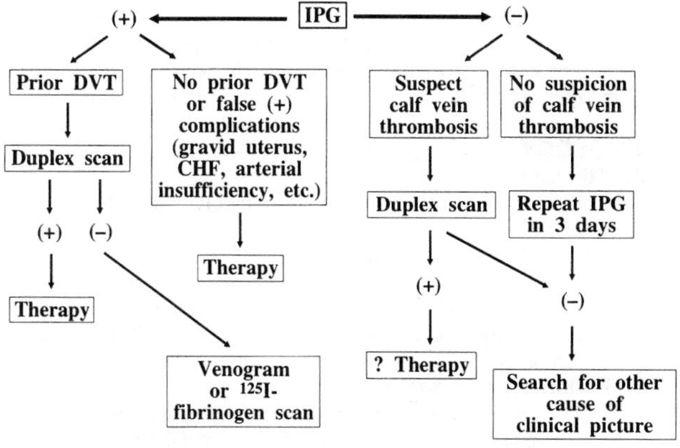

55

The Diabetic Foot

Robert C. Bass, M.D.

There are approximately 10 million diabetics in the United States (20% type I and 80% type II). Diseases of the foot are responsible for 20% of hospitalizations in diabetics, and lower extremity disease is the most common disorder requiring operation. Approximately two-thirds of all nontraumatic lower extremity amputations are performed on diabetics.

I. ETIOLOGY

A. Atherosclerosis.

1. Peripheral vascular disease tends to be bilateral and multisegmental.
2. "Small vessel disease" in diabetics can result in ischemic tissue, despite the presence of strong dorsalis pedis or posterior tibial pulses, and probably results from abnormal formation of capillary basement membranes during periods of hypoglycemia. There are no obstructive lesions.

B. Peripheral neuropathy.

1. Occurs in diabetics with disease of 10 years or more duration.
2. May be related to deposition of sorbitol metabolites in nerves.
3. Affects the motor, sensory, and sympathetic nerve supply to the lower limbs.
4. Resultant motor weakness and sensory loss leads to structural deformities (hammer toes, hallux valgus, Charcot joints) and improper weight bearing.

C. Impaired immunity.

1. Abnormal PMN function at blood glucose levels greater than 250 mg/dl.
2. Decreased leucocyte chemotaxis.
3. Impaired phagocytosis and intracellular killing.

D. Charcot joints.

1. Abnormal weight-bearing leads to painless osteoarthritis and joint deformities.
2. Resultant inflammation may mimic infection.
3. Can precipitate mal perforans ulcers.

II. PATHOLOGY

A. Foot or toe ulcer.

1. Results from injury, ischemia, foreign body.
2. Neuropathy prevents patient from noticing trauma, exacerbating injury.

B. Mal perforans ulcer.

1. Plantar ulcer with a long narrow tract that extends to the tarsal-metatarsal joint.
2. Abnormal weight-bearing over metatarsal heads leads to callous formation and plantar ulceration.
3. Usually requires ray amputation for complete healing.

C. Infection.

1. Begins with minor foot trauma or trivial break in the skin.
2. Inadequate circulation and impaired host defense permits spread of infection.
3. Continued ambulation causes spread of infection along fascial planes.
4. Infections are **polymicrobial,** with *B. fragilis, Proteus, Clostridium,* anaerobic *Streptococcus,* and enterococci.

III. TREATMENT

A. Treatment of non-infected foot ulcers.

1. Assess extent and severity.
2. Assess degree of neuropathy and vascular insufficiency.
3. Control blood glucose.
4. Judicious debridement of devitalized tissue and callouses.
5. Local wound care and wet to dry dressings.
6. Improve circulation, revascularization if indicated.
7. Careful follow-up and podiatric appliances.

B. Treatment of the infected diabetic foot.

1. *Failure to aggressively treat even trivial appearing diabetic foot infections places the patient's life and limb in jeopardy.*
2. Assess neuropathy, circulation.
3. Radiographs to rule out soft-tissue gas or osteomyelitis.
4. Wound and/or tissue cultures.
5. Broad-spectrum antibiotics (i.e., clindamycin/gentamicin, or Unasyn®/gentamicin or Unasyn®/ceftazidime).
6. For abscess or gangrene, operative intervention to drain abscess or amputate nonviable tissue.
7. Aggressive wound care and debridement.
8. Control metabolic abnormalities, glucose.
9. Absolutely no weight-bearing.
10. Revascularization may be indicated once infection has cleared.
11. May require skin graft or tissue flap for wound closure.

C. Prevention.

1. Most important aspect of diabetic foot care.
2. Non-constricting footwear.
3. Nail care, treat mycotic nail infections.

4. Keep web spaces clean and dry, inspect daily.
5. Daily examinations of plantar surface, with mirror, for injury or foreign bodies. Unrecognized injuries are common in diabetics with neuropathy.
6. Minor injuries should be brought to the physician's attention.

56

Acute Limb Ischemia

Kevin J. Ose, M.D.

I. ETIOLOGY

A. Arterial embolism.

1. Cardio-arterial embolization–most common source of peripheral emboli is the heart.
   a. Mural thrombus (previous myocardial infarction, atrial fibrillation, rheumatic heart disease, mitral stenosis, cardiomyopathy).
   b. Endocarditis.
   c. Atrial myxoma.
2. Arterio-arterial embolization–proximal arterial source.
   a. Aneurysmal source, in order of decreasing frequency–aortic, popliteal, femoral.
   b. Atheroembolism ("blue toe syndrome") from an ulcerating atherosclerotic plaque in a proximal large artery.
   c. Paradoxical embolus–venous embolic source that passes through an intracardiac shunt (ASD/VSD); rare.

B. Arterial thrombosis.

1. Atherosclerosis–clot on the surface of a plaque, hemorrhage beneath a plaque, stenosis, aneurysm.
2. Congenital anomaly.
   a. Popliteal entrapment.
   b. Adventitial cystic disease.
3. Infection.
4. Hematologic disorders (i.e., polycythemia).
5. Flow-related disorders (congestive heart failure, shock, dehydration).

C. Arterial trauma—iatrogenic *vs.* incidental.

1. Blunt (e.g., posterior knee dislocation).
2. Penetrating–direct injury to vessel, indirect through cavitation of a missile.
3. Iatrogenic–arterial monitor, angiography, cardiac catheterization, arterial blood sample.

D. **Drug-induced vasospasm**—with particular attention to illicit drug use and inadvertent arterial injection.
E. **Aortic dissection.**
F. **Severe venous thrombophlebitis**—phlegmasia alba dolens.
G. **Prolonged immobilization.**
H. **Idiopathic.**

II. INITIAL ASSESSMENT

A. **History.**
   1. Pain–onset, location, duration.
   2. History of previous claudication.
   3. Cardiac disease–valvular heart disease, atrial fibrillation, cardiomyopathy, myocardial infarction.
   4. Recent trauma.
   5. History of hypertension, chest or back pain.
   6. Drugs–ergotamines, dopamine, or history of IV drug use.
   7. Low-flow states–septic shock, dehydration, hemorrhage, congestive heart failure.

B. **Examination.**
   1. ***5 Ps*** of acute arterial insufficiency–**p**ain, **p**aralysis, **p**aresthesias, **p**allor, **p**ulseless. A 6th "P" that is sometimes added is "polar" (cold).
   2. Trophic skin and nail changes consistent with long-standing arterial insufficiency.
   3. ***Complete bilateral*** pulse examination, including auscultation for bruits and portable Doppler exam when unable to appreciate pulses by palpation.
   4. Assessment of limb viability.
      a. Muscle turgor (soft = viable, "doughy" = non-viable).
      b. Neurologic status–paralysis and anesthesia generally indicate a non-viable limb.
   5. Cardiac examination–rhythm, murmurs, rub.
   6. ***Chest radiograph*** and **abdominal radiographs**–look for wide mediastinum and vascular calcifications.
   7. ***EKG***—look for evidence of myocardial infarction, atrial fibrillation.

III. SECONDARY ASSESSMENT

A. **Duration—"golden period"** of 6 h before ischemia and myonecrosis may become irreversible.
B. **Non-invasive studies** can be helpful but must **not delay** definitive therapy.
C. **Indications for arteriography** (not necessary if diagnosis is readily apparent).
   1. Determine site of vascular obstruction, identify inflow.
   2. Suspected thrombosis.
   3. Suspected aortic dissection.
   4. Suspected multiple emboli.

D. Operative risk.

1. Most patients have underlying heart disease, which, in conjunction with the need for emergent surgery, make operative risk **high** in this setting.
2. Embolectomy under local anesthesia carries a lower operative risk than amputation or attempted revascularization.

IV. MANAGEMENT OF ACUTE ARTERIAL INSUFFICIENCY

A. Immediate heparinization in all cases to prevent further propagation of thrombus–bolus with 5,000-10,000 units of heparin, then start continuous infusion (~ 1,000 units/h) to maintain PTT at 1.5 to 2 times normal.

B. Arterial embolization.

1. Axial limbs 70-80% of sites.
2. Generally lodges at bifurcations of vessels:
   a. Common femoral–approximately 36%.
   b. Aortoiliac–approximately 22%.
   c. Popliteal trifurcation–approximately 15%.
   d. Upper extremity–approximately 14%.
3. Mortality is higher with more proximal location–aorta > iliac > femoral > popliteal.
4. After heparinization, emergent surgical embolectomy is treatment of choice.
   a. Local anesthesia.
   b. Isolation of artery (usually common femoral) with proximal and distal control.
   c. Fogarty® balloon-tipped catheter is introduced through an arteriotomy and passed beyond the area of clot. Balloon is inflated and catheter withdrawn, bringing clot out in front of it. May need to "milk" lower leg to remove small vessel clots. (Separate popliteal arteriotomy may be useful in some cases.)
5. Need **completion angiography** after removal of thrombus.
   a. "Back bleeding" and clinical examination are poor indicators of success.
   b. 20% of patients will have a good functional result after embolectomy despite absent distal pulses.
6. Continue heparin post-operatively; begin Coumadin® on day 3, continue until patient no longer at risk for further emboli; discontinue heparin when patient is adequately anticoagulated on Coumadin®.
7. ***Identify and treat the underlying cause*** (atrial fibrillation, mitral stenosis, myocardial infarction).
8. Watch for "reperfusion phenomenon."
   a. Ischemic muscle converts to anaerobic metabolism, with paralysis of the cellular Na^+-K^+ pump. The pH falls while concentrations of K^+, lactic acid, muscle enzymes, myoglo-

bin and oxygen free radicals all rise dramatically. Once the threatened muscle is reperfused, these toxic metabolites circulate throughout the body and can cause renal failure as well as multi-organ system failure.

b. Myoglobin precipitates in the renal tubules (acidic environment), leading to necrosis with a worsening spiral of oliguria, hyperkalemia, and metabolic acidosis.

c. Treatment–when myoglobin is present (red urine).
   (1) Correct hyperkalemia.
   (2) Alkalinize urine with intravenous $NaHCO_3$.
   (3) Give osmotic diuretic–mannitol (1 g/kg IV).
   (4) Fasciotomy to decompress compromised muscle.
   (5) Hemodialysis if necessary.

d. The mortality with this syndrome can be quite high.

C. Atheroembolism ("blue toe syndrome")–caused by occlusion of small digital vessels with palpable pulses in the major peripheral arteries.

1. Heparinization acutely–long-term anticoagulation is of no value.
2. Elective angiography to search for treatable embolic causes.
3. Thromboendarterectomy or complete arterial replacement with prosthetic graft if the source is identified.

D. Arterial thrombosis.

1. Generally suspected from history and exam (claudication, trophic skin changes, lack of palpable pulses on opposite side).
2. Previous collateralization may prevent development of myonecrosis.
3. Arteriography is key for identifying optimal surgical approach.

E. Arterial trauma.

1. Generally results from intimal flap with resultant thrombosis.
2. Penetrating injuries are most common (missile, blast, fracture, severe ligament tears and dislocation at the knee).
3. Arteriography mandatory–embolectomy and repair or bypass of damaged vessel.

F. Venous thrombosis (see also "Thromboembolic Prophylaxis and Management of DVT").

1. Major venous thrombosis involving the deep venous system of the thigh and pelvis produces characteristic clinical picture of pain, extensive edema, and blanching, termed **phlegmasia alba dolens**.
2. As impedance of venous return from the extremity progresses further, there is danger of limb loss from cessation of arterial flow leading to congestion, cyanosis, and distended veins, termed **phlegmasia cerulea dolens.**
3. Risk of venous gangrene if pulses are absent mandates heparinization and venous embolectomy with protective distal arteriovenous fistula.

G. Drug-induced vasospasm—treat by discontinuing drug; occasionally use of IV nitroprusside drip (vasodilatation), phentolamine (alpha blockade), or topical nitropaste is of value.

H. Aortic dissection.

1. Identify by history (hypertension, back/chest pain) and exam (absent pulses throughout).
2. Aortography (including thoracic arch) if suspected.

I. Thrombolytic therapy.

1. Lysis of clot by continuous arterial infusion of streptokinase or urokinase.
2. Should be considered when the morbidity and mortality of the surgical alternative are higher than the anticipated risks of thrombolytic therapy (i.e., acute myocardial infarction).
3. May be of use with occlusion of tibial and popliteal vessels, where surgical results are less successful.
4. Patients with "blue toe syndrome" or "trash foot" may also be candidates.
5. Use in patients with thrombosis of previous bypass grafts may be particularly effective.
6. May only be used when limb is *clearly viable* because it may take 24-36 h for circulation to be restored.

J. Compartment syndrome.

1. Caused by severe ischemia for an extended period.
2. Ischemia causes cell membrane damage and leakage of fluid into the interstitium.
3. Tissue swelling within a closed fascial compartment causes muscle necrosis and nerve ischemia.
4. If suspect, compartment pressures should be measured immediately. If > 40 mm Hg $\Rightarrow$ fasciotomy.
5. Fasciotomies allow muscles to expand and relieve high pressure.

K. Peri-operative management.

1. Extremity pulses checked frequently.
2. Neurological checks of extremities.
3. Follow motor function.
4. Monitor electrolytes, urinary output, etc.

V. PROGNOSIS

A. Mortality rate for arterial occlusion is 10-20%.

B. 5-15% of patients with arterial embolism require **amputation.**

C. Amputation is procedure of choice in patients with irreversible ischemia or those unable to tolerate extensive reconstruction.

D. The major factor in mortality is underlying cardiac disease.

57

Abdominal Aortic Aneurysm

Kevin J. Ose, M.D.

I. ETIOLOGY

A. **Atherosclerosis** in aneurysm patients is usually not causative.

B. **Inflammatory—**possibly autoimmune phenomenon.

C. **Infection—**mycotic or bacterial etiology–rare. Tertiary syphilis and *Salmonella* have been implicated.

D. **Traumatic—**rare cause; usually occurs in the thoracic aorta.

E. **Marfan's syndrome—**cystic medial necrosis.

F. **Genetic factors (?)—**The formation of abdominal aortic aneurysms is probably a multi-factorial degenerative process.

II. ANATOMY

A. **Abdominal aorta** from diaphragmatic hiatus at T-12 to bifurcation at L-4.

B. **Celiac axis** at the upper portion of L-1, superior mesenteric artery (SMA) at the lower one-third of L-1, inferior mesenteric artery (IMA) at L-3, and renal arteries at the upper portion of L-2.

C. **Normal diameter—**approximately 2 cm.

III. PATHOLOGY

A. **Location.**

1. Below origin of renal arteries in 95% of cases.
2. May extend to involve common iliac arteries, rarely beyond.

B. **Size—**from 3 to 15 cm, usually fusiform aortic dilation. Mycotic aneurysms are typically saccular in nature.

C. **Other manifestations** of diffuse atherosclerosis associated with abdominal aortic aneurysm (AAA).

1. Coronary artery disease–30%.
2. Hypertension–40%.

3. Associated occlusive arterial disease.
   a. Carotids–7%.
   b. Renals–2%.
   c. Iliac–16%.
4. Associated with other clinically significant aneurysms–thoracic aorta (4%), femoral (3%) and popliteal (2%) arteries.

IV. NATURAL HISTORY

A. 5-year rate of rupture of untreated AAA.

1. 7 cm or larger = 75%.
2. 6 cm = 35%.
3. 5-6 cm = 25%.

B. 5-year survival of untreated AAA.

1. < 6 cm = 48%.
2. ≥ 6 cm = 6%.

C. Autopsy studies—5% of aneurysms < 5 cm had ruptured, 39% of aneurysms 5-7 cm, and 65% of aneurysms > 7 cm had ruptured.

D. Increased size = increased risk of rupture.

V. CLINICAL PRESENTATION

A. Typical presentation—Most aneurysms are asymptomatic and are found on routine abdominal examination or ultrasound/CT scan done for other reasons.

B. Actively leaking AAA may present with abdominal, back, or flank pain due to tension on peritoneum from aneurysm or blood. Complaints may be mild or severe; requires a high index of suspicion. A leaking AAA may rapidly result in exsanguination due to free intraperitoneal rupture.

C. With leakage or free rupture, patients may present in shock.

VI. PHYSICAL EXAMINATION

A. Presence of pulsatile mass on deep palpation—5 cm aneurysm palpable in most patients.

B. Tortuous aorta may mimic AAA, presenting as a pulsating, expansile abdominal mass different from other abdominal masses that merely transmit aortic pulsations (pseudocyst, pancreatic carcinoma, etc.).

C. In thin individuals, aortic pulsations may be unusually prominent; however, careful bimanual palpation should confirm normal diameter.

D. Important to evaluate other peripheral arteries for associated occlusive disease (pulses and bruits) or further aneurysmal disease.

VII. DIAGNOSTIC STUDIES

A. Abdominal plain films are often diagnostic. Calcific rim ("egg shell") is often visible projecting anterior to the spine on cross-table lateral view.

B. Ultrasound (B-mode) is the simplest, least expensive method of detecting and following aortic aneurysms.

C. Abdominal CT scan is the most accurate but most expensive means of diagnosing and following AAA.

D. Aortography.

1. Poor study for diagnosis or assessment of size, as mural thrombus within AAA can obscure actual aneurysm size. Aortography provides important information regarding associated vascular lesions, however.
2. Indications for aortography.
   a. Hypertension–to rule out renovascular causes.
   b. Unexplained impairment of renal function.
   c. Aneurysm near renal arteries.
   d. Symptoms compatible with visceral angina.
   e. Evidence of peripheral artery occlusive disease.
   f. Evidence of "horseshoe" kidney.
   g. Angiogram being performed in another vascular bed (coronary/carotid/vertebral arteries).

VIII. CARDIAC WORK-UP OF ELECTIVE AAA REPAIR

Owing to high incidence of concomitant coronary artery disease and post-operative cardiac complications, the cardiac work-up is an essential part of the pre-operative evaluation. The following diagram may be useful:

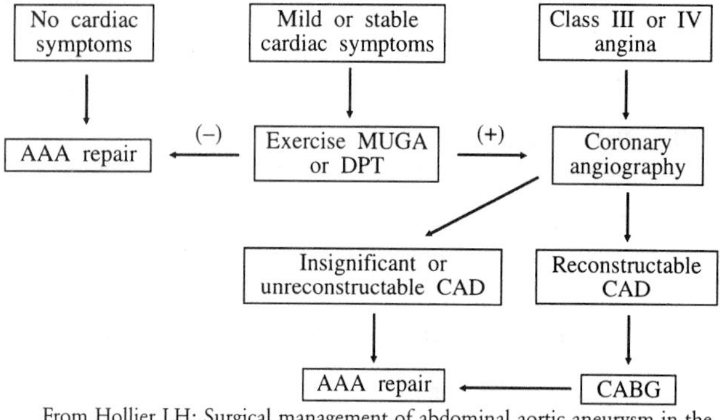

From Hollier LH: Surgical management of abdominal aortic aneurysm in the high-risk patient. *Surg Clin North Am* 66:2:269–279, 1986, with permission.

IX. OPERATIVE INDICATIONS

A. Patients with aneurysms > 4-5 cm are candidates for elective operation unless concomitant medical problems increase the operative risk or a 2nd pathological process markedly reduces the patient's life expectancy.

B. Size increase of > 0.5 cm/6 months.

C. When aneurysm becomes symptomatic, operation becomes imperative regardless of aneurysm size.

X. MANAGEMENT OF RUPTURED AAA

A. Diagnosis.

1. Abdominal pain–may be associated with back or flank pain and shock of varying degree (may be very mild).
2. Pulsatile mass–may be palpable in 50%; may be absent owing to hypotension.
3. Rupture–contained *vs.* free. Free rupture is usually associated with hemodynamic instability.
4. Clinical exam is most important–hemodynamically unstable patients go directly to the O.R. Stable patients with questionable presence of AAA may undergo emergent abdominal CT scan or ultrasound.
5. May simulate other intra-abdominal or medical conditions (renal colic, pancreatitis, myocardial infarction, muscular backache, etc.); therefore, a high index of suspicion is needed.

B. Therapy.

1. Rapid and maintained replacement of blood loss with crystalloid and blood transfusion to correct hypotension.
2. Midline approach used with rapid isolation of the aorta just below diaphragm for proximal control (approach via the gastro-hepatic omentum); clamping for approximately 30 min is possible without significant visceral ischemia.
3. Infra-renal clamp placed after aneurysm incised and surrounding hematoma evacuated, providing better visualization and avoiding damage to renal vasculature.
4. Low-porosity woven or PTFE graft should be used with ruptured AAA, as pre-clotting is not possible.
5. Renal insufficiency most common complication postoperatively. May be prevented in part by mannitol (12.5 g) or furosemide (40 mg) infusion prior to anesthesia induction.
6. Mortality rate is approximately 50%.

XI. ELECTIVE MANAGEMENT OF AAA

A. Pre-operative preparation.

1. Optimize cardiovascular function and fluid volume.
2. Mechanical +/− antibiotic bowel preparation. Paregoric® given orally pre-operatively reduces size of small bowel.
3. Establish water diuresis with adequate IV hydration before anesthesia and maintain during surgery. A thermodilution pulmonary artery catheter (Swan-Ganz®) may be helpful

during pre-operative hydration and peri-operative maintenance of adequate filling pressures and cardiac output. Mannitol (50 g) IV prior to cross-clamping aorta helps maintain adequate glomerular filtration rate.

4. Peri-operative parenteral antibiotics.

B. **Via midline or transverse incision,** aorta is mobilized and infrarenal clamp is placed for proximal control.

C. **Iliac arteries clamped** for distal control.

D. **IMA ligated** from within the aneurysm to avoid injury to collateral vessels to the left colon. (In patients with decreased visceral blood supply and patent IMA, it may be necessary to reimplant artery into graft.)

E. **Anterior portion of aneurysm wall** is opened and thrombus is removed.

F. **Posterior wall** is left in place and lumbar vessels suture ligated.

G. **Prosthetic graft** sewn in place.
   1. Tube graft if iliac arteries are normal.
   2. Bifurcation graft if iliac arteries are aneurysmal.

H. **Non-resective surgical therapy.**
   1. In a high-risk patient, axillo-bifemoral graft with induced aortic aneurysm thrombosis via catheter deposition of thrombogenic material or coil is a *rarely* used option.
   2. High complication rate, including thrombus extension into renal or mesenteric arteries and rupture of aorta, have caused most surgeons to abandon this form of therapy.

XII. COMPLICATIONS

A. **Atheroembolism** ("trash foot").
   1. Results from occlusion of small distal lower extremity arteries from embolization of aneurysmal sac fragments, or from thrombosis due to extended aortic clamp time.
   2. Large emboli above the ankle can be removed with an embolectomy catheter.

B. **Myocardial ischemia, arrhythmia, and infarction.**
   1. Arrhythmias–very common.
   2. Fatal myocardial infarction in 3% of elective patients, 10% of symptomatic patients, and 16% of ruptured AAA cases.
   3. Coronary artery disease is responsible for 50-60% of all deaths secondary to AAA repair.

C. **Renal insufficiency.**
   1. Causes.
      a. Hypovolemia.
         (1) Pre-operative dehydration.
         (2) Blood loss from leaking or ruptured aneurysms.
         (3) Intra-operatively when aortic cross-clamp is removed; can be prevented by adequate hydration.
         (4) Inadequate operative fluid replacements.

b. Atheromatous debris or thrombus dislodged during the procedure and embolizing to the kidney (renal atheroembolism).
c. Renal artery occlusion from aortic cross-clamping must be considered.

2. Oliguric renal failure–$< 3\%$, but $> 20\%$ of patients with ruptured aneurysms. Mortality rate of patients with renal failure and ruptured AAA is approximately 50%.

D. Stroke—can be embolic or secondary to hypotension.

E. Colon ischemia.

1. Normally there are two prominent collaterals between the SMA and the IMA: (1) marginal artery of Drummond; (2) meandering mesenteric artery (not normally present in the absence of SMA or IMA stenosis). These may be stenosed or occluded by the general atherosclerotic process.
2. Prevent ischemia and assure adequate perfusion by several intra-operative maneuvers.
   a. Palpate the root of the SMA–determine whether it is pulsatile.
   b. Examine the IMA orifice from within the opened aneurysm sac–determine whether it is open (retrograde bleeding). A large, wide-open IMA suggests the need to reimplant the artery.
   c. Doppler ultrasound–presence of audible Doppler flow over the base of the large bowel mesentery and serosal surface appears to be at higher risk of ischemic colitis.
   d. Fluorescein–ultraviolet luminescence should show bowel viability.
3. Suspect ischemia if patient has bowel movement during the first 24-72 h post-operatively. Stool is usually positive for blood (grossly or by heme test).
   a. Mucosal ischemia most common and usually manifested by mucosal sloughing; resolves spontaneously in most cases.
   b. Requires immediate sigmoidoscopy for diagnosis.
   c. Transmural involvement will require re-exploration and colonic resection with colostomy.

F. Spinal cord ischemia—rare after AAA repair; more common with thoracic aneurysm repair.

1. Syndrome–paraplegia with loss of light touch and pain sensation and loss of sphincter control. Proprioception and temperature sensation are spared.
2. Pathology.
   a. Anterior spinal artery is formed in the neck and supplies the spinal cord.
   b. Several "anterior radicular arteries" feed into the anterior spinal artery.
   c. The lowest (and largest) anterior radicular artery usually

arises at the T8-L1 level, but occasionally the origin is lower, leading to obliteration with abdominal aortic surgery (0.5% of cases).

G. Chylous ascites—can occur as a result of inadequate ligation of lymphatics during proximal aortic dissection.

H. Late complications.

1. Aortoenteric fistula.
   a. *De novo* or more commonly from proximal suture line of aortic graft.
   b. Distal portion of duodenum most common location–82% duodenum, 8% small bowel, 6% large bowel, 5% stomach.
   c. Presentation–GI bleeding with associated abdominal and back pain; may have "herald bleed" of more minor degree followed by exsanguinating hemorrhage.
   d. Diagnosis–endoscopy to rule out other source; if no definitive site is found, graft-enteric fistula must be assumed.
   e. Treatment–remove graft, oversew aorta, repair enteric defect; drain retroperitoneum (with or without antibiotic irrigation); extra-anatomic bypass (axillo-bifemoral).
2. Late infection of prosthetic graft material requires extra-anatomic bypass and removal of infected graft material and oversewing the aortic stump.
3. Sexual dysfunction.
   a. Retrograde ejaculation and/or inability to maintain erection in 30-40% of men due to aorto-iliac surgery.
   b. Caused by injury to sympathetic plexus around the aorta and failure to maintain hypogastric perfusion.

XIII. PROGNOSIS

A. Surgical repair has been shown to double survival time of patients with abdominal aortic aneurysm.

B. Operative mortality for elective repair is 1-2%.

C. Mortality for emergent repair of ruptured AAA ranges from 20% to 80% (mean = 50%) depending on the condition of the patient at presentation.

58

Cerebrovascular Disease

Kevin J. Ose, M.D.

Unrecognized carotid disease remains a major source of morbidity and mortality. Not every bruit requires invasive work-up and surgical intervention. On the other hand, some symptoms require aggressive investigation.

I. GENERAL CONSIDERATIONS

A. **Stroke** is the third leading cause of death in the U.S.

B. **Mortality of stroke** in the U.S. is approximately 188,000 deaths per year.

C. **Incidence of stroke** in the U.S. is approximately 160 per 100,000 population.

D. **Surgical goal** with cerebrovascular disease is the relief of symptoms of cerebral dysfunction and the prevention of stroke.

II. ANATOMY

A. **Anterior circulation**—carotid artery distribution; posterior circulation–vertebrobasilar system. Collateral flow between the circulations is dependent upon the circle of Willis.

B. **Right common carotid artery** originates from innominate artery; left common carotid artery originates from aortic arch.

C. **Internal carotid artery** originates at common carotid bifurcation–divided into four distinct anatomic portions.
1. Cervical–no branches.
2. Petrous–no branches.
3. Cavernous–ophthalmic artery.
4. Cerebral–cerebral arteries.

D. **External carotid artery** originates at common carotid bifurcation. In the face of extracranial internal carotid artery occlusive lesions, the external system will provide collateral circulation to the intracranial supply via the ophthalmic artery. External carotid artery branches (caudad–cephalad).
1. Superior thyroid.
2. Ascending pharyngeal.
3. Lingual.
4. Facial.

5. Occipital.
6. Posterior auricular.
7. Maxillary.
8. Superficial temporal.

E. Vertebral arteries—first branch off the subclavian artery, they pass through foramen in the transverse processes of the cervical vertebrae and enter the skull in the foramen magnum. The vertebral arteries unite within the skull to form the basilar artery. The basilar artery bifurcates into the two posterior cerebral arteries.

III. CLINICAL MANIFESTATIONS

A. Transient ischemic attack (TIA).

1. Episode of neurologic dysfunction lasting from a few minutes to no more than 24 h with no residual deficit.
2. Commonly affects vision of ipsilateral eye–**amaurosis fugax,** a transient blindness of one eye ("Like a shade closing over my eye").
3. Ipsilateral hemispheric symptoms–transient paresis and/or paraesthesias of contralateral extremity.
4. Risk of stroke–10% to 15% within the first year of onset of symptoms, then 2-4% per year thereafter.
5. Crescendo TIA–repeated neurologic events without interval neurologic deterioration. An indication for *emergent* cerebral angiography.

B. Reversible ischemic neurologic deficit (RIND)—neurologic dysfunction lasting > 24 h, but resolves in less than 2 weeks.

C. Stroke—acute neurologic deficit lasting longer than 24 h.

1. ***Stroke with minimal residual deficit*** (minimal or no residual neurologic dysfunction).
   a. Patients with completed stroke continue to have risk of further strokes at a rate of 5-9% per year, with a 5-year cumulative risk of 25-45%.
   b. Patients with severe deficits with minimal improvement should not be considered for carotid endarterectomy.
2. ***Stroke in evolution***—neurologic deficit gradually worsens over a period of hours or days.

D. Vertebrobasilar system disease causes "posterior" symptoms–headaches, vertigo, equilibrium changes, "drop attacks", bilateral visual disturbances, pharyngeal sensory loss, vasomotor and respiratory center changes.

E. Subclavian steal syndrome.

1. Proximal subclavian artery stenosis (proximal to vertebral artery).
   a. Subclavian artery unable to supply adequate blood flow to the arm during exertion.
   b. The blood flows retrograde down the ipsilateral vertebral artery to supply the subclavian artery distal to the stenosis. Exercise or use of the arm decreases vascular resistance

in the arm, leading to increased blood flow via the vertebral artery, decreased cerebral flow, and cerebral symptoms.

c. Most patients are asymptomatic.

d. Concurrent carotid disease may predispose to symptoms.

2. Symptoms–vertigo plus syncopal episodes; rarely (< 10%) correlated with arm exercise.
3. Stroke uncommon with this disorder.

F. **Asymptomatic carotid stenosis**—pre-occlusive plaque in internal carotid artery that has not yet produced monocular or hemispheric symptoms.

1. Associated with an increased incidence of a neurologic event (TIA and/or stroke).
2. Stenosis is significant if the lumen is compromised by 60% or more, and these patients should be considered for carotid endarterectomy (ACAS study–*JAMA,* May 10, 1995).

IV. PATHOLOGY

A. Etiology.

1. In Western countries, atherosclerosis is the primary pathologic event (> 90%).
2. Non-atherosclerotic causes of carotid stenosis (10%) include inflammatory angiopathies, fibromuscular dysplasia, kinking secondary to arterial elongation, extrinsic compression, traumatic occlusion, and spontaneous dissection.

B. **Obstruction at the carotid bifurcation** with proximal internal carotid involvement is most common location for atherosclerotic disease.

C. Carotid ulceration.

1. Loss of endothelium in the central portion of the lesion exposes loose atheromatous material and leads to platelet aggregation. This may result in distal embolization of debris.
2. Classification of ulcers.
   a. "A"–minimal discrete cavity within atheromatous plaque.
   b. "B"–large cavity with higher stroke rate.
   c. "C"–multiple cavities or cavernous appearance, causing high stroke and death rate.

D. Risk factors.

1. Age–individuals > 70 years old have 8 times greater incidence of stroke than those < 50 years old.
2. Atherosclerosis risk factors, including hypertension, smoking, diabetes, hyperlipidemia.
3. Associated factors–coronary artery disease, peripheral vascular disease.

V. DIAGNOSIS

A. Physical exam.

1. Bilateral upper extremity blood pressure.
2. Peripheral pulses–indicates peripheral vascular disease.
3. Neck bruits–very high-grade stenoses may not have audible bruits.

4. Neurologic exam.
5. Ophthalmic exam.

B. Noninvasive (see also "Non-invasive Vascular Laboratory Studies").

1. ***Doppler ultrasonic peri-orbital examination.***
   a. Internal carotid stenosis or occlusion is collateralized by flow via the connections between the external carotid and ophthalmic arteries.
   b. Doppler measures the direction and velocity of flow through the superficial temporal artery.
   c. Highly technician-dependent (subjective test results).
   d. No anatomic visualization.
2. ***Oculopneumoplethysmography.***
   a. Determine and compare ophthalmic artery pressure in both eyes.
   b. Ophthalmic artery pressure is unilaterally decreased.
   c. Suggests > 70% stenosis of the ipsilateral internal carotid artery, but does not localize lesion.
3. ***Duplex scanning***—combines B-mode image plus Doppler spectral analysis. This has largely replaced all other forms of testing.
   a. Best non-invasive test to identify carotid bifurcation disease.
   b. Provides accurate anatomic and flow information.
   c. Can determine the following.
      (1) Percent stenosis.
      (2) Nature of plaque.
      (3) Surface irregularity.
   d. High-grade stenosis is often misread as occlusion.
   e. Can identify flow reversal (i.e., subclavian steal syndrome).
4. ***Color-flow imaging.***
   a. Can evaluate flow in large areas and multiple vessels simultaneously.
   b. Effective for evaluating areas of flow disturbances (kinks, coils, occluded vessels, etc.). This technique does not improve accuracy, but it helps ensure more accurate placement of the Doppler flow sample.
   c. Evaluates vertebral arteries as well as other cervical vessels.

B. Cerebral angiography—not for screening purposes alone (work-up should start with non-invasive tests).

1. Indications–surgical candidates only:
   a. TIAs, stroke with minimal residual deficit.
   b. Significant carotid artery stenosis indicated by non-invasive testing.
   c. Acute stroke–use is controversial.
2. Arteriography.
   a. Visualization of all 4 neck vessels (carotids and vertebrals) and aortic arch.

b. 75% of patients with strokes have angiographically demonstrable lesions (40% of these are extracranial).
3. Digital subtraction imaging–contrast may be administered IV or intra-arterial. Contrast load is usually reduced. Resolution and visualization of small lesions may be less than conventional arteriography.

C. CT/MRI—obtain pre-operatively for the following reasons.
1. Rule out abnormalities other than cerebral infarction (i.e., intracerebral hemorrhage).
2. Determine the extent and nature of an infarction, identify previous silent infarct.

VI. OPERATIVE INDICATIONS

Procedure of choice is carotid endarterectomy (CEA).

A. TIA.
1. Multiple TIAs in the distribution of a diseased carotid artery (high-grade stenosis, ulcerated plaques, or mixed consistency plaques).
2. Single TIA with carotid bifurcation stenosis in excess of 50%.
3. Recurrent TIAs while patient is on anti-platelet drugs (along with lesion amenable to repair by CEA).

B. Stroke with minimal residual deficit.
1. Patients who have had a hemispheric stroke with good recovery (have obtained recovery plateau).
2. Carotid artery lesions amenable to operation.
3. Surgical team with low combined morbidity/mortality rate.

C. Asymptomatic carotid stenosis.
1. Carotid artery stenosis > 60%.
2. Patient is otherwise healthy with a life expectancy > 5 years.
3. Surgical team with combined morbidity/mortality rate < 3%.

D. Global ischemic symptoms—patients with evidence for combined vertebral-basilar and severe carotid disease may be candidates for CEA.

E. Acute stroke—generally considered a contraindication to CEA, but there are a few individual exceptions.

F. Stroke-in-evolution—indicated only in carefully selected patients by highly competent surgeons.

VII. CONTRAINDICATIONS TO SURGERY

A. Overall poor general condition.

B. Acute stroke—controversial.

VIII. SURGICAL COMPLICATIONS

Patients should be closely monitored in an ICU for 24 h postoperatively.

A. Wound hematoma—procedure performed under full heparinization. Potential for airway compromise.

B. Hypertension/hypotension.

1. Interference with baroreceptor mechanisms of the carotid sinus results in blood pressure lability.
2. Treatment–adequate fluid volume, nitroprusside, dopamine, and neosynephrine drips as needed.

C. Cranial nerve injury.

1. Recurrent laryngeal–vocal cord paralysis, hoarseness, poor cough mechanism.
2. Hypoglossal–unilateral tongue paralysis; tongue points to the side of the injury.
3. Marginal mandibular–drooping at corner of mouth.
4. Superior laryngeal–early voice fatigability, loss of high-pitch phonation.

D. Post-operative stroke, worsening of neurologic deficits, death.

1. Embolization of debris secondary to operative manipulations.
2. Intimal flap created at time of surgery.
3. Current accepted standards for peri-operative mortality < 2%, peri-operative stroke rate < 5% for symptomatic patients, < 3% for asymptomatic patients.

E. Post-operative myocardial infarction—leading cause of death following surgery.

59

Mesenteric Ischemia

Kevin J. Ose, M.D.

Mesenteric ischemia is an uncommon entity that carries a high mortality rate, usually as a result of delay in diagnosis. Successful treatment requires a high index of suspicion and recognition of both the chronic and acute forms.

I. ANATOMY AND PHYSIOLOGY

A. Circulation deficits in GI tract are uncommon due to abundant collateral circulation between:

1. Celiac axis.
2. Superior mesenteric artery (SMA).
3. Inferior mesenteric artery (IMA).

B. Collateral vessels.

1. Pancreaticoduodenal arcade (celiac and SMA).
2. Branch of left colic artery (SMA and IMA).
3. Marginal artery of Drummond–often small, not continuous, especially at splenic flexure (SMA and IMA).
4. Arc of Riolan (SMA and IMA).

C. Physiology.

1. Circulation increases with digestion, decreases with exercise.
2. Mesenteric vessels undergo *vasoconstriction* due to the following.
   a. Sympathetic stimulation.
   b. Decreased blood flow.
   c. Drugs (e.g., digitalis).

II. ACUTE MESENTERIC ISCHEMIA

A. Clinical presentation—hallmark is severe acute midabdominal pain *out of proportion* to physical findings.

1. Early–prominent symptoms of GI emptying (i.e., nausea, vomiting, diarrhea). Diffuse abdominal tenderness without peritoneal signs; active bowel sounds may be present.
2. Late–symptoms of intestinal infarction. Hypotension, acidosis, eventually leading to shock. Fever, bloody diarrhea, and

peritonitis develop late and are ominous findings. Mortality at this point 80-85% despite intervention.

3. Early diagnosis improves survival.

B. Etiology.

1. Embolization of SMA (40%)–one-third of patients have antecedent embolic episodes (lower extremity embolus, cerebrovascular accident). Patients with potential sources of emboli (atrial arrhythmias, atrial myxoma, mural thrombi) are at risk.
2. Thrombosis of SMA (40%)–thrombus formation on atherosclerotic plaque. Often preceded by symptoms of chronic mesenteric ischemia (postprandial pain, weight loss, bloating, diarrhea).
3. Non-occlusive ischemia (20%)–vasoconstriction of mesenteric vasculature due to low cardiac output ("low flow state"). Common predisposing conditions are myocardial infarction, congestive heart failure, renal or hepatic disease, medications such as digoxin, trauma, or operation leading to hypovolemia or hypotension.

C. Management—simultaneous fluid and electrolyte resuscitation and evaluation should be conducted *expeditiously.* Mesenteric angiography (with lateral views of aorta) is the *definitive* diagnostic test.

1. If peritonitis is present or there is evidence of intestinal infarction, immediate abdominal exploration should be performed.
2. Embolus–arteriography shows occlusion of SMA, with embolus lodged just beyond inferior pancreaticoduodenal and middle colic arteries ("meniscus sign").
   a. Systemic heparinization should be initiated.
   b. Angiography catheter may be used to infuse papaverine both pre- and post-operatively.
   c. Following adequate resuscitation, immediate exploration should be performed. Embolectomy is performed via transverse arteriotomy in SMA. Arteriotomy may be closed with or without vein patch.
   d. Assess bowel viability by direct inspection and/or fluorescein examination. Administer sodium fluorescein (1 g IV) and inspect the bowel under ultraviolet (Wood's) lamp. Viable bowel has a smooth, uniform fluorescence.
   e. Consider "second-look" operation to re-inspect bowel if there is questionable viability.
3. Thrombosis–arteriogram shows complete occlusion of SMA at origin. Usually very little collateralization.
   a. *Immediate* operation is necessary. Diagnosis is often made late, and extensive bowel necrosis is present. At exploration, bowel is often gray and pulseless.
   b. Revascularization should be attempted with aortomesenteric bypass graft (prosthetic or saphenous vein).

c. Resect non-viable bowel *after* revascularization. Consider a "second-look" operation.

4. Non-occlusive–arteriography shows marked narrowing and "pruning" of distal mesenteric vessels, but not large vessels.
   a. Treatment is primarily non-operative. Patients are often extremely ill and poor surgical risks.
   b. Optimize cardiac output (if possible).
   c. Angiographic catheter should be left in place in SMA and infuse papaverine
   d. Repeat angiography is performed after 24 h.
   e. Laparotomy indicated if peritoneal signs are present.

III. CHRONIC MESENTERIC ISCHEMIA

A. **Atherosclerotic involvement** of 2 of 3 main visceral arteries.

B. **Diagnosis**—symptoms often applicable to multiple etiologies (i.e., gallbladder disease, occult GI cancer, etc.).
   1. Chronic epigastric abdominal pain, colicky in nature, occurring 30-60 minutes after meal. May be relieved by defecation.
   2. Involuntary weight loss ("food fear").
   3. Presence of abdominal bruit.
   4. Angiography–used after other disease entities ruled out. Should include lateral view of aorta and take-off of vessels.

C. **Treatment**—surgical revascularization is indicated.
   1. Nutritional repletion.
   2. Bypass grafting.
      a. 2-vessel aortomesenteric graft (saphenous vein or prosthetic).
      b. Combined infra-renal aortic implant and aortomesenteric graft.
   3. Transaortic endarterectomy–for multiple-vessel disease.

D. **Prognosis**—relief of pain in 90% of cases.
   1. Best long-term results with multiple-vessel revascularization.
   2. Recurrence 10-30% with multiple-vessel revascularization *vs.* 50% for single-vessel.

IV. MESENTERIC VENOUS THROMBOSIS

A. **Clinical presentation**—In contrast to that of acute arterial ischemia, onset of symptoms is usually insidious in nature.
   1. Abdominal pain *out of proportion* to physical findings. Usually sudden in onset.
   2. May show the following.
      a. Signs of hypovolemia.
      b. Low-grade fever.
      c. Active bowel sounds.
      d. Abdominal distension.
      e. Localized tenderness (if infarction has occurred).
      f. Heme-positive stools are common.

B. Etiology.

1. Association with another pathological process (malignancy, visceral infection, pancreatitis, portal hypertension, trauma, etc.).
2. Hypercoagulable states due to coagulation disorders.
3. Idiopathic.

C. Diagnosis.

1. Leukocytosis.
2. Radiographs–may show distended small bowel loops, portal venous gas, or gas in bowel wall.
3. Barium enema–thumbprinting, lumenal narrowing.
4. Angiography–prolonged arterial phase; non-visualization of the venous phase, reflux of contrast into the aorta.
5. CT scanning–visualization of intraluminal thrombus, enlargement of thrombosed vein.
6. Duplex scanning of the mesenteric and portal veins has also been used.

D. Treatment—begins with fluid and electrolyte resuscitation.

1. Early heparinization for suspected thrombosis.
2. Antibiotics.
3. Laparotomy for peritonitis or suspected infarction.
   a. Wide resection followed by re-anastomosis usually recommended.
   b. Thrombectomy considered for large segments of compromised bowel.
   c. Consider second-look operation.
4. Post-operative care–continue anticoagulation, possibly for life.
5. Evaluate the etiology of thrombosis, including work-up for hypercoagulable state.

60

Renovascular Hypertension

Robert A. Cusick, M.D.

I. DEFINITION—Systemic hypertension resulting from decreased renal blood flow and subsequent activation of the renin-angiotensin system.

- **A. Most common surgical cause of hypertension.** Other surgical causes include coarctation of the aorta, primary aldosteronism, Cushing's syndrome, pheochromocytoma, renal parenchymal disease.
- **B. Found in < 5% of individuals with hypertension.**
- **C. The activation of the renin-angiotensin system** is protective to prevent renal parenchymal injury during times of inadequate perfusion.

II. PHYSIOLOGY (Figure 1).

- **A. Background**—Originally described by Goldblatt 50 years ago. He demonstrated that hypertension could be produced by 80% narrowing of the renal artery.
- **B. Renin is released from the juxtaglomerular apparatus** in response to a decrease in Na^+ concentration or decreased perfusion. Renin proteolytically cleaves angiotensinogen to angiotensin I and has a half-life of 20-30 min. Angiotensin-converting enzyme causes cleavage of angiotensin I (a decapeptide) to angiotensin II (an octapeptide) in the lung.
- **C. Angiotensin II** is the most potent vasoconstrictor known and causes contraction of smooth muscle in all vascular beds. Angiotensin II causes hypertension and stimulation of aldosterone secretion from the adrenal gland. Angiotensin II (half-life 4 min) is cleaved to form angiotensin III, which also causes aldosterone release.
- **D. Aldosterone** is produced by the zona glomerulosa of the adre-

nal gland. It increases intra-vascular volume by the reabsorption of sodium and water accompanied by the loss of potassium.

III. PATHOLOGY.

A. Atherosclerosis.

1. This represents 70% of renovascular hypertension.
2. Primarily occurs in elderly males (sixth decade of life).
3. The proximal one-third is usually affected, and this plaque is continuous with aortic plaque in 75% of cases.
4. 30-50% are bilateral; the left renal artery is more often affected.

B. Arterial fibrodysplasia—heterogenous disorder, accounting for 20-25% of renovascular hypertension.

1. Intimal fibrodysplasia.
   a. Accounts for 5% of dysplastic disease. There is no gender predominance; it occurs primarily in young people.
   b. Etiology–thought to be related to persistence of embryonic myointimal cushions, trauma, or abnormal flow patterns.
   c. The lesion can be focal, diffuse, or even form a web.
2. Medial fibroplasia.
   a. Accounts for 85% of dysplastic lesions and occurs primarily in young (30-50) women.
   b. Other arteries, such as the internal carotids and iliacs, can be affected.
   c. Etiology–unknown, may be related to changes in smooth muscle cells under the influence of estrogens or damage caused by stretching during pregnancy.
   d. Forms focal stenosis surrounded by microaneurysms in the mid and distal renal artery, which resembles a "string of beads" on angiogram.
   e. 85% involve the right renal artery, 70% are bilateral.
3. Peri-medial fibrodysplasia.
   a. Accounts for 10% of dysplastic lesions, usually affects young women.
   b. More progressive than medial fibrodysplasia. Etiology is unknown.
   c. Solitary or multiple areas of stenosis without dilatations in the distal renal artery.

C. Developmental renal artery disease.

1. Rare cause of renovascular hypertension; affects males and females equally.
2. Arteries are hypoplastic at their origin from the aorta and have an hourglass shape.
3. Accounts for 40% of renovascular hypertension in children.
4. Etiology–may result from abnormal fusion of the dorsal aorta during development. Can be associated with coarctation of the abdominal aorta or aortic hypoplasia.

D. Other causes of renovascular hypertension–aneurysms, arteriovenous malformations, dissections, renal artery thrombosis, cholesterol emboli from renal arterial plaques.

IV. CLINICAL MANIFESTATIONS

A. **Upper abdominal bruits** (found in > 50% of patients with renovascular hypertension (RVH), only 5% of patients with essential hypertension).
B. **15% of individuals with diastolic hypertension > 115 mm Hg** have renovascular hypertension.
C. **Sudden worsening of stable hypertension.**
D. **Hypertension before age 35** or rapid onset of hypertension after age 50.
E. **Malignant or drug-resistant hypertension.**
F. **Decreased renal function** after starting patient on an ACE inhibitor.

V. DIAGNOSIS

A. **Labs**—urinalysis with culture, creatinine, potassium, peripheral renin.
B. **Arteriography.**
   1. The "gold standard"–other tests only help determine who will undergo angiogram.
   2. Demonstration of collateral vessel indicates physiologically significant stenosis.
   3. A pressure gradient of 10% is adequate to cause increased renin secretion.
C. **Other tests.**
   1. Renin activity–peripheral renin normal in 25% of patients with RVH.
   2. Renal vein renin ratio.
      a. Affected renal vein renin divided by unaffected renal vein renin level.
      b. In renovascular hypertension, ratio is > 1.5.
      c. In 15% of patients, disease is bilateral, so ratio will be <1.5.
   3. Renal Systemic Renin Index (RSRI).
      a. $$\frac{\text{renal vein renin - systemic renin}}{\text{systemic renin}}$$
      b. Indicative of RVH if > 24% for one kidney or > 48% for both.
   4. Intra-arterial digital subtraction angiography–less contrast and renal toxicity.
   5. Rapid-sequence intravenous pyelogram (1, 2, 3 minutes after contrast injection).
      a. Affected kidney > 1.5 cm smaller than contralateral kidney.
      b. Sensitivity 70%, 10% false-positive results, 75% false negatives in children.
   6. Isotopic renography.

a. Used to assess both renal blood flow and excretion.
b. Sensitivity and specificity 75%.

VI. TREATMENT

A. Medical therapy.

1. Requires close follow-up, compliant patient, and life-long medications. Even with control of hypertension renal mass and function can be lost in up to 40% of patients.
2. Reported mortality from surgical and medical therapy is 30% and 70%, respectively.
3. Beta-blockers are the first line of therapy. ACE inhibitors are the most effective therapy, but may worsen renal function (especially patients with atherosclerotic disease).

B. Percutaneous transluminal renal angioplasty.

1. Developed in 1978 by Gruntzig. Involves a controlled disruption of the vessel wall. Treatment of choice for medial fibromuscular dysplasia and short segments of stenosis in the main renal artery.
2. Atherosclerotic lesions, especially involving the ostia and aorta, have a higher complication and recurrence rate.
3. > 90% of patients improve, but long-term results are still unclear.

C. Surgical therapy.

1. Has been associated with an increased survival as compared with medical therapy. Must be initiated prior to irreversible parenchymal loss.
2. Pre-operative preparation–patients are often hypovolemic and hypokalemic from excessive diuretic use.
3. Nephrectomy–rare (< 10% of patients), only in severe unilateral disease with uncontrollable hypertension, renal artery < 7 cm, complete occlusion, nephrosclerosis.
4. Endarterectomy–can be used for renovascular disease involving the aorta and both renal arteries.
5. Renal artery revascularization.
   a. Initial revascularization is critical, re-operation associated with a high nephrectomy rate (50%).
   b. Transverse, supraumbilical incision usually used.
   c. Saphenous vein grafts (SVG), PTFE (Gortex), and Dacron all used with similar patency in adults.
   d. Renal artery bypass often accompanies aortic repairs for occlusive or aneurysmal disease.
   e. Special procedures–splenic, gastroduodenal, or hepatic artery all used.
4. Results.
   a. Nephrectomy is very successful.
   b. Patients with fibrodysplastic disease and lateralizing renins do better. Older patients with atherosclerosis do worse.
   c. Mortality 1-2%.

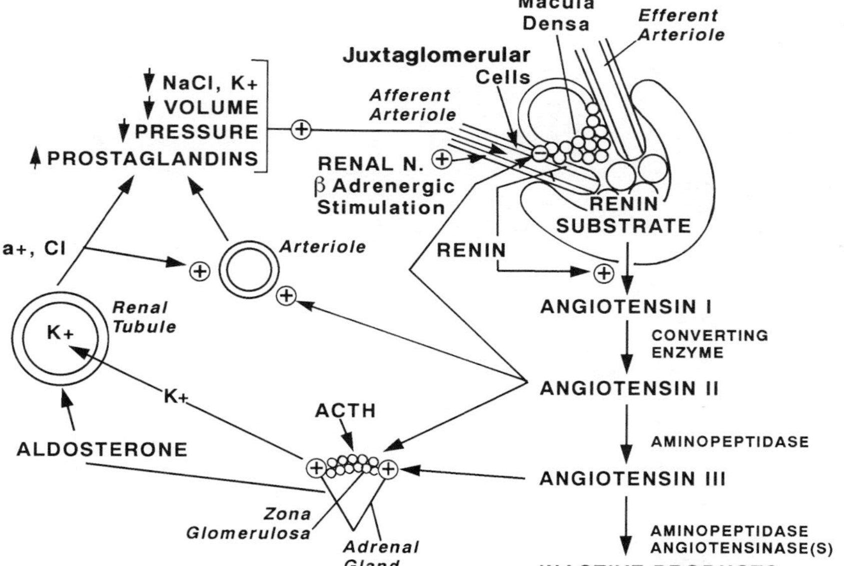

FIG. 1 Renin-Angiotensin-Aldosterone System

d. Overall, 80-90% better or cured in carefully selected patient groups:
   (1) Pediatric fibrodysplasia: 97%.
   (2) Adult fibrodysplasia: 94%.
   (3) Adult focal atherosclerosis: 91%.
   (4) Adult diffuse atherosclerosis: 72% (but only 24% cured).

61

Pediatric Surgery

David A. Rodeberg, M.D.

Children, particularly neonates, are not simply little adults. They have their own particular diseases and physiologic responses. In general, however, surgical philosophy and the approach to surgical disorders are similar to those in adults.

I. FLUID AND ELECTROLYTE REQUIREMENTS

A. Maintenance fluids.

1. Body weight method:

Body Weight	Free Water / Hour	Free Water / Day
0-10 kg	4 ml/kg/h	100 ml/kg/d
11-20 kg	40 ml for 1st 10 kg + 2 ml/kg/h for each kg > 10 kg	1000 ml + 50 ml/kg/d for each kg > 10 kg
> 20 kg	60 ml for 1st 20 kg + 1 ml/kg/h for each kg > 20 kg	1500 ml + 20 ml/kg/d for each kg > 20 kg

2. Body surface area method: 2000 ml/m^2/24 h (not accurate for infants < 10 kg body weight; requires calculation of body surface area from nomogram using height and weight).

B. Maintenance electrolytes.

1. Na^+–3-5 mEq/kg/24 h.
2. K^+–2-3 mEq/kg/24 h.
3. Ca^{++}–2 mEq/kg/24 h.
4. Mg^{++}–0.15-1 mEq/kg/24 h.

C. Resuscitation fluids.

1. Crystalloid–lactated Ringer's or normal saline solutions, 10-20 ml/kg.
2. Blood products.
   a. Whole blood–10-20 ml/kg.
   b. Packed RBC's–5-10 ml/kg.
   c. Plasma–10-20 ml/kg.
   d. 5% albumin–10-20 ml/kg.
   e. 25% albumin–2-4 ml/kg.

II. TOTAL PARENTERAL NUTRITION

Indicated in states of prolonged ileus, gastrointestinal fistulas, supplementation of oral feeds (short bowel syndrome, malabsorption states), catabolic wasting states (malignancy or sepsis), treatment of necrotizing enterocolitis. Children, particularly neonates, have little nutritional reserve, so parenteral nutrition must be considered early.

A. **Total maintenance rates for IV fluids** typically are calculated first, then the concentration of nutrients in the TPN is gradually increased daily.

B. **Estimate maintenance water requirements** (section I.A).

C. **Caloric requirements** (include allowance for stress, growth):
   1. 0-1 years–90-120 kcal/kg/day.
   2. 1-7 years–75-90 kcal/kg/day.
   3. 7-12 years–60-75 kcal/kg/day.
   4. 12-18 years–30-60 kcal/kg/day.

D. **Protein calories** (approximately 15% of total calories):
   1. 0-1 years–2.0-3.5 g/kg/day.
   2. 1-7 years–2.0-2.5 g/kg/day.
   3. 7-12 years–2.0 g/kg/day.
   4. 12-18 years–1.5 g/kg/day.

E. **Lipid calories** (approximately 30-40% total calories, should not exceed 50%):
   1. Lipid formulations:
      a. 10% = 10 g/100 ml = 1.1 kcal/ml.
      b. 20% = 20 g/100 ml = 2.0 kcal/ml.
   2. Begin with 0.5 g of lipid/kg/day and increase by 0.5 g/kg/day to a maximum of 3.0 g/kg/day.

F. **Carbohydrate calories** (approximately 50% total calories)–Minimum glucose infusion rate of 4-6 mg/kg/min for neonates.

III. TRAUMA (see "Trauma," section III.J.).

IV. LESIONS OF THE HEAD AND NECK

A. **Branchial cleft anomalies.**
   1. Branchial sinuses and cysts are remnants of embryologic structures.
   2. Most common anomaly arises from second branchial cleft (fistula from tonsillar fossa to anterior border sternocleidomastoid).
   3. Fistulas are usually discovered in childhood; cysts frequently are not seen until adulthood.
   4. Fistulas present with mucoid discharge; cysts present as mass anterior and deep to the upper third of the sternocleidomastoid. May become infected; 10% are bilateral; risk of *in situ* carcinoma in adults.
   5. Treatment–if infected, require incision and drainage; otherwise, excised during formal neck dissection under general anesthesia.

B. Thyroglossal duct remnants.

1. Thyroid develops from an evagination in the base of the tongue (foramen cecum) to the anterior larynx. If thyroglossal duct persists, the tract forms a cyst(s), which may become enlarged and symptomatic.
2. Most frequently occurs as a rounded, cystic mass of varying size in midline of the neck inferior to the hyoid that moves with swallowing and protrusion of the tongue.
3. Document presence of remaining normal thyroid tissue separate from the cyst prior to excision.
4. Symptoms include dysphagia, pain, or simple mass; may become infected. Symptoms of hypothyroidism may be present. Rarely a site for adult carcinoma.
5. Treatment involves total excision of the cyst, the central body of the hyoid bone, and the tract to the foramen cecum. If total excision of all thyroid tissue is unavoidable, thyroxine supplementation will be required.

C. Cystic hygroma.

1. Benign tumor of lymphatic origin.
2. Most located in the posterior triangle of the neck. Can cause respiratory insufficiency in infancy or when the glottic structures is involved.
3. 90% diagnosed by second year of life.
4. Sudden enlargement usually due to hemorrhage in the lesion.
5. Treatment is by excision, although radical surgery (i.e., excising involved blood vessels and nerves) is contraindicated. An initial trial of sclerotherapy may be effective.

V. THORACIC DISORDERS

A. Pulmonary sequestration.

1. Lung tissue that lacks bronchial communication to the normal tracheobronchial tree; blood supply derived from systemic arterial source.
2. Extra-lobar–2/3 diagnosed in infancy.
   a. 90% located in left posterior costophrenic sulcus.
   b. Rarely manifests as respiratory insufficiency, most frequently is asymptomatic and found incidently on chest radiograph. Feeding difficulty may be common, but infection is uncommon unless in communication with GI tract.
   c. Arterial supply usually low thoracic or abdominal aorta; venous drainage into azygos or hemiazygos system.
   d. Commonly have coexisting congenital anomalies (15-40%).
   e. Invested in its own visceral pleura.
3. Intralobar–majority diagnosed after age 1, often in adulthood.
   a. Should suspect in patients with recurrent pneumonias within the same bronchopulmonary segment.

b. 60% in left hemithorax; communicates with normal lung only via the pores of Kohn; become infected as a result of inadequate drainage.
c. Arterial supply similar to extralobar; venous drainage via pulmonary vein of affected lobe, causing a left-to-right shunt that can progress to CHF.
d. Incorporated within normal pulmonary parenchyma.

4. Diagnosis by plain radiograph and arteriography.
5. Symptomatic sequestrations require resection; extralobar by simple excision; intralobar frequently requires formal lobectomy; life-threatening hemorrhage possible if systemic vascular supply not recognized and controlled intra-operatively.

B. Bronchogenic cysts.

1. Derived from abnormal budding of the primitive tracheobronchial tube; most commonly seen in mediastinum or pulmonary parenchyma.
2. Produces symptoms of bronchial or esophageal obstruction, but may also be asymptomatic incidental discovery on chest radiograph.
3. Has mucoid central core surrounded by wall of cartilage and smooth muscle; lined with ciliated columnar epithelium.
4. 70% located within lung tissue; 30% located within mediastinum, extrinsic to lung.
5. Should be excised regardless of symptoms, usually by simple excision, although formal lobectomy may be required.

C. Cystic adenomatoid malformation.

1. Hamartomatous development of pulmonary parenchyma.
2. May present from asymptomatic mass to fetal hydrops (fatal), but most common presentation is respiratory distress in the newborn. Can present in later life as a result of recurrent pulmonary infection.
3. Symptoms produced by progressive air trapping with enlargement of mass and compression of normal lung and airways; may have associated pulmonary hypoplasia and pulmonary hypertension.
4. Treatment is formal lobectomy; rarely, systemic arterial supply may be present as in pulmonary sequestration. *In utero* resection and/or aspiration if symptomatic.

D. Congenital lobar emphysema.

1. Progressive obstructive emphysema, leading to massive distension of the involved lobe.
2. Affects left upper lobe and right middle lobe most commonly.
3. Two-thirds of patients male; rare in blacks and premature infants.
4. Greater than 50% develop symptoms within first few days of life; symptoms include dyspnea, wheezing, cough, tachypnea, and cyanosis. Neonates often trap fetal lung fluid in lobe, so appearance on chest radiograph may look like pneumonia until fluid clears.
5. Caused by partial airway obstruction due to abnormal carti-

laginous support of the bronchial wall ("ball valve effect"); leads to progressive air trapping with compression of normal lung and mediastinal shift.

6. First, must perform bronchoscopy to rule out external compression of bronchus producing air trapping and alveolar distension.
7. Primary treatment is lobectomy.

E. Congenital diaphragmatic hernia (Bochdalek).

1. Occurs as a result of failure of fusion of the transverse septum and the pleuroperitoneal folds during the eighth week of development.
2. Incidence up to 1:2000 live births; posterolateral defects account for 75-85%; majority on left side.
3. Excluding malrotation and patent ductus arteriosus, incidence of associated congenital defects between 10-20%.
4. Pathophysiology related to development of ipsilateral (and to varying degrees contra-lateral) pulmonary hypoplasia and to the development of persistent fetal circulation (PFC) also called persistent pulmonary hypertension of the newborn (PPHN); this produces right-to-left shunting with failure of oxygenation and ventilation. Prognosis dependent upon severity of pulmonary hypoplasia.
5. Present with respiratory distress (dyspnea, cyanosis, hypoxemia); scaphoid abdomen, decreased breath sounds, cardiac dextroposition; symptoms may develop immediately or several hours after birth ("honeymoon period"–better prognosis).
6. Chest radiograph–usually confirms diagnosis by findings of loops of gas-filled bowel within chest (may be confused with cystic adenomatoid malformation); may require GI contrast study in the stable patient to confirm diagnosis.
7. Pre-operative preparation: patient must first be stabilized.
   a. Decompress stomach (10 Fr Replogle® nasogastric tube).
   b. Intubate; mechanical ventilation maintaining high P_aO_2 and moderate hypocapnia ($PaCO_2 \approx 30$) using low airway pressures; high-frequency ventilation may be useful. Avoid mask ventilation of patient.
   c. Correct acidosis and alkalinize to pH of 7.5 - 7.6 with $NaHCO_3$ or THAM. Maintain tissue perfusion.
   d. Place monitoring catheters (postductal arterial line, adequate venous access).
8. After infant has been stabilized medically, surgical repair using transabdominal primary closure of diaphragmatic defect or patch closure with prosthetic material.
9. If patient remains unstable, extracorporeal membrane oxygenation (ECMO) has been shown to improve survival in infants with congenital diaphragmatic hernia and reversible pulmonary hypertension. Repair may then occur in 3-6 days or at completion of ECMO.

10. Inhalation of nitric oxide to reverse pulmonary hypertension may be useful.

F. Esophageal atresia and tracheoesophageal fistula.

1. Embryonic failure of separation of the trachea from the esophagus.
2. Usually present in the neonatal period with excessive salivation, feeding intolerance, drooling, or gagging; maternal polyhydramnios. H-type fistula may present at later age with recurrent pneumonias.
3. Diagnosis.
   a. Clinical suspicion in newborn with above findings.
   b. Inability to pass catheter beyond proximal esophagus.
   c. Obtain upright chest radiograph; absence or presence of gas in stomach and GI tract (determines esophageal atresia *vs.* tracheoesophageal fistula, respectively).
   d. Obtain ultrasound to determine position of aortic arch, presence of associated cardiac (> 30%) and genitourinary (12%) anomalies.
4. Types of atresias/tracheoesophageal fistulas (Figure 1):
   a. Type A (6-7%)–isolated esophageal atresia without fistula; gasless abdomen on radiograph.
   b. Type B (1%)–esophageal atresia with proximal tracheoesophageal fistula.
   c. Type C (86%)–esophageal atresia with distal tracheoesophageal fistula.
   d. Type D (1-5%)–esophageal atresia with proximal and distal tracheoesophageal fistula.
   e. Type E (5%)–tracheoesophageal fistula without atresia (H-type).
   f. Type F (1%)–esophageal stenosis without fistula.
5. Pre-operative preparation.
   a. 10 Fr Replogle catheter into proximal segment to prevent aspiration.
   b. Elevate head of bed.
   c. Avoid mask or pressure ventilation.
   d. Supportive fluid, electrolyte, and nutritional therapy; broad-spectrum antibiotics.
6. Surgical treatment–depends on cardiopulmonary stability of patient.
   a. Stable patient, no life-threatening anomaly, weight > 2500 g.
      (1) Immediate primary extrapleural thoracotomy, ligation/division of fistula, primary repair of esophageal atresia.
      (2) Extrapleural chest drainage, with or without gastrostomy.
   b. Unstable patient, life-threatening anomaly, weight < 1500 g.

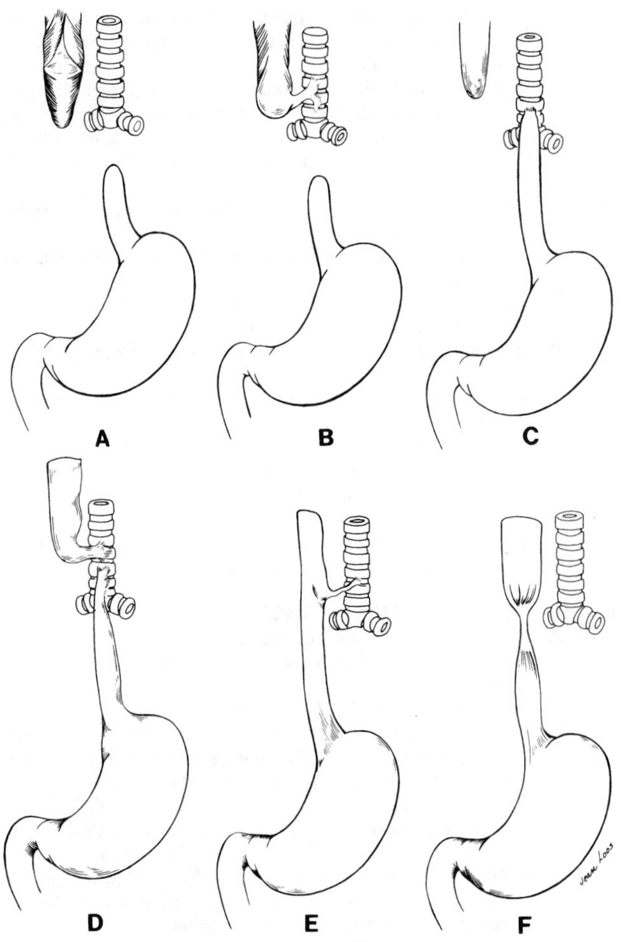

FIG. 1 **Types of Tracheoesophageal Fistulas**

(1) Decompressive gastrostomy.
(2) Delayed primary repair (1-2 weeks) when stable.

c. Unstable patient, persistent pulmonary distress (usually due to continued aspiration) and need for ventilatory support.
(1) Decompressive gastrostomy.

(2) "Staged repair"–extrapleural ligation/division of fistula, followed by transpleural primary repair of atresia when stable.

d. Isolated atresia without fistula–lower esophageal segment frequently too short for primary repair; initially requires cervical esophagostomy with a stomach, colon, or small bowel interposition at a later date (around 1 year of age).

7. Outcome.
   a. Anastomotic leak occurs in 11% of patients, and anastomotic stricture in 26%.
   b. Survival largely dependent upon associated congenital defects.
   c. High incidence of gastroesophageal reflux (44%), may require eventual fundoplication.

G. Mediastinal masses—divided into four anatomic subdivisions.

1. Superior–thymoma, thymic cyst, lymphoma, thyroid mass, parathyroid mass.
2. Anterior–thymoma, thymic cyst, teratoma, dermoid, lymphangioma, hemangioma, lipoma, fibroma.
3. Middle–pericardial cyst, bronchogenic cyst, lymphoma, granuloma.
4. Posterior–neurogenic tumors (neuroblastoma, ganglioneuroma), foregut duplications and cysts.

VI. GASTROINTESTINAL TRACT

A. Hypertrophic pyloric stenosis.

1. Gastric outlet obstruction due to hypertrophied pyloric muscle.
2. Affects 3 in 1000 infants; male:female ratio 5:1.
3. Occurs in first 2 months of life, with average age of clinical presentation 3-6 weeks. Nonbilious vomiting that increases in volume and frequency is seen. Dehydration is present, with classic electrolyte picture of "contraction" alkalosis (hypokalemia, hypochloremia, and metabolic alkalosis). Unconconjugated hyperbilirubinemia is also present.
4. 90% have palpable pyloric tumor ("olive") in the midepigastrium to right upper quadrant; examination is facilitated by nasogastric decompression and sedation.
5. Contrast upper GI study and/or ultrasound useful for confirming diagnosis when pyloric tumor not palpable or equivocal; should not be routinely obtained if symptoms and palpable mass present.
6. Pre-operative management.
   a. Operation is never an emergency, and adequate preoperative preparation is necessary for low morbidity.
   b. Nasogastric decompression.
   c. Fluid resuscitation and electrolyte correction, including

potassium repletion (once urine output assured), mandatory before operative repair. Correct HCO_3 to < 30.

7. Surgical treatment–classic operation is Fredet-Ramstedt pyloromyotomy (reported mortality approximately 0.3%) via RUQ, periumbilical or laproscopic approach.
8. Post-operative management.
   a. Nasogastric tube removed in OR.
   b. Continued intravenous hydration.
   c. Oral fluids (electrolyte solution) begun 6-12 h postoperatively, gradually advanced over 1-2 days to full volume formula feeds.

B. Intestinal obstruction in the neonate.

1. Should suspect with history of maternal polyhydramnios, bilious emesis, abdominal distension, or failure to pass meconium within first 24 hours of life.
2. *Bilious vomiting in an infant is a SURGICAL EMERGENCY and requires emergent evaluation to rule out malrotation and midgut volvulus.*
3. ***Intrinsic duodenal obstruction.***
   a. Frequent association with other anomalies.
   b. May be due to duodenal web, atresia, or stenosis.
   c. Presents with bilious vomiting, minimal abdominal distension.
   d. Abdominal radiographs reveal "double-bubble" sign.
   e. Surgical treatment includes excision of webs or duodenoduodenostomy for atresia and evaluation of distal bowel for other atresias.
4. ***Extrinsic duodenal obstruction: malrotation.***
   a. Malrotation of the midgut results in a narrow base for the small bowel mesentery, with predisposition to volvulus and intestinal infarction.
   b. Presents with sudden onset of bilious vomiting as newborn.
   c. Volvulus frequently results in significant vascular compromise and intestinal obstruction.
   d. Most reliably diagnosed by UGI to visualize malpositioned ligament of Treitz.
   e. Treatment includes emergent laparotomy and Ladd's procedure. This consists of evisceration, reduction of volvulus by counter-clockwise rotation, division of "Ladd's bands" thereby widening the mesenteric base between the duodenum and the colon, appendectomy, and placement of the small bowel in the right side and the colon in the left side of the peritoneal cavity.
   f. Nonviable bowel should be resected; questionably viable bowel should remain with a planned 24-h "second-look" laparotomy.
5. ***Jejunoileal obstruction: atresia and stenosis.***

a. Result of late mesenteric vascular accidents *in utero*.
b. Abdominal radiographs show dilated loops of small bowel; contrast enema usually demonstrates small unused "microcolon" although may be normal.
c. Martin-Zerella classification.
   (1) Type I–single mucosal atresia, bowel wall and mesentery in continuity, and normal bowel length.
   (2) Type II (most common)–single atresia with discontinuity of bowel and gap in mesentery.
   (3) Type III–multiple atresias.
   (4) Type IV–"apple peel" or "Christmas tree" deformity with markedly decreased bowel length.
d. Operative management is individualized, depending on number and length of atresias; includes resection with anastomosis, tapering enteroplasty, and exteriorization in the presence of compromised bowel.

6. ***Meconium ileus.***
   a. Obstruction of the distal ileum from inspissated meconium–associated with cystic fibrosis.
   b. Simple meconium ileus–bowel is impacted with pellets of meconium, with proximally dilated ileum packed with thick, tar-like meconium.
   c. Complicated meconium ileus–associated with meconium cysts, atresia, perforation, or meconium peritonitis.
   d. Presents with progressive abdominal distension and failure to pass meconium; abdominal radiograph shows obstruction with no air/fluid levels, soap bubble appearance in proximal colon; contrast enema shows microcolon with inspissated plugs of meconium.
   e. May respond to non-operative therapy with gastrografin enemas.
   f. Operative intervention indicated for complicated cases and where non-operative therapy fails; ranges from simple enterotomy and irrigation of bowel with N-acetylcysteine (Mucomyst®) to bowel resection with 1° anastomosis or temporary diverting colostomy.
   g. Survival predominantly based on associated pulmonary complications of cystic fibrosis.

7. ***Hirschsprung's disease.***
   a. Absence of parasympathetic ganglion cells in the affected segment of intestine; rectum and rectosigmoid most common.
   b. Suspected in any infant who does not pass meconium in the first 24 h of life, has newborn intestinal obstruction, or who has chronic constipation during the first year of life.
   c. Diagnosis obtained from barium enema (rectum of small to normal size with proximal colorectal dilatation) and rectal biopsy (absence of ganglion cells in Meissner's (sub-

mucosal) and Auerbach's (intermuscular) plexi; increase in acetylcholinesterase staining.

d. Initial treatment is immediate diverting colostomy proximal to the transition zone (determined by biopsies at time of operation).

e. Definitive pull-through operation at 9-12 months of age, or in some centers in the newborn period. New laproscopic techniques allow pull-through as infant without colostomy.

C. Intestinal obstruction in the infant (2 months - 2 years).

1. ***Intussusception.***
   a. Most common cause of bowel obstruction in 2-month to 2-year age range; > 50% have documented recent viral infection.
   b. Caused by telescoping of one segment of bowel (intussusceptum) into another (intussuscipiens). Ileocecal occurs most commonly.
   c. Sudden onset of recurring severe, cramping abdominal pain, vomiting, drawing up of legs; 60% have bloody ("currant jelly") stools. An elongated mass may be palpable in RUQ with an "empty" RLQ.
   d. Diagnosis by air or barium enema–"coiled spring" appearance.
   e. Initial treatment by attempted hydrostatic reduction during air enema if peritonitis or free air have been ruled out first (70 - 80% success rate).
   f. Requires surgical exploration if air enema reduction unsuccessful or if peritonitis present; manual reduction is performed distal to proximal, followed by appendectomy if bowel remains viable. If manual reduction is not possible or if lead point is identified, resection is indicated.
2. ***Incarcerated hernia*** (see "Hernia").

D. Necrotizing enterocolitis (NEC).

1. Most common GI emergency in the premature neonate.
2. > 90% in premature or low birthweight infants.
3. Etiology not known–appears to be related to ischemic intestinal damage, bacterial colonization, and intraluminal substrate (feedings).
4. Early clinical findings include ileus, gastric retention, bilious vomiting, and bloody stools; progressive findings include lethargy, apnea, bradycardia, hypothermia, shock, acidosis, and neutropenia.
5. Radiographic findings–pneumatosis intestinalis; late findings include "fixed" loop of bowel (suggests gangrenous changes), portal vein air or free air.
6. Medical management.
   a. Gastric decompression, NPO.
   b. Systemic antibiotics.

c. Fluid resuscitation, correction of acidosis, parenteral nutrition.
d. Close monitoring–serial CBC, platelet count and upright abdominal films (every 6 h).

7. Indications for surgery:
   a. Free air or portal vein air on radiograph (absolute indication).
   b. Clinical deterioration–persistent acidosis, thrombocytopenia, leukopenia.
   c. Diffuse peritonitis, abdominal wall erythema or induration.
   d. Paracentesis suggestive of non-viable bowel if fluid brown and cloudy, extracellular bacteria on gram stain, large number of WBCs with differential > 80% neutrophils.

E. Meckel's diverticulum.

1. The most common form of persistent vitelline duct remnant; less commonly persistent vitelline duct with sinus, persistent omphalomesenteric band, and vitelline duct cyst.
2. Occurs on antimesenteric border of ileum within 60 cm of ileocecal valve.
3. Complications.
   a. Bleeding (22%)–usually painless, due to ulceration of adjacent tissue from ectopic gastric mucosa; usually stops spontaneously, but can be massive.
   b. Obstruction (13%)–secondary to internal hernia around persistent omphalomesenteric band.
   c. Inflammation (2%)–mimics acute appendicitis.
   d. Intussusception (1%).
4. Diagnosis–high degree of suspicion, confirmed by ^{99m}technetium-pertechnate scan (can have false-positive result with enteric duplications or false-negative with H_2 blockers) if ectopic gastric mucosa present.
5. Treatment by wedge resection of diverticulum or segmental ileal resection with primary anastomosis; include appendectomy.
6. Incidental Meckel's diverticulum–generally recommend resection in patient under 18 years old, particularly if heterotopic tissue present; not indicated in asymptomatic adults.
7. Remember the "rule of 2s"–occurs in 2% of the population, symptomatic in 2% of cases, approximately 2 feet from the ileocecal valve, 2 inches in length, 2 types of mucosa (gastric/pancreatic), 2 x as often in male : female, 2 presentations (bleeding/obstruction).

F. Appendicitis (see also "Appendicitis").

1. Most common emergent abdominal operation in children.
2. Ruptured in 30-50% of children at presentation.

G. Gastroesophageal reflux (see "Esophagus").

1. Differs from adult GER.

a. Emesis is the most common presentation; malnutrition/failure to thrive; aspiration pneumonia and asthma; esophagitis; laryngospasm.
b. Frequently associated with mental retardation, which causes esophageal motility disorders.
c. Pre-operative evaluation:
   (1) UGI to exclude gastric outlet obstruction.
   (2) EGD to rule out Barrett's and grade esophagitis.
   (3) pH probe is most sensitive and specific for pathologic reflux (pH < 4 for $> 4\%$ of the time).
   (4) Obtain technetium gastric-emptying scan to rule out delayed gastric emptying or outlet obstruction.
d. Initial treatment is non-operative for 6-8 weeks–has a 80% response rate.
   (1) Upright position, thickened feedings, metoclopramide, H_2 blockers.
   (2) Frequently spontaneously resolves.
   (3) Contraindicated in patients with esophageal stricture or near-miss SIDS.
e. Operative therapy.
   (1) Usually not performed in children < 6 months of age.
   (2) Indications–failed medical therapy, severe esophagitis, Barrett's metaplasia, stricture, bleeding, neurologically impaired patient that needs a G-tube.
   (3) Two most common repairs: Nissen (360°) and Thal (270°), 10% and 20% recurrence, respectively.
   (4) Pyloroplasty in patients with delayed gastric emptying.

VII. ABDOMINAL WALL DEFECTS

A. Omphalocele.

1. A covered defect of the umbilical ring into which abdominal contents herniate; sac composed of an outer layer of amnion and an inner layer of peritoneum.
2. More than 50% of infants have serious associated congenital defects (genitourinary, cardiac, GI); always associated with malrotation.
3. Sac may contain only intestine, but usually contains liver as well; may be associated with loss of abdominal domain, with contracted abdominal cavity.
4. Management includes covering sac with sterile dressing, protection from hypothermia, gastric decompression, parenteral nutrition, and broad-spectrum antibiotics.
5. Surgical treatment–small defects can be closed primarily; moderate defects can have the skin closed and the subsequent hernia repaired later; larger defects require staged closure using silastic silo.

6. Overall survival depends on the size of the defect as well as the severity of associated congenital defects; mortality averages 30-35%.

B. Gastroschisis.

1. Defect of the anterior abdominal wall just lateral and usually to the right of the umbilicus.
2. No peritoneal sac, with resulting antenatal evisceration of bowel through the defect; resulting chemical irritation of bowel wall leads to thick edematous membrane on bowel surface, foreshortened bowel.
3. Always associated with nonrotation; 15% associated with intestinal atresias; other congenital defects unusual.
4. Management.
   a. Prevention of excessive insensible fluid and heat loss through exposed bowel; gastric decompression.
   b. Large amounts of intravenous fluids to maintain perfusion; initiation of total parenteral nutrition; broad-spectrum antibiotics.
   c. Primary repair successful in 70% of cases; if not possible, is treated with gradual decompression using a silastic silo.

C. Umbilical hernia.

1. Defect of the umbilical ring; more common in females and blacks.
2. Spontaneous closure in 80% of patients, usually if < 2 cm in diameter; if > 2 cm, less chance of spontaneous closure.
3. Observation recommended until child is 3 to 4 years of age; if persistent, undergo elective repair; large defects are repaired earlier.

D. Inguinal hernia.

1. Caused by persistence of the embryonic processus vaginalis.
2. Incidence varies with gestational age (9% to 11% in premature infants, 3.5% to 5% in term infants).
3. Approximately 10% bilateral; contralateral exploration indicated if patient is < 1 year old (60% bilateral).
4. Vast majority are indirect.
5. Examination reveals immobile, tender mass in groin, with mass extending along spermatic cord up to the internal ring.
6. Major complication is bowel incarceration with strangulation and possible infarction; significantly higher in pre-term infant (31%) and in infants in first year of life (15%).
7. High ligation of sac is adequate repair; may repair bilateral hernias simultaneously.
8. ***Incarcerated hernia***—in the absence of signs of compromised bowel (fever, peritonitis, leukocytosis) or obstruction, attempt reduction when diagnosed; achieved by placing firm pressure in the direction of the inguinal canal; facilitated by sedation and elevation of the legs and torso. If unreducible, or strangulation is suspected, urgent repair is indicated.

VIII. NEOPLASMS

A. Neuroblastoma—usually in children < 4 years old.

1. Origin–neural crest tissue.
2. Metabolically active–catecholamines (90%).
3. May mature to benign ganglioneuroma or spontaneously regress.
4. Presentation–70% disseminated at presentation.
   a. Abdominal mass–retroperitoneal, adrenal, medulla, or paraspinal ganglia. Posterior mediastinal mass. Spinal cord compression. Symptoms of catecholamine or VIP excess. Cerebellar ataxia–mostly with mediastinal involvement.
5. Diagnosis.
   a. Urinary catecholamine breakdown products–VMA and HVA screening 92% accurate.
   b. CT or MRI (may demonstrate spinal involvement more accurately).
   c. Bone scan and bone marrow aspiration.
   d. MIBG nuclear scan will show boney involvement and primary tumor.
6. Treatment–usually resistant to chemotherapy.
   a. Stage 1 or 2–operative resection with node removal.
   b. Stage 3 or 4–primary or delayed operative resection, chemo- and radiotherapy.
7. Prognosis–inversely related to age.
   a. Tumor stage and location.
   b. N-myc gene amplification, stroma poor or nodular rich pathology, elevated serum ferritin or LDH associated with poor prognosis.

B. Nephroblastoma (Wilm's Tumor).

1. Embryonal renal neoplasm–mesenchymal origin. Two related but separate tumors–clear cell sarcoma and malignant rhabdoid tumor.
2. Etiology unclear.
3. Presentation.
   a. Maximal incidence 1 - 5 years of age.
   b. 10% associated with congenital abnormalities–anidria, genitourinary malformations, hemihypertrophy, skin hamartoma's, mental retardation, Beckwith-Wiedemann syndrome.
   c. Symptoms–fever, abdominal pain, firm irregular painless abdominal mass, hematuria, hypertension.
   d. Diagnosis–ultrasound (cystic *vs.* solid, invasion of vena cava), CT or MRI, chest radiograph to screen for pulmonary metastases.
4. Treatment.
   a. Operative–tumor removal even with distant metastases, 10% of cases have bilateral involvement.

b. Solitary lung metastases may be excised.
c. Adjuvant chemo- and radiation therapy beneficial. Preoperative chemo- and radiation therapy may enable operative therapy for tumors initially too large for resection.

5. Prognosis–worse with anaplasia, sarcomatous changes, positive nodes, increased staging, older age.
   a. Favorable histology > 80% survival for 4 years.
   b. Unfavorable histology 50-70% survival for 4 years.

62

Carcinoma of the Lung

Christopher S. Meyer, M.D.

I. EPIDEMIOLOGY

A. **Most common cancer** in highly industrialized nations.
B. **Male:Female ratio**—2:1.
C. **150,000 new cases** in U.S. each year.
D. **Leading cause of cancer deaths** in men and women.
E. **Incidence**—higher among urban residents and the lower economic class.

II. ETIOLOGY

A. **Cigarette smoking.**
   1. Overall risk of lung cancer in smokers is 10 times that of nonsmokers.
   2. Possible association of lung cancer with exposure to passive smoking.
   3. Cigarette smoke acts synergistically with environmental pollutants in carcinogenesis.

B. **Occupational exposure.**
   1. Asbestos.
   2. Ionizing radiation.
   3. Arsenic.
   4. Nickel.
   5. Chromium.
   6. Chloromethyl ethers.
   7. Mustard gas.

C. **Atmospheric pollution** due to industrial expansion.
D. **Genetic predisposition.**

III. PATHOLOGY

A. **Histological classification** of malignant epithelial lung tumors according to World Health Organization, 1981.
   1. Squamous cell carcinoma–spindle cell (squamous) carcinoma.

2. Small cell carcinoma.
   a. Oat cell carcinoma.
   b. Intermediate cell type.
   c. Combined oat cell carcinoma.
3. Adenocarcinoma.
   a. Acinar adenocarcinoma.
   b. Papillary adenocarcinoma.
   c. Bronchiolo-alveolar adenocarcinoma.
   d. Solid carcinoma with mucus formation.
4. Large cell carcinoma.
   a. Giant cell carcinoma.
   b. Clear cell carcinoma.
5. Adenosquamous carcinoma.
6. Carcinoid tumor.

B. Location of primary tumors.

1. "Central" tumors–squamous and small cell carcinomas.
2. "Peripheral" tumors–adenocarcinoma and large cell carcinomas.

C. Method of spread.

1. Invades lymphatics and blood vessels, resulting in early metastasis.
2. Oat cell carcinoma is most aggressive.
3. 30-50% of patients with lung cancer have lymphatic or hematogenous spread at initial presentation.
4. Metastases in order of preference–regional lymph nodes, liver, adrenals, brain, bone, and kidneys.
5. Contralateral pulmonary metastases at post-mortem exam–10-14%.

IV. FOUR MAJOR TYPES OF MALIGNANT EPITHELIAL LUNG TUMORS

A. Adenocarcinoma.

1. 40% of malignant epithelial lung tumors.
2. Relative incidence appears to be increasing.
3. Often a "peripheral" tumor.
   a. Arises mostly in the periphery of lung parenchyma.
   b. May be related to focal scars or regions of fibrosis.
4. Early metastasis because of early invasion of lymphatics and blood vessels.

B. Squamous cell carcinoma.

1. 30% of primary malignant epithelial lung tumors.
2. Occur in the segmental, lobar, or mainstem bronchi.
3. Relatively slow-growing and late to metastasize.
4. Spread pattern.
   a. Direct invasion of peribronchial lymph nodes and replacement of adjacent pulmonary parenchyma.
   b. Peripheral tumors commonly invade chest wall.

5. Microscopically.
   a. Well-differentiated tumors produce keratin, epithelial pearls, and squamous pattern.
   b. Poorly-differentiated tumors with less obvious keratinization.

C. Small cell carcinoma (oat cell carcinoma)
1. 20% of malignant epithelial lung tumors.
2. Originate in the major bronchus at or near the hilum.
3. Noted for its rapid growth and early metastasis via lymphatic and hematogenous spread.
4. Staging (not based on TNM).
   a. Limited–disease limited to one hemithorax.
   b. Extensive–spread beyond one hemithorax.
5. Precise diagnosis required because treatment and prognosis of small cell carcinoma differs considerably from non-small cell.

D. Large cell carcinoma.
1. 10% of malignant epithelial lung tumors.
2. "Peripheral" tumor.
3. Heterogeneous group.
   a. *Not* showing squamous or glandular differentiation.
   b. *Not* being of small cell type.
   c. Ultrastructurally–most are poorly-differentiated adenocarcinomas.
4. Rapid growth and early metastasis.

V. METASTATIC TUMORS IN THE CHEST

A. Lungs are one of the most frequent sites for metastases.

B. Lungs are first organ to filter many venous-borne metastases.

C. May present as diffuse pulmonary involvement or solitary pulmonary nodule.

D. Common malignancies metastatic to lung—breast, melanoma, renal cell, prostate, thyroid, pancreatic, soft tissue sarcoma, and osteosarcoma.

VI. CLINICAL FEATURES

A. Local manifestations may be nonspecific, since most patients also suffer from chronic bronchitis and emphysema due to cigarette smoking.
1. Cough and sputum.
   a. Evaluate for change of an established cough.
   b. Evaluate for change in quality or quantity of sputum.
2. Dyspnea–sudden onset may indicate obstruction of a main bronchus.
3. Hemoptysis.
4. Wheezing.

5. Chest pain–constant, debilitating, and localizing pain may be due to metastatic bony erosion.

B. Metastatic manifestations.

1. Intrathoracic manifestations.
   a. Pleural effusion.
   b. Pleuritic pain.
   c. **Superior vena cava syndrome.**
      (1) Compression or direct invasion of great veins of the thoracic outlet.
      (2) Dyspnea, severe headaches, and periorbital, facial, and neck edema.
   d. Pericardial effusion.
2. Extrathoracic manifestations.
   a. Brachial neuritis–tumor invading the brachial plexus.
   b. **Horner's syndrome.**
      (1) Tumor invading cervical and first thoracic segment of sympathetic trunk.
      (2) Ptosis, myosis, and enophthalmos on affected side.
   c. Hoarseness–tumor spread involving the ipsilateral recurrent laryngeal nerve.
   d. Metastases in order of preference–liver, adrenals, brain, bones, and kidneys.
   e. Bone metastases usually osteolytic; most frequently ribs and vertebrae involved.

C. Non-metastatic systemic manifestations.

1. Endocrine-related syndromes.
2. Metabolic (weight loss).
3. Thrombophlebitis.

VII. DIAGNOSIS

A. Radiology.

1. Chest radiograph is usually abnormal when patient is symptomatic.
2. Chest radiograph abnormalities suspicious of malignancy.
   a. Atelectasis or lobar emphysema.
   b. Enlarged hilum or hilar mass.
   c. Atelectasis or lobar emphysema.
   d. Enlarged upper or middle mediastinum.
   e. Evidence of bony erosion due to metastases.
3. CT scan.
   a. Search for additional pulmonary nodules.
   b. Evaluate spread to pleura and mediastinal structures.
   c. Direct percutaneous transthoracic needle biopsy.

B. Sputum cytology.

1. 70-80% sensitive.
2. Multiple specimens increase accuracy.
3. Best sputum specimens within 36 h of bronchoscopy.
4. Most helpful in patients with central tumors.
5. Disappointing results for early screening of lung cancer.

C. Pleural fluid cytology.

1. When effusion present on chest radiograph.
2. 40-75% sensitivity.
3. Highest yield for adenocarcinoma.

D. Bronchoscopy.

1. Higher yield in patients with central tumors; can evaluate for synchronous lesions.
2. Complications rare with fiberoptic bronchoscope.
3. Allows transbronchial biopsies, brush cytology, and bronchial washings for cytology.

E. Mediastinoscopy.

1. 50% of patients have involved mediastinal lymph nodes at initial presentation.
2. Mediastinoscopy may be used prior to thoracotomy to evaluate resectability.
3. Tumor yield approximately 30-40% of exams.

F. Percutaneous needle biopsy.

1. Negative result does not rule out carcinoma.
2. Indications.
   a. When surgery is most likely *not* in the treatment plan (small cell).
   b. Patients who cannot tolerate a thoracotomy.
3. Contraindications.
   a. Bleeding diathesis.
   b. Bullous disease near the lesion.
4. 96% sensitivity with two attempts.
5. Complications.
   a. Pneumothorax–24%; only 10% require chest tube placement.
   b. Minor hemoptysis–6%.

VIII. T-N-M CLASSIFICATION

Primary Tumor (T)	Nodal Involvement (N)	Distant Metastasis (M)
T0: no tumor	N0: no nodes	M0: no metastasis
TX: positive cytology	NX: unable to assess	MX: unable to assess
TIS: carcinoma *in situ*	N1: ipsilateral nodes (peribronchial or hilar)	M1: metastasis
T1: <3 cm, no bronchial invasion	N2: ipsilateral nodes (mediastinal)	
T2: >3 cm, invades hilum pleura or bronchus	N3: contralateral nodes (mediastinal)	
T3: invades parietal pleura, chest wall, diaphragm, mediastinum		
T4: invades unresectable structures—aorta, atrium, vertebral body		

IX. STAGING FOR LUNG CANCER

Occult Carcinoma	Tx/N0/M0
Stage I	TIS/N0/M0, T1/N0/M0, T2/N0/M0
Stage II	T1/N1/M0, T2/N1/M0
Stage IIIa	T1/N2/M0, T2/N2/M0, T3/N0/N1, T3/N1/M0, T3/N2/M0
Stage IIIb	any T/N3/M0, T4/any N/M0
Stage IV	metastasis (any T, any N, M1)

X. TREATMENT OF NON-SMALL CELL CARCINOMA

A. Surgical.

1. Assessment of pulmonary reserves.

Resection	Pneumonectomy	Lobectomy	Wedge/Segmental
MVV	> 55% predicted	> 40%	> 35%
FEV1	> 2.0 L/min	> 1.0 L/min	> 0.61/min

   a. Pulmonary Function Test (PFT):
   b. Clinical assessment by stair climbing at a normal rate without significant increase in pulse or respiratory rate.
      (1) One flight–tolerate thoracotomy.
      (2) Two flights–tolerate lobectomy.
      (3) Three flights–tolerate pneumonectomy.
2. Thoracotomy with resection of tumor.
   a. Non-small cell carcinoma cases.
      (1) 65% inoperable at time of diagnosis.
      (2) 15% inoperable at thoracotomy.
      (3) 20% will undergo resection (of these, 15% will die within 2-3 years after surgery from local or distant metastases).
   b. Wedge resection or segmentectomy.
      (1) Indications–peripheral tumor < 3 cm, patient with marginal pulmonary reserve or metachronous or synchronous tumors.
      (2) High recurrence rate reported in some series, especially with adenocarcinoma.
   c. Lobectomy.
      (1) Procedure of choice for disease confined to one lobe.
      (2) Includes entire first-level lobar lymphatics.
      (3) Mortality rate of 0-5%.
   d. Pneumonectomy.
      (1) Indications–hilar involvement or tumor extension across oblique fissure.
      (2) Can result in poor pulmonary reserve with *significant* change in lifestyle.
      (3) Mortality rate of 5-10%.

B. Non-surgical.
1. Radiation.
   a. Palliation–often helpful in relieving symptoms of superior vena cava obstruction and mediastinal invasion, as well as cough, hemoptysis, and pain (especially bone pain).
   b. Pre-operative irradiation.
      (1) No improvement in survival, but increased post-operative complications.
      (2) Exception is superior sulcus tumor (Pancoast); improved survival (45% *vs.* 30%) with pre-operative irradiation and *en bloc* resection.
   c. Post-operative irradiation–controversial, under study.
2. Chemotherapy–used to treat patients with advanced disease; response rates to single-agent and combined-drug chemotherapy are low.
3. Immunotherapy–under investigation.
4. Laser therapy–may be useful to relieve endobronchial obstruction in unresectable tumors.

XI. TREATMENT OF SMALL CELL CARCINOMA

A. Surgical intervention rarely indicated.

B. Multiple drug regimens are more effective than a single agent.
1. Many combinations have been shown to extend survival.
2. Side-effects are worse with multiple agents.

C. Tumor response seen in 75-95% of patients.
1. 50% of patients with limited disease (disease limited to one hemithorax) see complete response.
2. 20% of patients with widespread disease see complete response.

XII. PROGNOSIS

A. Overall 5-year survival for patients with non-small cell carcinoma of the lung.
1. Stage I, resected–80%.
2. Stage II, resected–50%.
3. Stage III–< 10%.

B. 5-year survival by cell type.
1. Squamous–68%.
2. Adenocarcinoma–25%.
3. Small cell–0% (few patients survive 2 years from diagnosis).

XIII. WORK-UP OF SOLITARY PULMONARY NODULE (SPN)

A. Definition—peripheral pulmonary nodule less than 6 cm in diameter.

B. Incidence of SPN representing metastatic disease from an asymptomatic primary malignancy is exceedingly low. Extensive metastatic work-up is unnecessary.

C. **Consider SPN metastatic** if occurs in patient with current or previous extrapulmonary primary malignant tumor.

D. **Incidence of diseases** that may present as SPN.
   1. Malignant nodules–40%.
      a. Bronchogenic carcinoma–30%.
      b. Solitary metastatic lesions–8%.
      c. Bronchial adenoma (mainly carcinoid)–2%.
   2. Benign nodules–60%.
      a. Infectious granulomas–50%.
      b. Non-infectious granulomas–3%.
      c. Benign tumors–3%.
      d. Miscellaneous–4%.

E. **Radiographic characteristics of benign nodules.**
   1. Small, smooth, with sharply circumscribed margins.
   2. Calcification–only 0.5% malignant.
   3. No increase in size in 2 years–doubling time is 20 to 400 days for malignant tumors.

F. **Management of SPN.**
   1. Further radiographic evaluation of the nodule, and evaluation for other pulmonary nodules (chest CT, tomography).
   2. Radiographic evidence of benignity–follow with yearly chest radiograph.
   3. Suspected malignancy.
      a. Attempt needle biopsy for diagnosis.
      b. Bronchoscopy.
      c. Evaluate for thoracoscopy or thoracotomy with nodule resection.

63

Peri-Operative Management of the Cardiac Surgery Patient

Arthur B. Williams, M.D.

I. PRE-OPERATIVE EVALUATION

A. History and physical examination.

1. It is important to realize that symptoms of heart disease are usually late findings. Surgical intervention often is optimal before symptoms arise.
   a. Control of angina, recent myocardial infarction.
   b. Signs or symptoms of congestive heart failure.
   c. Arrhythmias, presence of a pacemaker.
   d. Neurologic symptoms; presence of carotid bruits; syncope.
   e. Claudication, rest pain; documentation of peripheral pulses.
   f. History of peptic ulcer disease or gastrointestinal bleeding.

B. Pre-operative testing.

1. Electrocardiogram–arrhythmias, ischemic changes, conduction delays.
2. Laboratory–as per usual pre-op, include coagulation studies, type and crossmatch for 2 units of packed RBCs.
3. PA and lateral chest radiograph.
4. Review of cardiac catheterization and echocardiogram results.
   a. Distribution of coronary artery disease.
   b. Evaluation of ventricular wall motion and ejection fraction.
   c. Presence of valvular dysfunction.

C. Medications—A comprehensive list of both pre-admission and pre-operative medications should be included in the pre-operative note. In general, medications are continued until surgery, **especially anti-anginal agents, nitroglycerine and heparin**

drips, and anti-arrhythmics. Peri-operative steroid and insulin coverage is per routine.

D. Pre-operative orders.

1. Accurate height and weight recorded in chart in order to calculate BSA.
2. Hibiclens® scrub the night before surgery.
3. NPO after midnight.
4. Antibiotics on call–cefuroxime 1.5 g IVPB.

II. OPERATIVE PROCEDURES

A. Coronary artery bypass grafting (CABG).

1. Indications.
   a. Chronic stable angina, unrelieved by medication.
   b. Unstable angina, despite full treatment.
   c. Acute myocardial infarction–if significant coronary disease exists beyond the area of infarction, ongoing angina post-infarction, or unstable hemodynamic status. Controversy exists on the timing of surgical intervention.
   d. Ventricular arrhythmias with coronary disease.
   e. Failed percutaneous transluminal coronary angioplasty (PTCA).
2. CABG shown to be superior to medical treatment of coronary disease in the following situations:
   a. In patients with asymptomatic/mild angina and:
      (1) Significant left main disease.
      (2) 3-vessel coronary artery disease with proximal left anterior descending (LAD) disease and/or decreased LV function.
   b. In patients with chronic moderate to severe angina.
   c. Unstable angina despite full medical therapy.
   d. Failed PTCA.
   e. Persistent ventricular arrhythmias in patients with CAD.
3. Internal mammary artery grafts conduit of choice due to superior patency rates compared to saphenous vein grafts (*in situ* and free grafts) (90-95% vs. 50-60% at 10 years).

B. Valve replacement or repair.

1. Aortic stenosis.
   a. Commonly due to bicuspid valve, rheumatic disease, or calcific aortic stenosis.
   b. Symptoms include triad of dyspnea, angina, and syncope.
   c. Indications for surgery include symptomatic patients with valve gradient of > 50 mm Hg or valve area < 0.8 cm^2/m^2. Asymptomatic patients with significant stenosis and LVH should also be considered.
   d. Coronary angiography is performed owing to high rate of concomitant coronary artery disease.
2. Aortic insufficiency.
   a. Causes include rheumatic disease, annular ectasia, endocarditis, and aortitis.

   b. Frequently asymptomatic, but symptoms of congestive heart failure may be present.
   c. Indications for surgery include symptomatic patients and patients with cardiomegaly or deteriorating systolic function as assessed by echocardiography.
3. Mitral stenosis.
   a. Primarily rheumatic in origin.
   b. Symptoms include dyspnea, orthopnea, and paroxysmal nocturnal dyspnea. Radiograph may demonstrate left atrial enlargement and pulmonary venous hypertension.
   c. Indications for surgery are the presence of chronic symptoms or several acute episodes of pulmonary venous hypertension.
   d. Chronic atrial fibrillation is a complication of progressive left atrial enlargement.
4. Mitral regurgitation.
   a. Causes include rheumatic disease, myxomatous valve structure, endocarditis, ischemia or papillary muscle dysfunction, and congenital structural defects.
   b. Severity and development of symptoms varies with the etiology; rheumatic disease is more insidious in onset, whereas ischemic mitral regurgitation is often acute in onset.
   c. As with mitral stenosis, indications for surgery depend on the severity of symptoms.
   d. Ischemic mitral regurgitation is usually corrected at the time of coronary bypass, either with valve replacement or annuloplasty. Often mild ischemic mitral regurgitation improves by coronary bypass only. Depending on the structural defect present, rheumatic or myxomatous valve disease may be corrected by valve repair or replacement. The advantages of repair *vs.* replacement are the low rate of endocarditis and lack of need for long-term anticoagulation.

C. Aortic dissection.

1. DeBakey Classification:
   a. Type I–intimal disruption of ascending aorta, which dissects to involve the descending aorta and abdominal aorta.
   b. Type II–involving the ascending aorta only (stops at the innominate artery).
   c. Type III–descending aorta only. (Distal to left subclavian artery.)
2. Stanford Classification:
   a. Type A–dissection involves ascending aorta.
   b. Type B–dissection involves only the descending aorta.
3. Multiple causes–atherosclerosis, cystic medial necrosis (i.e., Marfan's syndrome), infectious, trauma.
4. Diagnosis is usually made by aortogram or chest CT. Preoperative control of hypertension with nitroprusside and beta-blockers is an essential part of management.

5. Dissection may advance proximally to disrupt coronary blood flow or induce aortic valve incompetence, or distally, causing stroke, renal failure, or intestinal ischemia.
6. Operative repair involves replacement of the affected aorta with a prosthetic graft. Cardiopulmonary bypass is required for repair of Type A dissections, and hypothermic circulatory arrest is often used for transverse arch dissections. Aortic valve replacement and coronary reimplantation may be required for Type A aneurysms that involve the aortic root. Type B dissections can be medically managed unless expansion, rupture, or compromise of branch arteries develops or hypertension becomes refractory.
7. Post-operative complications include renal failure, intestinal ischemia, stroke, and paraplegia.

D. Traumatic aortic disruption.

1. This injury results from deceleration injury, and usually occurs just distal to the left subclavian artery, at the level of the ligamentum arteriosum.
2. Chest radiograph findings include widened mediastinum, pleural capping, associated first and second rib fractures, loss of the aortic knob, hemothorax, deviation of the trachea or NG tube, and associated thoracic injuries (scapular fracture, clavicular fracture).
3. Definitive diagnosis is made by aortogram, but chest CT and transesophageal echocardiography also aid in the diagnosis.
4. Imperative that immediate life-threatening injuries (i.e., positive diagnostic peritoneal lavage) be treated prior to repair.

E. Congenital heart surgery—Numerous congenital anomalies have been described, but in general most congenital heart disease can be broken down according to the physiologic disturbances.

1. Obstructive lesions–include valvular stenoses and coarctation of the aorta. Long-term sequelae include concentric cardiac hypertrophy and subsequent failure due to ventricular pressure overload. Repair or replacement of the involved valve or segment is the mainstay of operative treatment.
2. Left-to-right shunts (acyanotic)–the majority of patients in this group have atrial and ventricular septal defects. Also included are patent ductus arteriosus and truncus arteriosus. Symptoms are due to chronic volume overload of the pulmonary circulation, which eventually leads to pulmonary hypertension. Cyanosis is a very late finding in these anomalies, due to right-sided heart pressures exceeding left-sided heart pressures (Eisenmenger's syndrome). Operative repair involves patch closure of the septal defect or ductal ligation.
3. Right-to-left shunts (cyanotic)–these defects include tetralogy of Fallot, transposition of the great arteries, tricuspid atresia, total anomalous pulmonary venous drainage, and Ebstein's anomaly. These defects involve complex repairs that are usu-

ally performed during infancy. Palliative procedures include Blalock-Taussig shunts (subclavian artery to pulmonary artery) and aortopulmonary artery shunts.

III. POST-OPERATIVE CARE

A. Hemodynamics.

1. Invasive monitors include arterial lines, pulmonary artery catheters, and, occasionally, left atrial catheters.
2. Every effort should be made to optimize ventricular filling pressures and systemic blood pressures. In general, up to 3 L of crystalloid is used; after that, blood or colloid is used to increase filling pressures. Hypertension aggravates bleeding along suture lines and is controlled by a nitroprusside drip. In general, lower blood pressures are preferred as long as a mean blood pressure > 60 mm Hg is maintained. There are numerous causes for hypotension post-operatively; before beginning specific treatment, know the filling pressures, cardiac rhythm, cardiac index, and systemic vascular resistance.

B. Antiarrhythmics.

1. Digoxin can be given prophylactically to most CABG and valve patients. Contraindications include pre-existing conduction defects.
2. Atenolol has been shown to be a useful adjunct to digoxin. Contraindications include conduction defects, recent myocardial infarction, poor ventricular function, and diabetes mellitus.

C. Anticoagulation—Antiplatelet agents are given to all CABG patients. Patients with mechanical valve replacements are given warfarin starting POD#1, and dosage adjusted to maintain protime INR within recommended levels.

D. Hardware.

1. Mediastinal tubes are discontinued when drainage is less than 200 cc/8 h and no air leak is present.
2. Antibiotics are discontinued after the mediastinal tubes are removed.
3. Pacing wires are by convention atrial on right side and ventricular on left side. They are removed at 4 days or the day prior to discharge.

IV. POST-OPERATIVE COMPLICATIONS

A. Arrhythmias.

1. Ventricular ectopy–most common.
   a. For frequent (> 6-10/min) or multifocal PVCs, treat with lidocaine bolus of 1 mg/kg, followed by drip at 2-4 mg/min.
   b. Cardioversion needed if progresses to symptomatic ventricular tachycardia or if patient develops ventricular fibrillation.

c. Atrial or atrioventricular pacing at a slightly higher rate may suppress ectopy.
2. Nodal or junctional rhythm.
   a. Treatment may not be necessary (assure no hypotension).
   b. Rule out digoxin toxicity, make certain serum $K^+ > 4.5$, rule out hypomagnesemia.
   c. May require A-V sequential pacing if loss of atrial kick has significant hemodynamic sequelae.
3. Supraventricular tachycardia (SVT)–includes atrial fibrillation and flutter.
   a. Onset may be heralded by multiple PACs.
   b. Atrial ECG using atrial pacing leads often helpful in distinguishing fibrillation from flutter during rapid rates.
   c. Atrial fibrillation–digoxin used to control rate.
   d. Treatment of atrial flutter.
      (1) Rapid atrial pacing > 400 bpm.
      (2) Digitalization followed by IV beta blocker.
      (3) IV verapamil followed by digitalization. Calcium channel blockers must be given judiciously as wide complex SVT can mimic V-tach.
   e. In both instances, if any significant drop in blood pressure or cardiac output, the arrhythmia should be treated with synchronous DC cardioversion at 25-50 joules. This should be done prior to digitalization, however, to prevent onset of ventricular arrhythmias.
   f. Adenosine can be used initially as a diagnostic and therapeutic intervention. Transient bradycardia/asystole allows interpretation of rhythm and may be therapeutic.
   g. Diltiazem may also be used if adenosine fails to convert. Load with 15-25 mg initially (may repeat if no effect in 15-20 min), and start drip at 5-10 mg/h.

B. Bleeding.

1. Causes–include medications, clotting deficits, reoperation, prolonged operation, technical factors, hypothermia, and transfusion reactions.
2. Treatment.
   a. Assure normothermia.
   b. Measurement of clotting factors–PT, PTT, fibrinogen, platelet count, activated clotting time.
   c. Correction.
      (1) Fresh frozen plasma, cryoprecipitate, platelets.
      (2) Protamine for continued heparinization.
   d. Transfusion reaction protocol if suspected.
3. Exploration for post-operatuve hemorrhage–indications: mediastinal tube output of > 300 cc/h despite correction of clotting factors. Technical factors found as cause > 50% of time.

C. Renal failure—incidence is 1-30%.

1. Diagnosis–renal *vs.* pre-renal azotemia.

2. Management.
   a. Optimize volume status and cardiac output.
   b. Discontinue nephrotoxic drugs.
   c. Maintain urine output > 40 cc/h (low-dose dopamine, furosemide, ethacrynic acid as indicated; lasix or lasix/mannitol drips if persistent oliguria).
   d. Dialysis–either peritoneal or hemodialysis may be used.
   e. Outcome–mortality rates 0.3-23% depending upon the degree of azotemia; if dialysis is required, mortality ranges from 27-53%.

D. Respiratory failure.

1. Mechanical–mucous plugging, malpositioned endotracheal tube, pneumothorax.
2. Intrinsic–volume overload, pulmonary edema, atelectasis, pneumonia, pulmonary embolus (uncommon).

E. Low cardiac output syndrome—cardiac index < 2.0 L/min/m^2.

1. Signs–decreased urine output, acidosis, hypothermia, altered sensorium.
2. Assessment–heart rate and rhythm (EKG: possible acute myocardial infarction), pre-load and afterload states (pulmonary artery catheter readings), measurement of cardiac output.
3. Treatment.
   a. Stabilize rate and rhythm.
   b. Optimize volume status, systemic vascular resistance.
   c. Correct acidosis, hypoxemia if present (chest radiograph for pneumothorax).
   d. Inotropic agents if necessary.
   e. Persistent low cardiac output despite inotropic support requires placement of intra-aortic balloon pump.

F. Cardiac tamponade.

1. Onset–suggested by increasing filling pressures with decreased cardiac output; decreasing urine output and hypotension; quiet, distant heart sounds, and eventual equalization of right- and left-sided atrial pressures.
2. High degree of suspicion when coincides with excessive postoperative bleeding.
3. Chest radiograph may demonstrate wide mediastinum. Echocardiogram if readily available or diagnosis uncertain.
4. Treatment–emergent re-exploration is treatment of choice and may be needed at bedside for sudden hemodynamic decompensation. Transfusion to optimize volume status and inotropic support; avoid increased PEEP.

G. Peri-operative myocardial infarction—incidence 5-20%.

1. Diagnosis–new onset Q waves post-operatively; serial isoenzymes, increased MB fractions; segmental wall motion abnormalities by transthoracic or transesophageal ECHO.
2. Treatment–vasodilation (IV nitroglycerine is preferred to ni-

troprusside). Continued hemodynamic deterioration should be treated with immediate intra-aortic balloon counterpulsation. This "unloads" the ventricle and may preserve non-ischemic adjacent myocardium.

3. Outcome–associated with increased morbidity and mortality as well as poorer long-term results.

H. Post-operative fever.

1. Common in the first 24 h post-operatively; etiology unknown, may be associated with pyrogens introduced during cardiopulmonary bypass. Treat pyrexia with acetaminophen and cooling blankets, as associated hypermetabolism and vasodilation can be detrimental to hemodynamic status, and increase myocardial work.
2. Post-operative fevers for valve patients should be considered for culture. CABG patients should have full fever work-up on 5th post-operative day if still febrile, as most post-operative fevers are due to atelectasis.
3. Special attention should be paid to invasive monitors, and lines used longer than 3 days should be changed.
4. Peri-operative antibiotics should be continued until all invasive monitors and drainage tubes have been removed.
5. Sternal wound–daily inspection for drainage and stability. Sternal infections are disastrous in the cardiac patient, and early evidence of post-operative infection should be treated with operative debridement.
6. Post-pericardiotomy syndrome–characterized by low-grade fever, leukocytosis, chest pain, malaise, and pericardial rub on auscultation. Usually occurs 2 to 3 weeks following surgery, and is treated with NSAIDs. Steroids are sometimes necessary.

I. CNS complications.

1. Causes–pre-existing cerebrovascular disease, prolonged cardiopulmonary bypass, intra-operative hypotension, and emboli (either air or particulate matter).
2. Transient neurologic deficit–occurs in up to 12% of patients. Improvement usually occurs within several days.
3. Permanent deficit–suspect in patients with delayed awakening post-operatively; may have pathologic reflexes present.
4. Post-cardiotomy psychosis syndrome–incidence 10-24%. Starts around post-operative day 2 with anxiety and confusion; may progress to disorientation and hallucinations. Treat with rest and quiet environment; antipsychotics may be given as necessary. It is essential to rule out organic cause of delirium: substance withdrawal, hypoxemia, hypoglycemia, electrolyte abnormality, etc.
5. CT scan early for suspected localized lesions; EEG in patients with extensive dysfunction.
6. Treatment–optimize cerebral blood flow, avoid hypercapnia.

a. Post-operative seizures treated with lorazepam and loading with diphenylhydantoin.
b. Mannitol may be needed in presence of increased intra-cranial pressure, depending on hemodynamic status.

64

Thoracoscopy

Rebeccah L. Brown, M.D.

The first operative thoracoscopy was reported in 1910 by H.C. Jacobaeus, who performed closed intrapleural pneumonolysis for the treatment of pulmonary tuberculosis using a cystoscope and two-cannula technique. Interestingly, Jacobaeus was a professor of medicine, not surgery. With the introduction of streptomycin in 1945, interest in thoracoscopy waned, and its use was essentially confined to biopsy. The advent of video-assisted thoracoscopy (VATS) and refinement of ancillary instrumentation has launched a new interest in thoracoscopy, and its applications are rapidly expanding.

I. INDICATIONS

A. Treatment of primary spontaneous pneumothorax.

1. Allows for bleb and bullae resection, mechanical pleural abrasion, instillation of sclerosing agents, and assessment of lung re-expansion.
2. Indications.
   a. Persistent air leak for longer than 48-72 h after chest tube insertion for initial spontaneous pneumothorax.
   b. First recurrence of a spontaneous pneumothorax.
   c. Initial pneumothorax in patients with history of pneumothorax on contralateral side.
   d. Initial pneumothorax in patients whose geographic distance from medical care or occupation (i.e., pilots, scuba divers) places them at extreme risk.

B. Diagnosis and treatment of pleural masses and effusions, benign or malignant.

1. Definitive diagnosis of pleural effusion.
2. Determination of pleural involvement in lung cancer.
3. Biopsy for diffuse pleural processes.
4. Pleurodesis to prevent recurrent malignant effusion.
5. Debridement and decortication in early empyema.
6. Traumatic hemothorax.
7. Management of chylothorax.

C. Lung biopsy for diagnosis of diffuse lung disease.

1. Open lung biopsy still preferred in critically ill, ventilator-dependent patient.

D. Resection of peripheral indeterminate pulmonary nodule.

1. Non-calcified, < 3 cm diameter.
2. Indeterminate etiology after appropriate workup.
3. Location in outer third of lung parenchyma.
4. Absence of endobronchial extension.

E. Evaluation of mediastinal disease.

1. Resection or biopsy of mediastinal mass.
2. Adjunctive measure in staging of primary lung cancer–usually in combination with cervical mediastinoscopy. Allows assessment of subcarinal, aortopulmonary window, and para-aortic lymph nodes. Has essentially replaced the Chamberlain procedure in some institutions.

F. Evacuation and drainage of early empyema.

G. Pericardiectomy for effusive disease.

H. Applications in trauma—only in hemodynamically stable patients.

1. *Definitely helpful:*
   a. To assess integrity of diaphragm.
   b. To control bleeding intercostals.
   c. To evacuate residual hemothorax.
   d. To evacuate empyema and decorticate.
2. *Potentially helpful:*
   a. To assess mediastinal injury.
   b. To assess pericardial injury.
   c. To treat lung and bronchial lacerations.
   d. To treat esophageal injury.

II. CONTRAINDICATIONS

A. Obliterated pleural space.

B. Inability of patient to tolerate single lung ventilation.

C. Hemodynamic instability.

D. Coagulopathy.

E. Should be condemned for treatment of cancer.

III. TECHNIQUE

A. General anesthesia.

B. Single-lung ventilation using double-lumen endotracheal tube or bronchial blocker incorporated into single-lumen endotracheal tube.

C. Position patient in lateral decubitus position as for posterolateral thoracotomy with appropriate padding of pressure points.

D. Inject proposed port sites with local anesthetic with epinephrine to decrease bleeding from sites.

E. Placement of port sites depends on procedure performed. At least three ports are usually required for full exploration. Optimal position of the camera and accessory ports often described with reference to a baseball diamond. Camera site generally at "home plate" in 6th or 7th intercostal space between mid and posterior axillary line, vertically aligned with iliac crest. Area of interest is at "second base", and additional ports are at "first and third bases".

F. **Standard Carlens mediastinoscope** may be used for a thoracoscope. Zero degree scope typically used, but 30-degree angled scope provides superior visualization of dome and lateral recesses of the diaphragm.

G. **Standard rigid bronchoscopy or mediastinoscopy instruments** are used for suctioning, manipulating the lung, or for biopsies. Specialized endoscopic staplers are available.

H. **Be prepared** for conversion to open thoracotomy.

IV. COMPLICATIONS

A. **Overall incidence of complications**—10%.

B. **Prolonged air leak**—most common complication.

C. **Wound infection.**

D. **Bleeding.**

E. **Need for conversion to open thoracotomy.**

V. COST CONSIDERATIONS

Currently there is no procedure that can be performed more cheaply by video-assisted thoracoscopy than by conventional open technique. Theoretical advantages of decreased post-operative pain and decreased hospital stay are yet to be proven.

65

Renal Transplantation

Scott R. Johnson, M.D.

I. PATIENT SELECTION

A. Patient selection.

1. Criteria.
   a. ESRD from a variety of etiologies.
   b. Patient life expectancy longer than graft half-life.
2. Absolute contraindications.
   a. Malignancy.
   b. Current infection.
   c. Hepatitis.
   d. HIV.
3. Relative contraindications.
   a. History of noncompliance.
   b. Malnutrition.
   c. Severe cardiovascular disease.
   d. Substance abuse.
   e. High likelihood of recurrent renal disease.

B. Patient evaluation.

1. History and physical.
   a. Original disease, previous transplant history.
   b. Transfusion history.
   c. Cardiovascular history; claudication, angina.
   d. Urinary tract dysfunction; obstruction, BPH, chronic pyelonephritis.
   e. Malignancy.
   f. COPD, asthma, smoking.
   g. Diabetes mellitus.
   h. Liver disease, jaundice, biliary colic.
   i. Alcohol or substance abuse.
   j. HIV, exposure.
2. Pre-transplant studies.
   a. Routine screening labs; renal, hepatic, CBC, coagulation screen, UA, calcium, phosphorous, magnesium.

b. Hepatitis screen, HIV, VDRL, viral titers (CMV, EBV, varicella), throat and urine cultures, TB skin test.
c. Chest radiograph, EKG.
d. Blood typing, HLA, panel reactive antibodies (PRA).

3. Specific evaluations.
   a. Atherosclerosis–dipyridamole thallium scan, consider catheterization or CABG.
   b. Peptic ulcer disease–EGD, consider H_2 blockers or highly selective vagotomy.
   c. Cholelithiasis–cholecystectomy.
   d. Colonic disease–barium enema, colonoscopy; consider colectomy if diverticulosis present.
   e. VCUG.

II. INDICATIONS

A. Primary renal diseases.

1. Focal and segmental glomerulosclerosis.
   a. Recurrence rate in graft 20-30%.
   b. High risk of recurrence: age < 15 years, protracted time course from diagnosis to ESRD or when mesangial proliferation is present in a biopsy specimen.
   c. 40-50% with recurrence will lose graft.
2. IgA nephropathy.
   a. Recurrence in 50%.
   b. Up to 80% recurrence with LRD graft.
   c. Graft loss with recurrence is less than 10%.
3. Membranoproliferative glomerulonephritis (MPGN) Type I.
   a. Recurrence in 20-30%.
   b. Graft loss with recurrence in 40%.
4. MPGN type I.
   a. Recurrence in up to 80%.
   b. Graft loss in 10-20%.
5. Membranous glomerulonephritis.
   a. Recurrence is unusual 3-7%.
   b. Graft loss is rare.
6. Anti-glomerular basement membrane disease.
   a. Histologic recurrence in 50%.
   b. Clinical recurrence in 25%.
   c. Graft loss is rare.

B. Systemic diseases.

1. SLE.
   a. Recurrence in less than 1%.
   b. May reflect burned-out disease when ESRD develops or use of immunosuppression.
2. Hemolytic uremic syndrome.
   a. Recurrence in 10-25%.
   b. Graft loss due to recurrence in 50%.
   c. Risk factors for recurrence.
      (1) Transplant < 3 months from diagnosis.
      (2) Use of ALG or OKT3.

3. Henoch-Schonlein Purpura.
   a. Histologic recurrence in 30% of adults and up to 75% of children.
   b. Clinical recurrence in less than 10%.
   c. Graft loss is rare.
4. Diabetes mellitus.
   a. Leading cause of ESRD leading to renal transplant.
   b. Histologic recurrence in up to 100%.
   c. Graft loss due to diabetes mellitus in about 5%.
5. Mixed cryoglobulinemia.
   a. Recurrence in about 50%.
   b. Graft loss may occur.
6. Multiple myeloma.
   a. Recurrence appears to be common.
   b. Death due to underlying disease appears to precede graft loss.
7. Wegener's granulomatosis.
   a. Recurrence has been noted to occur in the graft.
   b. Recurrence can be treated with cyclophosphamide and steroids.
8. Primary hyperoxaluria Type I.
   a. Recurrence and graft loss are the usual clinical course.
   b. Combined liver-kidney transplant provides the deficient enzyme and appears to be the therapy of choice.
9. Cystinosis.
   a. Recurrence histologically is common, but graft dysfunction is unusual.
   b. Cystine accumulation continues in other organ systems and leads to morbidity.
10. Fabry disease–recurrences have been reported.
11. Sickle cell disease.
12. Progressive systemic sclerosis.
13. Alport syndrome.
   a. Defect in collagen assembly resulting in sensorineural deafness and renal dysfunction.
   b. Renal transplants have been performed; results match those of controls.
   c. Presence of new collagen antigen in graft has led to development of anti-GBM disease in recipients, which may lead to graft loss.

III. DONOR SELECTION – ANTIGEN MATCHING

A. ABO antigens.

1. Matching required for renal transplant, otherwise hyperacute rejection ensues.
2. Isoagglutinins are present in sera of individuals to A or B antigens.
3. Several successful A2 to O renal transplants have been performed.

4. ABO-incompatible transplants may be performed if isoagglutinins are removed by splenectomy and plasmapheresis.

B. HLA class I or class II antigens.

1. Class I antigens consist of A, B, or C loci antigens located on the surface membranes of all nucleated cells.
2. Class II antigens consist of DP, DQ, and DR loci found primarily on immune cells, dendritic cells and endothelial cells.

C. Living donors.

1. Six antigen match, HLA-identical, implies that both haplotypes for class I A and B loci and the DR loci of class II antigens are identical between donor and recipient.
2. Long-term graft survival in HLA identical transplants is 90%.
3. As HLA antigen disparity increases, graft survival worsens; the use of cyclosporine and donor-specific transfusions will improve the graft survival in HLA disparate transplants.

D. Cadaveric donors.

1. HLA-A and B antigen matching in cadaveric transplantation may provide a long-term benefit.
2. HLA-DR matching provides a greater benefit than class I antigen matching.
3. The use of cyclosporine-based regimens appear to be responsible for the success without strong antigen matching.

IV. TRANSPLANT PROCEDURE

A. Donor nephrectomy.

1. Left kidney is preferred because of longer renal vein and better access to arteries.
2. Oblique flank incision over the 12th rib from the rectus to the parasternal line.
3. Muscle layers are divided, exposing the peritoneum, which is retracted and Gerota's fascia is exposed.
4. Gerota's fascia is incised, and the kidney is exposed. The ureter is followed to a point beyond the iliac vessels and divided. A cuff of areolar tissue surrounding the ureter is also removed to ensure a vascular supply.
5. The artery is divided at the aorta, followed by the renal vein.
6. The kidney is flushed with preservation solution (UW or Euro-Collins), placed on ice, and transported to the recipient room.

B. Transplant.

1. Oblique incision cranial to inguinal ligament–muscles are divided, the peritoneum is exposed and retracted medially to expose the iliac vessels.
2. Vascular anastomoses are performed as follows.
   a. Renal artery to external iliac artery (end-to-side).
   b. Renal artery to hypogastric artery (end-to-end).
   c. Renal vein to external iliac vein (end-to-side).
   d. Accessory renal arteries can be anastomosed end to side to the largest renal artery and then anastomosed to the recipient vessels. Usually done *ex vivo* on ice.

3. Ureteroneocystostomy.
   a. Requirements.
      (1) Tension-free repair.
      (2) Water-tight repair.
      (3) 1 cm submucosal tunnel to prevent reflux.
   b. Methods.
      (1) Leadbetter-Politano–uses a transvesical approach, bladder is entered, and the distal donor ureter is sewn mucosa to mucosa from within the bladder.
      (2) Litch–extravesical approach ureteropyelostomy–recipient proximal ureter is anastomosed to the donor renal pelvis.

C. Post-operative care.

1. General post-operative care does not differ from that of the general surgical patient.
2. Beware of volume depletion due to post-transplant diuresis. This can be avoided by replacing urine output cc per cc q 4 h with IV fluid of similar electrolyte composition.
3. Sutures or wound clips are generally left in place for 21 days because of delayed wound healing in renal failure patients and immunosuppressed patients.
4. Foley catheters are left in place for 2-5 days post-operatively.

D. Assessment of graft function.

1. Urine output–non-specific, decreased urine output may indicate hypovolemia, urinary obstruction, ureteral compromise, vascular compromise, ATN, rejection.
2. Creatinine and BUN–as above, non-specific.
3. Ultrasound–demonstrates patency of artery and vein, detects fluid collection and hydronephrosis.
4. Radionucleotide imaging–can image flow and function.
5. Renal biopsy–may yield definitive pathologic diagnosis in cases of dysfunction, difficult to assess CSA nephrotoxicity.

V. IMMUNOSUPPRESSION

A. Immunosuppressive drugs.

1. Azathioprine.
   a. Imidazole derivative of mercaptopurine.
   b. Inhibits lymphoid proliferation by blocking DNA/RNA synthesis.
   c. Initial dose 3-5 mg/kg and tapered to 1-3 mg/kg.
   d. Complications–leukopenia, nausea, and vomiting, pancreatitis and hepatitis.
2. Glucocorticoids.
   a. Inhibit IL-1 and IL-6 production by macrophages.
   b. High doses at induction and tapered to a maintenance dose.
   c. Complications–Cushing's disease, osteoporosis, cataracts, hyperlipidemia.
3. Cyclosporine A.
   a. Cyclic polypeptide.

b. Prevents production of IL-2 by T helper cells.
c. Metabolized by hepatic cytochrome P-450; levels are affected by many commonly prescribed medications.
d. Complications–renal toxicity, hypertension, tremors, paresthesia, hypertrichosis.

4. Antithymocyte globulins.
a. MALG, ATGAM, ALG, RATS.
b. Polyclonal sera to human lymphocytes/thymocytes produced in animals.
c. Function to deplete these cells from the recipient (lysis or RES uptake).
d. Complications–fever, chills, anaphylaxis, serum sickness, and ARDS.

5. Monoclonal antibodies (OKT3).
a. Murine monoclonal antibody to the pan T cell receptor CD3.
b. Deplete CD3 cells from circulation.
c. Complications–fever, chills, pulmonary edema.

6. FK506.
a. Similar to cyclosporine.
b. Also prevents IL-2 production by T helper cells.
c. Also metabolized by hepatic P-450 system.
d. Complications are similar to cyclosporine, including nephro- and neurotoxicity.

B. Therapeutic regimens.

1. Cyclosporine monotherapy–CSA alone.
2. Cyclosporine dual therapy–CSA and glucocorticoids or azathioprine.
3. Cyclosporine triple therapy–CSA, glucocorticoids and azathioprine.
4. Sequential therapy.
a. Induction therapy with antilymphocyte preparation, azathioprine, and glucocorticoids.
b. CSA administration is delayed until renal function improves.
c. Allows recovery from preservation injury prior to CSA introduction.
d. Results in delayed time to first rejection and lower Cr at 3 months.

VI. REJECTION

A. Hyperacute rejection.

1. Occurs promptly after revascularization of the graft.
2. Caused by presence of pre-formed antibodies–repeated transfusions, pregnancy, previous transplants.
3. Graft thrombosis follows, requiring transplant nephrectomy.
4. Usually identified by a positive crossmatch.

B. Accelerated rejection.

1. Occurs around day 3-5 post-transplant.
2. Reflects recipient sensitization to donor.

3. Can be treated with antilymphocyte preparations but represents a risk factor for graft loss.

C. Acute rejection.

1. Accounts for 85% of rejection episodes in first 3 months post-transplant.
2. May be related to non-compliance or to medications that reduce CSA levels.
3. Symptoms–fever, malaise, oliguria, graft tenderness, elevated Cr.
4. Treated with glucocorticoids; if resistant, with antithymocyte preparations.

D. Chronic rejection.

1. Diagnosis is difficult, can be based upon biopsy or Cr increase after 6 months.
2. Biopsy demonstrates obliterative fibrosis of vasculature and tubules.
3. Risk factors for chronic rejection include acute rejection episodes, low CSA dosage, and infection.
4. No effective therapy is currently available.

VII. COMPLICATIONS

A. Surgical complications.

1. Vascular complications
   a. Renal artery thrombosis.
      (1) Incidence about 1%.
      (2) Presents with a sudden decline in urine output.
      (3) Diagnosis with US, technetium scan, angiogram.
      (4) Emergent revascularization is mandatory to prevent graft loss.
      (5) Causes include intimal dissection, kinking, hyperacute rejection, irreversible acute or accelerated rejection, and hypercoagulable states.
   b. Renal artery stenosis.
      (1) Incidence is 2-10%.
      (2) Presents with refractory hypertension, unexplained rise in Cr, or a change in graft bruit.
      (3) Diagnosis with Doppler sonography or angiography.
      (4) Management may include hypertension control, percutaneous transluminal angioplasty, resection and reanastomosis, or bypass graft.
   c. Renal vein thrombosis.
      (1) Incidence of 0.3-4.2%.
      (2) Symptoms include oliguria, graft swelling and tenderness, and hematuria.
      (3) Diagnosis with angiography, Doppler sonography, technetium scan.
      (4) Attempts at thrombectomy are usually unsuccessful at salvaging the graft; success with thrombolytics have been reported.

(5) Causes include vessel kinking, compression due to hematoma, lymphocelea or urinoma.

d. Hemorrhage.

(1) Very rare occurrence.

(2) Often related to the development of a mycotic aneurysm.

(3) Nephrectomy is usually indicated.

2. Urinary tract complications.

a. Ureteral leakage.

(1) Incidence of 3-10%.

(2) Related to ureteral ischemia, anastomotic tension.

(3) Usually in first month after transplant.

(4) Symptoms–pain and graft swelling, fever, and sepsis.

(5) Urine fistula.

a) Diagnosis.

b) CT, US may demonstrate fluid collection.

c) Nuclear renography is less sensitive.

(6) Management.

a) Percutaneous nephrostomy and stenting.

b) Ureteroneocystostomy revision.

c) Boari flap, donor-recipient pyeloureterostomy.

b. Ureteral obstruction.

(1) Most common urinary complication.

(2) Etiology includes hematoma, kinking, or edema.

(3) Late onset obstruction is related to fibrosis from ischemia.

(4) Presentation depends upon degree of obstruction.

(5) Oliguria, elevated Cr, sepsis, anuria.

(6) Diagnosis by sonography, antegrade pyelography (most sensitive), renal venography (less sensitive).

(7) Management.

a) Percutaneous nephrostomy and surgical correction.

b) Percutaneous transluminal dilatation and stenting.

c. Urinary bladder complications.

(1) Occur early after transplant.

(2) Present with palpable mass, rise in Cr, pain in graft bed.

(3) Usually related to extravasation from anterior cystotomy.

(4) Diagnosis made with sonography (fluid collection), cystography.

(5) Management–exploration and primary repair with bladder decompression.

3. Miscellaneous complications–Lymphoceles.

a. Incidence ranges from 0.6-18%.

b. Many are asymptomatic and eventually are resorbed, some present with mass effects (vascular compression), lymph fistula.

c. Diagnosis is made with sonography (fluid collection).

d. Management.
   (1) Percutaneous drainage: high recurrence rate and potential for infection.
   (2) Intraperitoneal window permits lymph drainage into peritoneal cavity.

B. Medical complications.

1. Infections.
   a. General considerations.
      (1) Influenced by degree of immunosuppression.
      (2) 80% of transplant recipients develop infection.
      (3) 40% of transplant deaths are due to infection.
   b. 1st month.
      (1) Etiology related to surgical procedure.
      (2) Wound infections, UTI, infections related to indwelling catheters.
      (3) Pneumonia.
      (4) Also infections transmitted with graft (HIV, CMV, hepatitis).
   c. 1st to 6th month–high mortality due to degree of immunosuppression; viral infections are common.
   d. Beyond 6 months–risk is reduced because of reduced immunosuppression.
2. Malignancy.
   a. General considerations.
      (1) Immunosuppression predisposes to the development of malignancy.
      (2) Incidence of *de novo* malignancy is 1-16% in renal transplant recipients.
   b. Lymphoproliferative disease (LPD).
      (1) Strong association with EBV infection.
      (2) 1% incidence in renal transplant recipients.
      (3) 80% are non-Hodgkin's lymphomas.
      (4) B cell origin.
      (5) Extranodal (graft and CNS are common).
      (6) Usually appear in the first 4 months post-transplant.
      (7) OKT3 appears to increase risk of LPD.
      (8) Reduction of immunosuppression is usually required.
   c. Skin cancer.
      (1) Non-melanoma forms predominate.
      (2) Squamous cell is most common.
      (3) More aggressive than in general population.
      (4) Increased incidence of regional metastasis.
      (5) Present about 5 years post-transplant.
   d. Cervical cancer.
      (1) 3rd most common post-transplant malignancy.
      (2) HSV-2 and HPV have been implicated in pathogenesis.
      (3) Conventional therapy is appropriate.
      (4) Reduction of immunosuppression is not mandated.

66

Liver Transplantation

MARTHA A. FERGUSON, M.D.

I. HISTORY

A. **1967**—Starzl performed first successful liver transplant.
B. **1983**—Venovenous bypass introduced for use during anhepatic phase.
C. **1984**—Broelsch *et al* introduced split-liver transplantation.

II. INDICATIONS FOR TRANSPLANTATION

Liver transplantation is generally reserved for the patient with end-stage liver disease (ESLD) who has a life expectancy of less than 1 year and for whom no other therapy is suitable. More specific indications include the following.

A. **Progressive jaundice.**
B. **Ascites** refractory to diuretic control.
C. **Spontaneous hepatic encephalopathy.**
D. **Recurrent sepsis** (including spontaneous bacterial peritonitis).
E. **Recurrent variceal hemorrhage.**
F. **Coagulopathy** unresponsive to Vitamin K replacement.
G. **Severe fatigue** that interferes with activities of daily living.

III. SPECIFIC DISEASES NECESSITATING TRANSPLANTATION

A. **Alcoholic cirrhosis**—most common cause of liver failure in this country and associated with a low recidivism rate following transplantation.
B. **Hepatitis**—virtually all patients with chronic Hepatitis B or C will ultimately become re-infected, with variable outcomes.
C. **Acute fulminant hepatic failure**—secondary to drug toxicity or hepatitis. Transplantation for acute viral hepatitis has a better outcome than for chronic hepatitis.
D. **Inborn errors of metabolism**—this category includes gly-

cogen storage disease, Wilson's disease, alpha-1-antitrypsin deficiency, and Protein S deficiency, among others.

E. Primary hepatic malignancy—controversial indication, associated with high likelihood of recurrent disease.

IV. ORGAN SELECTION

In general, standard criteria apply–hemodynamically stable donor with no evidence of sepsis or non-CNS primary malignancy; normal MegX (lidocaine metabolism); and ABO compatibility.

A. Cadaveric whole organ.

B. Cadaveric reduced-sized grafts—full right, full left, or left lateral lobe graft. With a left lateral lobe, a size discrepancy of 10:1 can be overcome.

C. Living related liver donation—increases the limited pool of pediatric-sized livers. Graft and patient survival rates as high as 95%.

V. URGENCY OF NEED

Because of limited availability of organs, potential recipients are ranked according to clinical status:

Status	Definition
1	ICU patient, life expectancy < 7 days
2	ICU patient, not on life support
3	Hospitalized, non-ICU
4	At home, functioning normally
07	Temporarily inactive

VI. OPERATIVE PROCEDURE (Figure 1)

A. Bilateral subcostal incision with midline extension to xiphoid process.

B. Establishment of veno-venous bypass lines for splanchnic bed and lower extremity decompression during vena caval and portal cross-clamping. Cannulas from the portal and femoral veins drain blood into the axillary vein.

C. Simultaneous graft preparation and reduction if appropriate.

D. Mobilization of native liver and isolation of superior/inferior vena cava, portal vein, hepatic artery, and hepatic duct.

E. Recipient hepatectomy.

F. Vascular anastomoses of donor organ—Supra-hepatic cava, infrahepatic vena cava, hepatic artery, and finally portal vein anastomoses.

G. Biliary continuity by end-to-end bile duct anastomosis or choledochojejunostomy. A T-tube stent may be placed for monitoring of bile output.

H. Abdominal closure with non-absorbable fascial sutures.

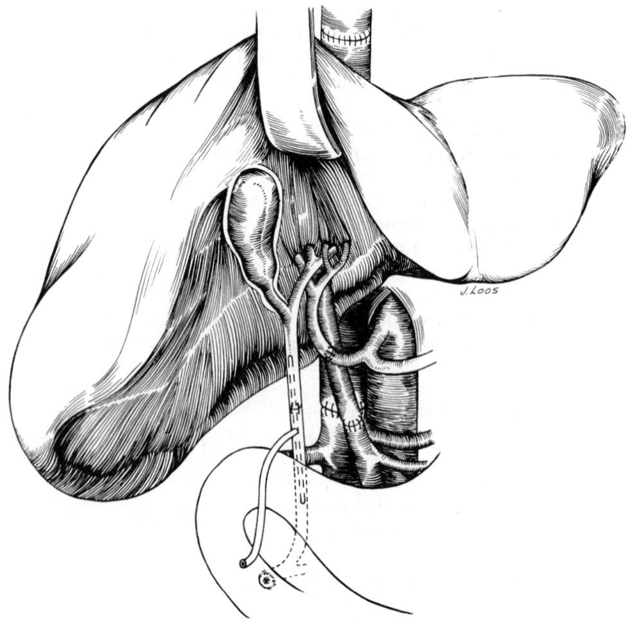

FIG. 1 Hepatic Transplantation

VII. POST-OPERATIVE CARE

A. Hemodynamic monitoring and resuscitation with the aid of pulmonary artery catheter.

B. Ventilatory support often for 24 to 48 h post-transplantation.

C. Electrolyte management—correction of glucose, calcium, potassium, magnesium, and phosphate are particularly important.

D. Infection surveillance and prophylaxis—TMP/SMX, nystatin, and ganciclovir (if transplantation from CMV-positive to CMV-negative).

E. Immunosuppression—protocols vary among institutions.

1. OKT3–used in some centers for induction and in most centers for acute rejection.
2. Azathioprine.
3. Steroids–usually begun at high dose and tapered over the ensuing months. Weaning completely from steroids has been accomplished in selected liver transplant patients.
4. Cyclosporin (CsA) or (FK506)–a new formulation of CsA, Neosporin, has achieved more consistent levels with open biliary drainage and impaired hepatic function.

VIII. ASSESSMENT OF GRAFT FUNCTION

A. **Routine laboratory tests**—transaminase levels, alkaline phosphatase, serum bilirubin, and coagulation parameters are very non-specific, but usually used to follow trends in graft function.

B. **Bile output from T-tube**—volume will decrease with rejection or biliary stricture.

C. **Radionuclide imaging** can be used to assess hepatocellular function and continuity of biliary drainage.

D. **Liver biopsy**—most specific for differentiating rejection from recurrent hepatitis, steatosis, ischemia, or other causes of graft dysfunction.

IX. COMPLICATIONS

A. **Primary non-function**—has become relatively rare cause of graft dysfunction since the introduction of UW solution. Manifested by failure to regain hepatic function in the early postoperative period. Urgent re-transplantation is usually indicated.

B. **Rejection**—occurs at some time in up to 60% of patients. OKT3 induction decreases the incidence of early rejection (within the first two weeks).

C. **Hepatic artery thrombosis.**

D. **Portal vein thrombosis**—usually requires retransplantation, but may respond to thrombolytic therapy.

E. **Biliary complications**—manifested by fever, rising bilirubin, and alkaline phosphatase. Diagnosed by cholangiogram. Biliary stricture is managed by conversion to choledochojejunostomy.

F. **Vena caval obstruction.**

G. **Renal dysfunction.**

H. **Infection and immunosuppressive drug complications.**

X. RESULTS (1994 UNOS DATA)

A. **Patient survival at 1 year**—81%.

B. **Graft survival at 1 year**—76%; at 3 years, 70%.

67

Pancreas Transplantation

Martha A. Ferguson, M.D.

I. HISTORY

A. 1921—Banting and Best report discovery of insulin.

B. 1966—Kelly and Lillehei perform first pancreas transplant.

C. 1986—Corry and associates develop technique of urinary bladder diversion of exocrine secretions.

II. INDICATIONS FOR PANCREAS TRANSPLANTATION

Insulin-dependent diabetes mellitus is associated with increased risk of blindness (25X), kidney disease (17X), gangrene (20X), and heart disease or stroke (2X) compared to non-diabetic patients. Pancreas transplant is performed in 3 categories of patients:

A. Patient with functioning renal transplant, to prevent the development of nephropathy in the transplanted kidney.

B. Insulin-dependent diabetic with end-stage renal disease (ESRD) in need of simultaneous kidney-pancreas transplantation.

C. Nonuremic diabetics with other secondary complications of their disease. Not as commonly performed. The risks of surgery and immunosuppression must be balanced against the likelihood of developing secondary complications of diabetes.

III. SPECIFIC INDICATIONS AND CONTRAINDICATIONS

A. IDDM documented by absence of circulating C-peptide.

B. Microalbuminuria with a creatinine clearance of less than 60 ml/min.

C. Proteinuria with a projected dialysis requirement.

D. Autonomic neuropathy.

E. Retinopathy.

F. Labile diabetes and failure of medical management.

G. Absence of coronary artery disease.

H. **Absence of gangrene** or ongoing sepsis.
I. **Age** between 18 and 50 years.

IV. ORGAN SELECTION

Most are performed from cadaveric donors. In addition to standard criteria for donor selection, there are specific contraindications to pancreas transplantation.

A. **Presence of diabetes mellitus.**
B. **Chronic pancreatitis.**
C. **Pancreatic damage** secondary to trauma.
D. **History of alcohol abuse** or relapsing pancreatitis (relative).

V. OPERATIVE PROCEDURE (Figure 1)

A. The recipient bed is prepared in the right iliac fossa.
B. Venous drainage is first established by portal vein-external iliac vein anastomosis.
C. Arterial inflow is determined by manner of donor harvest. With the whole graft, the celiac axis and SMA are preferentially removed together on an aortic patch which is anastomosed end-to-side to the recipient external iliac artery.
D. Management of exocrine secretions:
   1. Diversion to the urinary bladder by anastomosis to second portion of duodenum, harvested *en bloc* with the pancreas. This technique is associated with the highest patient and graft survival, and has the advantage of using urinary amylase to monitor graft function.
   2. Diversion into the bowel is more physiologic but associated with fistula formation.
   3. Pancreatic duct occlusion with injectable synthetic polymer completely blocks exocrine secretion, but can lead to severe inflammation and fibrosis.

VI. POST-OPERATIVE CARE

A. **Since vascular thrombosis is the most common cause of early graft loss,** some form of peri-operative anticoagulation is recommended. Suggested protocols include aspirin, systemic heparinization, and low-molecular weight dextran.
B. **Graft function** can be monitored by urinary amylase levels and glucose homeostasis. Since 90% of the pancreas may be lost before glucose homeostasis is impaired, this is not very sensitive.
C. **There is no reliable technique for the diagnosis of rejection.** In the patient undergoing simultaneous kidney-pancreas transplant, rejection is usually monitored by following serum creatinine levels. Rejection demonstrated on biopsy of the renal allograft is also an indication of pancreatic rejection.
D. **Immunosuppressive regimens** vary, but most centers use induction with ALG or OKT3 and maintenance with cyclosporin or FK506, prednisone, and azathioprine.

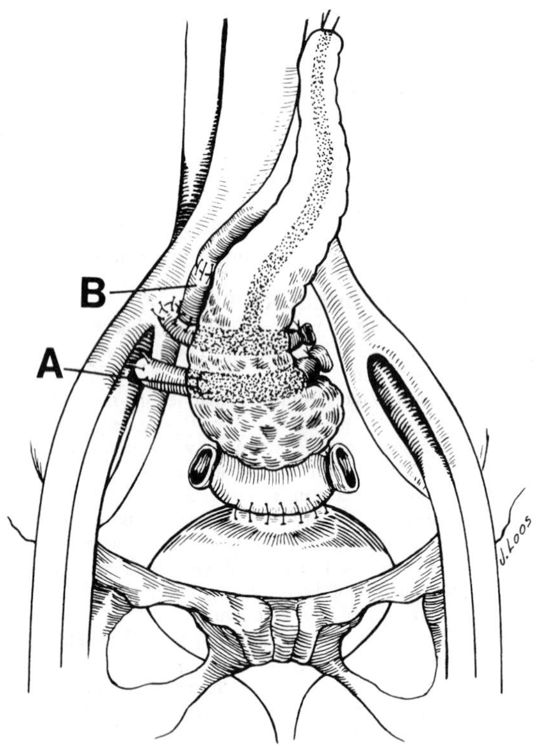

FIG. 1 Pancreas Transplantation (**A**, venous anastomosis; **B**, arterioal anastomosis)

E. **Radionuclide perfusion scans** can be used to evaluate blood flow to the allograft.

VII. COMPLICATIONS

A. Graft pancreatitis.

1. Secondary to preservation injury and ischemia.
2. Suggested by hyperamylasemia and local graft pain.
3. May require drainage of peri-pancreatic collections or operative debridement of necrotic pancreas.

B. Graft thrombosis.

1. Most common cause of sudden early graft loss (10-20%).
2. Attributed to the fact that the pancreas is a low-flow organ.

3. If confirmed by radionuclide scan, the graft must be removed urgently to prevent septic or vascular complications.

C. Anastomotic failure.

1. Presents with fever, leukocytosis, and drainage of clear fluid from the operative wound.
2. Rare with bladder drainage of the exocrine pancreas, but can be fatal if not addressed early.

D. Sepsis—almost always related to the development of graft pancreatitis or anastomotic failure.

E. Bleeding.

1. Site is usually gastrointestinal tract.
2. Usually related to the use of anticoagulation in perioperative period.

VIII. RESULTS

A. Percent patient survival at 1 year 91%.

B. Percent graft survival at 1 year 75%; at 3 years 65%.

68

The Hand

Khang N. Thai, M.D.

Hand injuries and infections should never be underestimated, because a seemingly "minor" problem can result in prolonged recovery, loss of employment, or permanent disability. It is important to recognize when a hand specialist is required and which conditions require emergent treatment.

I. HAND INJURIES

A. History.

1. Mechanism of injury (laceration, crush, bite, etc.), degree of contamination.
2. Time elapsed since injury or onset of infection, previous treatment.
3. Associated injuries.
4. Past medical history.
5. Age, occupation, tetanus status, allergies.
6. Hand dominance, pre-injury function.

B. Assessment—Since many hand injuries are work-related or involve long-term disability, documentation of the injury, including a thorough neurovascular exam, is of extreme importance. Photographs should be taken if convenient.

1. ***Vascular assessment.***
   a. Control bleeding with local pressure and elevation. *Never blindly clamp bleeding vessels.*
   b. Assess brachial, radial, and ulnar pulses.
   c. Assess capillary refill.
2. ***Sensory assessment.***
   a. Assess each nerve by its distribution (Figure 1).
   b. Use pinprick and 2-point discrimination along longitudinal axis (6 mm distinction at fingertip).
   c. *Never* administer anesthetic before completing sensory exam.

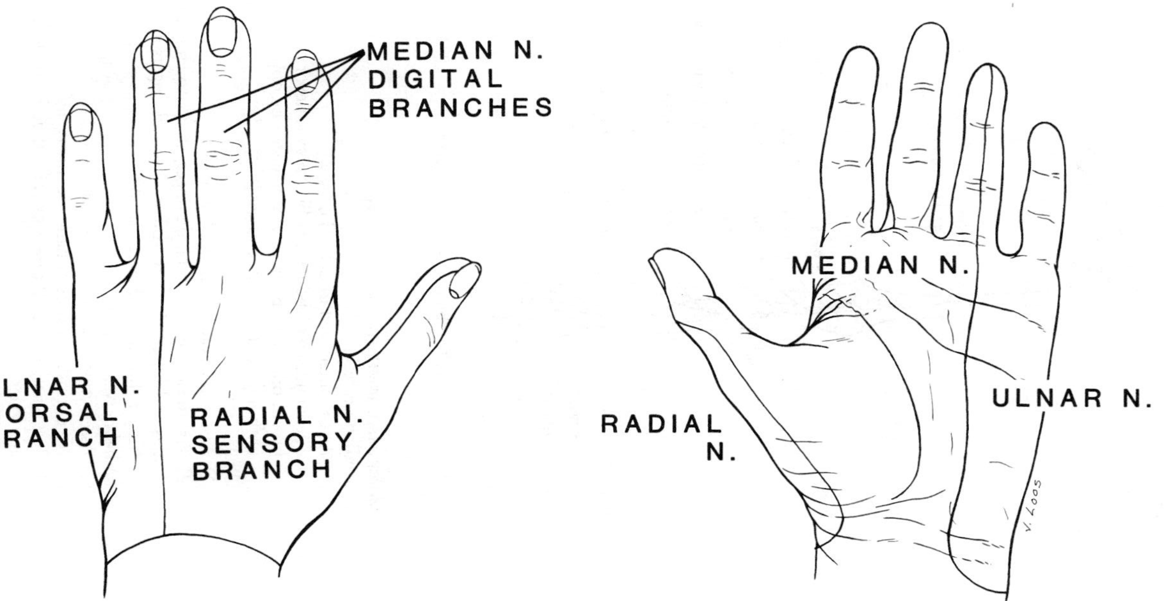

FIG. 1 Sensory Areas of the Left Hand

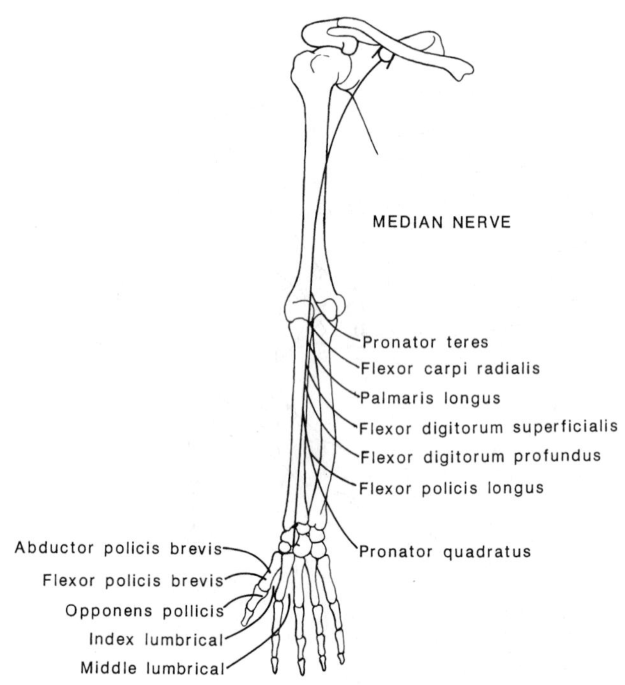

FIG. 2 **Motor Distribution of Median Nerve**

3. ***Motor assessment.***
   a. **Median** nerve.
      (1) Assess innervated muscles (Figure 2).
      (2) Thenar muscles (abductor pollicis brevis, flexor pollicis brevis, opponens pollicis) can be tested by opposition of thumb to ring or little finger (Figure 3).
   b. **Ulnar** nerve.
      (1) Assess innervated muscles (Figure 4).
      (2) Test flexion of ring and little finger, ability to cross index and long fingers, or ability to spread fingers apart (finger abduction) (Figure 5).
   c. **Radial** nerve.
      (1) Assess innervated muscles (Figure 6).
      (2) *No* intrinsic muscles of hand are innervated.
      (3) Test wrist and MCP extension, also thumb abduction and extension.

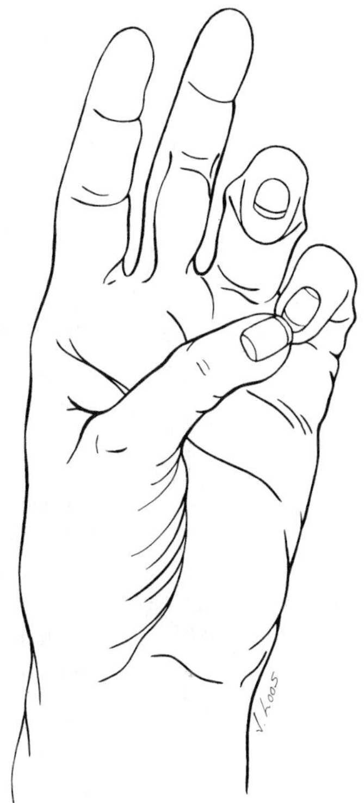

FIG. 3 **Thumb Opposition**

4. Musculotendon assessment.
   a. **Flexors.**
      (1) Flexor digitorum profundus (FDP)—stabilize proximal interphalangeal (PIP) joint and have patient flex distal joint (Figure 7).
      (2) Flexor digitorum superficialis—block FDP by placing all but the finger being tested in extension, and have patient flex individual finger at PIP joint (Figure 8).
   b. **Extensors.**
      (1) Extensor tendons can be tested by having patient extend each finger independently.
      (2) Extensor indicis proprius and extensor digiti quinti ten-

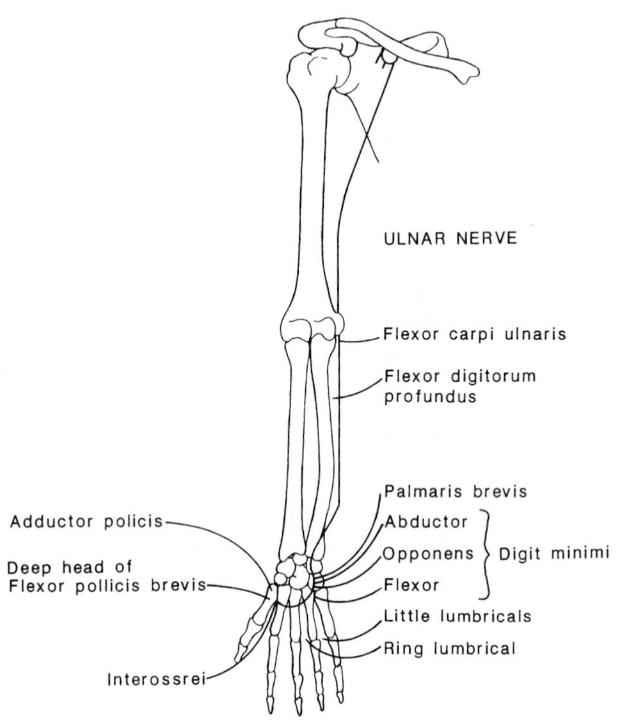

FIG. 4 Motor Distribution of Ulnar Nerve

dons can be tested by having patient make a fist and extending index and little finger independently.

5. ***Skeletal assessment.***
   a. If there is *any* question about a foreign body, dislocation, or fracture, obtain radiographs.
   b. A fracture is highly suspected if **hematoma, deformity,** or **persistent local tenderness** follows any closed injury.
   c. Always examine the entire extremity. Beware of associated elbow and shoulder trauma, and obtain radiographs accordingly.
   d. Obtain anteroposterior, lateral, and true oblique radiographs to avoid missing small fractures.

C. Treatment.

1. Basic rules.
   a. Irrigation and debridement of devitalized tissue.

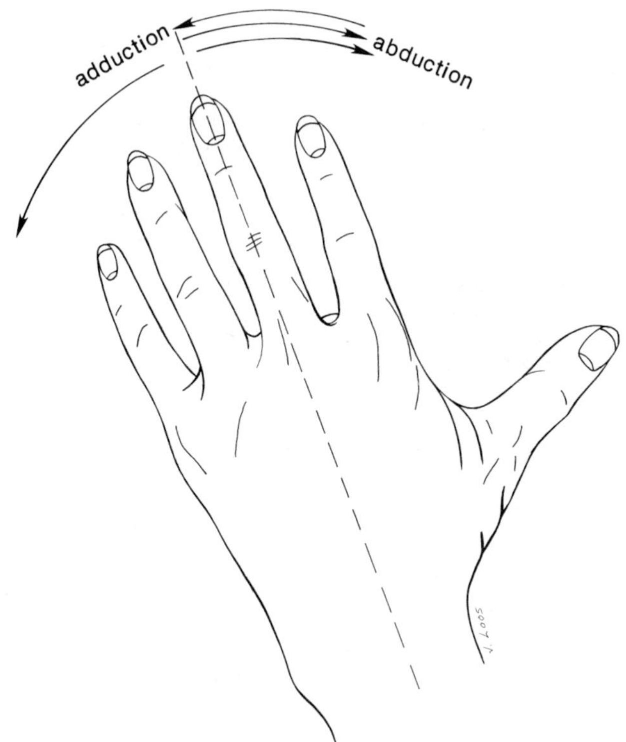

FIG. 5 Finger Abduction

b. Control bleeding with pressure, always elevate the extremity.
c. Antibiotics and tetanus prophylaxis as needed.
d. Dressings and splints should be comfortable, conforming, and not circumferential.

2. ***True emergencies***—these injuries require definitive treatment urgently. Referral to a hand specialist is recommended.
   a. Vascular compromise–poor capillary refill, pale white or bluish color, absent pulses.
   b. Hemorrhage that cannot be controlled by direct pressure.
   c. Open fracture or dislocation.
   d. Heavy contamination of an open wound.
   e. Compartment syndrome.

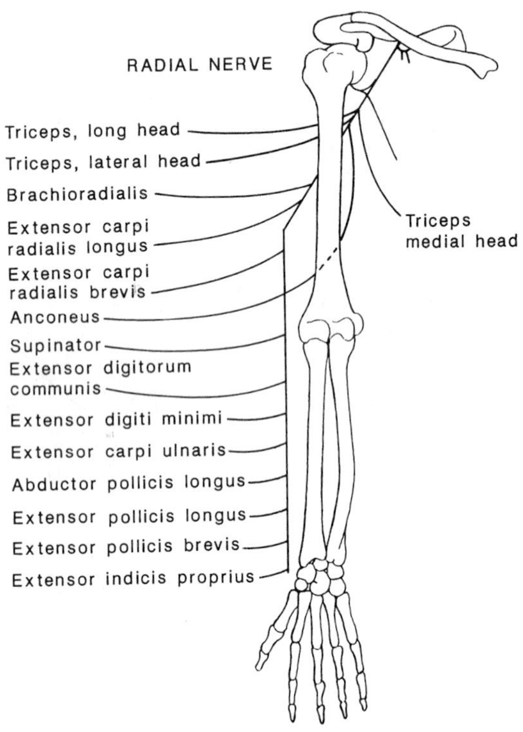

FIG. 6 Motor Distribution of Radial Nerve

f. Amputation–see below.
g. Emergency cases–NPO, start IV, send type and screen, antibiotic (cephalosporin) and tetanus prophylaxis, elevate the injured extremity.

3. Injuries that require urgent care, but definitive treatment may be delayed.
   a. Tendon and/or nerve injuries in clean wounds.
      (1) Anesthetize, irrigate thoroughly.
      (2) Close the skin.
      (3) Splint in neutral position.
      (4) Schedule for definitive repair in 5-7 days.
   b. Closed fractures.
      (1) Splint and elevate.
      (2) Return for evaluation within 24 h.
4. ***Special injuries***—In general, non-absorbable monofilament

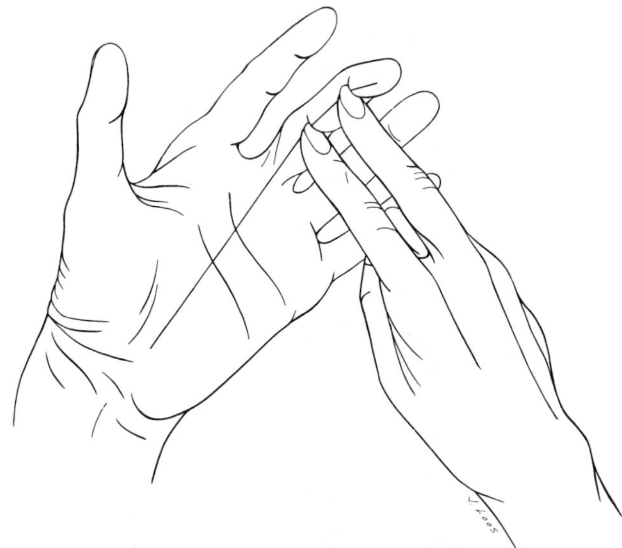

FIG. 7 **Examination of Flexor Digitorum Profundus**

sutures should be used for skin closure. The exception is in infants/children, in whom chromic sutures may be used to avoid suture removal. Absorbable sutures are used for reapproximation of deeper tissues.

a. **Puncture wounds.**
   (1) Check for foreign body by radiographs and exploration (if indicated).
   (2) Ellipse skin around wound to debride; avoid probing the wound.
   (3) Leave open for drainage.

b. **Flap wounds.**
   (1) Proximally based flaps usually have good blood supply. Distally based flaps have greater risks of tip necrosis.
   (2) A flap sutured under tension is likely to become ischemic.
   (3) A long flap has a greater chance of survival if the subcutaneous fat is trimmed away and the skin then used as a full-thickness skin graft (FTSG).

c. **Avulsed flap.**
   (1) May be sutured in place after defatting as a FTSG.
   (2) Usually does better with a formal split-thickness skin graft (STSG).

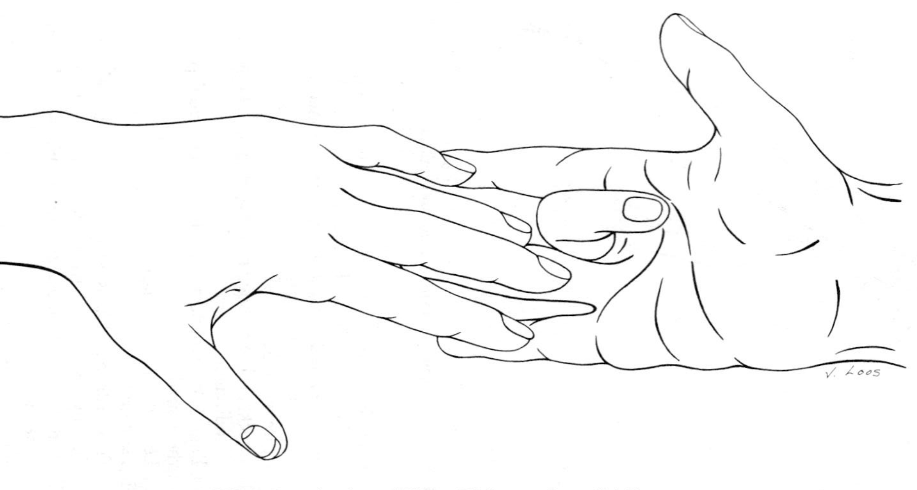

FIG. 8 Examination of Flexor Digitorum Superficialis

d. **Fingertip avulsion**—requires surgical treatment if there is an open joint or exposed bone after debridement. Should obtain radiograph to rule out epiphyseal plate injury.

e. **Bite wounds.**
   (1) Human or animal bites are prone to severe infection despite innocuous appearance.
   (2) Usually on dorsal surface of MCP joints when due to punching mouth. Do not suture lacerations over MCP joints if human bite wound cannot be excluded.
   (3) Requires thorough wound debridement and irrigation.
   (4) Leave wound open with wet dressing, splint, and elevate.
   (5) For human bites, admit patient for treatment with systemic antibiotics and hand soaks.
   (6) Most common pathogens in human bites *Eikenella corrodens,* animal bites *Pasteurella multocida.* Both are sensitive to penicillin.

f. **Nailbed injury.**
   (1) Drain subungual hematoma with needle-tip electrocautery. May need to remove nail plate if hematoma involves more than 30% of the matrix.
   (2) For a fractured nail or visible extension of laceration into matrix, remove loose nail and repair matrix with fine chromic suture, replace nail (with holes for drainage) as splint or pack edges of epo- and perionychium with non-adherent dressing.
   (3) Rule out growth plate injuries in children.

II. HAND INFECTIONS

Hand infections can have devastating sequelae if not treated properly. These infections require an aggressive approach of thorough debridement, irrigation, intravenous antibiotic(s), and splinting.

Infections in diabetic patients are caused by mixed flora and require broad-spectrum antibiotics, whereas injuries that are treated in the emergency room require only covering of gram-positive organisms (e.g. penicillin, erythromycin, oxacillin, or the cephalosporin groups).

Immobilization is important in the majority of hand injuries and infections. Most commonly the hand is splinted in the "position of safety". The proper position is as follows.

(1) Wrist in **dorsiflexion** (15-30 degrees).
(2) Metacarpal-phalangeal (MP) joints at 90 degree **flexion.**
(3) Interphalangeal (IP) joints in **full extension.**
(4) Thumb in **abduction.**

A. Cellulitis.

1. Presents with fever, swelling, lymphangitis.
2. *Streptococcus/Staphylococcus* usual organisms.
3. Rule out a deep infection.
4. Treat with elevation, antibiotics.

B. Paronychia—localized infection at the base of the fingernail.
1. Clinical presentation consists of erythema, marked tenderness, and purulent drainage around the margins of the nail.
2. Treat with incision and drainage of the eponychia, or partial/total nail removal, antibiotic, and elevation.
3. Bacteriology–*Staphylococcus* or mixed organisms.
4. Chronic paronychia results from destruction of the nail matrix, usually as a result of infection. Nail fragments act as foreign bodies. Chronic drainage may be due to fungal infection or carcinoma.

C. Felon (distal pulp space infection).
1. Tender, tense distal finger.
2. Usually caused by *Staphylococcus aureus.*
3. Treatment–incision and drainage early; do not wait for fluctuance.
4. Incise directly over the most superficial aspect of the infected area.
5. Late complications include osteomyelitis of the distal phalanx.

D. Suppurative tenosynovitis.
1. Flexor tendon sheath infections are characterized by **Kanavel's four cardinal signs.**
   a. Finger held in slight flexion.
   b. Finger is uniformly swollen and red.
   c. Intense pain on passive extension.
   d. Tenderness along line of sheath.
2. Treat with incision and drainage of tendon sheath emergently in the operating room; antibiotics, and elevation postoperatively.
3. If untreated, may spread to other tendon sheaths and the deep palmar space.

E. Cat-scratch disease.
1. Infection tends to be aggressive and spread rapidly.
2. Diagnosis is made by history.
3. Primary organism is *Pasteurella multocida* (also known as *Pasteurella septica*).
4. Clinical presentation includes painful swelling and serosanguineous drainage.
5. Antibiotic of choice is penicillin. Alternative regimens include cephalosporins or tetracycline.

F. Aquatic injuries.
1. Typically hand lacerated while cleaning a fish tank.
2. The usual organism is *Aeromonas hydrophila,* of the *Pseudomonadaceae* family.
3. The drug of choice is 2nd or 3rd generation cephalosporins. Gentamicin may be added to the regimen if organism is resistant.

G. Herpetic infections.
1. Commonly found among health-care personnel.
2. Diagnosis based on clinical findings of Tzank smear of aspirate

from vesicles. Immunofluorescent titers may be used for confirmation.

3. Clinical signs include erythema, and painful swelling over the dorsum of affected finger(s), presence of small vesicles of clear fluid.
4. Therapy consists of immobilization and elevation. Blebs may be unroofed if symptomatic, and nail may be removed for comfort. Oral acyclovir or topical acyclovir may be beneficial. *Never* incise or drain due to high incidence of superinfection.
5. Course usually lasts about 2-3 weeks.

III. TECHNIQUES FOR NERVE BLOCKS (see "Anesthesia," section X).

IV. TREATMENT OF THE PATIENT AND AMPUTATED PART FOR POSSIBLE REIMPLANTATION

Always obtain, at minimum, a telephone consultation with a hand specialist prior to making any decisions regarding reimplantation.

A. Strong contraindications.

1. Associated injuries that make the patient too unstable for the prolonged initial reimplantation procedure and/or multiple subsequent procedures.
2. Multilevel, crush, or degloving injury to the amputated part precluding functional recovery.
3. Severe chronic illness.

B. Relative contraindications.

1. Single digit amputation, especially proximal to flexor digitorum superficialis insertion.
2. Avulsion injuries, as evidenced by the following.
   a. Nerves and tendons dangling from the part.
   b. "Red streaks"–bruising over the digital neurovascular bundles indicating vessel disruption.
   c. Previous injury or surgery to the part.
   d. Extreme contamination.
   e. Lengthy warm ischemia time (applicable to macro-reimplantation in which the part contains significant muscle mass).
   f. Age–very advanced.

C. Handling of an amputated part.

1. Cleanse gross debris with saline-moistened gauze.
2. Wrap in a moist saline sponge. Do *not* place directly in saline, as dessication and maceration of tissues will occur.
3. Place in plastic bag in iced saline bath with several layers of gauze between part and ice. Do *not* immerse part in ice or ice-cold saline; freezing and thawing of cells can occur.

D. Care of the patient.

1. Examine carefully for life-threatening associated injuries, which can be overlooked, particularly in the macro-reimplantation candidate.
2. Use direct pressure, not tourniquets, to control bleeding.

69

Urologic Problems in Surgical Practice

M. Ryan Moon, M.D.
Michael B. Rousseau, M.D.

I. UROLOGIC INFECTIONS

A. Cystitis.

1. Female cystitis is typically an ascending bacterial infection associated with sexual activity, pregnancy, and the post-partum period.
2. Male cystitis is usually associated with urologic pathology such as obstruction (benign prostatic hypertrophy, cancer, stricture), urine stasis (neurogenic bladder), foreign body (calculus, indwelling catheter) and inadequate treatment of persistent urinary pathogens (chronic bacterial prostatitis).
3. Etiology–most uncomplicated infections acquired outside hospital caused by coliform bacteria; nosocomial infections caused by more resistant pathogens; gram-negative organisms predominate (*E. coli, Proteus, Enterobacter, Klebsiella, Pseudomonas*); occasionally *Streptococcus faecalis* and *Staphylococcus* species are cultured.
4. Clinical presentation–dysuria, frequency, urgency, incontinence, hematuria, suprapubic pain.
5. Laboratory findings–a catheterized urine specimen from the female and a clean-catch midstream-voided specimen from the male are equivalent. Urinalysis shows at least 5-10 WBCs per high-power field, often with hematuria and bacteriuria; nitrite, leukocyte esterase positive, but not conclusive. Urine culture typically grows > 100,000 CFU/ml.
6. Treatment–consists of empirical use of broad-spectrum oral antibiotics with gram-negative organism coverage (organism-specific antibiotics can be begun when cultures are complete) for 3-7 days.

   a. Nitrofurantoin macrocrystals 50 mg PO QID.
   b. Trimethoprim 160 mg/sulfamethoxazole 800 mg PO BID.
   c. Ciprofloxacin 500 mg PO BID.
7. If symptoms and cultures clear on antibiotics in sexually active females, no further work-up is necessary. Males require further urologic evaluation to rule out urologic pathology.
8. Patients with chronic indwelling urinary catheters or those on intermittent self-catheterization have urine colonized with bacteria, typically two or more pathogens. If these patients are asymptomatic, treatment is not necessary and only rarely successful in clearing the bacteria. Adequate hydration and good bladder emptying are essential in preventing the progression of colonization to infection.

B. Acute bacterial prostatitis.

1. Clinical findings–typically an acute febrile illness, urgency, frequency, dysuria, chills, low back pain, perineal or rectal pain. Rectal examination reveals an exquisitely tender, firm, and indurated prostate. Vigorous rectal exam or massage should be *avoided* because of the risk of causing bacteremia and septicemia.
2. Laboratory findings–leukocytosis with differential left shift. Urinalysis shows pyuria, microscopic hematuria, and bacteriuria.
3. Urethral instrumentation should be avoided. Patients may require placement of suprapubic catheter.
4. Complications–acute bacterial cystitis is frequently associated. Also associated are acute urinary retention, prostatic abscess, pyelonephritis, epididymo-orchitis, bacteremia, or septic shock.
5. Treatment–broad-spectrum antibiotics against gram-negative bacilli. In the stable patient, oral antibiotics can be used (trimethoprim/sulfamethoxazole attains adequate prostate tissue levels as well as the newer quinolones–ciprofloxacin, norfloxacin), for total of 20 to 30 days. In the unstable patient showing signs of sepsis, combination therapy of intravenous aminoglycoside and ampicillin is indicated.

C. Acute epididymo-orchitis.

1. Etiology–two major groups.
   a. Sexually transmitted organisms–associated with younger men; usually *Chlamydia trachomatis* and *Neisseria gonorrhea.*
   b. Infection associated with concomitant urinary tract infections (UTI) or prostatitis. Associated with urinary tract obstruction in older men. Usually *E. coli, Proteus, Klebsiella, Enterobacter, Pseudomonas.*
2. Clinical findings–symptoms may follow an acute lifting or straining activity. Typically a painful, swollen, tender epididymis and testicle are found. Overlying scrotal skin may be red, swollen, and warm. A tense, reactive hydrocele may be present, which makes testicular palpation difficult. The spermatic

cord is often thickened and painful, with radiation to the flank.

3. Laboratory findings–leukocytosis with left shift often present. Urinalysis shows pyuria and bacteriuria in non-standard epididymo-orchitis. Urine culture may grow gram-negative bacilli listed above. Special cultures are usually required for isolation of *Chlamydia* and *Neisseriae* (often unsuccessful) from urethral discharge.
4. Treatment.
   a. Bed-rest during the acute phase.
   b. Scrotal elevation–athletic supporter, ice pack to scrotum.
   c. Avoidance of sexual activity and physical activity.
   d. Analgesia, antipyretics, and antibiotics.
      (1) Sexually transmitted organisms–ceftriaxone 250 mg with 1 cc lidocaine IM followed by doxycycline 100 mg PO BID for 21 days or tetracycline 500 mg PO QID for 21 days. Both patient and partner should be treated. Use of condom in sexual activity is encouraged.
      (2) Non-sexually transmitted organisms–antibiotics are determined by urine culture and sensitivity results. Usually those listed for prostatitis are appropriate empirically.

D. Acute pyelonephritis.

1. An acute bacterial inflammation of the renal parenchyma initiated by ascending bacteria (reflux), and far less commonly by hematogenous and lymphatogenous routes of infection.
2. Organisms–*E. coli, Proteus, Enterobacter, Klebsiella.*
3. Clinical findings–fever, chills, severe costovertebral angle pain and tenderness, frequency, urgency, dysuria, nausea, and vomiting.
4. Laboratory findings–significant leukocytosis with left shift. Urinalysis is significant for pyuria, bacteriuria, occasional hematuria, and occasional leukocyte or granular casts. Urine culture is typically positive for greater than 100,000 CFU/ml.
5. Differential diagnosis–includes pancreatitis, basal pneumonia, appendicitis, cholecystitis, diverticulitis, pelvic inflammatory disease, and renal or perirenal abscess.
6. Treatment–minimally symptomatic patients who are tolerating their diet can be treated expectantly with oral broad-spectrum antibiotics against gram-negative bacilli. In the severely ill patient, prompt treatment is essential to prevent sepsis, renal scarring, and loss of renal function. Initial empiric treatment should consist of an intravenous aminoglycoside and ampicillin. Antibiotics should be guided by urine culture results and intravenous therapy is continued for at least 1 week or until patient is afebrile for 24 h. Conversion to appropriate oral antibiotics can then be initiated and is usually continued for at least 2 weeks.

7. If symptoms and fever persist after 72 h of appropriate antibiotic and fluid therapy, urologic evaluation is required to investigate other pathology (i.e., renal abscess, stones, obstruction).

II. UROLOGIC EMERGENCIES

A. Trauma.

1. Hematuria following trauma.
   a. Degree of hematuria has no correlation to severity of urologic injury. In general, > 50 RBCs/hpf should be investigated.
   b. All acceleration/deceleration, or flank trauma associated with any hypotension should have renal radiologic evaluation regardless of the degree of hematuria. Up to 20% of patients with significant upper urinary tract injury have no hematuria.
   c. Rapid evaluation of the kidneys can be done by bolus injection of IV contrast material (at a dose of 2 mg/kg) with the initial resuscitation fluids, followed by 5 and 10 minute abdominal films.
2. Renal trauma.
   a. Etiology.
      (1) Blunt renal trauma–usually MVAs. Accounts for 70-90% of renal trauma; 80% will have injuries to other organ systems. Any patient sustaining injury to the flank, abdomen, or lower chest should be suspected of having renal trauma.
      (2) Penetrating renal trauma–usually knife or gunshot wounds; 80% will involve other organ systems.
   b. Classification.
      (1) Minor injuries–85% of cases.
         a) Renal contusion–contusion of renal parenchyma.
         b) Cortical laceration–superficial laceration of parenchyma not associated with collecting system.
      (2) Major injuries–10-15% of cases.
         a) Deep laceration–renal parenchymal laceration extending into collecting system. Includes renal rupture in which multiple lacerations separate portions of parenchyma.
         b) Renal pedicle injury–involves renal veins and/or artery.
   c. Diagnosis.
      (1) Intravenous pyelography yields definitive diagnosis in 90% of renal injuries. Failure to visualize a kidney suggests a pedicle injury or congenital absence of a kidney. Prompt function without extravasation of contrast material suggests a minor injury such as renal contusion or cortical laceration. Extravasation of contrast indicates a laceration involving the collecting system.

(2) CT scan–can show all of the above plus evidence of retroperitoneal hematoma, define the vascular perfusion, and evaluate other organ systems.
(3) Angiography–useful when renal pedicle injury is suspected as long as the patient is hemodynamically stable.

d. Treatment.
(1) Prior to any operative attempt at renal exploration, the function of the uninjured kidney must be known.
(2) Penetrating renal trauma almost always requires immediate exploration.
(3) Blunt renal trauma.
a) 85% of cases can be managed nonsurgically (i.e., renal contusion, cortical laceration, and some deep lacerations).
b) Renal pedicle injuries always require exploration and repair or nephrectomy.
c) Intermediate injuries may involve surgical or nonsurgical treatment depending on the patient's overall condition and severity of injury.

e. Late complications–urinomas, hydronephrosis, arteriovenous fistulas, renovascular hypertension, bleeding.

3. Ureteral trauma.
a. Ureters are rarely injured due to blunt trauma; however, the "blast effect" from projectiles can injure the ureter even in the absence of actual transection. Most injuries are iatrogenic from pelvic surgery with transection or ligation of the ureter.
b. Treatment depends on the mechanism of injury and location (lower, middle, or upper). Excretory urograms, retrograde pyelograms, and CT scans often define the injury.
(1) Simple ureteral ligation–prompt recognition may be treated by release of ligature. Late recognition may require partial ureterectomy and ureteral reimplantation into the bladder. Prevention is the best treatment.
(2) Simple surgical transection–requires immediate uretero-ureterostomy and stent placement.
(3) Gunshot wounds–require exploration and wide debridement of injured segment because of potential "blast effect." Ureteroureterostomy or transuretero-ureterostomy may be required, depending on severity of injury.

4. Bladder trauma.
a. Etiology–external blunt trauma (blow to lower abdomen), pelvic fracture (account for 90%), penetrating injury, iatrogenic (gynecologic or pelvic surgery).
b. Presentation–bony pelvis generally protects the bladder from external violence. Nevertheless, 10 to 15% of patients with pelvic fracture will have a bladder or urethral injury.

Bladder rupture may present as an acute abdomen with extravasation of urine into the peritoneal cavity (intraperitoneal rupture). Alternatively, bony spicules from a fractured pelvis may penetrate the bladder with pelvic extravasation of urine (extraperitoneal rupture).

c. Diagnostic evaluation.
   (1) History of lower abdominal trauma (steering-wheel blow in MVA) or pelvic fracture. Significant bladder injury in the absence of a pelvic fracture is highly unlikely in blunt trauma.
   (2) Patients may be unable to urinate or may have lower abdominal pain, gross hematuria, or pelvic hematoma. Diagnostic peritoneal lavage may return urine.
   (3) Radiographic examination.
      a) Abdominal/pelvic plain film–examine for pelvic fractures, soft tissue masses, deviated bowel gas pattern suggesting pelvic hematoma or urinoma.
      b) Excretory urogram–documents function of kidneys and may show bladder extravasation, but is often inadequate.
      c) Cystogram–urethral injury in males must be **ruled out by retrograde urethrogram** (see section A.5 below) prior to inserting urethral catheter. Cystography is performed after catheterization of the bladder. Fill the bladder with 50-75 cc of contrast material and examine x-ray film for gross extravasation. If no extravasation is seen, follow with additional 200-300 cc contrast. Repeat radiograph, again examine for extravasation. Finally, completely drain bladder and repeat pelvic radiograph. Final film is essential for identifying posterior bladder rupture and extravasation. It is helpful to obtain AP as well as oblique films when evaluating pelvis and bladder. Cystogram should *always* precede excretory urogram.

d. Treatment.
   (1) Penetrating injuries–usually require prompt exploration, debridement, and repair. Most patients with penetrating injuries are at high risk for concomitant rectal injury.
   (2) Blunt injuries.
      a) Extraperitoneal bladder ruptures with sterile urine and no intra-abdominal injuries can be managed with catheter drainage. If free bony spicules are seen on work-up, the injury will require exploration and removal of the penetrating foreign bodies.
      b) Intraperitoneal bladder ruptures require immediate exploration, repair, and drainage.
      c) Manipulation of pelvic hematoma is to be avoided.

5. Urethral trauma.
   a. Anatomy–the urethra in the male is divided into anterior and posterior divisions. The anterior urethra consists of the urethra distal to the urogenital diaphragm. The posterior urethra extends from the inferior edge of the urogenital diaphragm to the proximal bladder neck. Anterior injuries are often associated with straddle-type trauma to the perineum or urethral instrumentation. Posterior urethral injuries most often occur with pelvic fractures. Female urethral injuries are unusual.
   b. Anterior urethral injuries may extravasate blood along fascial planes. An injury to the urethra limited by Buck's fascia (i.e., urethral instrumentation injury) will result in blood extravasation along the penis. An injury through Buck's fascia will demonstrate extravasation of blood along the fascial planes of the abdomen (Scarpa's fascia) and scrotum, penis, and perineum (Colles' fascia).
   c. Posterior urethral injuries almost always occur with pelvic fractures and are usually associated with pelvic hematoma. Blood at the urethral meatus, inability to void, and high-riding prostate on rectal exam is highly suggestive of a posterior injury.
   d. Diagnostic procedures–**all suspected urethral injuries in males must be evaluated by a retrograde urethrogram prior to insertion of a bladder catheter.** Urethral catheterization can easily convert a partial tear into a complete urethral transection. Retrograde urethrogram is simply performed by injecting 10-15 cc of contrast material into the urethra with a syringe and taking oblique pelvic x-ray films. If no extravasation is seen with complete filling of the urethra into the bladder, a catheter can be passed gently. If any obstruction or difficulty in passing the catheter is encountered, the procedure should be terminated, and immediate urology consult obtained.
   e. Treatment.
      (1) Minor anterior urethral lacerations can be managed with bladder catheter drainage alone. Penetrating injuries require exploration, debridement, and repair.
      (2) More severe anterior urethral injuries, usually straddle-type injuries, may require exploration.
      (3) Management of posterior urethral injuries is controversial. Two options exist.
         a) Immediate exploration with primary urethral re-anastomosis.
         b) Suprapubic catheter placement for urinary diversion. In general, due to the severity of other life-threatening injuries with pelvic fracture, the conservative approach of suprapubic urinary catheter diversion is preferred.

B. Acute scrotum.

1. Definition–the acute scrotum refers to the swollen, tender scrotum associated with a testicular, epididymal, or spermatic cord abnormality, usually a diagnostic dilemma in the pediatric population.
2. Differential diagnosis–includes testicular torsion, torsion of testicular appendages, acute epididymo-orchitis, tense hydrocele, or acute incarcerated inguinal hernia. Correct diagnosis and expeditious treatment are essential to prevent organ loss.
   a. Testicular torsion is the spontaneous twisting of the testicular pedicle, causing acute testicular ischemia. Most commonly presents as an acute onset of testicular or unilateral scrotal pain, swelling, and tenderness in the 10-18 year-old age group. Pain is severe, and urinalysis is normal. Many patients complain of a similar event within the past year that resolved spontaneously. The testicle is usually elevated in the scrotum and is exquisitely tender. If the diagnosis is in doubt, a radionuclide testicular scan can be obtained; however, delay in treatment for greater than 6 h may result in further organ damage. Surgical treatment consists of exploration, detorsion, and orchiopexy. The contralateral testicle is sutured in place as well to prevent torsion. Orchiectomy is performed if a nonviable testicle is found.
   b. Acute epididymo-orchitis occurs in patients ranging from the sexually active pubertal male on up into the elderly male age groups. The onset of pain is gradual and may be accompanied by irritative voiding complaints. Urinalysis may show pyuria. Scrotal elevation may decrease the pain, and the opposite testis is normal. Treatment consists of symptomatic relief and appropriate antibiotics (see section I).
   c. Torsion of testicular or epididymal appendages–vestigial remnants of the müllerian ductal system persist as small, pedunculated appendages from the testis and epididymis. Occasionally, these appendages can spontaneously twist on their pedicles, causing acute ischemia and a painful scrotum. Patients are usually pre-pubertal, and voiding complaints are absent. Urinalysis is normal. Examination reveals exquisitely tender, pea-sized mass near the head of the epididymis. The testicle is usually not tender. A "blue dot" sign is described on scrotal transillumination; however, it may be obscured by localized scrotal edema and redness. Treatment is conservative: bed-rest, ice packs, and analgesics. If the diagnosis is in doubt, surgical exploration may be necessary to rule out testicular torsion, and excise the appendage.
   d. Incarcerated inguinal hernia–usually only confused with testicular torsion in young male patients. May be acute on-

set, severe pain with scrotal swelling and hyperemia. Nausea and vomiting may be present. Urinalysis is normal.

III. URINARY RETENTION

A. Etiology—bladder emptying requires a coordinated bladder contraction in the absence of bladder outlet obstruction.

1. Factors that inhibit a coordinated bladder contraction.
   a. Neurogenic dysfunction–results from a neurologic process that gives a hyporeflexic ("flaccid") neurogenic bladder, such as injury to the sacral spinal cord, cauda equina, or the pelvic nerves. Also present during the initial stages of any level of spinal cord injury (spinal shock).
   b. Decompensated bladder–overdistention of the bladder can overstretch the detrusor muscle and inhibit its ability to contract (i.e., long-term diabetes, prolonged use of antipsychotics or anticholinergics).
2. Factors that cause bladder outlet obstruction.
   a. Male–benign prostatic hypertrophy, prostate cancer, urethral stricture, bladder neck contracture, bladder calculi.
   b. Female (very uncommon causes of urinary retention)–urethral stenosis, urethral trauma, urethral diverticulum, cystourethroceles, urethral coveinoma.

B. Presentation and diagnosis.

1. Acute symptoms–urgency and suprapubic pain.
2. Chronic symptoms–progressive obstructive voiding symptoms leading eventually to anuria or **overflow incontinence.**
3. Asymptomatic and present with an abdominal mass, renal insufficiency, or bilateral hydronephrosis.
4. Diagnosis usually confirmed by placement of a Foley catheter with return of a large quantity of urine.

C. Treatment.

1. Attempt is made to pass an 18 Fr Foley catheter.
   a. Common causes for inability to pass a Foley catheter:
      (1) Inadequate lubrication (lubrication can be injected up the urethra with a small syringe).
      (2) Young male patient who overtightens external sphincter (will fatigue after about 30 sec).
      (3) Urethral strictures (scar tissue occluding urethral lumen).
      (4) Enlarged median lobe of the prostate or defect from a previous TURP (transurethral resection of the prostate) can create an acute angulation in the prostatic urethra. A **coude catheter** may be successful because of its angulated tip.
   b. If initial attempts at passing an 18 Fr Foley or coude tip catheter are unsuccessful, a urologist should be consulted. The use of filiforms and followers, percutaneous cystotomy, or formal cystoscopy may be required.
2. Definitive treatment of urinary retention varies with the causative factors.

a. Benign prostatic hypertrophy–usually managed with TURP or open prostatectomy (removal of only the inner adenoma of the prostate through a surgical incision).
b. Prostate cancer–prostate cancer that has progressed to urinary obstruction often has metastasized to bone or lymph nodes; therefore, usually treated hormonally (orchiectomy, LHRH agonist). Prostate cancer can also cause urinary retention by spinal cord compression from vertebral metastasis (neurogenic hyporeflexic bladder).
c. Bladder neck contracture–caused by scarring at the bladder neck, usually following TURP. Managed by transurethral incision of the bladder neck.
d. Urethral stricture–managed by transurethral incision or urethroplasty.
e. Hyporeflexic neurogenic bladder–usually managed with ISC (intermittent straight catheterization).
f. Decompensated bladder–also managed by ISC.

3. Post-obstructive diuresis–following relief of urinary retention, there may be a significant diuresis.
   a. Post-obstructive diuresis is primarily due to excess water and solute retained during period of urinary retention (physiologic diuresis).
   b. Rarely, a diuresis will occur due to a tubular defect with loss of the kidney's ability to concentrate urine. A hypovolemic state can result from this pathologic diuresis. The patient's vital signs should be closely monitored for orthostatic changes and IV fluid replacement as needed.

IV. UROLITHIASIS

A. Etiology.

1. ***Calcium oxalate*** or mixed calcium oxalate/calcium phosphate stones.
   a. Account for 70-80% of urolithiasis.
   b. Usually 30-50 years of age; calcium-containing stones three times more common in men.
   c. Untreated patient has 60% chance of forming second stone in 7 years.
   d. Usually they are "idiopathic" and due to either excessive absorption (in GI tract) or excretion (by kidney) of calcium, causing hypercalcuria.
   e. Approximately 5% have hyperparathyroidism with hypercalcemia.
   f. Less than 1% of calcium stones are caused by other metabolic diseases such as Type 1 renal tubular acidosis (distal RTA) or primary hyperoxaluria.
   g. Radiopaque.
2. ***Struvite*** or infection stones.
   a. Contain magnesium ammonium phosphate.
   b. Account for 15% of urolithiasis.
   c. Usually infected with urease-producing bacteria (usually

Proteus but also *Klebsiella, Pseudomonas,* and *Staphylococcus*), which produce an alkaline urine (urine pH 7.0 or greater).
   d. Less radiopaque than calcium-containing stones.
3. ***Uric acid stones.***
   a. Account for about 5-10% of stones.
   b. May be associated with hyperuricemia or gout or may result from the hyperuricuria during the acute stages of chemotherapy for myeloproliferative diseases.
   c. Most are idiopathic and associated with normal serum and urine uric acid levels.
   d. Often, the urine pH is persistently low, which will precipitate uric acid stones.
   e. Radiolucent.
4. ***Cystine stones.***
   a. Accounts for less than 3% of stones.
   b. Result from an inherited defect of the renal tubule causing loss of cystine, ornithine, arginine, and lysine in the urine.
   c. Urinalysis shows characteristic hexagonal microscopic crystals.
   d. Faintly radiopaque.

B. Presentation.

1. Stones may be asymptomatic or may cause symptoms from obstruction at the ureteropelvic junction, at the neck of a calyx, or along the course of the ureter.
2. Renal colic is caused by distention of the urinary tract and is related to the rapidity of development, not to the degree of distention.
3. Pain may be referred to the flank, the abdomen, the testicle, or into the scrotum or labia.
4. Distal ureteral stones often cause irritative bladder symptoms of urinary urgency and frequency.
5. Differential diagnoses include appendicitis, small bowel obstruction, diverticulitis, ovarian torsion, and ectopic pregnancy.
6. Bladder stones cause irritative symptoms of urgency, frequency, dysuria, and, occasionally, bladder outlet obstruction. Usually caused by bladder outlet obstruction with urinary stasis.
7. Occasionally obstructing calculi are associated with infected urine causing pyohydronephrosis. This can produce life-threatening sepsis and is considered a *surgical emergency,* requiring prompt drainage (percutaneous or endoscopic).

C. Diagnosis.

1. Urinalysis shows microscopic hematuria and occasionally pyuria. Struvite stones are associated with alkaline urine, and uric acid stones are associated with acidic urine.
2. IVP (intravenous pyelogram)–best method to diagnose urolithiasis and should demonstrate the size and location of the stone as well as the degree of obstruction.

3. Retrograde pyelograms (done through cystoscope)–sometimes necessary in patients who cannot tolerate an IVP (patients with renal insufficiency or allergy to IV contrast).
4. Serum calcium, uric acid, and phosphorous levels should be obtained. BUN and creatinine are important to evaluate renal function.
5. Strain urine to obtain any passed calculi for stone analysis.

D. Treatment.

1. Usually patients with small, uncomplicated ureteral or renal calculi can be managed with oral analgesics and followed as outpatients.
2. Patients with an obstructing calculus associated with a solitary kidney, persistent vomiting, fever, suspected urinary tract infection, or pain uncontrolled with oral analgesics should be admitted.
3. Patients with pyohydronephrosis (obstructing calculus with urinary tract infection) who are septic should have emergent placement of a ureteral stent by cystoscopy or placement of a percutaneous nephrostomy.
4. Current urologic management of ureteral stones usually involves transurethral endoscopic manipulation, either fragmenting and extracting the stone, or pushing it up into the kidney for ESWL (extracorporeal shock wave lithotripsy).
5. Most renal stones are now managed with ESWL. Larger renal calculi are sometimes managed with percutaneous nephroscopy (endoscopic manipulation through a percutaneous flank approach) or open surgical removal (pyelolithotomy, nephrolithotomy, partial nephrectomy or nephrectomy).
6. Bladder calculi are usually removed transurethrally with simultaneous correction of the underlying bladder outlet obstruction.

PART III

Procedures

70

Vascular Access Techniques

Susan E. MacLennan, M.D.

I. PERIPHERAL VENOUS ACCESS

A. Sites.

1. The veins of the hands and arms are most often used for intravenous catheter placement. Phlebotomy is most easily done in the antecubital fossa, whereas IV catheters function best in the veins on the dorsum of the hand, forearm, and upper arm. Distal veins should be utilized first, but when unsuccessful, choices in order of preference are as follows.
   a. Cephalic vein ("intern's vein").
   b. Basilic vein.
   c. Median vein.
   d. Greater saphenous vein.
2. IV access or phlebotomy may be obtained in the saphenous veins under certain circumstances such as major trauma, cardiac arrest, etc., but generally should be avoided because of the risks of phlebitis or infection (especially in patients with diabetes or peripheral vascular disease). The saphenous vein may be found ~ 1 cm anterior and superior to the medial malleolus.

B. Technique of peripheral venous cannulation.

1. In patients who need rapid volume expansion, use the largest gauge catheter available (14-ga. or 16-ga.). Blood should be administered through an 18-ga. IV or larger.
2. In circulatory collapse, the antecubital veins are used for rapid access.
3. Apply tourniquet proximally.
4. Locate vein and cleanse the overlying skin with alcohol or betadine.
5. Local anesthesia may be considered but is not usually necessary.

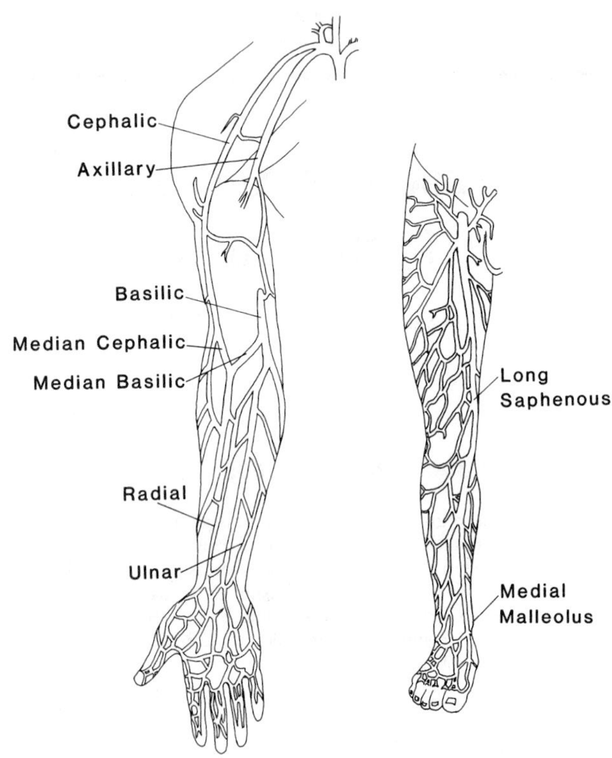

FIG. 1 **Anatomy of Veins of Upper and Lower Extremities**

6. Hold the vein in place by applying pressure on the vein distally.
7. Puncture the skin with the needle bevel upward; enter the vein from either side or from above.
8. When blood return is noted, advance approximately 1 mm further, stabilize the needle, and slide the catheter into place.
9. Remove the tourniquet and needle, attach IV tubing, and apply a sterile dressing.

II. CENTRAL VENOUS ACCESS

A. Indications.

1. Inadequate peripheral venous access.
2. Total parenteral nutrition.

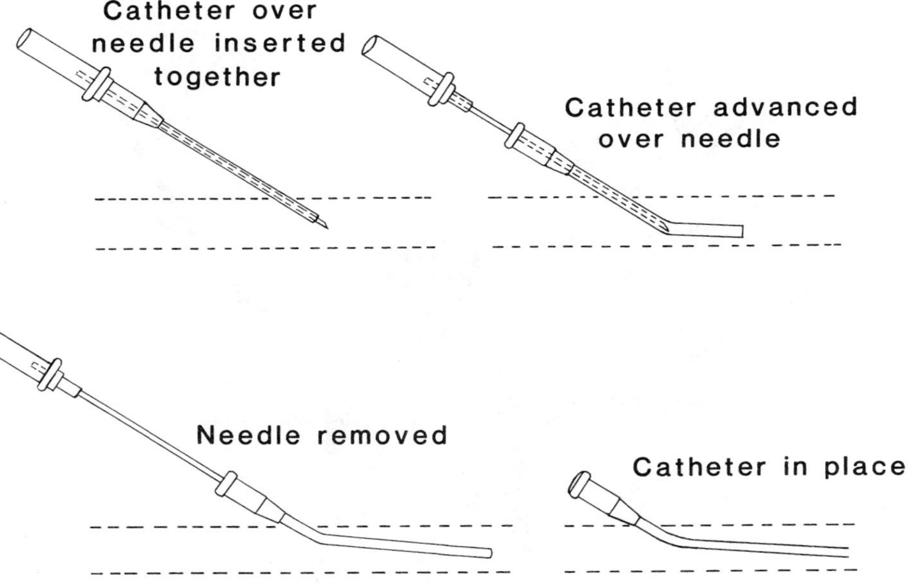

FIG. 2 Insertion of the Over-Needle Catheter

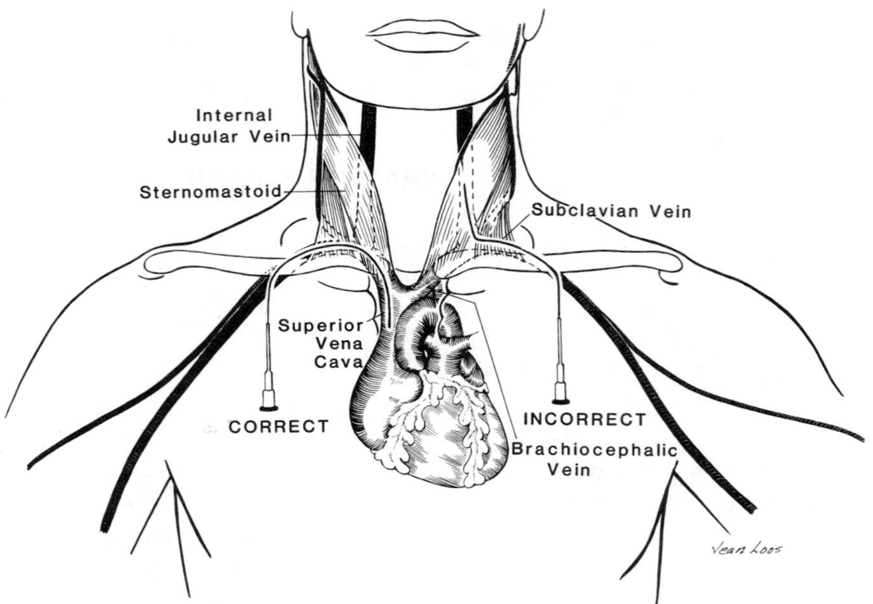

FIG. 3 Venous Anatomy of Thoracic Inlet

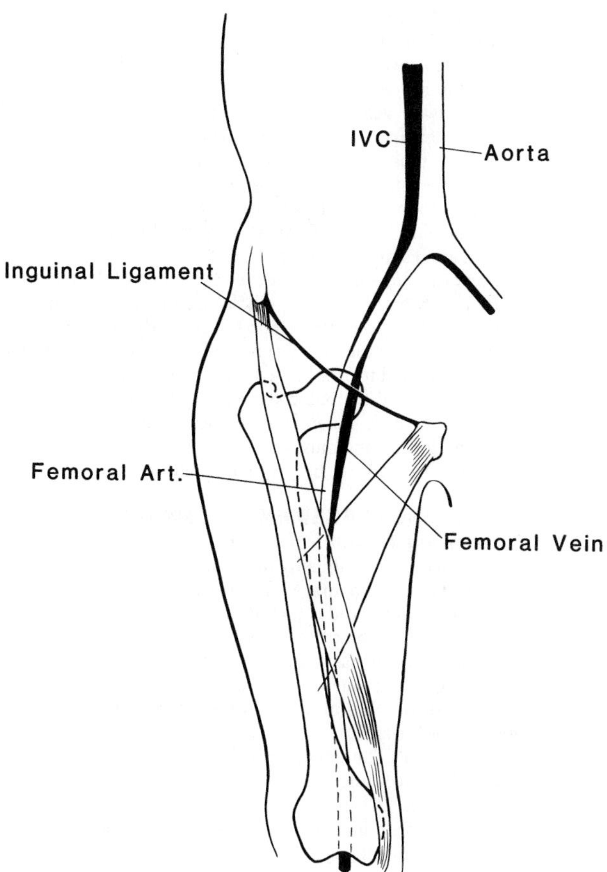

FIG. 4 Anatomy of Femoral Vein

3. Chemotherapeutic administration.
4. Central venous and pulmonary artery pressure monitoring.

B. Anatomy for central venous catheter placement.

1. ***External jugular vein***—formed at the angle of mandible by the posterior facial veins and the posterior auricular vein, passes caudally over the sternocleidomastoid (SCM) to enter the subclavian vein lateral to the anterior scalene muscle.
2. ***Internal jugular vein***—arises from base of skull in the carotid sheath *posterior* to internal carotid artery and terminates

in subclavian vein anterior and lateral to common carotid artery. Runs medial to SCM in its upper part, posterior in triangle between two heads of SCM, and behind clavicular head in its lower part.

3. ***Subclavian vein***—continuation of axillary vein at lateral border of first rib, passes over first rib anterior to anterior scalene muscle, continues *behind medial third* of clavicle, where it is fixed to the rib and clavicle. Joins the internal jugular to form the innominate vein behind sternocostoclavicular joint. Subclavian artery and apical pleura lie behind vein at medial third of the clavicle.
4. ***Femoral vein***—used as a last resort because of the increased frequency of thrombosis, embolism, and infection. The vein is located *medial* to the femoral artery in the femoral sheath inferior to the inguinal ligament. The artery may be found at the midpoint of a line connecting the anterior superior iliac spine and the pubic symphysis; the vein is one fingerbreadth medial. A useful mnemonic is NAVEL, which refers to the formal anatomy in a lateral to medial orientation: Nerve, Artery, Vein, Empty Space, and Lymphatics.

III. CENTRAL LINE PLACEMENT TECHNIQUES

A. External jugular vein—not a preferred site owing to positional function and difficulty maintaining a dressing.

1. Patient is prepped, draped, and placed in Trendelenburg position. Patient's head is turned to opposite side.
2. The vein at the base of the neck is compressed to distend it.
3. Standard peripheral IV catheter or central catheter placed by Seldinger technique may be used.

B. General principles of internal jugular and subclavian vein catheterization.

1. Check PT, PTT, and platelet count before puncture attempts to rule out coagulopathy.
2. Equipment.
   a. Povidone-iodine or Hibiclens® prep solution.
   b. 4 x 4 gauze sponges.
   c. Sterile towels.
   d. Local anesthesia (1% lidocaine/carbocaine) with 22- and 25-ga. needles for administration.
   e. 2-0 silk suture.
   f. #11 scalpel blade.
   g. 3-cc, 5-cc, or 10-cc syringe.
   h. 18-ga. thin-walled needle at least 6 cm long with Seldinger wire.
   i. Single or multilumen catheter (15-20 cm long).
   j. Rolled towel or sheet.
   k. IV sedation–optional.
3. Place a rolled towel vertically between the shoulder blades, put patient in Trendelenburg position with neck extended.

If the patient is anxious and hemodynamically stable, consider sedation.

4. Wear gown, mask, and gloves, prep with 3 applications of betadine followed by a single application of alcohol. Drape patient to expose both internal jugular and subclavian veins.
5. Infiltrate local anesthesia at puncture site with 25-ga. needle, then 22-ga. needle; infiltrate tract toward the vein, aspirating prior to instilling anesthetic. In subclavian venipuncture, it is especially important to anesthetize the clavicle edge. The vein should be localized with the 22-ga. needle if possible.
6. Flush catheter with sterile saline, estimate length to sternomanubrial junction to place in superior vena cava.
7. Mount 18-ga. thin-walled needle on non-Leure Lock syringe.
8. Insert slowly, while aspirating, until blood returns; the needle should always be parallel to the floor. Bright red blood usually means arterial puncture; remove needle and apply pressure for 10 min.
9. If no blood returns, withdraw needle *slowly* under negative pressure; blood may still return into syringe. If still no blood return, re-attempt directed in a more cephalad direction.
10. After blood returns, stabilize needle, carefully remove syringe, occluding needle with finger to prevent air embolism.
11. Place guide wire through needle gently; it should advance *easily.* Withdraw needle, holding the wire in position.
12. Nick skin with #11 blade, slide dilator over wire to enlarge skin site and tract, remove dilator, then advance catheter over wire into desired position (17.5 cm for left subclavian and left internal jugular; 15 cm for right subclavian, and 12.5 cm for right internal jugular).
13. Remove wire, attach IV tubing with 500 ml bag of D5W. Lower fluid bag below atrial level to observe free return of blood into the IV tubing.
14. Suture at skin, place sterile occlusive dressing.
15. Obtain STAT portable chest radiograph. Acceptable sites for catheter tip are SVC or innominate-vena cava junction. Do not leave catheter tip in right atrium, contralateral subclavian, or retrograde in internal jugular.

IV. SPECIFIC SITES

A. Internal jugular-central approach (Figure 5).

1. Locate the triangle formed by the 2 heads of SCM and the clavicle.
2. Insert 22-ga. localizing needle at apex of triangle formed by two heads of SCM.

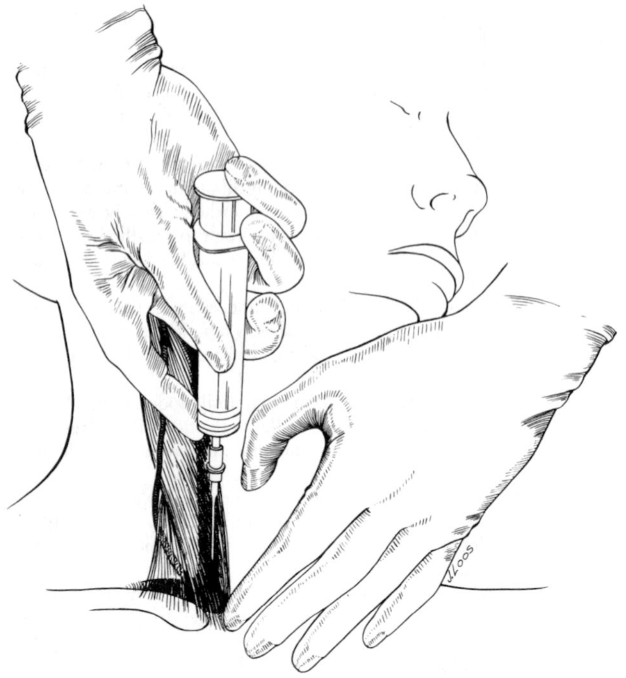

FIG. 5 Central Approach for Internal Jugular Venipuncture

3. Aim needle parallel to clavicular head toward ipsilateral nipple at 45-60° angle until vein is entered.
4. If needle is inserted 3 cm without blood return, attempt new puncture in slightly more lateral position.
5. Do *not* proceed medially, as carotid artery may be punctured.
6. Right Internal jugular (IJ) lines have straightest course to right atrium and lowest overall complication rate.

B. Internal jugular—posterior approach (Figure 6).

1. Insert needle under SCM 3 fingerbreadths above the clavicle, aiming anteriorly to suprasternal notch at 45° angle to sagittal and horizontal planes.
2. Vein should be entered within 5-7 cm of needle penetration.

C. Subclavian vein catheterization (infraclavicular) [Figure 7].

1. Insert needle 1-2 cm below junction of medial and middle third of clavicle.
2. Advance needle parallel to chest wall until clavicle is encountered.

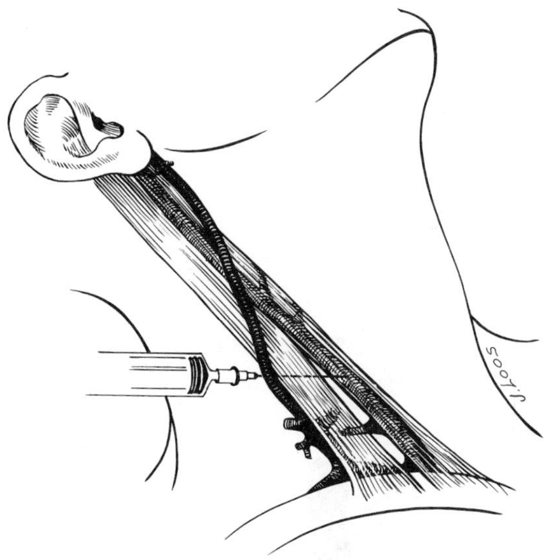

FIG. 6 Posterior Approach for Internal Jugular Venipuncture

3. With index finger in the sternal notch and thumb on the clavicle, march down the clavicle until the needle passes beneath. Aim just above the notch and advance the needle.
4. When the vein is entered, carefully rotate the needle 90° to aim the bevel caudally so the wire will pass into the innominate vein.
5. Vein can also be entered via supraclavicular approach, but with higher incidence of arterial puncture.

D. Contraindications to central venous catheterization.

1. Thrombosis of central veins.
2. Coagulopathy–a relative contraindication. Many coagulopathies can be temporarily overcome with transfusion of fresh frozen plasma, cryoprecipitate, or platelets, followed by immediate venipuncture. It is preferable to place deep lines in areas that are compressible in the event of bleeding (i.e., internal jugular, femoral, brachial). Also consider cutdown of antecubital veins.
3. Bullous emphysema–avoid subclavian approach.

E. Complications.

1. Catheter misplacement–poor blood return, cardiac irritability, pain in neck or ear. Corrective options include the following.

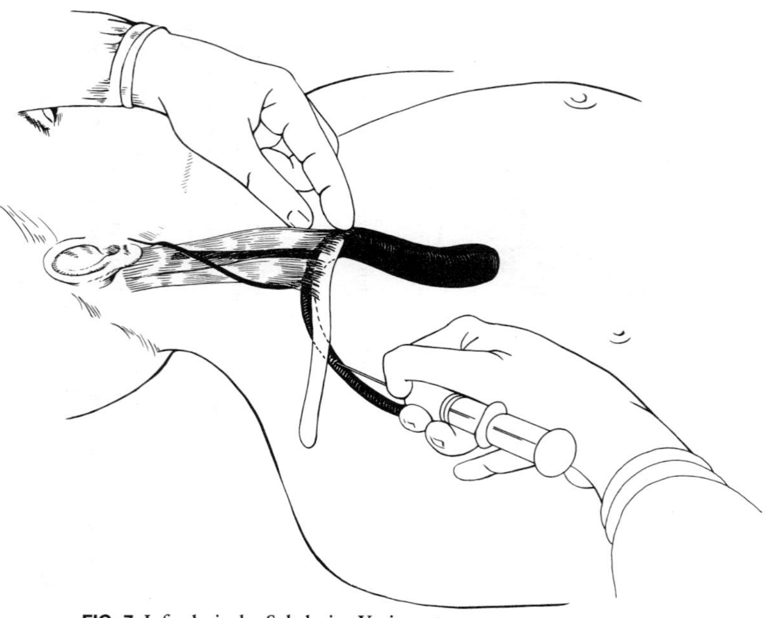

FIG. 7 Infraclavicular Subclavian Venipuncture

   a. Reposition under fluoroscopy.
   b. Re-attempt entire procedure.
2. Arterial puncture (subclavian, carotid, femoral).
3. Hemorrhage–venous or arterial.
4. Pneumothorax–always check chest radiograph after failed attempts and prior to re-attempting central venipuncture on contralateral side.
5. Thoracic duct injury, with or without chylothorax (left IJ).
6. Extravasation of fluid, hyperalimentation, etc.
7. Brachial plexus injury.
8. Air embolism.
9. Catheter or wire embolization.
10. Hydrothorax.
    a. Primary–placement of catheter into pleural or mediastinal spaces.
    b. Secondary–erosion of catheter through SVC after successful placement.
11. Infection.
    a. Cellulitis at puncture site.
    b. Bacteremia from catheter colonization (catheter sepsis).
    c. Increased incidence with use of multilumen catheters.
12. Thrombosis (central venous)–clinical signs include unilateral upper extremity edema, upper extremity and neck venous distention and neck pain. There is a well-described incidence of pulmonary embolism following subclavian vein thrombosis. **Treatment** is similar to that of lower extremity DVT: remove catheter, heparinize, then administer long-term warfarin.

V. LONG-TERM CENTRAL ACCESS

A. Silastic catheters (Hickman, Groshong, Broviac)–single-, double-, or triple-lumen catheters, which may be attached to an implantable port or may exit percutaneously through the skin.

B. Placed through a break-away sheath via Seldinger technique using internal jugular (IJ) or subclavian approach. An alternate method is venous cut-down on the internal jugular or cephalic veins.

C. Implantable ports are more appropriate for long-term access, where cannulation is intermittent. They can be difficult to access by the patient because of their position and the pain associated with cannulation. Implanted ports, however, allow participation in physical activities such as swimming. They require an operating room for removal. For daily access or short-term therapy (weeks), percutaneous catheters are more desirable. They are easy for patients to access and cannulation is not painful. They limit activities, however, but can be removed in the office or at the bedside.

VI. PERCUTANEOUS ACCESS FOR HEMODIALYSIS

A. **Long-term access** is achieved by surgically created arteriovenous fistulas.

B. **Temporary access** is primarily achieved using a specific dual-lumen catheter (Quinton-Mahurkar)–intake is on side of catheter, blood returns through distal side and end ports.

C. **Standard Seldinger technique** for placement.

D. **Site of placement** is generally subclavian or femoral. The complications of placement are similar to standard central access.

E. **Femoral placement** decreases mobility, increases risk of iliofemoral deep venous thrombosis, and is prone to bleeding and infection. Despite risks, femoral catheters may be indicated in unstable, bedridden, or ventilator-dependent patients, as well as in instances in which the operator is unfamiliar with the subclavian approach. Femoral access should not be placed ipsilateral to a present or proposed renal transplant.

F. **Following placement,** catheters must be charged with heparin (5,000 U/ ml) each time they are accessed.

VII. PERIPHERALLY INSERTED CENTRAL (PIC) CATHETERS

A. **Provide central venous access** to distal subclavian vein from antecubital fossa of non-dominant arm.

B. **Lower cost**—do not require operative placement, can be placed by trained RN or technician, require post-placement chest radiograph.

C. **Requirements**—long catheter length (30-50 cm) and small lumen (2-3 Fr).

D. **Catheters** are more fragile, more prone to clot, and long-term placement leads to risk of thrombophlebitis.

E. **No risk** of pneumothorax or serious hemorrhage.

VIII. ARTERIAL ACCESS

A. **Indications.**

1. Continuous blood pressure measurement.
   a. Shock from hypovolemia, hemorrhage, burns, trauma.
   b. Use of IV vasopressors or vasodilators.
   c. Major operations in which major fluid shifts can be expected.
   d. Severe cardiac or respiratory disease.
   e. Patients in whom changes in blood pressure could be deleterious: cardiovascular, cerebrovascular disease.
   f. Patients in whom non-invasive monitoring is unreliable (obese, shock, bypass).
2. Need for frequent blood sampling.
   a. Blood gases for ventilator management.
   b. Serial electrolytes, blood counts in ICU setting.
   c. Avoids discomfort, difficulty, complications of frequent arterial and venous puncture.

B. Sites of cannulation (in order of preference):
1. Radial.
2. Axillary.
3. Dorsalis pedis.
4. Femoral.
5. Brachial should not routinely be used because of high risk of embolic and ischemic hand complications.

C. Radial artery cannulation.
1. Begin with an assessment of collateral circulation–modified Allen's test (Figure 8).
   a. Compress radial and ulnar arteries.
   b. Patient clenches fist to exsanguinate palmar skin.
   c. Release pressure over ulnar artery.
   d. Return of skin color in ≤ 6 sec indicates patency of ulnar artery and superficial palmar arch, suggesting adequate collateral flow in the event of complicated radial artery cannulation.
2. ***Technique (Figure 9).***
   a. Apply arm-board to hand and forearm dorsally.
   b. Place roll of gauze behind wrist to dorsiflex hand 60°.
   c. Prep as per central venous access.
   d. Infiltrate local anesthetic without epinephrine into proposed insertion site.
   e. Use a 20-ga., 1.25-2 inch long, Teflon(™)-coated angiocath (options include self-contained over-wire catheters [Arrow®] and Seldinger technique).
   f. Palpate arterial pulse and insert catheter/needle at 30-45° angle to skin. Advance catheter slowly towards pulse until blood returns in needle hub.
   g. Tilt needle and catheter down slightly and, while holding needle in place, slide catheter over needle into artery.
   h. Remove needle, attach T-piece extension and pressure tubing, flush catheter, and make certain good waveform is present.
   i. Suture catheter securely with 2-0 or 3-0 silk.
   j. Apply sterile dressing.

D. Axillary artery cannulation.
1. Shave axilla, hyperabduct and externally rotate arm.
2. Palpate pulse just below biceps muscle.
3. Use 20-ga., 5 cm long needle with guide wire, 16 cm long catheter.
4. Insert needle as high as possible within axilla, 35° angle to skin.
5. Insert guide wire, remove needle.
6. Place catheter and suture to skin.

E. Dorsalis pedis artery cannulation (Figure 10).
1. Best used in younger patients. Not to be used in patients with diabetes or peripheral vascular disease.
2. Same technique as radial artery.

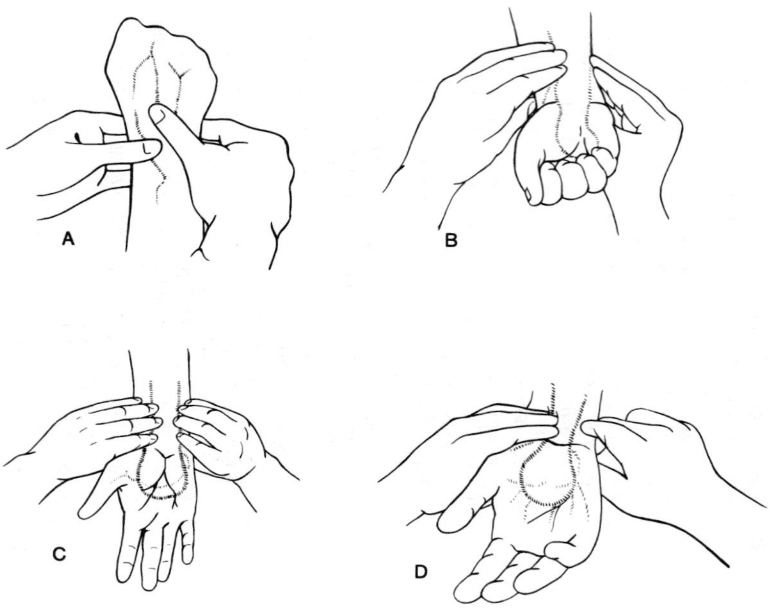

A

B

C

D

FIG. 8 Allen's Test (see section VIII.C.1.)

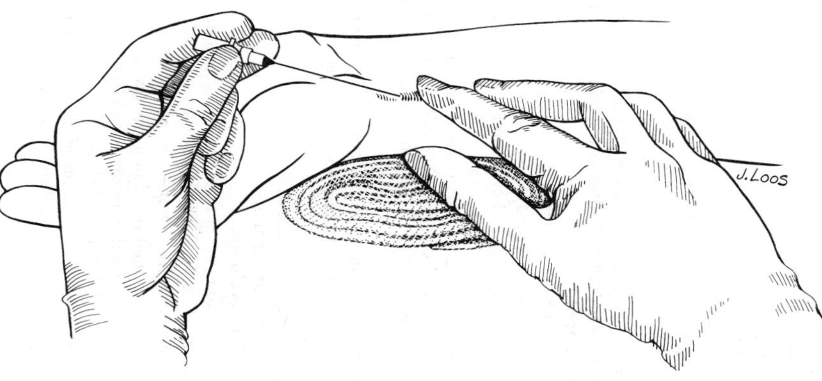

FIG. 9 Cannulation of Radial Artery

F. Femoral artery cannulation.

1. Same rate of complications as radial cannulation.
2. Safer than a difficult radial cannulation.
3. Longer average catheter duration than radial (about 2 days more).
4. Twice the rate of complications of radial cannulation in patients with peripheral vascular disease (17% *vs.* 8%).
5. Should be reserved for hemodynamically unstable patients for speed and facility of procedure.
6. ***Technique:***
   a. Shave groin.
   b. Use 19- to 20-ga., 16 cm long catheter.
   c. Insert needle/catheter 2 cm below inguinal ligament at 45°.
   d. Secure catheter to skin with 2-0 silk.

G. Disparities between A-line and cuff pressure measurements.

1. Variance of 5-20 mm Hg is within expected range. Peak central pressures are slightly lower than peak peripheral pressures owing to inertia of entrainment of a column of blood meeting resistance.
2. Cuff pressure > 20 mm Hg over A-line pressure.
   a. Improper cuff size (usually cuff too small) or placement.
   b. Severe peripheral vascular disease with catheter in a distal artery.
   c. Improperly calibrated sphygmomanometer or transducer.
   d. Dampened waveform–look for tubing problems.
      (1) Air bubbles or blood in line.
      (2) Clotting at catheter tip.
      (3) Loose connections.
      (4) Line occlusion.
      (5) Kinked catheter from dressing position.
3. A-line pressure > 20 mm Hg over cuff pressure.
   a. Severe vasoconstriction–use cuff pressure.
   b. Catheter in small vessel in high-flow state.
   c. Resonance of catheter system–use larger, more compliant tubing with length ≤ 36″.

H. Complications—overall incidence of A-line-related complications is about 7% for radial and femoral lines. In the presence of peripheral vascular disease, however, this doubles to 17%. The incidence of complications is also increased with different percutaneous or cutdown techniques. Catheter size and material appear to have little or no effect on complication rates.

1. ***Ischemia/thrombosis***—most common complication.
   a. Radial artery is occluded in 25% of all cannulations, yet ischemic damage to hand is uncommon.
   b. Increased incidence with peripheral vascular disease, use of vasopressors.
   c. Not predicted by Allen's test.

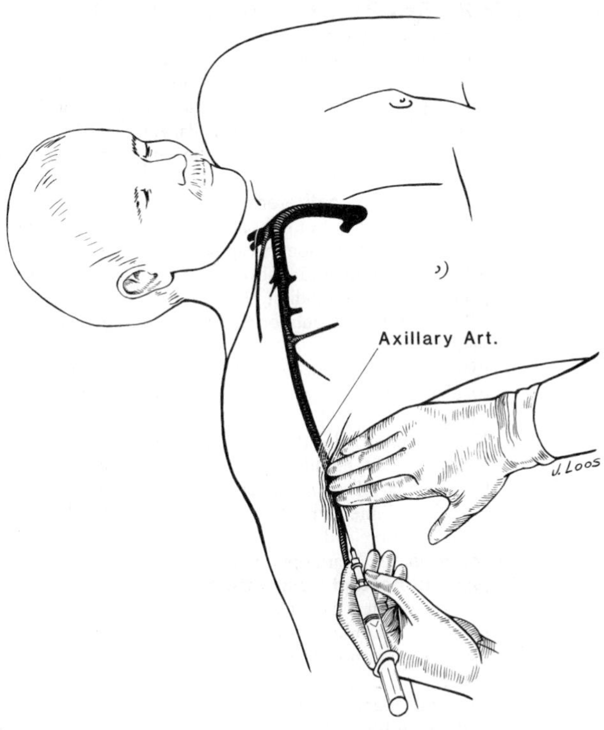

FIG. 10 Cannulation of Axillary Artery

d. Use continuous line flush with heparin at 2-4 U/ml.

2. ***Infection***—catheter-related sepsis. Change catheter when erythema develops at the insertion site or positive blood cultures are drawn through the catheter.
3. ***Embolism.***
   a. From clots in catheter tip or air in tubing.
   b. Increased incidence with intermittent line flush.
4. ***Hemorrhage.***
   a. Rapid blood loss/exsanguination may follow any disconnection in system between patient and transducer.
   b. Decreased incidence with ≥ 5-10 min. of direct pressure post decannulation.
5. ***Pseudoaneurysm.***
   a. May occur when periarterial hematoma develops.
   b. If present–arterial repair indicated.

IX. PULMONARY ARTERY CATHETERIZATION

The pulmonary artery catheter was designed to provide a clinical means for frequent and reliable assessment of left ventricular preload. In the absence of severe cardiopulmonary dysfunction, the pulmonary capillary wedge pressure provides an index of the left atrial pressure and, hence, the left ventricular end-diastolic pressure (preload). Starling's law describes the relationship of preload to cardiac function.

A. Pulmonary artery catheters.

1. Allow measurement of right atrial, right ventricular, pulmonary artery, and pulmonary capillary wedge pressure.
2. Allow calculation of cardiac output and other hemodynamic parameters by thermodilution.
3. Allow sampling of pulmonary arterial (mixed venous) and right atrial blood.
4. Extra lumens are added on some catheters for atrial or ventricular pacing, or for continuous cardiac output monitoring.
5. Newer, specialized catheters are equipped with continuous fiberoptic SvO_2 monitoring, as well as intraventricular EKG leads, which allow measurement of left ventricular end-diastolic **volume,** rather than pressure–theoretically a better indicator of preload.

B. Indications (see "Cardiopulmonary Monitoring").

C. Equipment needed for insertion.

1. Pulmonary artery catheter.
2. Pressure monitoring lines.
3. Two 3-way stopcocks to connect to proximal and distal ports.
4. 3 cc syringe for balloon inflation (comes with Swan-Ganz®).
5. Equipment for central venous cannulation, catheter sheath (Cordis® introducer) and optional Swan-Ganz® plastic sheath that allows catheter adjustment under sterile conditions.
6. Transducers, pressure monitors.
7. Sterile gowns, gloves, mask, drapes.
8. An assistant, preferably an experienced SICU nurse.

D. Preparing for catheter insertion.

1. Peripheral IV line must be in place for fluids and emergency medications.
2. Lidocaine, atropine, and defibrillator must be available.
3. Continuous ECG monitoring.
4. Set up transducer and connecting tubing.
5. Zero and calibrate transducer.
6. Prep area as per central venous catheter insertion.

E. Insertion sites.

1. Subclavian vein (left is preferred over right).
2. Internal jugular vein (right preferred over left).
3. Femoral vein.

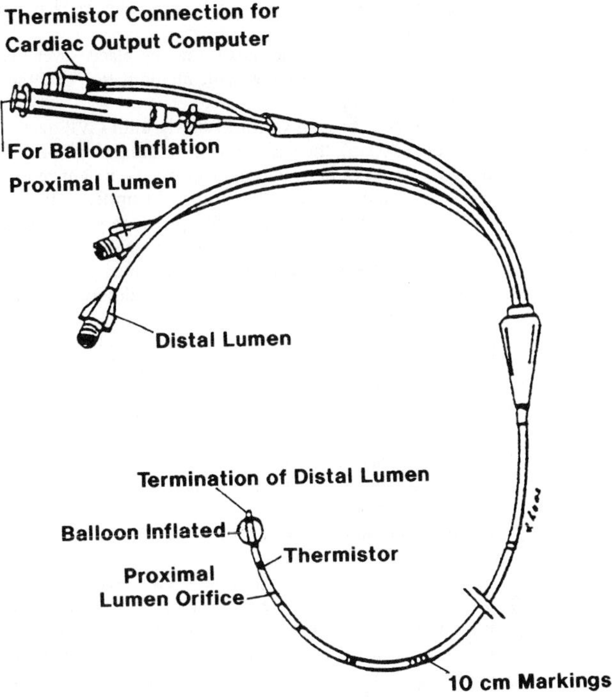

FIG. 11 Triple-Port, 4-Lumen, Swan-Ganz® Catheter

4. Brachial vein via antecubital cutdown–only as last resort; highest risk of complications.

F. Insertion of catheter.

1. Use meticulous aseptic technique.
2. Cannulate central vein, introduce catheter sheath (Cordis®) and suture in place after blood return is confirmed.
3. Attach IV tubing to Cordis® line. After this, catheter is brought into the sterile field, set up and tested:
   a. Flush the proximal, distal lumens with sterile saline containing 2-4 units heparin/cc to eliminate air bubbles and test system.
   b. Test balloon with 1.5 cc air inflation to rule out leaks.
   c. Connect thermistor to cardiac output computer, note increase in temperature after warming the thermistor between fingertips. If thermistor is non-functional, replace Swan-Ganz® catheter before insertion.

   d. Shake the catheter tip to confirm pressure wave changes on the monitor.
4. A clear plastic collapsible sheath may be placed over the catheter at this time to allow sterile manipulation of catheter after insertion.
5. Insert catheter through Cordis® slowly until CVP tracing is seen (15-20 cm), then ask assistant to inflate balloon.
6. Slowly advance catheter into right atrium, then right ventricle; when right ventricle waveform is identified, advance catheter smoothly and quickly into pulmonary artery (see Section G and Figure 12). While advancing, hold catheter firmly and close to Cordis® to avoid kinking.
7. Slowly advance to wedged position in pulmonary artery and deflate balloon.
   a. If pulmonary artery waveform returns–good position.
   b. If wedge waveform persists ("over-wedged")–withdraw slightly and re-check.
8. *Always deflate balloon before withdrawing catheter, and inflate before advancing.*
9. Confirming wedge position.
   a. Catheter flushes easily before inflating balloon (excludes catheter obstruction).
   b. Loss of pulmonary artery tracing with balloon inflation; returns with deflation.
   c. PCWP $\leq$ PAD pressure (normal PCWP 6-12 mm Hg).
10. To determine wedge, inflate balloon slowly while monitoring waveform. To prevent pulmonary artery rupture, stop inflation when wedged waveform is achieved. Always disconnect inflation syringe and unlock port prior to reconnecting and inflating the balloon. This avoids inadvertent overdistention or rupture of balloon and pulmonary artery.
11. Conditions of low cardiac output, tricuspid regurgitation, or pulmonary hypertension may require multiple attempts or fluoroscopy to pass the catheter. Mitral regurgitation may make waveforms difficult to interpret, also making catheter placement difficult. Changes in patient position (Trendelenburg's or left or right decubitus) are sometimes helpful.
12. If internal jugular or subclavian vein is used, pulmonary artery should be within 50-60 cm of catheter insertion; 70-80 cm for femoral or antecubital sites.
13. Document location of catheter tip and rule out pneumothorax with chest radiograph, preferably upright.
14. Monitor the waveform continuously to recognize inadvertent wedging ("over-wedging") which can cause pulmonary infarction. If catheter is noted to be over-wedged, adjust immediately.

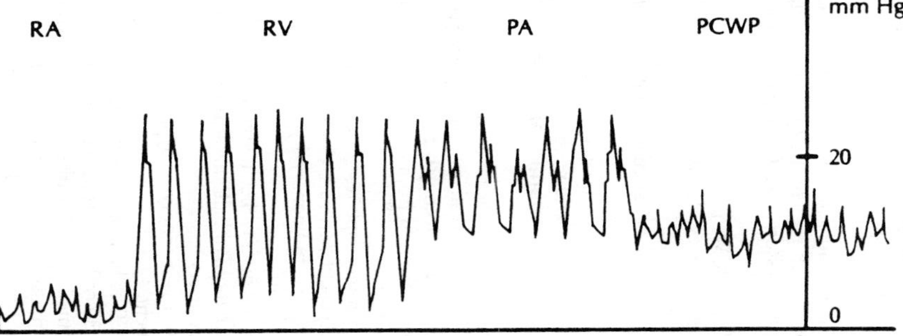

FIG. 12 Characteristic Waveform Changes (From Shuck JM, Nearman HS: Technical skills in patient care. In Davis JH: Clinical Surgery, St. Louis, C.V. Mosby, 1987, p. 711, with permission)

G. Waveforms seen during passage of pulmonary artery catheter.

1. Vena cava–dampened waveform, gentle sinusoidal motion with breathing. Abrupt increase with cough.
2. Right atrium–similar to vena cava, but less dampened.
3. Right ventricle–an abrupt increase in systolic pressure, which rapidly falls toward zero in diastole. Diastolic waveform has appearance of square root sign.
4. Pulmonary artery.
   a. Systolic pressure same as right ventricle (RV).
   b. Dicrotic notch present (best distinguishing factor).
   c. Diastolic pressure rises (tracing does not fall to zero as in RV).
5. Wedge (PAO, PCWP).
   a. Small A, V waves; fluctuates with ventilation.
   b. Mean pressure ≤ PAD.
   c. Read mean number at end-expiration, preferably off ventilator.
   d. Rising, flattened wedge tracing indicates "over-wedge"–deflate, withdraw, and re-check.

H. Complications of pulmonary artery catheter placement

1. ***Catheter kinks/knots***—if a knot is suspected, confirm with chest radiograph and call invasive angiographer to untie knot via femoral vein deflecting wire.
2. Pulmonary infarction from prolonged balloon occlusion of pulmonary artery.
3. Pulmonary artery rupture.
   a. Incidence–.06%.
   b. Risk factors–pulmonary hypertension, anticoagulation, hypothermia.
   c. Caused by tip if catheter advanced too far, eccentric balloon inflation, or balloon overinflation that ruptures pulmonary artery.
   d. Symptoms–hemoptysis, hypotension.
   e. Treatment.
      (1) < 30 cc hemoptysis–observe.
      (2) > 30 cc hemoptysis–consider wedge angiogram performed through catheter to show extravasation.
      (3) If massive, bronchoscopy with/without a double-lumen endotracheal tube may be indicated.
4. ***Sepsis***—site cellulitis/positive blood cultures. Infection rate related to duration of catheter being in place:
   a. If ≤ 3 days–5%.
   b. If 4 days–10%.
   c. If 5 days–15%.
5. ***Dysrhythmia***
   a. Related to passage of catheter through right ventricle.
   b. Transient PVCs develop in majority of patients (75%).

c. Persistent PVCs in 3-13%.
d. Risk factors for ectopy–acidosis, hypokalemia, hypothermia, hypoxia, prolonged time to pass catheter.
e. Advanced ventricular arrhythmias 3-12%; however, prophylactic lidocaine rarely indicated.
f. Treatment.
   (1) Intravenous lidocaine.
   (2) Withdraw catheter if unable to suppress (sometimes a large loop in the RV may be the cause).

6. Balloon rupture–replace catheter.
7. Transient right bundle branch block (RBBB) may occur; therefore, patients with pre-existing left bundle branch block (LBBB) are at risk for developing complete heart block. Consider placement of transvenous pacemaker prior to pulmonary artery catheter insertion or use a pacing Swan-Ganz® catheter (less reliable).
8. Endocarditis–from sepsis; more common in burn patients.

X. LINE CHANGE PROTOCOL (University of Cincinnati Surgical Intensive Care Unit)

A. Triple-lumen catheter and arterial line.
   1. Over-wire for one positive blood culture.
   2. New site for second positive culture, cellulitis at site, positive tip culture, or sepsis.

B. Pulmonary artery catheter–catheter and Cordis® every 72 h; one change over wire if cultures negative.

C. Surveillance cultures.
   1. Cultures for increased temperature, WBC count, clinical picture.
   2. All catheter tips are cultured when lines are removed.

71

Airways

Timothy D. Kane, M.D.

I. INDICATIONS FOR USE OF ARTIFICIAL AIRWAYS

A. Absolute indications.

1. Inadequate ventilation.
   a. Apnea.
   b. Increasing $PaCO_2$ (> 50 mm Hg).
2. Inadequate oxygenation–decreasing PaO_2 (< 55 mm Hg on room air) unresponsive to supplemental O_2.
3. Penetrating neck trauma with expanding hematoma.
4. Acute airway obstruction.

B. Strong relative indications.

1. Inadequate airway protection–CNS disorders.
2. Shock.
3. Severe chest wall injury (e.g., flail segment diaphragmatic rupture, open pneumothorax).
4. Massive retroperitoneal hemorrhage.
5. Severely injured, combative patient.

C. Relative indications.

1. Maxillofacial trauma.
2. Pulmonary contusion.
3. Inadequate pulmonary toilet.
4. Augment work of breathing for patients with acutely elevated ventilatory workloads, or decreased ventilatory capacity.

II. INITIAL MEASURES

A. Foreign body removal.

B. Chin-lift, jaw-thrust (with in-line cervical traction).

C. Oropharyngeal airway.

1. Relieves upper airway obstruction by elevating the base of the tongue off the posterior wall of the pharynx.
2. May prevent inadvertent laceration of the tongue in the incoherent or seizing patient and can be used as a bite block with oral endotracheal tubes.
3. Poorly tolerated in alert patient because of gag reflex.

D. Nasopharyngeal airway.

1. Used to relieve upper airway obstruction caused by tongue or soft palate falling against posterior wall of the pharynx.
2. Suctioning via this airway is less traumatic than nasal suctioning.
3. Better tolerated than oropharyngeal airway.
4. Alternate every 24 h between right and left nares to minimize sinusitis, otitis media, and nasal necrosis.
5. Avoid if coagulopathy present.

III. INVASIVE MEASURES OF AIRWAY MANAGEMENT—ENDOTRACHEAL INTUBATION

A. Methods.

1. Orotracheal intubation.
   a. Primarily for unconscious or anesthetized patients.
   b. Passed orally using direct laryngoscopy.
   c. Advantages—rapid introduction, can accommodate larger endotracheal tube.
   d. Disadvantages—patient discomfort, easily dislodged.
2. Nasotracheal intubation.
   a. Passed via nasopharynx blindly or with laryngoscopy. More difficult to place.
   b. Method of choice in trauma patients with possible cervical spine injury.
   c. Advantages—better tolerated, easier stabilization.
   d. Complications—same as nasopharyngeal airway.

B. Technique.

1. Preparation.
   a. Obtain permission if patient's condition allows.
   b. Equipment—ambu bag, laryngoscope, endotracheal tubes (various sizes), 10 cc syringe, lubricant, tube stylet, and anesthetic spray. Do not attempt endotracheal intubation without adequate suction set-up.
   c. Select tube size (rule of thumb)—in adults, the diameter of fifth digit approximates tube size (usually a 7- or 8-mm diameter endotracheal tube). Tube size of 8 or greater facilitates bronchoscopy.
2. Orotracheal intubation.
   a. Pre-oxygenate patient with mask ventilation of 100% O_2 while monitoring oxygen saturation.
   b. Place in sniffing position (neck flexed, head extended)—*contraindicated* in patients with possible cervical spine injury.
   c. Anesthetize posterior pharynx with spray.
   d. Open mouth widely using crossed finger technique with the right hand (thumb on lower incisors, index finger on upper incisors).
   e. Insert laryngoscope using left hand in right-hand corner of mouth and advance, sweeping the tongue to the left.
   f. Have assistant apply cricoid pressure, especially in emergent intubation.

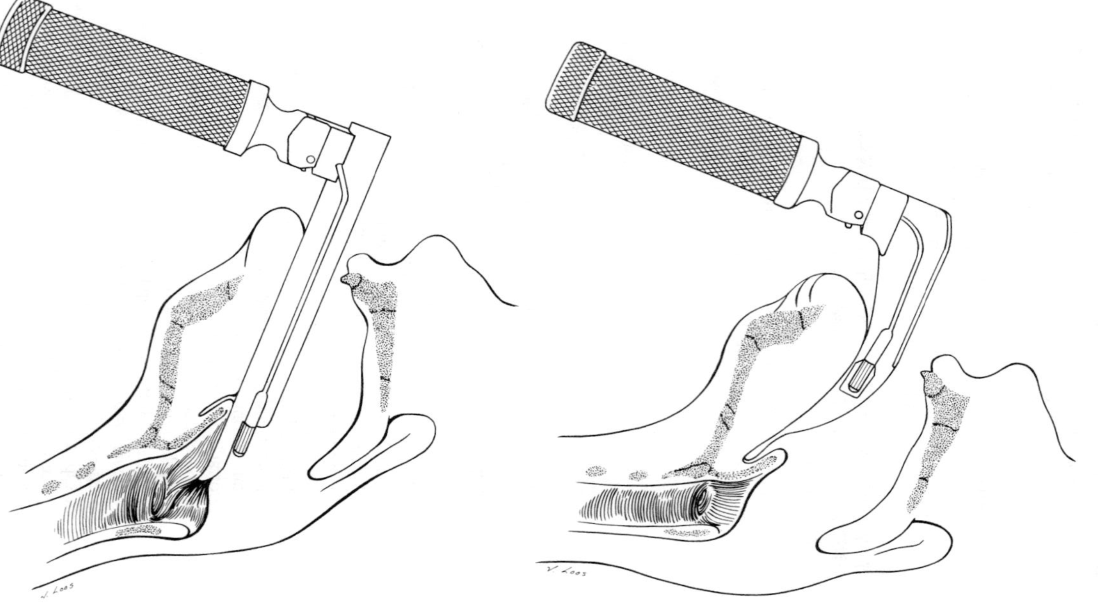

FIG. 1 Straight *vs.* Curved Blade Laryngoscopy Positioning

g. When the epiglottis is visualized, the tip of the laryngoscope is placed above (for curved laryngoscope blades) or below (for straight blades) the epiglottis (Figure 1). The laryngoscope is then lifted, not tilted, to visualize cords. Pharynx may require suctioning for adequate visualization of cords (Figures 2 & 3).
h. Insert tracheal tube under direct vision *through* vocal cords. Time insertion with patient's inhalation.
i. If unsuccessful, after 15 sec remove laryngoscope and return to step (a).

3. Post-intubation.
   a. Check for adequate and symmetric ventilation by inspection and auscultation of the chest.
   b. If cuff is present, inflate with minimal amount of air that will prevent leakage during ventilation. Cuff pressures ideally should be maintained at less than 20 mm Hg to prevent tracheal necrosis.
   c. Secure tube with adhesive or trach-tape.
   d. Check tube position by chest radiograph.
   e. After 10-20 min, obtain arterial blood gas and adjust ventilator accordingly.
4. Nasotracheal intubation.
   a. Patient should be breathing spontaneously.
   b. Prepare and position patient as for orotracheal intubation.
   c. Anesthetize nasal mucosa with cocaine or lidocaine and small dose of phenylephrine for anesthesia and vasoconstriction to avoid epistaxis.
   d. Pre-oxygenate patient.
   e. Gently advance tube through well-lubricated nares, going cephalad from nostril (to avoid the large inferior turbinate) and then posterior and caudad into the nasopharynx. Rotate tube to facilitate passage.
   f. Listen for patient breath sounds *through* the nasotracheal tube. Gently advance tube into trachea, during inspiration.
   g. If unable to pass tube, use laryngoscope and Magill forceps to introduce nasotracheal tube into the larynx under direct vision.
   h. Follow post-intubation procedures as for orotracheal intubation.

D. Complications of intubation.

1. Aspiration during attempted intubation.
2. Malposition–esophageal intubation, extubation, endobronchial intubation (most common lethal error is esophageal placement; most common malposition is intubation of the right mainstem bronchus).
3. Tube obstruction–kinking, compression, foreign body, secretions.
4. Traumatic intubation; tracheal erosion due to long-term intubation.

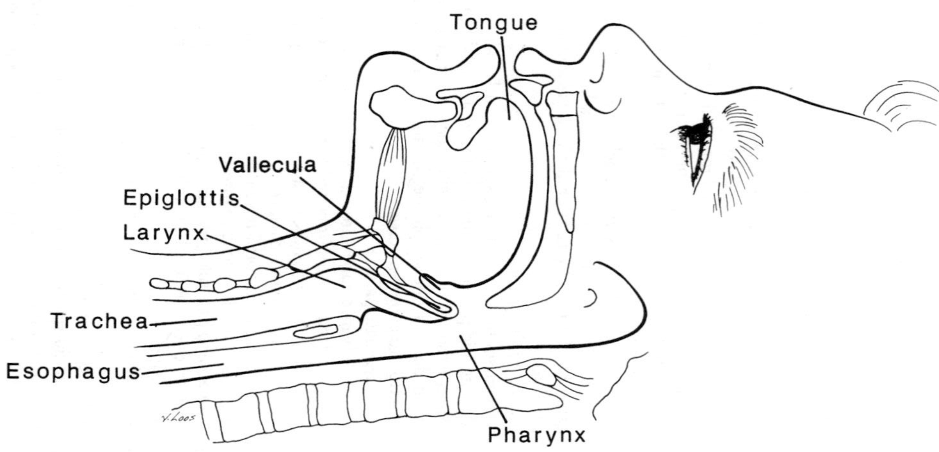

FIG. 2 Cervical Anatomy (Sagittal View)

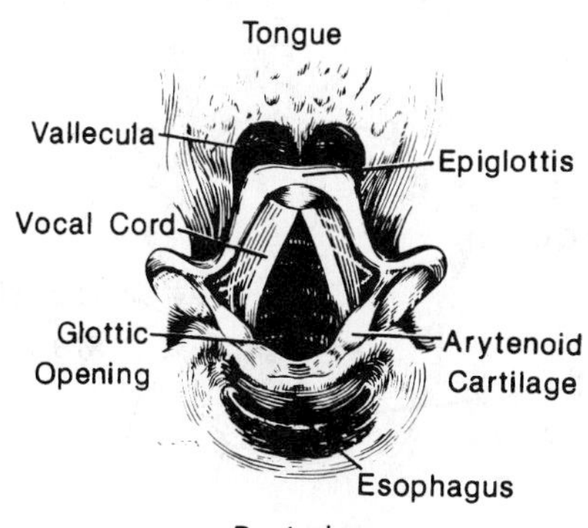

FIG. 3 Anatomy During Direct Laryngoscopy

5. Tracheoesophageal fistula–results from tracheal ischemia due to excessive cuff pressure.
6. Spinal cord injuries from hyperextension of neck in patients with unstable cervical spine.
7. If any question about tube placement, tube patency, or tube obstruction, remove tube and re-intubate.

IV. CRICOTHYROTOMY

A. Definition—surgical transtracheal intubation through the cricothyroid membrane.

B. Indications—urgent need for airway in a patient who cannot be intubated nasally or orally.

C. Technique.

1. Palpate thyroid and cricoid cartilage to define anatomy and identify cricothyroid membrane (Figure 4).
2. Make a vertical midline incision and expose cricothyroid membrane. If no scalpel is available, a 14 gauge IV catheter attached to oxygen source may provide temporary oxygenation. (*Caution:* Prolonged ventilation via the small catheter will result in hypercarbia due to inadequate exhalation of CO_2.)
3. Incise cricothyroid membrane with scalpel (horizontal incision) and enlarge ostomy by turning scalpel handle 90°.
4. Insert appropriate size (usually 6 or 7 mm) tracheostomy or endotracheal tube through ostomy into trachea.

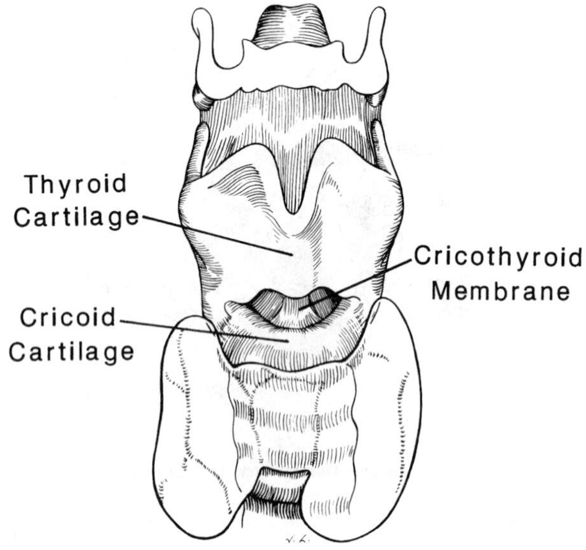

FIG. 4 Anatomy of Cricothyroid Membrane

5. Check position of tube by auscultation and obtain chest radiograph to confirm position.
6. Consider converting cricothyroidotomy to formal tracheostomy or endotracheal intubation when patient's condition allows. This should be performed within 24 h due to risk of inadvertent loss of airway.

D. Complications.

1. Early–hemorrhage, creation of false passage, subcutaneous emphysema, perforation of esophagus, and mediastinal emphysema.
2. Late–tracheal stenosis, especially in pediatric age group. Consider converting to formal tracheostomy early in children.

V. TRACHEOSTOMY

A. Definition—operative placement of an artificial airway through the anterior portion of the 2nd or 3rd tracheal ring.

1. Techniques.
   a. Open operative procedure–standard of care, minimal complication rate.
   b. Percutaneous dilatational tracheostomy–newer technique, does not require OR (no travel), inexpensive, rapid, and comparable to open method for complication rate.

B. Indications.

1. When procedures in upper airway may cause airway compromise, tracheostomy is performed electively (head and neck surgical patients).
2. Prolonged intubation.
   a. Tracheostomy is indicated if the patient remains intubated for 2-3 weeks. Tracheostomy should be postponed if high levels of PEEP are required.
   b. Early tracheostomy (< 7 days of mechanical ventilation) is associated with shorter ICU stay and decreased hospital stay, duration of mechanical ventilation, and incidence of pneumonia.
   c. Tracheostomy provides better patient comfort and mobility.
3. Upper airway obstruction.
   a. Not recommended for emergent airway control. This is better accomplished by a cricothyroidotomy.
   b. Anticipated obstruction or inability to perform elective intubation (i.e., a large goiter, pharyngeal or neck mass causing tracheal compression, laryngeal tumor, previous head and neck irradiation, etc.).

C. Complications.

1. Hemorrhage–Early bleeding due to inadequate hemostasis usually managed with direct pressure. Late hemorrhage from erosion into major vessel, usually innominate artery. Temporary control of tracheo-innominate fistula can be obtained by placing a finger anterior to the trachea into the mediastinum through the tracheostomy incision and compressing the innominate artery against sternum while patient is returned to OR for emergent ligation via median sternotomy.
2. Pneumothorax, pneumomediastinum, pneumoperitoneum.
3. Accidental extubation–in the early post-operative period, it may be difficult to replace the tracheostomy tube, since a mature tract has not yet developed. It is often preferable to place an oral endotracheal tube until the situation is stabilized. Intra-operative placement of "tag" sutures in trachea facilitate replacement. Replacement may be facilitated by passing a small, red rubber catheter through the skin incision into the trachea as a guide. (Remember, a clamp can be used to hold soft tissues apart to allow air exchange.)
4. Tube malposition–insertion into bronchi or mediastinum may occur. Confirm position with chest radiograph.
5. Obstruction–foreign body, blood, inspissated secretions, and floppy cuffs.
6. Swallowing dysfunction–resolves with removal of tube or deflation of cuff.
7. Tracheoesophageal fistula–incidence as high as 0.5%, results from tracheal ischemia due to pressure from tracheostomy tube and cuff.

8. Tracheomalacia–due to cuff overinflation, high PEEP.
9. In the obese patient, a standard tracheostomy tube becomes displaced into the pretracheal soft tissues. A spiral-flexible endotracheal tube (Anode tube) or custom-length tracheostomy tube may be required.

VI. CRITERIA FOR EXTUBATION (see "Respiratory Care").

72

Tube Thoracostomy

MICHAEL J. GORETSKY, M.D.

I. DRAINAGE APPARATUS

A. The 3-bottle system (Figure 1)–trap, underwater seal, and suction regulation.

1. Bottle 1–the trap. Fluid drained from pleural cavity remains in bottle.
2. Bottle 2–underwater seal. Air is forced out from the pleural space during expiration, when intrapleural pressure is positive.
3. Bottle 3–suction control. Suction intensity is controlled by placing tip of tube below a given distance from the surface of the water in bottle 3 (i.e., suction of −10 cm H_2O achieved by placing tip of tube 20 cm below surface) and increasing suction from vacuum source until air bubbles gently through the water.
4. Can be placed on water seal by disconnecting bottle 3 from bottle 2 and leaving short tube open to atmosphere.

B. Compartmental plastic chest drainage units (Figure 2)–analogous to the bottles of the 3-bottle system.

II. CHEST TUBE INSERTION

A. Indications—pneumothorax, effusion, or instillation of intrapleural sclerosing agents.

1. For suspected hemothorax or empyema, larger chest tubes (32 - 36 Fr) are placed through the 5th intercostal space in the midaxillary line and positioned posteriorly.
2. Simple pneumothoraces or malignant pleural effusions can be decompressed with smaller chest tubes (20 - 28 Fr) placed in a similar fashion.

B. Insertion of the chest tube.

1. Position patient by placing a folded towel beneath the scapula and abducting the arm, with the hand placed behind the head.
2. Provide sedation with parenteral narcotic and/or benzodiazepine.

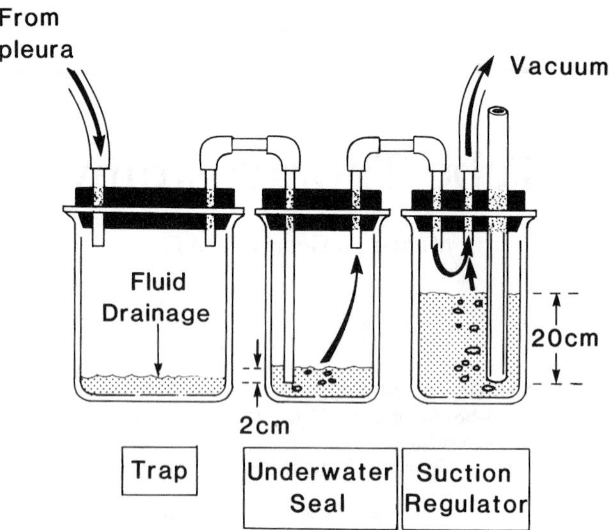

FIG. 1

3. Using sterile technique, prepare a wide operative field with bactericidal solution (povidine-iodine and alcohol) and sterile drapes.
4. Infiltrate a wide area of skin and subcutaneous tissue over the 6th rib in the midaxillary or anterior axillary line with local anesthetic (i.e., 1% lidocaine), down to the periosteum of the rib. Do not place chest tube below the 6th intercostal space, and avoid placement in areas adjacent to previous thoracostomy incisions.
5. Advance the needle through the intercostal space superior to the 6th rib (this avoids the neurovascular bundle) until the pleural space is entered; this is confirmed by aspiration of the pleural air or fluid. Slowly withdraw the needle until it is out of the pleural space, then inject anesthetic to provide pleural anesthesia.
6. Make a skin incision down to the 6th rib; incision should be large enough to admit the index finger.
7. Tunnel above the 6th rib in to the 5th intercostal space using a Kelly clamp. Gently spread the intercostal muscles to the level of the pleura.
8. Once the pleura is reached, close clamp and carefully push the tip through the pleura in to the pleural space (Figure 3).

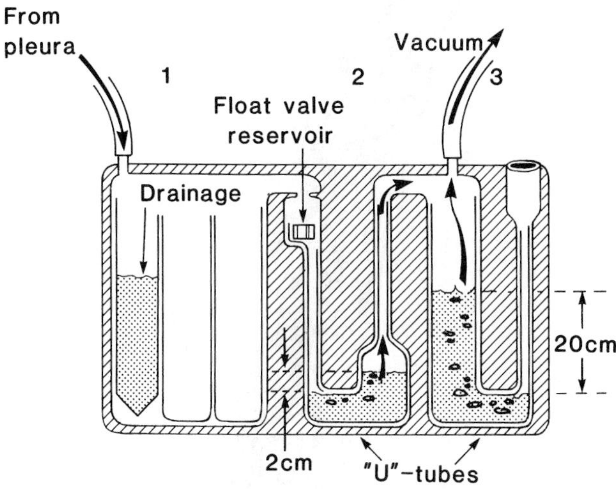

FIG. 2

This is usually accompanied by a rush of air, blood, or other pleural fluid.

9. Spread the jaws of the clamp to create a passage large enough to admit the index finger, which is then placed in to the pleural space to check for the presence of adhesions. The lung should be palpable during inspiration, ensuring entrance into the pleural cavity.
10. Grasp the chest tube at the tip with a Kelly clamp and guide the tube into the pleural space in an apicoposterior direction. Ensure that the last hole in the chest tube (always located on the radiopaque marker line) is within the pleural cavity.
11. Secure the tube to the skin with a large suture (i.e., 0 silk) and connect to a drainage apparatus. Intrapleural location of the chest tube can be confirmed by noticing the development of condensation on the inner surface of the tube during respiration and by noting the movement of fluid within the tubing during respiration.
12. Apply an occlusive dressing to the thoracostomy wound, using petroleum gauze or a Tegaderm®.
13. Obtain a portable chest radiograph to document proper positioning of the tube, evacuation of air and/or fluid, and expansion of the lung.

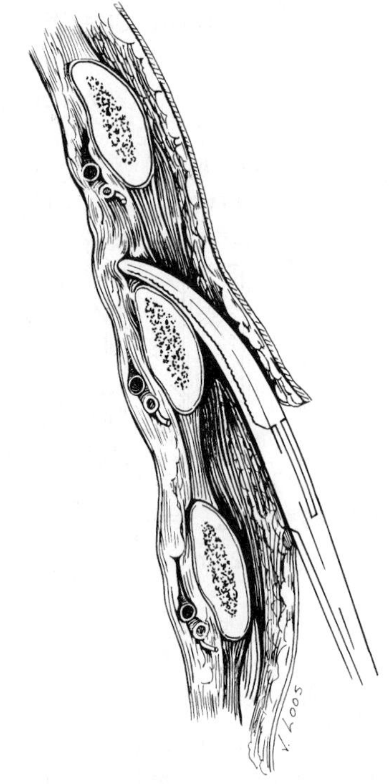

FIG. 3

C. Maintenance.

1. Obtain daily portable chest radiographs until tube removed.
2. Change dressing periodically to inspect the thoracostomy site.
3. *Never clamp a chest tube!!* This risks the development of a tension pneumothorax.

D. Complications.

1. Injury to intrathoracic and extrathoracic structures (intercostal vessels, pulmonary structures, diaphragm, great vessels, abdominal organs)–can be prevented by digital exploration prior to tube insertion, avoiding the intercostal bundle, and placement of the tube in the 5th to 6th intercostal space.
2. Tube malposition (major or minor fissure, subpleural).
3. Infection, empyema.
4. Tube displacement–if occurs, a new thoracostomy tube should be placed via a separate entrance site.

III. CHEST TUBE REMOVAL

A. **Chest tube should be removed** under the following conditions: (1) drainage is decreased to an acceptable amount (75 - 100 cc/24 h); and/or (2) "air leak" is not detectable for 24 h.

B. **Iatrogenic pneumothorax** is the most common complication.

C. **Procedure.**

1. Sedation with narcotic and/or benzodiazepine.
2. Remove all dressings, cut the anchoring suture, and cleanse skin with bactericidal solution.
3. Wearing a sterile glove, pinch the skin around the chest tube.
4. Have the patient perform the Valsalva maneuver, and rapidly remove the chest tube while pinching the skin around the tube to avoid the introduction of air.
5. Apply a generous amount of antibiotic ointment to the exit wound, and cover with an occlusive dressing (gauze and tape, Tegaderm®, or Duoderm®).
6. Dressing should remain in place for 24 - 48 h.

73

Thoracentesis

Arthur B. Williams, M.D.

I. INDICATIONS

A. Diagnostic evaluation of pleural fluid.

B. Therapeutic aspiration of fluid or air to return lung volume.

II. MATERIALS

A. Thoracentesis kit—become familiar with the set available. Most are based on a catheter-over-needle design.

B. Without a kit.

1. Local anesthetic, sterile drapes, prep kit, gloves.
2. 25-ga. needle, 22-ga. 1.5″ needle, 5 cc syringe.
3. 16- to 18-a. angiocath, 20-60 cc syringe.
4. Three-way stopcock.
5. IV pressure tubing, collection container, hemostat.

C. 500-1000 cc evacuated bottle.

III. PROCEDURE

A. Review upright chest radiograph, along with percussion of dullness to localize fluid. Blunting of the costophrenic angle on PA view indicates > 250 cc is present. Loculated effusions should be localized by ultrasound.

B. Obtain informed consent.

C. The patient should be sitting comfortably, leaning forward with arms resting over 1-2 pillows on a bedside table. In critically ill patients, the lateral decubitus position is used.

D. Thoracentesis is generally performed along the **posterior axillary line** from the back. The correct site is 1-2 interspaces *below* the level of the effusion, but *not* below the 8th intercostal space (Figure 1).

E. Using sterile technique, the area is prepped and draped. Local anesthetic is infiltrated intra-dermally over the superior margin of the rib below the chosen interspace. This is continued with the 1.5″ needle through the subcutaneous tissue to infiltrate the periosteum and intercostal muscles. Care is taken to aspirate with each move. When the pleura is entered and fluid returned, note depth with a clamp, withdraw the syringe 0.5 cm, and inject to anesthetize the pleura. Then remove needle.

F. Insert a 16- to 18-ga. angiocath through the anesthetized area to the previous depth while *continuously aspirating.* Care must be taken to avoid the neurovascular bundle (by advancing *over* the superior portion of the rib). The pleura has been entered when fluid returns. Advance the angiocath over the needle and withdraw the needle. Occlude the catheter lumen with a finger to prevent a pneumothorax. Interspace a 3-way stopcock between the angiocath and large syringe. The third lumen is directed to the collecting chamber.

G. Confirm position by aspirating into syringe with the stopcock "off" to the collection chamber. If good return is noted, turn the stopcock "off" to the patient and expel the contents of the syringe into the collection chamber. Repeat this procedure until the

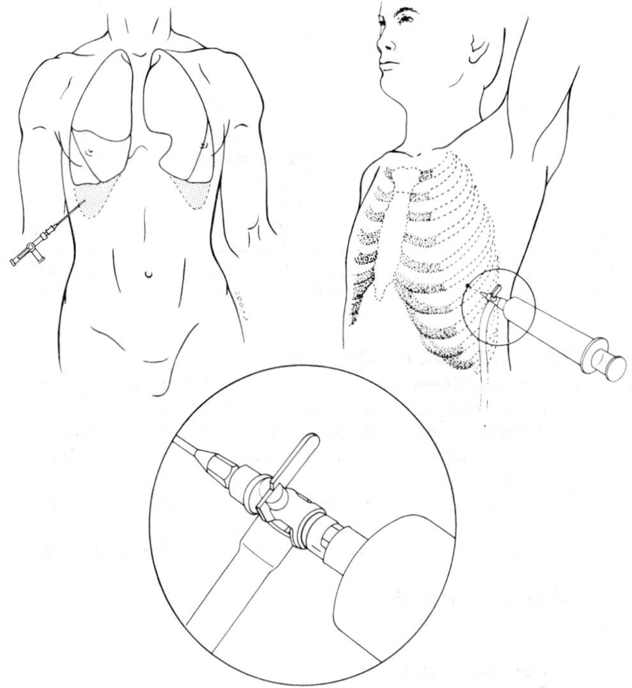

FIG. 1 Thoracentesis

desired amount of fluid is removed or no further fluid is obtained. When an evacuated bottle is used, after confirming position of the catheter, turn the stopcock "off" to the syringe and allow free aspiration.

H. Remove the angiocath and apply a sterile dressing.

I. Recommended pleural fluid studies.

1. Hematology–cell count and differential.
2. Chemistry–specific gravity; pH; LDH; amylase; glucose; protein.
3. Microbiology–gram stain; bacterial, fungal, and acid-fast bacillus cultures.
4. Pathology–cell cytology to rule out malignancy (in heparinized bottle).

J. Obtain a chest radiograph to confirm the efficacy of the aspiration and to rule out a pneumothorax.

IV. INTERPRETATION OF THE RESULTS

Labs	Transudate	Exudate
Protein	< 3 g/dl	> 3 g/dl
Protein ratio (effusion:serum)	< .6	> .6
Specific gravity	< 1.016	> 1.016
LDH	Low	High
LDH ratio (effusion:serum)	< .6	> .9
Glucose	2/3 serum glucose	Low
Amylase	< 200 IU/ml	> 500 IU/ml
RBC	< 10 k/mm^3	> 100 k/mm^3
WBC	< 1000/mm^3	> 1000/mm^3

When using the criteria of protein ratio > .6; LDH > 280 IU/L; and LDH ratio > .9, the sensitivity of determining exudate *vs.* transudate is 94% and specificity is 93%.

V. DIFFERENTIAL DIAGNOSIS

A. Transudate—cirrhosis, nephrotic syndrome, congestive heart failure, lobar atelectasis, viral infection.

B. Exudate—empyema, malignant effusion, intra-abdominal infection, pancreatitis, tuberculosis, trauma, pulmonary infarction, chylothorax.

C. Grossly bloody—iatrogenic injury, pulmonary infarction, trauma, tumor, hepatic or splenic puncture.

D. Extremely low glucose consistent with rheumatoid process.

VI. COMPLICATIONS

A. Pneumothorax.

B. Hemothorax.

C. Hepatic or splenic puncture.

D. Parenchymal tear.

E. Empyema.

74

Bladder Catheterization

John J. Bruns, Jr., M.D.
Michael B. Rousseau, M.D.

I. URETHRAL CATHETERIZATION

A. Continuous catheterization—indications.

1. Monitor urine output (UOP) accurately.
2. Relieve urinary retention due to infra-vesicle obstruction or neuropathic/myopathic loss of bladder tone with the following possible complications.
   a. Post-obstructive diuresis, if > 200 cc/hr, watch UOP.
   b. Hemorrhage secondary to bladder mucosal disruption.
   c. Hypotension with vasovagal response.
3. Urinary incontinence–temporary therapy, not long term.
4. Perineal wounds (burns, operative, traumatic) to prevent soilage.
5. Remove clots with hematuria (24-28 Fr.).
6. Aid in healing post GU lower procedure used as stents.
7. Medication induced urinary retention.

B. Intermittent catheterization indications; Robinson catheter.

1. Determine post-void residuals.
2. Sterile diagnostic urinalysis and cultures.
3. Management of neurogenic bladder and chronic urinary retention.
4. Psychogenic urinary retention.

C. Contraindications.

1. Psychogenic urinary retention (relative).
2. Trauma–approximately 10% of ER injuries.
3. Posterior urethral disruption of concern in males > females with pelvic fractures from deceleration accidents (see "Urologic Problems in Surgical Practice").
4. Anterior urethral injury primarily caused by perineal or straddle trauma.
5. Prostatic or urethral infection and epididymitis (relative).
6. Recent urethral or bladder neck surgery (variable).

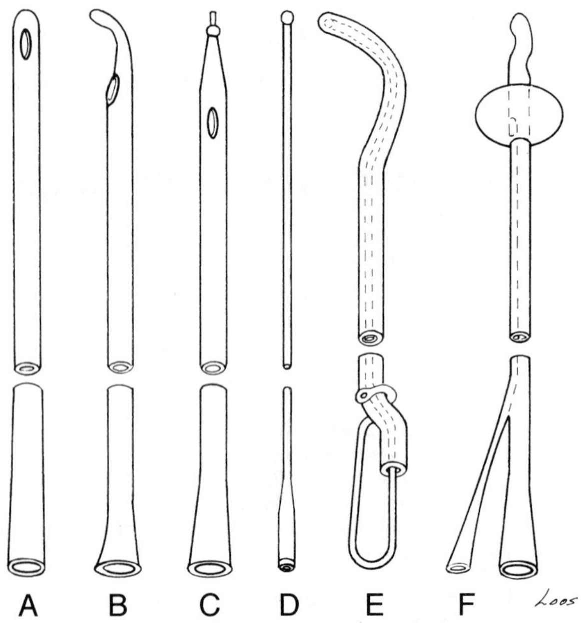

FIG. 1 **Urethral catheters—*A*,** soft rubber; ***B*,** coudé; ***C*,** Phillips, which attaches to ***D*,** filiform, which may be threaded over ***E*,** wire stylet; ***F*,** Foley self-retaining urethral catheter.

D. Materials (Figures 1 & 2):

1. 16-20 Fr. Foley catheter with 5 cc balloon (18 Fr. most common, smaller in females).
2. 5-8 Fr. pediatric feeding tube in infants (no balloon), don't use in adults secondary to coiling within urethra (1 Fr = .33 mm Ex diameter, luminal diameter may vary).
3. Sterile catheterization kit with water-soluble lubricant, gloves, prep solution, cotton balls, drapes, and water for balloon inflation.
4. Closed drainage system.
5. Normal saline irrigation and a catheter syringe.

E. Technique—males (Figures 3 & 4).

1. Position patient in the supine position, legs spread slightly. Lay out equipment in a convenient array, with both hands in sterile gloves. Confirm integrity of Foley balloon. Drape field with opening in drape over the penis.
2. Grasp the penis with non-dominant hand. If right-handed, stand on patient's right and hold perpendicular to body erect with modest tension (this hand is now contaminated and must

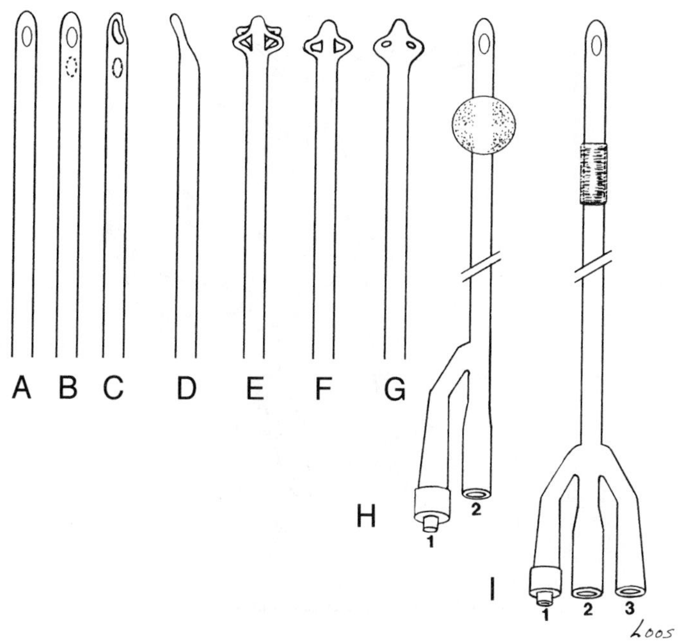

FIG. 2 Large-diameter catheters—*A,* conical tip urethral catheter; ***B,*** Robinson urethral catheter; ***C,*** Whistle-lip urethral catheter; ***D,*** coudé hollow olive-tip catheter; ***E,*** Malecot self-retaining, four-wing urethral catheter; ***F,*** Malecot self-retaining, two-wing urethral catheter; ***G,*** Pezzer self-retaining drain, open-end head, used for cystostomy drainage; ***H,*** Foley-type balloon catheter; ***I,*** Foley-type, three-way balloon catheter, one limb of distal end for balloon inflation (**1**), one for drainage (**2**), and one to infuse irrigating solution to prevent clot retention within the bladder (**3**).

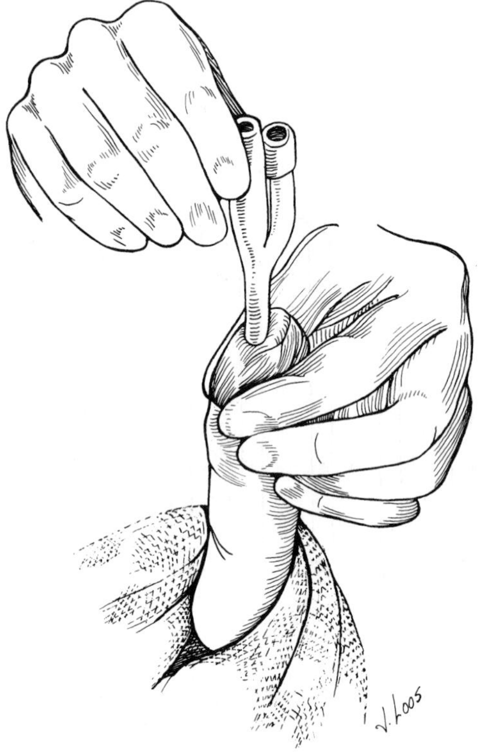

FIG. 3 Urethral Catheterization in Male Patient

remain in place). Prep the glans, foreskin, and meatus with antiseptic solution. Foreskin is retracted in an uncircumcised male to allow for an adequate prep.

3. Insert the well-lubricated catheter into the meatus while maintaining slight stretching tension on the penis with gentle, constant pressure. There will be some resistance as the catheter passes the prostate and sphincter. Have the patient take slow, deep breaths to aid in passage. The catheter should be inserted to the balloon sidearm; urine return confirms the catheter tip is within the bladder. If no urine is obtained, apply constant suprapubic tension and irrigate with 20-30 cc of normal saline to clear the ports. If there is free return of irrigation, it is unlikely that the catheter resides in the urethra.
4. When confident that the balloon lies within the bladder, inflate

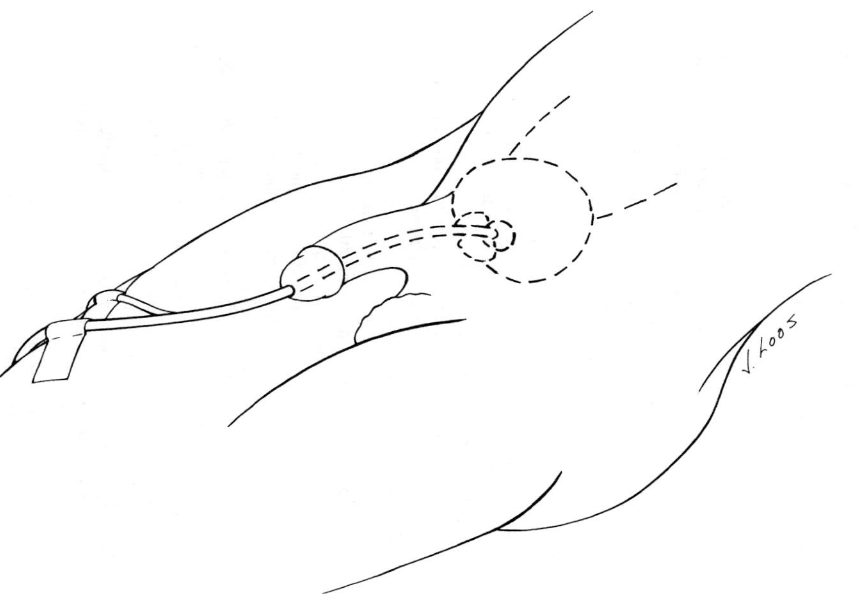

FIG. 4 Proper Position of Urethral Catheter in Bladder

the balloon with 5 cc of sterile water. If excessive resistance exists, deflate balloon and reattempt passage. Withdraw catheter to seat the balloon against the bladder neck. Connect the catheter to a sterile closed-drainage system.

5. Advance foreskin to prevent paraphimosis. Secure the catheter to the patient's thigh or abdomen with some slack to prevent accidental dislodgment and prevent catheter pull.

F. Technique—females (Figure 5).

1. Position patient supine with knees flexed and legs fully abducted ("frog-leg" position) and drape patient.
2. Spread labia with fingers of non-dominant hand to expose the urethral meatus (this hand is now contaminated and must remain in position). Prep introitus from anterior to posterior. An assistant can help with retraction.
3. Using sterile technique, insert well-lubricated catheter into urethral meatus to approximately 10-15 cm. Return of urine confirms position in the bladder. Again, if no urine returns, apply suprapubic pressure, then irrigate.
4. Inflate balloon with 5 cc of sterile water. Withdraw catheter gently to seat against the bladder neck. Tape to thigh with some slack and connect to sterile closed-drainage system.

G. Difficult urethral catheterizations.

1. Causes–meatal stricture, urethral stricture, prostatic hypertrophy, urethral disruption, urethral obstruction, anxious patient.
2. Possible solutions.
   a. Assure that catheter is well lubricated, and repeat attempt.
   b. If pain limits procedure, instill 20 cc xylocaine (2%) jelly–if resistance is met, abort; fat embolus has been reported.
   c. If anxiety limits procedure, ativan or morphine sulfate administration and continual, gentle catheter pressure to bypass the external sphincter.
   d. Attempt intubation with larger catheters (20-24 Fr.) or smaller catheters (5-8 Fr. pediatric feeding tube, may bypass urethral obstruction, but may coil in urethra).
   e. Meatal strictures can be dilated with a hemostat.
   f. Coude® catheter–most useful.
      (1) Tip forms an obtuse angle with the catheter body.
      (2) If catheter is not passable, often the tip has become obstructed by the following.
         a) The floor of the bulbous urethra.
         b) A pocket formed by hypertrophied prostatic lobes.
         c) Urethral stricture.
      (3) The Coude® tip is directed against the roof of the urethra.
      (4) If the Coude® tip becomes engaged in a pocket or fold, long axis rotation causes disengagement.
   g. The use of filiform and Phillips' catheters may be necessary if a Coude® catheter is impassable. This should always be attempted by a urologist.

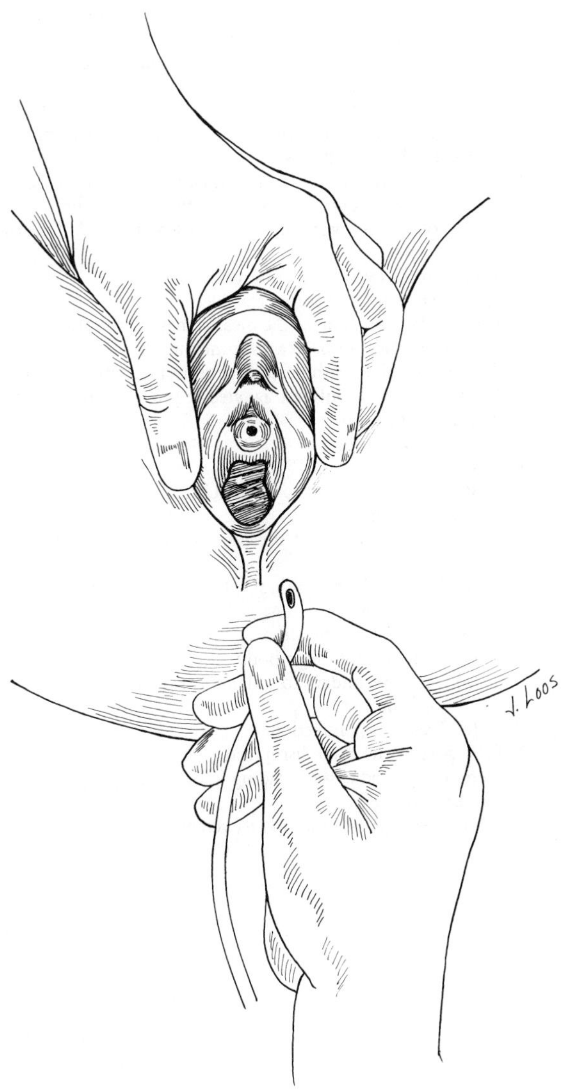

FIG. 5 Urethral Catheterization in Female Patient

h. If still unable to pass a catheter by these methods, consider the following.
   (1) Consider the possibility of urethral disruption and obtain a retrograde cystourethrogram.
   (2) Consider urologic placement of a catheter with cystoscopic aid or placement of a suprapubic catheter.

H. Care of urethral catheters.

1. Closed drainage system is the primary concern. If necessary to open, gloves should be employed with aseptic technique.
2. Urine collection bag should remain below the level of the catheter insertion.
3. Aseptic technique during insertion.
4. Remove catheter as soon as feasible.
5. Careful daily washing of the meatus may inhibit infection.
6. Flush or replace for decreased urine output.
7. Tape to medial leg with flexibility for normal patient movement.
8. Restrain patients confused/agitated to prevent catheter removal with intact balloon.

I. Complications.

1. Infection.
   a. Primary source of nosocomial UTIs.
   b. Possible causes.
      (1) Contamination at the time of insertion due to a break in technique.
      (2) Retrograde (ascending) infection, break in closed drainage system.
      (3) Bacterial colonization of meatus.
      (4) Presence of foreign body.
      (5) Sepsis secondary to inflation of the balloon in the prostatic urethra.
      (6) Pre-existing infection.
2. False passage, urethral disruption.
3. Hemorrhage and cystitis leading to hematuria.
4. Urethral stricture.
5. Obstructed catheter and urinary retention.

75

GI Intubation

M. Ryan Moon, M.D.

I. STOMACH

A. Nasogastric (NG) tubes—used for gastric decompression. Pass the largest size tolerable to the patient. Feeding is best accomplished by nasoduodenal tubes.

1. ***Levin tube***—a soft tube with a single lumen. Connect to low intermittent suction to prevent the gastric mucosa from occluding the tube.
2. ***Salem sump tube***—dual-lumen tube.
   a. The main lumen should be placed on low continuous suction. A sideport (blue) vents the tube to allow continuous sump suction.
   b. The vent should be flushed with 15 cc of air and the main lumen with 30 cc of saline every 3-4 h to ensure patency. The vent is patent when it "whistles" continuously.
3. ***Method of insertion.***
   a. Elevate the head of the patient at least 30°, then flex neck.
   b. Lubricate the tube with water-soluble lubricant or lidocaine jelly.
   c. Insert the tube into a nostril and pass it into the nasopharynx (a small bend in the tip of the tube will aid passage). The patient should swallow when the tube is felt in the back of the throat. Sips of water will facilitate passage of the tube into the esophagus in an awake patient.
   d. Advance into the stomach.
   e. A series of four black marks are on the main lumen. The proximal mark, at the nares, indicates insertion to the distal esophagus, the middle two marks to the body of the stomach, and the distal mark to the pylorus/duodenum.
   f. Inadvertent nasotracheal intubation is confirmed by the patient gasping for air, coughing, or unable to speak.
   g. Confirm tube position by instilling 20-30 cc of air while listening over the stomach with a stethoscope and by aspi-

ration of gastric contents. Aspiration of gastric contents is a more reliable method. Always confirm with radiograph if used for feeding.

h. Use of viscous lidocaine and Cetacaine® spray minimizes patient discomfort.

i. Secure the tube with tape. Tubes taped tightly to the nostril or nasal septum may lead to pressure necrosis (Figure 1).

j. Patient with Zenker's diverticulum may need endoscopic guidance for safe insertion.

B. Orogastric tubes.

1. Preferred if NG intubation is contraindicated (anterior basilar skull fracture, nasopharyngeal trauma).
2. ***Ewald tube***—especially suited for lavage of the stomach and emergency evacuation of blood, toxic agents, medications, or other substances.
   a. Large (18-36 Fr) double-lumen tube.
   b. The 36 Fr lumen is connected to continuous suction, the 18 Fr lumen is used for irrigation.
   c. **Method of insertion**—in patients with loss of consciousness or loss of the gag reflex, insertion of a cuffed endotracheal tube prior to orogastric tube insertion is preferred.
      (1) Lubricate the tube.
      (2) Insert the tube into the mouth and down the esophagus into the stomach. If the patient is conscious, have him/her sip water.
      (3) Verify position of the tube by aspiration of gastric contents and by auscultation.
      (4) Connect to suction; begin irrigation when the stomach is empty. The amount of irrigant used should be monitored. The large bore of this tube may allow rapid overdistention of the stomach with the resultant risk of aspiration.

II. DUODENAL/SMALL BOWEL TUBES

A. Nasoduodenal feeding tubes.

1. Tubes are smaller, softer, and more flexible than NG tubes.
2. Fluoroscopic placement preferred.
3. ***Prior to institution of tube feedings, the tube position must be verified by radiograph.***
4. Types of tubes.
   a. **Corpak®**—unweighted, has a bullet at the tip to prevent passage of tube into regions of the tracheobronchial tree that lack cartilaginous support; a wire stylet may be used to pass tube into duodenum under fluoroscopic guidance.
   b. **Frederick-Miller®**—has a stylet with flexible and stiff ends. Must only be placed under fluoroscopic guidance to prevent inadvertent tracheobronchial placement. This tube is much easier to pass into the duodenum.

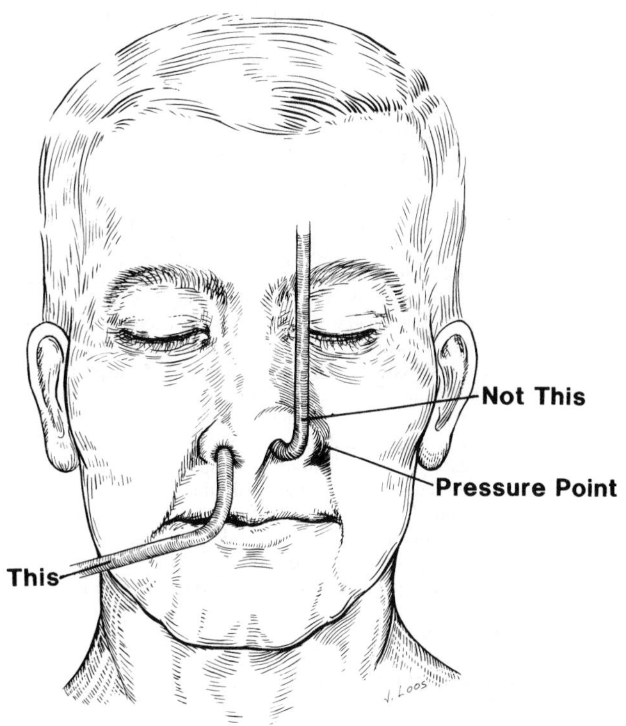

FIG. 1

5. Placement of the tube past the ligament of Treitz eliminates most of the potential for aspiration.
6. Nasoduodenal tubes allow for early institution of enteric feedings, prior to full resolution of ileus.
7. ***pH-Guided nasointestinal feeding tubes***—Advantages: decreased cost; rapid, easy placement; eliminates endoscopic/fluoroscopic requirements; decreased radiation exposure. Placement:
   a. Similar to that for standard bedside feeding tube placement; pH monitor allows for continuous pH readings.
   b. Flush tube with 10 cc tap water; insert guidewire; lubricate tip with water-soluble lubricant.
   c. Temporary ground pad attached to patient's skin; test tube by attaching monitor, and placing tip of tube in contact

with tube's ground wire (pH reading of 0.5 indicates functioning sensor and monitor).

d. Attach tube's ground wire to ground electrode pad; care must be taken to ensure reference electrode does not become detached, and that electrode gel does not dry.
e. Gently push tip of nose superiorly as tube is introduced; pass through naso- and oropharynx and into esophagus; initial readings average 6.5 to 6.6 (little variation).
f. Tube advanced until gastric pH (< 3.5) observed. (*Note:* The stomach is the only viscus in continuity with the nasopharynx that routinely has a pH < 5; if tube is advanced more than 45 cm without a drop in pH, then pulmonary placement or curling of tube in upper alimentary tract is likely.)
g. After observing gastric pH, cap gastric decompression tube if present, and insufflate 100-200 cc of air to distend stomach; insufflate 10 cc air boluses every 3-5 cm of tube advancement. (These maneuvers lessen the tube's chance of gastric rugal fold entrapment.)
h. Tube advanced until sudden, rapid increase in pH readings is encountered, signifying transpyloric passage. (*Note:* When rate of pH rise is gradual, tube is likely to be curled in stomach with the tip at the gastroesophageal junction.)
i. Obtain plain radiograph of abdomen after placement to confirm position prior to use.
j. When the pH changes of initial-to-lowest and lowest-to-final are both greater than 4 units, intestinal passage occurs in greater than 90% of attempts.
k. Anti-ulcer regimens do not interfere with placement.

B. Nasointestinal tubes for decompression of the small bowel.

1. Effectiveness is controversial. Used mainly for early postoperative bowel obstruction or obstruction secondary to carcinomatosis.
2. ***Cantor tube***—single-lumen tube with a mercury-filled balloon at the distal end.
   a. To prepare the balloon tip, inject 5 cc of mercury into the middle of the balloon tangentially with 21-ga. needle, then withdraw all air from the balloon.
   b. Lubricate the tube.
   c. While the patient is sitting upright, use a cotton-tipped applicator to help guide the balloon into the nasopharynx. When the tube falls into the back of the throat, have the patient swallow; the tube will travel by gravity into the stomach.
   d. Once the tube is in the stomach, aspirate stomach contents, then place to gravity.
   e. Tape the tube to side of face with 4-6″ loop. This permits the tube to advance by peristalsis.
   f. Place the patient on the right side and advance the tube to

the "P" position as marked on the outside of the tube. Have the patient remain in this position until the "D" mark is at external nares, indicating passage into the duodenum.

g. Confirm duodenal position by radiograph. The tube may be positioned at the pylorus under fluoroscopic guidance.
h. Place the patient on the left side until the tube has advanced several inches. Allow the patient to resume activity and the tube to be drawn downward by peristalsis. Leave a 4″ loop free. Pass the tube 3″ every 4 h. Irrigate with 15 cc saline before advancing the tube.
i. When the tube will no longer advance by peristalsis, place on low intermittent suction.
j. To remove the tube, slow, gentle withdrawal is necessary. The tube should be withdrawn approximately 1 ft/h to prevent intussusception.

3. ***Miller-Abbott tube***—dual lumen with 1 lumen for intermittent suction and the other to a balloon, which can be filled with mercury or water once the tube enters the stomach.

C. Tubes for intraoperative intestinal decompression.

1. ***Types***—Baker, Dennis, and Leonard tubes all have a suction port and a balloon to facilitate placement.
2. ***Placement.***
   a. Introduce tube into stomach via oral or nasogastric route.
   b. Inflate the balloon and pass manually through the duodenum into the small bowel.
   c. May be placed through an enterotomy at the risk of intra-abdominal enteric spillage.

III. SENGSTAKEN-BLAKEMORE TUBE

A. An oral gastric tube equipped with an esophageal and gastric balloon for tamponade and ports for aspiration.

B. Advantages—immediate cessation of bleeding in greater than 85% of patients; availability of device. **Disadvantages**—frequent recurrence of hemorrhage after deflation of balloon; high incidence of complications if used by inexperienced personnel (aspiration, esophageal perforation, ischemic necrosis).

C. Indication—acutely bleeding esophageal varices refractory to sclerotherapy and medical management.

D. Insertion.

1. Check the balloons under water to assure that no leaks are present and to verify patency of all 3 lumens of the tube.
2. Measures to prevent aspiration.
   a. Endotracheal intubation in virtually all patients.
   b. Gastric lavage to empty stomach.
   c. Have wall suction available.
   d. Pharynx is *not* anesthetized so as to maintain the gag reflex if the patient is not intubated.
3. Lubricate the tube and pass it into the stomach via the mouth.

4. The tube is advanced fully, and air is injected into the suction lumen while auscultating over the stomach region.
5. ***Confirm the intragastric location*** of the gastric balloon by instilling small amount of water-soluble contrast medium into the balloon and obtaining an radiograph *before* inflating balloon fully.
6. Inflate gastric balloon slowly with 200-300 cc of air and double clamp with rubber-shod surgical clamps. Stop air inflation *immediately* if the patient complains of epigastric pain or if insufflation of air is not audible over the epigastric region.
7. Apply gentle traction on the tube until resistance indicates that the balloon is at the esophagogastric junction.
8. Tape the tube to the facemask of a football helmet or attach to 1-2 lb of traction to maintain gentle traction of tube.
9. Aspirate the gastric tube (suction tube) or lavage with saline. If there is no evidence of continued bleeding, there is no need to inflate the esophageal balloon.
10. A second nasoesophageal tube is passed into the proximal esophagus to monitor continued bleeding above the gastric and/or esophageal balloons and to aspirate salivary secretions. The Minnesota tube is a modification that has an esophageal port to obviate the need for this extra tube.
11. If bleeding continues, the esophageal balloon is slowly inflated to 40 mm Hg. Use lowest pressure that stops bleeding. Double clamp the balloon inlet with rubber-shod surgical clamps. *Do not* inflate the esophageal balloon $>$ 40 mm Hg.
12. Gastric and esophageal lumens are connected to intermittent suction.
13. Tape scissors to the head of the bed in plain view if urgent transection and removal of the tube is required.
14. Irrigate the gastric lumen tube frequently and record the appearance of the return fluid.
15. Both balloons are inflated for 24 h, after which the esophageal balloon is slowly deflated and the patient is observed for signs of rebleeding. If rebleeding occurs, the esophageal balloon is reinflated.
16. If no rebleeding, the gastric balloon is deflated after 24 h, and the patient is observed.
17. If no further bleeding occurs 24 h after the gastric balloon is deflated, mineral oil should be given prior to removal. The tube is completely transected with scissors and removed. This ensures that balloons are deflated completely and that the tube is not re-used.
18. The esophageal balloon is always deflated first to prevent the risk of migration then asphyxiation.
19. Nursing supervision is essential. Complications are frequent and include aspiration, mucosal bleeding, and esophageal or gastric perforation.

76

Paracentesis

David L. Brown, M.D.

I. INDICATIONS

A. Diagnostic.

1. Etiology of ascites.
2. Suspicion of spontaneous bacterial peritonitis.

B. Therapeutic—to relieve dyspnea and/or anorexia.

1. Up to 2 L of ascitic fluid can be drawn off every 24 h.
2. Colloid replacement is indicated with therapeutic paracentesis to prevent complications associated with rapid loss of volume: Give 100 cc of Dextran-70 IV for each L of fluid removed or 12.5 g albumin per L removed.
3. Consider peritoneovenous shunt if repeated paracentesis is required in a patient who is refractory to medical therapy.

II. TECHNIQUE

A. Ensure that a large-bore, functional IV is in place.

B. Empty urinary bladder.

C. Examine abdomen and choose site.

1. Ultrasound guidance may be needed in a scarred abdomen to avoid inadvertent bowel injury.
2. The preferred site is halfway between the ASIS and the umbilicus, lateral to the rectus abdominus muscle (Figure 1).

D. Position patient—supine, slight reverse Trendelenburg, with a pillow under the opposite side.

E. Prep and drape sterilely.

F. Infiltrate with local anesthesia down to peritoneum using a 25-ga. needle.

G. Switch to a 16-ga. angiocath, and while aspirating, advance until free fluid is encountered. (Make a 'z-track' when traversing the subcutaneous tissues and musculature to prevent an ascitic leak from a straight entry track.)

H. Remove needle from catheter; attach 3-way stopcock, and withdraw desired amount of fluid. Connect IV tubing and a ster-

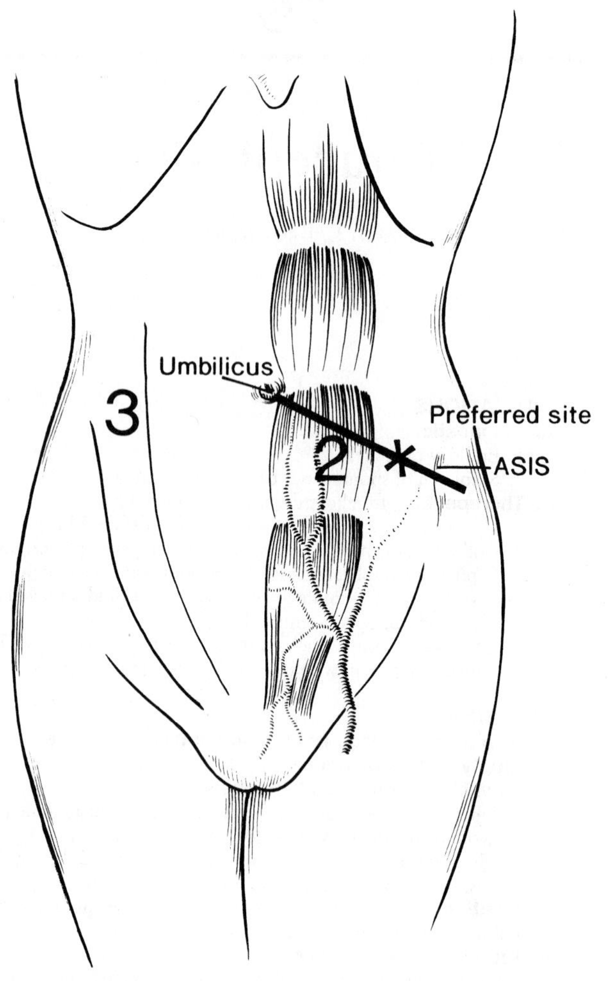

FIG. 1

ile bag or vacuum bottle if a large amount of fluid is to be withdrawn.

I. **When finished,** apply betadine ointment and dressing.

III. POTENTIAL COMPLICATIONS

A. **Persistent leakage of ascites** from paracentesis site.
B. **Intra-abdominal bleeding.**
C. **Infection** of ascitic fluid.
D. **Perforated viscus** (bowel or bladder).
E. **Hemodynamic instability** (hypotension).
F. **Hepatorenal syndrome or hepatic coma** if too much fluid is removed without appropriate replacement therapy.
G. **Electrolyte abnormalities.**

IV. FLUID ANALYSIS

A. **Send fluid for the following tests.**
   1. Cell count (RBC, WBC).
   2. Gram stain, culture (bacterial, fungal, acid-fast bacillus).
   3. Cytology.
   4. Chemical analysis–specific gravity, total protein, amylase, fibrinogen, LDH, glucose and pH.

B. **Diagnosis.**

	Protein (g/dl)	Albumin ratio: serum/ ascites	Cytology (/mm^3)	Specific gravity	LDH ratio: ascites/serum	Other
Cirrhosis	< 2.5	> 1.1	——	< 1.016	——	——
Peritoneal cancer	> 2.5	< 1.1	> 500 (all types)*	> 1.016	> 0.6	——
Infection	> 2.5	——	WBC > 300	> 1.016	> 0.6	pH < 7.3
Pancreatic disease	> 2.5	——	——	> 1.016	——	Amylase

* Malignant cells may be found in 50% of patients with cancer; however, about 4% of patients with cirrhosis will have malignant-appearing cells in their ascitic fluid.

77

Diagnostic Peritoneal Lavage (DPL)

David A. Rodeberg, M.D.

I. INTRODUCTION

A. **Mainstay of evaluation** of **unstable** blunt abdominal trauma and selected cases of penetrating trauma.

B. **Ideally, should be performed by the surgeon caring for the patient** since it is a surgical procedure that alters subsequent examination of the patient.

C. **Unreliable** in assessment of most retroperitoneal injuries.

D. **Usually performed early in patient evaluation,** typically during secondary survey. If free intraperitoneal air is suspected, perform abdominal films prior to DPL (DPL can introduce air).

E. **Nearly half of patients with hemoperitoneum will not have positive abdominal findings.**

F. **May also be used for evaluating critically ill patients for intra-abdominal process.**

II. INDICATIONS

A. **DPL—**history of blunt abdominal trauma and manifestations of hypovolemia–hypotension and tachycardia.

B. **DPL and/or CT,** depending on availability of CT and time available for patient evaluation. CT scan should be performed with both IV and GI contrast. *The patient must be hemodynamically stable!*

1. Depressed sensorium or altered pain response leading to possible false-negative physical examination (ethanol intoxication, head injury, drug abuse, spinal cord injury).
2. Equivocal abdominal findings–often a result of lower rib fractures, pelvic fractures, and lumbar spine fractures.
3. Positive abdominal findings–localized tenderness, guarding.
4. Unavailability of patient for continued monitoring–patient

undergoing general anesthetic for other injuries, DPL needed to definitively clear abdomen.

5. Low rib fractures, particularly on left side.

C. Controversial indications for DPL and/or CT.

1. Penetrating injury to surrounding areas.
   a. Lower chest–below nipples or 4th intercostal space.
   b. Flank.
   c. Buttocks and perineum.
2. Abdominal stab wounds or low-caliber gunshot wounds with negative physical signs–controversial.

III. CONTRAINDICATIONS

A. Absolute contraindication—obvious indications for exploratory laparotomy–free air, peritonitis, penetrating trauma.

B. Relative contraindications.

1. Multiple abdominal operations or midline scars–appendectomy or Pfannenstiel's scar alone does not preclude DPL.
2. Gravid uterus–use supra-umbilical open technique above fundus.
3. Inability to decompress bladder–use supra-umbilical open technique.
4. Inability to decompress stomach–use infra-umbilical open technique.
5. Pelvic fracture with possible hematoma–use supra-umbilical open technique to avoid false-positive results obtained by entering retroperitoneal hematoma.

IV. TECHNIQUES

A. Semi-open.

1. Insert nasogastric tube and urinary catheter–stomach and bladder must be decompressed to avoid injury.
2. Restrain patient, sedate if necessary.
3. Shave peri-umbilical region–above and below umbilicus.
4. Prep region widely with betadine, drape with sterile towels.
5. Decide on supra- or infra-umbilical incision.
6. Infiltrate proposed site (skin and subcutaneous tissue) with 1% xylocaine with epinephrine–enhances local hemostasis to minimize false-positive results, use even in comatose or anesthetized patient.
7. Incise skin (1-5 cm vertical incision needed depending on body habitus) and subcutaneous tissue down to midline fascia.
8. Place towel clips on both sides of the fascial incision for traction.
9. Using #11 scalpel blade, make a 2-3 mm stab incision in fascia.
10. With strong upward traction on the towel clips by the assistant, the operator places the trochar-catheter apparatus through the fascial opening and then pushes it through the

peritoneum (and posterior fascia). This initial push should be done perpendicular to the skin and must stop after one feels the "pop" of the peritoneum. At this point, the trochar-catheter apparatus is tilted down, the catheter alone is advanced toward the pelvis, and the trochar removed.

11. Attach the aspirating device and aspirate using a 12 cc syringe.
    a. If ≥ 10 cc is positive.
    b. If < 10 cc the aspirate is returned to the abdomen with the lavage fluid.
12. If aspirate is negative for blood, instill 1 L (10 cc/kg in children) lactated Ringer's or normal saline solution from a pressure bag. Shake the patient's abdomen periodically or move patient into and out of Trendelenburg. Use warm fluid in hypothermic patients.
13. When only a small level of fluid remains in the bag, drop the nearly empty bag to the floor to drain the fluid. The fluid drains by siphon action; hence, if all the fluid is allowed to run in along with some air, the siphon is lost and must be restarted by applying suction via a needle and syringe to a port in the tubing. Tubing used must *not* have a one-way filter device.
14. While the fluid is draining, keep a sponge packed into the wound for hemostasis and constantly hold the catheter in place.
15. After the fluid has returned (300-500 cc minimum), clamp the tubing and withdraw catheter (avoids siphoning blood from wound into bag).
16. Wound closure–a heavy suture may be placed to close the small fascial defect (optional), skin closure with skin staples (hold ends of wound taut with towel clips).

B. **Percutaneous**—closed, Seldinger technique–uses needle/trochar, guide wire, and advancing catheter.

C. **Open technique**—midline fascia is incised over 3-4 cm, posterior fascia/peritoneum is held with hemostats and opened under direct vision, catheter without trochar is advanced into peritoneal cavity. Fascial closure is required at completion.

V. TECHNICAL PROBLEMS

A. **Poor fluid return**—adjust catheter position, twist catheter, place patient in reverse Trendelenburg position, apply manual pressure to abdomen, instill an additional 500 cc fluid, have patient take deep breaths, make sure there is not a one-way valve in the IV tubing, fluid may exit the chest tube or Foley catheter.

B. **Air in tubing**—check all connections, make certain catheter is advanced far enough to avoid exposed side holes, reestablish siphon as described above.

C. **Infusion into abdominal wall**—recognize immediately and repeat DPL.

VI. COMPLICATIONS

A. Bowel injury.

B. Bladder laceration.

C. Injury to major blood vessels (aorta, inferior vena cava).

D. Hematoma.

E. Wound infection.

VII. INTERPRETATION

A. Grossly positive—≥ 10 cc of blood on initial aspirate.

B. Microscopic/chemistry criteria—positive on lavage (blunt trauma).

1. ≥ 100,000 RBC/mm^3 (97% sensitivity, 99.6% specificity) (≥ 10,000-20,000 for penetrating trauma–controversial)
2. ≥ 500 WBC/mm^3 (≥ 25-100 for penetrating trauma).
3. Presence of particulate (fecal, vegetable) matter.
4. Presence of bacteria on gram stain.
5. Elevated amylase, bilirubin.
6. Fluid exiting the chest tube or Foley catheter.

78

Principles of Abscess Drainage

Betty J. Tsuei, M.D.

I. SUPERFICIAL ABSCESSES

Usually subcutaneous and easily accessible. Includes hidradenitis suppurativa, small breast abscesses, infected sebaceous cysts, and perianal abscesses.

A. Technique.

1. IV pain control (i.e., morphine, demerol) and sedation (diazepam, midazolam). Narcan® should be available.
2. Localization of fluid collection by palpation. This may be difficult if extensive induration and edema is present.
3. Sterile prep and drape.
4. Field block with appropriate local anesthetic.
5. Aspiration of the fluctuant area with an 18-ga. needle to collect a sample for gram stain and anaerobic and aerobic cultures. This may also be useful in localizing the fluid collection if a fluctuant mass is not readily palpable.
6. Adequate incision over the fluctuant area, following skin lines when possible. Excision of a small skin ellipse may aid in keeping the wound edges open, especially if outpatient packing and dressing will be needed.
7. Swab for culture if sample was not previously obtained.
8. Break down loculations with finger or instrument.
9. Irrigate liberally with saline.
10. Pack cavity with thin strip gauze. Iodoform gauze can be used to help maintain hemostasis during the first 24 h.
11. Leave packing intact for 24 h, then remove and evaluate.

B. Antibiotics—Use of systemic antibiotics (PO or IV) depends upon degree of surrounding cellulitis and the condition of the patient. Most superficial abscesses are caused by *Staphylococcus* species, unless the patient is diabetic or the GI tract is involved. Diabetic patients often require more aggressive management of infections and glucose control.

II. DEEP ABSCESSES

Include intra-abdominal, intramuscular, deep breast abscesses, and perirectal abscesses.

A. These require drainage in the operating room for adequate exposure, analgesia, and equipment.

B. CT-guided aspiration and drainage may be feasible in specific cases, especially localized intra-abdominal collections. Antibiotic coverage should be provided peri-operatively.

79

Gram Stain Technique

DAVID L. BROWN, M.D.

I. Smear thin layer of material to be stained on slide using a wire loop that has been previously flame-sterilized and cooled.

II. Allow material to air-dry.

III. Heat-fix specimen to slide, using three *quick* passes through a flame (too much heat can destroy organisms due to protein denaturing).

IV. Normal prep:

Gentian violet	1 min
H_2O rinse	
Iodine	1 min
*Alcohol**	1-2 sec
H_2O rinse	
Safranin	1 min
H_2O rinse	

** Extensive decolorizing of slide with too much alcohol may make gram-positive organisms appear gram-negative.*

V. Quick prep: Violet, iodine, and safranin stains can be applied for only 15-20 seconds each and still produce a well-stained specimen.

VI. Under oil immersion:

A. Gram-positive organisms retain the Gentian violet and appear dark blue/purple.

B. Gram-negative organisms are decolorized, re-stain with Safranin, and appear red.

PART IV

Formulary

Clyde I. Miyagawa, Pharm.D.,
Robert E. Isemann, R.Ph., Carole Ebner, R.Ph.,
and Leslie A. Wermeling, RPh.

Categories

Generic Drugs

Ammonia Detoxifiers, Aids In Hepatic Encephalopathy

Drug	Supplied	Dose/Route	Remarks
Lactulose (Cephulac, Chronulac)	Solution: 3.33 g/5 ml	**Hepatic encephalopathy:** PO: 30-45 ml 3-4 times daily initially, then adjust dose to produce 2-3 soft stools per day or stool pH of 5. Usual dose is 90-150 ml/day. PR: 300 ml diluted with 700 ml water or 0.9% sodium chloride administered rectally and retained for 30-60 min every 4-6 h as necessary. **Constipation:** PO: 15-30 ml daily.	Indicated in hepatic encephalopathy, constipation. *Contraindicated* in low-galactose diet. Results comparable to those achieved with neomycin. Decreases blood ammonia concentration by 25-50% as a result of acidification of colon contents and formation of ammonium ion. May be used in renal failure or partial deafness. Less than 3% is absorbed from the small intestine following oral administration. Can be given concomitantly with oral neomycin.
Neomycin sulfate (Mycifradin)	Tabs: 0.5 g Solution: 125 mg/5 ml	**Hepatic coma:** PO: 4-12 g/day in 4 divided doses. **Bowel preps:** a. Condon Nichols: 1 g neomycin and 1 g erythromycin base PO at 1 pm, 2 pm, 11 pm day before surgery. b. Hunter: 1 g neomycin PO q 1 h for 4 h, then q 4 h for 36 h. Erythromycin base 1 g PO q 6 h for 36 h.	*Contraindicated* in intestinal obstruction and neomycin sensitivity; 97% unabsorbed. *Caution* with concurrent use of other nephrotoxic and ototoxic drugs. Its use in hepatic encephalopathy is based on hypothesis that GABA-mediated neurotransmission contributes to the CNS depression of the condition.

Flumazenil (Mazicon)	Vials: 0.1 mg/ml	See "Benzodiazepine Antagonists" for dosing.	

Angiotensin-Converting Enzyme Inhibitors (* Dose reduction in renal failure)

Benazepril* (Lotensin)	Tabs: 5,10,20,40 mg	**HTN:** 10-40 mg/day in single or or 2 divided doses.	See Enalapril for additional comments.
Captopril* (Capoten)	Tabs: 12.5,25,50,100 mg	**HTN:** 25-150 mg bid/tid up to 450 mg/day. **Heart Failure:** 25-100 mg tid up to 450 mg/day (May start with 6.25-12.5 mg in patients with normal/low blood pressure. **Diabetic Nephropathy:** 25 mg tid. **Left Ventricular Dysfunction after MI:** 6.25 mg single dose, increase to 12.5 mg tid and titrate up to 50 mg tid over several weeks.	Most common side-effects are rash, loss of taste perception, and cough. May cause neutropenia/agranulocytosis, especially in patients with renal dysfunction, SLE (reversible after discontinuation of drug). *Contraindicated* in pregnancy during 2nd and 3rd trimesters. Best given 1 h before meals.
Enalapril* (Vasotec)	Tabs: 2.5,5,10,20 mg	**HTN:** 5-40 mg/day in single or 2 divided doses. **Heart Failure:** 5-20 mg/day, usually in 2 divided doses. **Asymptomatic Left Ventricular Function:** 5-20 mg/day in 2 divided doses.	Most common side-effects are headache, dizziness, fatigue, renal insufficiency, hyperkalemia, cough. *Contraindicated* in pregnancy during 2nd and 3rd trimesters.
Enalaprilat* (Vasotec IV)	Injection: 1.25 mg/ml	**HTN Crisis:** 0.625-1.25 mg q 6 h. **HTN:** 1.25-5 mg q 6 h (0.625 mg initially when given concomitantly with diuretic).	See Enalapril for additional comments.
Fosinopril (Monopril)	Tabs: 10,20 mg	**HTN:** 10-40 mg/day in single or 2 divided doses.	See Enalapril for additional comments.

(continued)

Angiotensin-Converting Enzyme Inhibitors—*(cont.)*

Drug	Supplied	Dose/Route	Remarks
Lisinopril* (Prinivil, Zestril)	Tabs: 5,10,20,40 mg	**HTN:** 5-40 mg/day in single or 2 divided doses. **CHF:** 5-20 mg qd	See Enalapril for additional comments.
Quinapril* (Accupril)	Tabs: 5,10,20,40 mg	**HTN:** 10-80 mg/day in single or 2 divided doses. **CHF:** 10-40 mg/day in 2 divided doses. **CHF:** Adjunctive therapy along with diuretic or digitalis.	See Enalapril for additional comments.
Ramipril* (Altace)	Caps: 1.25,2.5,5,10 mg	**HTN:** 1.25-20 mg/day in single or 2 divided doses. **CHF:** 1.25-5 mg bid.	See Enalapril for additional comments.

Anti-Arrhythmics

Adenosine (Adenocard)	Injection: 6 mg/2 ml	IV: Rapid IV bolus only, 6 mg over 1-2 sec. If no response, repeat with 12 mg. May repeat 12 mg bolus a second time. Doses should be followed by rapid NS flush.	Conversion to sinus rhythm of paroxysmal supraventricular tachycardia including Wolfe-Parkinson-White syndrome. May need larger doses in the presence of methylxantrines. Facial flushing, chest pain are common. Not effective in atrial fibrillation.

Amiodarone (Cordarone)	Tabs: 200 mg Injection: 50 mg/ml (3 ml amps)	PO: Loading dose 800-1600 mg/day in divided doses for 1-3 weeks until therapeutic response occurs. Then decrease dose as tolerated to 600-900 mg/day for 1 month and then to the maintenance dose of 400 mg/day. IV: Rapid Load: 150 mg in 100 ml D5W over 10 min. Slow Load: Then add 900 mg to 500 ml D5W. Infuse at 1 mg/min (33.3 ml/h) for 6 h. Maintenance: Then decrease rate of slow load infusion to 0.5 mg/min (16.7 ml/h). This rate may be continued up to 3 weeks, regardless of age, renal or LV function. Breakthrough Arrhythmias: May give supplemental 150 mg boluses in 100 ml D5W over 10 min.	Class III anti-arrhythmic for life-threatening recurrent ventricular arrhythmias *that do not respond to other anti-arrhythmics*. Should only be used by physicians familiar with the drug. Will increase digoxin concentrations (decrease digoxin dose by 50%). Multiple adverse side-effects, including potentially fatal pulmonary and hepatic toxicity. IV form is indicated for treatment and prophylaxis of frequently recurring ventricular fibrillation and hemodynamically unstable ventricular tachycardia in patients refractory to other treatment. *Contraindicated* in patients with hypersensitivity to any of its components and in patients in cardiogenic shock, marked sinus bradycardia, and 2nd and 3rd degree A-V block in absence of functioning pacemaker. Most common adverse effect is hypotension, which should initially be treated by *slowing the infusion*. Other adverse effects include asystole, cardiac arrest, EMD, ventricular tachycardia, cardiogenic shock, AV block, and liver function test abnormalities. Infusion must be delivered by a volumetric infusion pump utilizing an in-line filter and PVC tubing. Drug

(continued)

Anti-Arrhythmics—*(cont.)*

Drug	Supplied	Dose/Route	Remarks
			should be mixed with D5W in a glass or polyolefin bottle.
Bretylium (Bretylol)	Amps, Vials, Syringes: 50 mg/ml	**Acute ventricular arrhythmias:** 5 mg/kg undiluted IVP over 1 min; may repeat with 10 mg/kg prn if no response. **Maintenance therapy:** 5-10 mg/kg IM/IV q 6-8 h or 1-2 mg/min via continuous infusion.	Class III anti-arrhythmic. Useful in ventricular fibrillation and ventricular tachycardia, but no better than lidocaine. Second drug of choice following lidocaine for treatment of ventricular fibrillation. Hypotension may develop within first hour of therapy.
Digoxin (Lanoxin, Lanoxicaps)	Tabs: 125,250,500 µg Caps: 50,100,200 µg Elixir: 50 µg/ml Amps: 100,250 µg/ml	**Digitalizing dose** (Adults): PO: 10-15 µg/kg, with 50% of dose given as first dose, then 25% of dose given at 6-8 h intervals until adequate response is achieved or total digitalizing dose is administered. IVP: 8-12 µg/kg, with 50% of dose given as first dose, then 25% of dose given at 4-8 h intervals until adequate response is achieved or total digitalizing dose is administered. Maintenance dose should be adjusted by creatinine clearance.	Usual therapeutic serum level range (adult) 0.8-2.0 ng/ml. Higher levels may be needed in control of ventricular rate in atrial flutter or fibrillation. Only 60-85% of tablet or elixir dose is absorbed. Capsules are 90-100% absorbed. Doses should be modified when changing from one route of administration to another.
Diltiazem (Cardizem IV)	Vials: 5 mg/ml	IV: 0.25 mg/kg bolus over 2 min. If inadequate response after 15 min, give 0.35 mg/kg over 2 min; infusion at 5-15 mg/h for 24 h; then convert to PO therapy.	Calcium channel blocker for atrial fibrillation/flutter and paroxysmal supraventricular tachycardia. May cause hypotension. Vials must be refrigerated.

Esmolol (Brevibloc)	Injection (for boluses): 10 mg/ml Concentrate for IV infusion (must be diluted): 250 mg/ml	IV: Loading dose of 500 μg/kg over 1 min, followed by maintenance infusion of 50 μg/kg/min for 4 min. If no response, repeat loading dose and increase infusion to 100 μg/kg/min. Repeat procedure until the desired response is obtained or a maximum infusion of 300 μg/kg/min is reached.	Short-acting β1 selective adrenergic blocker for supraventricular tachycardia. May cause hypotension. Useful for controlling intra-operative and post-operative hypertension.
Flecainide (Tambocor)	Tabs: 50,100,150 mg	PO: Initial dose 100 mg q 12 h; usual dose 100-200 mg q 12 h. Maximum 400 mg/day.	Class IC anti-arrhythmic for documented life-threatening ventricular arrhythmias (sustained ventricular tachycardia [VT]). Secondary to proarrhythmic effect, reserve for patients who do not respond to conventional therapy. Use cautiously in patients with congestive heart failure or myocardial infarction.
Lidocaine (Xylocaine)	For direct IV injection: amps, vials, syringes: 10,20 mg/ml For preparation of IV infusion (must be diluted): amps, vials, syringes: 40,100,200 mg/ml	IV loading dose: 1-1.5 mg/kg. If no response, may repeat in 5 minutes as needed to a total of 3 mg/kg. Infusion: 1-4 mg/min.	Class IB anti-arrhythmic. Drug of choice for ventricular tachycardia, fibrillation, and premature beats. Elevates fibrillation threshold. Therapeutic plasma concentration is 1-5 μg/ml.

(continued)

Anti-Arrhythmics—*(cont.)*

Drug	Supplied	Dose/Route	Remarks
Mexiletine (Mexitil)	Caps: 150,200,250 mg	PO: 200 mg q 8 h; usual dose 200-300 mg q 8 h. Maximum dose 1200 mg/day.	Class IB anti-arrhythmic for suppression of documented life-threatening symptomatic ventricular arrhythmias, including multifocal PVCs and ventricular tachycardia.
Moricizine (Ethmozine)	Tabs: 200,250,300 mg	PO: Usual dose 200-300 mg q 8 h.	Class I anti-arrhythmic for documented life-threatening sustained VT. Secondary to proarrhythmic effects, use in patients in whom benefits outweigh risks.
Procainamide HCl (Pronestyl)	Vial: 100,500 mg/ml Tabs and Caps: 200, 375,500 mg Tabs (sustained release): 250,500,750,1000 mg	100 mg IV over 2 min; repeat 100 mg every 5 min until arrythmia is controlled or to a total of 1 g. Infusion: 0.02-0.08 mg/kg/min, or 2-6 mg/min. PO: Total daily dose of up to 50 mg/kg given in divided doses.	Class IA anti-arrhythmic. Secondary drug for ventricular arrhythmias that are not digitalis induced. Therapeutic plasma concentration is 4-8 µg/ml. Decrease dosage in renal insufficiency, CHF, and elderly. Monitor NAPA levels. Rapid IV administration may cause severe hypotension.
Propafenone (Rhythmol)	Tabs: 150,300 mg	PO: 150 mg q 8 h initially; usual dose 150-300 mg q 8 h. Maximum 900 mg/day.	Class IC anti-arrhythmic for life-threatening ventricular arrhythmias (sustained VT). Due to proarrhythmic effects, not recommended for less severe ventricular arrhythmias.

Propranolol HCl (Inderal)	Tabs: 10,20,40,60, 80,90 mg. Amp: 1 mg/ml. Extended release caps: 60,80,120,160 mg. Solution: 20 mg/5 ml, 40 mg/5 ml. Solution Concentrate: 80 mg/ml.	Parenteral: 0.5-3 mg IV slowly (<1 mg/min), may repeat initial dose after 2 min; then wait at least 4 h before additional doses. Oral: **Hypertension:** 20-40 mg PO bid initially, then gradual increments up to 640 mg/day. Usual maintenance dose: 160-480 mg/day. **Angina pectoris:** 10-20 mg PO tid or qid initially, then gradual increments q 3-7 days up to 320 mg/day until optimal response. Usual maintenance dose: 160-240 mg/day. **Cardiac arrhythmias:** 10-30 mg tid or qid. **Migraine prophylaxis:** 80 mg/day in divided doses initially, then up to 240 mg/day by gradual increments. **Pheochromocytoma** (as adjunct to α-adrenergic blocking agents): 60 mg/day in divided doses for 3 days prior to surgery, or 30 mg/day in divided doses for inoperable tumors. **Myocardial infarction:** 180-240 mg daily, bid, tid, or qid beginning 5-21 days after infarction.	Contraindicated in sinus bradycardia, cardiogenic shock, heart block greater than first degree, bronchial asthma. Non-selective β-adrenergic blocking agent.
Quinidine gluconate (Quinaglute, Duraquin)	Extended release tabs: 324 mg Vial: 80 mg/ml	IM: 600 mg, then up to 400 mg q 2 h adjusting dose by the effect of the previous dose. IV: 800 mg diluted with 40 ml D5W and administered at rate of 16 mg/min.	Class IA anti-arrhythmic. Can decrease myocardial contractility. Comparable activity to procainamide in the treatment of atrial or ventricular arrhythmias. With IV administration, monitor blood pressure during infusion. May

(continued)

Anti-Arrhythmics—*(cont.)*

Drug	Supplied	Dose/Route	Remarks
			cause increase in digoxin levels. Therapeutic plasma concentrations 2-6 µg/ml.
Quinidine sulfate (Quinidex, Cin-Quin)	Tabs: 200,300 mg Extended release tabs: 300 mg	PAC's & PVC's: 200-300 mg tid/qid. PSVT: 400-600 mg q 2-3 h until paroxysm is terminated. Conversion of Atrial Fibrillation (after controlling ventricular rate with digoxin): 200 mg q 2-3 h for 5-8 doses. Maintenance: 200-300 mg tid or qid. Sustained release forms: 300-600 mg q 8-12 h. Do not exceed 3-4 g daily in any regimen.	
Solatol (Betapace)	Tabs: 80,160,240 mg	PO: Initial 80 mg bid. Usual maintenance: 160-320 mg/day in divided doses.	Non-selective beta blocker. Owing to its arrhythmogenic potential, it is indicated *only* for suppression and prevention of documented life-threatening ventricular arrhythmias. May cause or worsen CHF. Dosage must be reduced in renal insufficiency.
Tocainide (Tonocard)	Tabs: 400,600 mg	PO: initially 400 mg q 8 h; usual maintenance dose is 1.2-1.8 g daily in 3 divided doses.	Class IB anti-arrhythmic. Electrophysiologically and hemodynamically similar to lidocaine. Therapeutic plasma concentration usually 4-10 µg/ ml. Because of risk of blood dyscrasias and pulmonary toxicity, use only in treatment of life-threatening ventricular arrhythmias.

Verapamil (Calan, Isoptin Verelan)	Amps: 2.5 mg/ml Tabs: 40,80,120 mg SR tabs: 120,180, 240 mg	IVP: 5-10 mg slow IV bolus over 2-3 min; dose may be repeated after 30 min if unsatisfactory initial response. PO: **Angina:** Initial 40-80 mg q 6-8 h. Usual maintenance: 240-480 mg daily in 3-4 divided doses. **Hypertension:** Initial 40 mg bid to 80 mg tid. Usual maximum of conventional tablets: 360 mg/day in divided doses. Sustained release tablets: Maxiumum 480 mg/day.	Calcium channel blocker *contraindicated* in severe CHF and shock. Metabolized in liver; renal excretion. Onset of action is within 1-2 min, with peak effect occurring in 10-15 min. Used in rapid conversion to sinus rhythm of paroxysmal re-entrant SVTs that incorporate the AV node as part or all of the re-entrant circuit. Also used for temporary control of rapid ventricular rate in atrial flutter or atrial fibrillation. Can cause bradycardia, hypotension, high-degree AV block and asystole, and transient ventricular ectopy.

Antibiotics—Miscellaneous

Atovaquone (Mepron)	Tabs: 250 mg	PO: 750 mg tid with food for 21 days.	Antiprotozoal for treatment of *Pneumocystis carinii pneumonia*. Requires administration with food for maximal absorption.
Chloramphenicol (Chloromycetin)	Caps: 250 mg Susp: 150 mg/5 ml Parenteral: 1 g	PO/IV: 50 mg/kg/day in divided doses q 6 h.	Adverse effects: non-dose-related irreversible bone marrow depression leading to aplastic anemia; dose-related reversible bone marrow depression (plasma concentrations of greater than 25 µg/ml); Gray syndrome; GI disturbances. Owing to toxicity, should only be used for serious infections.

(continued)

Antibiotics—Miscellaneous—*(cont.)*

Drug	Supplied	Dose/Route	Remarks
Clindamycin (Cleocin)	Caps: 75,150,300 mg Solution: 75 mg/5 ml Parenteral: 150 mg/ml	IV/IM: 600 mg q 8 h; 900 mg q 8 h for PID. PO: 150-450 mg q 6 h.	Adverse side-effects: diarrhea; pseudomembranous colitis with toxic megacolon, rare (1:7500) due to *C. difficile* toxin; rash; neutropenia; eosinophilia; Covers gram-positives (not *Neisseria* or enterococci), *C. diphtheriae*, *Actinomyces*, anaerobes, 10-15% *B. fragilis* resistant. *Clostridia* variable sensitivity.
Metronidazole (Flagyl)	Tabs: 250, 500 mg Vials: 5 mg/ml (100 ml) for IV infusion. RTU: 500 mg/100 ml	PO (Adults): **Trichomoniasis:** 250 mg tid for 7 days or 2 g in a single dose. **Amoebic dysentery:** 750 mg tid for 5-10 days. **Pseudomembranous colitis:** 250 mg qid x 7 days. IV (Adults): 500 mg q 8 h. **Anaerobic bacterial infections:** IV: 500 mg q 8 h.	For oral use in treatment of *Trichomonas vaginalis* and asymptomatic consorts, as well as amebiasis. For IV use in the treatment of intraabdominal abscess, peritonitis, septicemia, CNS infections, and lower respiratory tract infections. Effective against obligate anaerobes. Should not be used with alcohol, in pregnancy, with known hypersensitivity, or liver dysfunction. Potentiates Coumadin effects on anticoagulation.

Pentamidine (Pentam 300 NebuPent)	Parenteral: 300 mg Aerosol: 300 mg	**Pneumocystis carinii:** IM: 4 mg/kg once daily for 14 days. IV: 4 mg/kg once daily for 14 days (infused over at least 1 h). Aerosol: 300 mg every 4 weeks via the Respirgard II nebulizer.	For use in patients with *Pneumocystis carinii pneumonia* (PCP) who are unresponsive to trimethoprim/sulfamethoxazole, trypanosomiasis, and visceral leishmaniasis. Prevention of PCP by inhalation. Nephrotoxicity (25%), hypotension, hypoglycemia (5-10%), leukopenia, and thrombocytopenia can occur.
Trimethoprim/ sulfamethoxazole (Bactrim, Septra)	Tabs: 80 mg trimethoprim, 400 mg sulfamethoxazole (available as D.S.) Susp: 40 mg trimethoprim/5 ml, 200 mg sulfamethoxazole/5 ml Parenteral: trimethoprim (16 mg/ml), sulfamethoxazole (80 mg/ml)	PO (Adults): 1 double strength or 2 regular strength tabs q 12 h. IV: For *Pneumocytosis carinii*: 15-20 mg/kg/day of the trimethoprim component in 3 or 4 divided doses. For urinary tract infections or *Shigella* enteritis: 8-10 mg/kg/day in 2-4 divided doses.	For use in urinary tract infections and traveller's diarrhea, acute otitis media, adult chronic bronchitis, *Pneumocystis carinii pneumonia*, and *Stenotrophomonas maltophilia* infections. *Contraindications*: hypersensitivity to trimethroprim or sulfa drugs, megaloblastic anemia secondary to folate deficiency, and pregnancy at term and nursing mothers. Excretion is renal. Adjust dose in renal failure.
Vancomycin	Parenteral: Various. Pulvules: 125,250 mg Susp: Various	IV: 500 mg—1 g q 12 h. PO: 125 mg qid x 7 days for pseudomembranous colitis.	Can cause hypotension if given IV push in 10 min or less ("red-neck" syndrome). Should be given over 1 h IV. Desired serum peak level 35-45 μg/ml, trough 5-10 μg/ml. Can cause phlebitis, fever, rash, nausea, neutropenia,

(continued)

Antibiotics—Miscellaneous—*(cont.)*

Drug	Supplied	Dose/Route	Remarks
			eosinophilia, flushing over upper chest, anaphylaxis, ototoxicity. Increased incidence of nephrotoxicity when administered concomitantly with aminoglycosides. Little nephrotoxicity when used alone. Not appreciably absorbed from GI tract.

Antibiotics—Aminoglycosides

Drug	Supplied	Dose/Route	Remarks
Amikacin (Amikin)	Parenteral: 50,250 mg/ml	IV/IM: 15 mg/kg/day divided q 8 h or 12 h; or 5-7 mg/kg per dose.	All aminoglycosides may cause or increase neuromuscular blockade. Use with caution in patients with myasthenia gravis, Parkinsonism, botulism, with neuromuscular blocking drugs or with massive transfusion of citrated blood. Avoid concurrent use with ethacrynic acid, furosemide, or methoxyflurane. Can cause nephrotoxicity; ototoxicity usually with high-frequency loss, especially with larger total dose. Toxicity is associated with greater than 10 days of therapy, prior aminoglycosides, peak serum level >32 µg/ml, trough level >10 µg/ml. Rare eosinophilia, arthralgia; fever; skin rash.

Gentamicin (Garamycin)	Parenteral: multiple strengths	IM/IV: 3 mg/kg/day in divided doses or 5 mg/kg/day as a single dose.	Can cause nephrotoxicity, ototoxicity, fever, skin rash,neuromuscular blockade. Serum peak levels: 5-10 μg/ml; serum trough levels <2.0 μg/ml. Not usually administered parenterally because of lack of assay availability.
Kanamycin (Kantrex)	Caps: 500 mg Injection: 37.5,250,333 mg/ml	IV/IM: 15 mg/kg/day divided q 8 or 12 h. Total daily dose not to exceed 1.5 g. PO: 8-12 g daily in divided doses as an adjunct in the treatment of hepatic encephalopathy.	Adjust dose in renal insufficiency. Can cause ototoxicity, nephrotoxicity, neuromuscular blockade, skin rash, fever. Serum peak levels: 15-25 μg/ml.
Neomycin sulfate (Mycifradin, Neobiotic)	Tabs: 500 mg Liquid: 125 mg/5 ml	**Hepatic coma:** PO 4-12 g/day in divided doses. **Enteropathogenic E. coli:** PO 50 mg/kg/day in divided doses.	Can cause nausea, vomiting, diarrhea; interferes with absorption of digoxin; about 3% of an oral dose is absorbed and if a sufficient amount is absorbed, ototoxicity, nephrotoxicity, and neuromuscular blockade can result.
Streptomycin	Injection: 400,500 mg, 1,5 g	IM/IV: **Tuberculosis:** 15 mg/kg/day. **Endocarditis:** 1 g bid for 1 week followed by 500 mg bid for 1 week.	Other aminoglycosides are more effective against gram-negatives. Major indications are treatment of TB and, with penicillin, treatment of endocarditis caused by *S. viridans*. Can cause vestibular damage, rash, peripheral neuritis, anaphylaxis, renal damage, rarely blood dyscrasias, neuromuscular blockade. IM injection should be deep to avoid pain and sterile abscesses. May be used as part of a

(continued)

Antibiotics—Aminoglycosides—*(cont.)*

Drug	Supplied	Dose/Route	Remarks
			multiple drug regimen for *Mycobacterium avium.*
Tobramycin (Nebcin)	Injection: Various.	IV/IM: 3 mg/kg/day in divided doses or 5 mg/kg/day as a single dose.	Serum peak levels: 5-10 μg/ml; serum trough levels <2.0 μg/ml. More active against *Pseudomonas* sp. than gentamicin.

Antibiotics—Carbapenems (Thienamycins)

Drug	Supplied	Dose/Route	Remarks
Imipenem and Cilastatin (Primaxin)	Parenteral: 250,500 mg	0.5-1.0 g IV over 30 min q 6 h.	Highly stable against beta lactamases. Can be associated with risk of suprainfection, especially fungal, emergence of resistant *P. aeruginosa*, pseudomembranous colitis, phlebitis, hypersensitivity, rash, elevated SGOT, SGPT, alk. phos., confusion, seizures, nausea, vomiting. Do not use in a true PCN allergy. Adjust dose in renal insufficiency.

Antibiotics—Cephalosporins

Drug	Supplied	Dose/Route	Remarks
ORAL:			
Cefaclor (Ceclor) (2nd generation)	Caps: 250,500 mg Susp: 125,187,250, 375 mg/5 ml	PO: 0.25 - 0.5 g q 8 h.	Can cause serum sickness-like reactions (1-2%), joint aches, erythema multiforme, rash, purpura. Effective against ampicillin-resistant strains of *Haemophilus influenzae*.

Cefadroxil (Duricef) (1st generation)	Caps: 500 mg Susp: 125,250, 500 mg/5 ml Tabs: 1 g	PO: 1-2 g qd for cystitis; 1 g q 12 h for other indications.	Can cause GI distress, rash. Can be administered once or twice a day because of a prolonged half-life (1-2 h).
Cefixime (Suprax) (3rd generation)	Tabs: 200,400 mg Powder for suspension: 100 mg/5 ml	PO: 400 mg qd or 200 mg bid.	Similar to cefaclor in spectrum of activity.
Cefpodoxime (Vantin) (2nd generation)	Tabs: 100,200 mg Susp: 50,100 mg/5 ml	PO: 200 mg q 12 h.	Similar to cefaclor in spectrum of activity.
Cefprozil (Cefzil) (2nd generation)	Tabs: 250,500 mg Powder for suspension: 125,250 mg/5 ml	PO: 250-500 mg q 12-24 h.	Similar to cefaclor in spectrum of activity.
Cefuroxime axetil (Ceftin) (2nd generation)	Tabs: 125,250,500 mg Powder for suspension: 125 mg/5 ml	PO: 250-500 mg q 12 h.	Similar to cefaclor in spectrum of activity.
Cephalexin (Keflex) (1st generation)	Caps: 250,500 mg Susp: 125,250 mg/5 ml; 100 mg/1 ml Tabs: 250,500 mg, 1 g	PO: 0.25 - 0.5 g q 6 h.	Can cause GI distress, skin rash, eosinophilia, leukopenia, and elevated SGOT. Comparable spectrum of activity and duration of action to that of cephradine.
Cephradine (Velosef, Anspor) (1st generation)	Caps: 250,500 mg Susp: 125,250 mg/5 ml	PO: 0.25 - 0.5 g q 6 h.	Delayed absorption when given with food. Comparable spectrum of activity and duration of action to that of cephalexin.

(continued)

Antibiotics—Cephalosporins—*(cont.)*

Drug	Supplied	Dose/Route	Remarks
ORAL—*(cont.)*			
Loracarbef (Lorabid) (2nd generation)	Caps: 200 mg Susp: 100 mg/5 ml	PO: 200-400 mg q 12 h.	Similar to cefaclor in spectrum of activity.
PARENTERAL:			
Cefamandole (Mandol) (2nd generation)	Injection: multiple strengths	IM/IV: 0.5-1.0 g q 6-8 h.	Can cause pain on IM injection, phlebitis, vasodilation, hypersensitivity, rash, urticaria, eosinophilia, fever, weakly + Coombs, neutropenia, thrombocytopenia, mild elevation of BUN/creatinine, SGOT, SGPT, and alk. phos. Rare disulfiram-like reactions after alcohol. Effective against ampicillin-resistant species of *Haemophilus influenzae*.
Cefazolin (Ancef, Kefzol) (1st generation)	Injection: multiple strengths	IM/IV: 0.5-1.0 g q 8 h.	Adverse side-effects: rash, elevated SGOT and alk. phos.; phlebitis, Coombs +, abnormal coagulation tests in uremia. Can be administered q 8 h because of an extended half-life. Similar spectrum of activity to cephalothin and cephapirin.
Cefoperazone (Cefobid) (3rd generation)	Injection: 1,2 g	IM/IV: 2-4 g q 8-12 h.	In severe infections should be administered q 6 h. Very high biliary concentrations can be obtained in unobstructed biliary disease. Can

			cause hypoprothrombinemia. Minimal anaerobic activity. Biliary excretion.
Cefotaxime (Claforan) (3rd generation)	Injection: 1,2 g	IM/IV: 1-2 g q 6-8 h.	Can be administered q 8 h in mild infections. Active metabolite has antibacterial activity similar to a 1st-generation cephalosporin. Good CNS penetration.
Cefotetan (Cefotan) (2nd generation)	Injection: 1,2 g	IM/IV: 1-2 g q 12 h.	Comparable spectrum of activity to that of cefoxitin at less frequent dosing interval.
Cefoxitin (Mefoxin) (2nd generation)	Injection: 1,2 g	IM/IV: 1-2 g q 6-8 h.	Adequate activity against anaerobic organisms.
Ceftazidime (Fortaz) (3rd generation)	Injection: multiple strengths	IM/IV: 1-2 g q 8 h.	Best activity of all 3rd-generation cephalosporins against *P. aeruginosa*.
Ceftizoxime (Cefizox) (3rd generation)	Injection: 1,2 g	IM/IV: 1-2 g q 8-12 h.	Similar in spectrum of activity to cefotaxime. Poor CNS penetration.
Ceftriaxone (Rocephin) (3rd generation)	Injection: multiple strengths	IM/IV: 1-2 g once or twice a day.	Extended half-life (5-10 h) allows for BID or qd dosing. Biliary excretion (40%).

(continued)

Antibiotics—Cephalosporins—*(cont.)*

Drug	Supplied	Dose/Route	Remarks
PARENTERAL—*(cont.)*			
Cefuroxime (Zinacef) (2nd generation)	Injection: 750 mg, 1.5 g	IM/IV: 0.75-1.5 g q 8 h.	Minimal anaerobic activity. Good CNS penetration. Drug of choice for prophylaxis in cardiac surgery patients.
Cephalothin (Keflin) (1st generation)	Injection: multiple strengths	IM/IV: 0.5-1.0 g q 4-6 h.	Can cause phlebitis, rash, fever, eosinophilia, elevated SGOT, neutropenia, anaphylactoid reaction, convulsions when given in high doses in renal failure, Coombs +, thrombocytopenia, nephrotoxicity, false + "clinitest", pain on IM injection. At 300 mg/kg/day, it may cause a defect in platelet function and coagulation with delayed fibrinogenfibrin polymerization. Similar spectrum of activity to cefazolin and cephapirin, but must be administered q 6 h.
Cephapirin (Cefadyl) (1st generation)	Injection: multiple strengths	IM/IV: 0.5-1.0 g q 4-6 h.	Can cause phlebitis, rash, eosinophilia, fever, pain on IM injection, elevated SGOT, neutropenia, anemia, Coombs +, elevated BUN in patients > 50. Similar spectrum of activity and duration of action to that of cephalothin and cefazolin, but must be administered q 6 h.

Antibiotics—Macrolides

Azithromycin (Zithromax)	Caps: 250 mg	500 mg as a single dose on the first day, followed by 250 mg qd on days 2 through 5.	Administer at least 1 h before or 2 h after meals. Increased anaerobic and gram-negative activity compared with erythromycin. Longer half-life, allowing for qd dosing.
Clarithromycin (Biaxin Film Tabs)	Tabs: 250,500 mg Susp: 125,250 mg/5 ml.	250-500 mg q 12 h.	Dosage adjustment in renal failure. Increased activity against *S. aureus streptococci*, *Legionella*, *Moraxella catarrhalis* and *Chlamydia trachomatis* than erythromycin. Also increased anaerobic activity. Active against mycobacterium avium complex. Longer half-life, allowing for bid dosing. Can take without regards to meals.
Erythromycin base (E-mycin, Ilotycin)	Caps: 125,250 mg Tabs: 250,333,500 mg	PO: 250 mg q 6 h *or* 333 mg q 8 h. **Prophylaxis of streptococcal infections:** Bacterial endocarditis (prior to dental procedure): 1 g 1 h before the procedure and 500 mg 6 h later. **Rheumatic heart disease:** 250 mg bid. **Syphilis:** 500 mg qid for 15 days. **Gonorrhea:** 500 mg qid for 7 days. **Chlamydia/mycoplasma:** 500 mg qid for 7 days.	Administer on an empty stomach.

(continued)

Antibiotics—Macrolides—*(cont.)*

Drug	Supplied	Dose/Route	Remarks
Erythromycin estolate (Ilosone)	Caps: 250 mg Susp: 125 mg/5 ml, 250 mg/5 ml Tabs: 500 mg	PO: 250 mg q 6 h.	May cause reversible cholestatic hepatitis, and is *contraindicated* in patients with hepatic dysfunction or pre-existing liver disease.
Erythromycin ethylsuccinate (EES)	Susp: 100 mg/2.5 ml, 200,400 mg/5 ml Tabs: 400 mg Chewable tabs: 200 mg	PO: 400 mg q 6 h.	Erythromycin ethylsuccinate (400 mg) is equivalent to erythromycin base, stearate, or estolate (250 mg). Less GI upset.
Erythromycin gluceptate (Ilotycin)	Parenteral: 250,500, 1000 mg	IV: 15-20 mg kg daily in 4 divided doses. **Legionnaires' disease:** 1-4 g in divided doses, alone or in conjunction with rifampin.	
Erythromycin lactobionate (Erythrocin, Lactobionate-IV)	Parenteral: 500, 1000 mg	IV: 15-20 mg/kg daily in 4 divided doses	Not administered IVP because of local irritative properties.
Erythromycin stearate (Erythrocin)	Tabs: 250,500 mg	PO: 250 mg q 6 h.	

Antibiotics—Monobactams

Drug	Supplied	Dose/Route	Remarks
Aztreonam (Azactam)	Parenteral: 500 mg, 1 g, 2 g	IV: 1.0 - 2.0 g q 8 h.	Highly stable against beta lactamases. Covers gram-negatives. Highly active against

			Neisseria, *H. influenzae*, *Enterobacteriaceae*; moderate against *P. aeruginosa*. Not active against acinetobacter, *P. maltophilia*, *P. capacia*, *Staph.*, *Strep.*, anaerobes. Can cause phlebitis, hypersensitivity, rash, mild elevation of SGOT in 1/3 of patients. Should not be used for surgical prophylaxis or treatment of suspected or documented gram-positive and anaerobic infections.

Antibiotics—Penicillins

AMINOPENICILLINS:

Amoxicillin (Amoxil, Larotid)	Caps: 250,500 mg Susp: 50,125,250 mg/ 5 ml Chewable tabs: 125,250 mg	PO: 250-500 mg q 8 h.	May be given with meals. Single doses of 3 g have been effective for initial treatment of acute, uncomplicated urinary tract infections in non-pregnant women. Drug of choice for prevention of bacterial endocarditis for dental, oral, or upper respiratory procedures.
Amoxicillin and clavulanic acid (Augmentin)	Susp: 125,250 mg/5 ml Chewable tabs: 125,250 mg Tabs: 250,500 mg	PO: 250-500 mg q 8 h.	May be given with meals. Clavulanic acid has very weak antibacterial activity when used alone. Use should be reserved for infections caused by beta-lactamase-producing bacteria. Two 250 mg tabs have twice the clavulanic acid of one 500 mg tab.

(continued)

Antibiotics—Penicillins—*(cont.)*

Drug	Supplied	Dose/Route	Remarks
Ampicillin (Omnipen, Polycillin)	Caps: 250,500 mg Susp: 100,125,250, 500 mg/5 ml Parenteral: multiple strengths	PO: 250-500 mg q 6 h.	May be administered with meals, but maximum absorption is obtained if given 1 h before or 2 h after meals.
Ampicillin/ sulbactam (Unasyn)	Injection: 1.5 g (1 g ampicillin, 0.5 g sulbactum); 3.0 g (2 g ampicillin, 1 g sulbactum)	IV: 1.5-3 g q 6 h.	Has good gram-positive and gram-negative activity. Has anaerobic activity. Not effective against pseudomonas. Stable against beta-lactamase-producing strains. Similar in spectrum of activity to cefoxitin. Includes enterococcus.
EXTENDED-SPECTRUM PENICILLINS:			
Carbenicillin disodium (Geopen)	Parenteral: multiple strengths	IV/IM: 5 g q 4 h.	May cause hypokalemia and functional thrombocytopenia with large doses in patients with severe renal impairment. One g of carbenicillin has 4.7-6.5 mEq of sodium. Dosage adjustment in renal failure is necessary.
Carbenicillin indanyl-sodium (Geocillin)	Tabs: 382 mg	PO: 382-764 mg 4 times daily.	Used only for the treatment of acute or chronic infections of upper and lower urinary tract.
Mezlocillin (Mezlin)	Parenteral: multiple strengths	IV/IM: 3-4 g q 4-6 h.	May cause hypokalemia and functional thrombocytopenia with large doses in patients

			with severe renal impairment. One g of mezlocillin has 1.75-1.85 mEq of sodium. Dosage adjustment in renal failure is necessary.
Piperacillin (Pipracil)	Parenteral: multiple strengths	IV/IM: 3-4 g q 4-6 h.	May cause hypokalemia and functional thrombocytopenia with large doses in patients with severe renal impairment. One g of piperacillin has 1.85 mEq of sodium. Dosage adjustment in renal failure is necessary.
Pipericillin Tazobactam (Zosyn)	Parenteral: multiple strengths: 2 g pipericillin/ 0.25 g tazobactam; 3 g pipericillin/ 0.375 g tazobactam; 4 g pipericillin/ 0.5 g tazobactam	IV: 3.375 g q 6 h.	Dosage adjustment in renal failure is necessary. Use in soft-tissue, intra-abdominal, or mixed infections. May cause hypokalemia and functional thrombocytopenia with large doses in patients with renal impairment.
Ticarcillin (Ticar)	Parenteral: multiple strengths	IV/IM: 3 g q 4 h.	May cause hypokalemia and functional thrombocytopenia with large doses in patients with severe renal impairment. One g of ticarcillin has 5.2-6.5 mEq of sodium. Dosage adjustment in renal failure is necessary.
Ticarcillin and clavulanic acid (Timentin)	Parenteral: 3 g ticarcillin, 100 g clavulanic acid	IV: 3 g q 4 h.	Dosage adjustment in renal failure is necessary. One g has 4.75 mEq of sodium.

(continued)

Drug	Supplied	Dose/Route	Remarks
NATURAL PENNICILLINS:			
Penicillin G benzathine (Bicillin, Bicillin L-A)	Parenteral: 300,000 units/ml, 600,000 units/ml	**Staphylococcal and Streptococcal infections:** IM: 1.2 mu as single dose. **Early syphilis** (primary & secondary): IM: 2.4 mu as a single dose. **Syphilis** (> 1 year's duration): IM: 2.4 mu once a week for 3 consecutive weeks. **Neurosyphilis:** IM: 2.4 mu once a week for 3 consecutive weeks. **Rheumatic fever prophylaxis:** IM: 1.2 mu once every 4 weeks, *or* 600,000 units once every 2 weeks.	IM administration only. IM penicillin G benzathine results in serum concentrations of penicillin G that are more prolonged but lower than those achieved with an equivalent IM dose of penicillin G procaine or pencillin G potassium or sodium. Used *only* in mild to moderate infections caused by organisms susceptible to *low* concentrations of pencillin G, for prophylaxis of infections, or as follow-up therapy to pencillin G potassium or sodium. Pencillin G potassium or sodium should be used when high concentrations of pencillin G are required.
Penicillin G potassium, **Penicillin G sodium**	Solution: 400,000 U/5 ml Tabs: 200,000 U 250,000 U, 400,000 U, 500,000 U, 800,000 U Parenteral: multiple strengths	**Staphylococcal and Streptococcal infections:** PO: 200,000-500,000 U q 6-8 h for 10 days. IV: 1-2 mu q 4 h. ***Neisseria meningitidis* infections:** IV: 1-2 mu q 2 h or 20-30 mu daily as a continuous infusion. ***Clostridium* infections:** IV: 20 mu daily in divided doses.	Susceptible to acid hydrolysis; only 15-30% of an oral dose is absorbed. Food will decrease the rate and extent of oral absorption. Should *not* be used for initial treatment of severe infections. Achieves rapid and high concentrations of pencillin G in the treatment of severe infections caused by organisms susceptible to pencillin G following IM or IV

		Neurosyphilis: IV: 2-4 mu q 4 h for 10 days, followed by benzathine penicillin 2.4 mu IM once weekly for 3 wks. **Bacterial endocarditis prophylaxis:** IV/IM: 2 mu 30 min prior to the procedure, followed by 1-2 mu IM or IV 6-8 h later. Gentamicin should also be administered 30 min prior to the procedure and again 6-8 h later in patients with prosthetic heart valves or a history of endocarditis.	administration. Dosage modification in renal failure is necessary.
Penicillin G procaine (Wycillin)	Parenteral: 300,000 units/ml, 500,000 units/ml, 600,000 units/ml	**Staphylococcal and Streptococcal infections:** IM: 600,000 units - 1.2 mu qd for 10 days. **Uncomplicated gonorrhea:** IM: 2.4 mu in each buttock as a single dose with 1 g of oral probenecid.	IM administration only. Serum concentrations are more prolonged but lower than those achieved with an equivalent IM dose of penicillin G potassium or sodium.
Penicillin V, Pencillin V potassium	Susp: 125,250 mg/5 ml Tabs: 125 mg (PEN VK), 250, 500 mg Film-coated tabs: 250, 500 mg (PEN VK)	**Staphylococcal and Streptococcal infections:** PO: 125-250 mg q 6-8 h for 10 days or 500 mg q 12 h for 10 days. **Prophylaxis of recurrent rheumatic fever:** PO: 125-250 mg twice daily. **Prophylaxis of bacterial endocarditis:** Dental procedures: 2 g 1 h prior to procedure and 1 g 6 h later.	Penicillin V is more resistant to acid-catalyzed inactivation than penicillin G. Administer 1 h before or 2 h after meals. 250 mg of penicillin V is equivalent to 400,000 units of the drug.

(continued)

Antibiotics—Penicillins—*(cont.)*

Drug	Supplied	Dose/Route	Remarks
		Prophylaxis of Pneumococcal infections: PO: 125 mg twice daily (age <5 years); 250 mg twice daily (age >5 years).	
PENICILLINASE–RESISTANT PENICILLINS:			
Cloxacillin	Caps: 250,500 mg Solution: 125 mg/5 ml	PO: 250-500 mg q 6 h.	Administered 1 h before or 2 h after meals.
Dicloxacillin	Caps: 125,250,500 mg Susp: 62.5 mg/5 ml	PO: 125-500 mg q 6 h.	Administered 1 h before or 2 h after meals.
Methicillin	Injection: multiple strengths	IM/IV: 1 g q 4-6 h	Acute interstitial nephritis is reported more frequently than with any other penicillinase-resistant penicillin. Dosage reduction in renal failure is recommended.
Nafcillin	Caps: 250 mg Tabs: 500 mg Injection: multiple strengths	PO: 250-500 mg q 4-6 h. IM: 500 mg q 4-6 h. IV: 500 mg - 1 g q 4 h. **Endocarditis/osteomyelitis:** 1-2 g IV q 4 h.	Orally at least 1 h before or 2 h after meals. Used primarily for *S. aureus* (not methicillin-resistant).
Oxacillin	Caps: 250,500 mg Solution: 250 mg/5 ml Injection: multiple strengths	PO: 500 mg - 1 g q 4-6 h. IM/IV: 250-500 mg q 4-6 h. **Severe infection:** 1 g q 4-6 h.	Adverse hepatic effects are reported more frequently than with any other pencillinase-resistant penicillin. Orally at least 1 h before or 2 h after meals.

Antibiotics—Quinolones

Ciprofloxacin (Cipro)	Tabs: 250,500,750 mg Inj: 200,400 mg	**UTI**: 250-500 mg q 12 h. **Other**: 500-750 mg q 12 h.	Give with or without meals. Avoid Mg/Al antacids and iron preparations 2 h before or after administration. Dose reduction in renal failure.
Enoxacin (Penetrex)	Tabs: 400 mg	PO: 400 mg bid.	Give 1 h before or 2 h after meals.
Lomefloxacin (Maxaquin)	Tabs: 400 mg	PO: 400 mg qd.	Give with or without meals.
Norfloxacin (Noroxin)	Tabs: 400 mg	**Complicated UTI**: 400 mg bid x 10-21 days. **Uncomplicated UTI**: 400 mg bid x 7-10 days.	Give 1 h before or 2 h after meals. Treatment of UTI only. Dose reduction in renal failure. Avoid magnesium/aluminum antacids and iron preparations 2 h before or after administration.
Ofloxacin (Floxin)	Tabs: 200,300,400 mg Inj: 200,400 mg	PO: 200-400 mg q 12 h IV: 200-400 mg bid.	Do not take with food. Avoid Mg/Al antacids and iron preparations 2 h before or after administration. Dose reduction in renal failure.

Antibiotics—Tetracyclines

Demeclocycline (Declomycin)	Caps: 150 mg Tabs: 150,300 mg	PO: 600 mg in 2 or 4 divided doses. SIADH: 600 mg in 3-4 divided doses.	Administer 1 h before or 2 h after meals. Adverse reactions: GI distress, skin rash, deposition in teeth, hepatotoxicity, phototoxicity (17-35%), benign elevated CSF pressure, anaphylaxis, vasopressin-resistant

(continued)

Antibiotics—Tetracyclines—*(cont.)*

Drug	Supplied	Dose/Route	Remarks
			diabetes insipidus (almost 100% at doses of 1200 mg/day). May be useful in "inappropriate" anti-diuretic hormone secretion (SIADH). Covers gram-positives and gram-negatives, *Mycoplasma pneumoniae*, and *Chlamydia*. Tetracycline of choice in patients with impaired renal function.
Doxycycline (Vibramycin, Doxycaps, Vivox, Doxy-100 or Doxy-200	Susp: 50 mg/5 ml Caps: 50,100 mg Tabs: 50,100 mg Parenteral: 100,200 mg	PO/IV: 0.1 g q 12 h on 1st day, then 0.1-0.2 g/day. 200 mg initially, then 100 mg q 2 h for both PO/IV.	Covers gram-positives and gram-negatives, *Mycoplasma pneumoniae*, *Chlamydia*, *Bacteroides*, and *Rickettsiae*. As with other tetracyclines, avoid administration with antacids and other drugs containing aluminum, calcium, iron, and magnesium.
Minocycline (Minocin)	Caps: 50,100 mg Susp: 50 mg Tabs: 50,100 mg Parenteral: 100 mg	PO/IV: 200 mg initially, followed by 100 mg q 12 h.	Covers gram-positives and gram-negatives, some acinetobacter, *Chlamydia*. Vestibular symptoms occur more often than with other tetracyclines (30-90%).

Anticoagulants and Thrombolytics, Coagulants, Antiplatelet and Antifibrinolytic Agents

Abciximab (Reopro)	Injection: 2 mg/ml, 5 ml vial	IV: Bolus of 0.25 mg/kg 10-60 min before start of PTCA, followed by continuous IV infusion of 10 µg/min for 12 h.	Monoclonal antibody antiplatelet agent used as adjunct to PTCA for prevention of acute cardiac ischemic complications in patients at high risk for abrupt closure of the treated

			coronary vessel. *Contraindicated* in active internal bleeding, recent history of GI or GU bleeding or CVA, thrombocytopenia, recent trauma or major surgery, severe HTN, use of IV dextran before or during PTCA, or use of oral anticoagulants within 7 days. Use with caution in patients >65 y.o., patients < 75 kg, those with history of prior GI disease, or patients receiving thrombolytics. May cause anaphylaxis. Most common adverse effects include bleeding, thrombocytopenia, hypotension, bradycardia, nausea/vomiting.
Alteplase (Activase)	Powder for injection: 20 mg (11.6 million IU/vial) 50 mg (29 million IU/vial) 100 mg (58 million IU/vial)	IV: **Myocardial infarction**: 60 mg 1st hour, 20 mg 2nd hour, 20 mg 3rd hour as an infusion; Adults <65 kg: 0.75 mg/kg 1st hour, then 0.25 mg/kg/hour x 2 hr. **Pulmonary embolism**: 100 mg over 2 h.	A tissue plasminogen activator produced by recombinant DNA. *Contraindicated* in patients with active internal bleeding, CVA, intracranial neoplasm, aneurysm, or recent intracranial or intraspinal surgery or trauma.

(continued)

Anticoagulants and Thrombolytics—*(cont.)*

Drug	Supplied	Dose/Route	Remarks
Aminocaproic acid (Amicar)	Tabs: 500 mg Syrup: 250 mg/ml Vials: 250 mg/ml	**ADULTS:** initially 5 g po or slow IVP, then after 1 h give 1 to 1.25 g/h for 8 h or until bleeding is controlled, up to 30 g/24 h. Rapid IV infusion may induce hypotension, bradycardia, or arrhythmias. Give initial IV dose of 4-5 g in 250 ml NS, LR or D5W over 1 h. Subsequent hourly doses of 1 g in 50 ml diluent over 1 h. In **primary hyperfibrinolysis,** platelet count is normal, precipitation does not occur when protamine is added to citrated blood, and the time required for lysis of a euglobin clot is less than normal, whereas in **disseminated intravascular coagulation (DIC)** the platelet count is usually decreased, precipitation occurs in the protamine test, and euglobin test is normal. Aminocaproic acid can be given to patients with DIC only if heparin is given concomitantly.	Antifibrinolytic. For treatment of excessive bleeding caused by systemic hyperfibrinolysis and urinary fibrinolysis. *Contraindicated* with evidence of active intravascular clotting process.

Anistreplase [anisoylated plasminogen streptokinase activator complex; APSAC] (Eminase)	Powder for injection: 30 units	IV: 30 units over 2-5 min.	Used for management of acute myocardial infarction. Use with caution after recent major surgery, internal bleeding, trauma, endocarditis and pericarditis, HTN, hemorrhagic ophthalmic conditions, and oral anticoagulant therapy. May not be as effective if given >5 days after prior anistreplase or streptokinase therapy because of possible resistance due to antistreptokinase antibody—antibody may also increase risk of allergic reaction.
Dalteparin sodium (Fragmin)	Injection: 2500 units anti-factor Xa/0.2 ml (deep SQ injection only)	**Prophylaxis of DVT** in patients undergoing abdominal surgery who are at high risk for thromboembolic complications: 2500 IU SQ qd, starting 1-2 h prior to surgery, then qd x 5-10 days postop.	A low-molecular-weight heparin. Use with caution in patients with increased risk of hemorrhage, renal and hepatic impairment, and history of heparin-induced thrombocytopenia.
Dextran 40 (LMD, Gentran 40, Rheomacrodex)	10% solution of dextran 40 in NS or D5W	**Prophylaxis of venous thrombus and pulmonary embolism:** 500-1000 ml continuous infusion (~ 10 ml/kg) on day of surgery then 500 ml (~5 ml/kg)/day x 2-3 days. 500 ml may be given every 2-3 days during period of risk, up to 2 weeks. **Shock:** Maximum dose of 20 ml/kg for first 24 h, then maximum of 10 ml/kg/day up to 5 days.	Plasma expander, retards rouleau formation and RBC sludging. Can cause severe allergic reactions; carefully monitor renal and cardiac function. May interfere with tests for blood cross-matching.

(continued)

Anticoagulants and Thrombolytics—*(cont.)*

Drug	Supplied	Dose/Route	Remarks
Dipyridamole (Persantine, Persantine IV)	Tabs: 25,50,75 mg Injection: 10 mg	PO: 75-100 mg qid. IV: 0.142 mg/kg/min over 4 min.	Adjunct to Coumadin anticoagulants in the prevention of post-operative thromboembolic complications of cardiac valve replacement. Potential use with or without aspirin in the prevention of myocardial reinfarction. IV dipyridamole as an alternative to exercise in thallium myocardial perfusion imaging for the evaluation of coronary artery disease in patients who cannot exercise adequately.
Enoxaparin sodium (Lovenox)	Injection: 30 mg/0.3 ml (SQ injection only)	**Prophylaxis of post-op DVT in patients undergoing hip replacement surgery:** 30 mg SQ bid (1st dose as soon as possible after surgery, but not more than 24 h post-op). Continue throughout post-op period until risk of DVT is diminished. Average duration 7-10 days.	A low-molecular-weight heparin. Has greater bioavailability, longer half-life, and less effect on thrombin than unfractionated heparin. Use with caution in patients with increased risk of hemorrhage, renal impairment, and history of heparin-induced thrombocytopenia.
Heparin sodium (Panheparin)	Parenteral: Available in a number of dosage strengths and dosage forms. *Be certain to check concentrations before administration*!	For venous thrombosis, atrial fibrillation, pulmonary embolism, DIC (controversial), prevention of cerebral thrombosis in evolving stroke, adjunctive treatment in coronary occlusion with acute MI, and in peripheral arterial embolism: 1. Continuous IV infusion: 5000 to 10,000 units	Regulate dosage by frequent testing of PTT. Aim for PTT 1.5 to 2 times the control value. Use with caution in subacute bacterial endocarditis (SBE), dissecting aneurysm, severe hypertension, hemophilia, thrombocytopenia, diverticulitis, ulcerative colitis, recent surgery, peptic ulcer disease,

		IVP bolus, followed by 1000-2000 units/h continuous infusion. 2. Intermittent IV injection: 10,000 units IV bolus, then 5000-10,000 units IV bolus q 4-6 h. 3. Intermittent SC injection: 5000 units IV bolus, then 8000-10,000 units SC q 8 h. For prevention of post-op deep venous thrombosis (DVT) and pulmonary embolism: 5000 units SC 2 h before surgery, followed by 5000 units SC q 8-12 h for 7 days or until patient is fully ambulatory, whichever is longer. **Treatment of overdosage:** give 1.0-1.5 mg of 1% protamine sulfate by slow IV infusion for every 100 units of heparin given in previous 4 h to be neutralized. Maximum dose 50 mg in any 10 min period.	severe hepatic or renal disease. Low-dose prophylaxis is usually ineffective in reducing incidence of thrombosis after orthopedic surgery.
Phytonadione (Vitamin K, Aquamephyton, Mephyton [oral], Konakion)	Tabs: 5 mg Parenteral: 2 mg/ml, 10 mg/ml Konakion (IM use only): 2 mg/ml, 10 mg/ml	**Treatment of oral anticoagulant-induced hypoprothrombinemia:** 2.5-10 mg up to 25 mg (rarely, up to 50 mg) PO/SQ/IM/IV initially. Redose in 6-8 h (12-48 h after PO administration) if patient has not been shortened satisfactorily. **Hypoprothrombinemia due to other causes in Adults:** 2.5-25 mg (rarely, up to 50 mg); route of administration depends on severity of condition and response obtained.	Will not antagonize anticoagulant effect of heparin. Keep dosage as low as possible so that refractoriness to further anticoagulant therapy is minimized and the patient is not decreased below the effective anticoagulant level. Give IM/SQ when possible to avoid possible severe adverse reactions associated with IV administration. **Maximum IV rate is 1 mg/min.** Use with caution in hepatic impairment.

(continued)

Anticoagulants and Thrombolytics—*(cont.)*

Drug	Supplied	Dose/Route	Remarks
Protamine sulfate	Amp: 10 mg/ml	**Heparin antidote:** 1-1.5 mg of 1% protamine sulfate solution for every 100 units heparin given in previous 4 h by IV infusion. Maximum dose 50 mg over 10 min period.	IV rate not to exceed 5 mg/min. *Monitor blood pressure continuously during administration.*
Streptokinase (Streptase, Kabikinase)	Vials: 250,000, 600,000, 750,000 and 1,500,000 IU/vial	**Pulmonary embolism, deep vein thrombosis, arterial thrombosis or embolism:** initially 250,000 IU IV infusion over 30 min, followed by 100,000 IU/h IV continuous infusion for 24-72 h. **Occluded arteriovenous cannulae:** Infuse 250,000 units in 2 ml solution into each occluded limb of cannula over 25-35 min, clamp x 2 h, then aspirate and flush with NS. Avoid in patients with recent streptococcal infections or recent administration of streptokinase secondary to antibody formation. To prevent recurrent thrombosis post-streptokinase treatment, administer heparin by IV infusion and follow with oral anticoagulant therapy. Special caution with: (1) recent surgical or obstetrical procedure (past 10 days), biopsies, or GI bleeding; (2) recent trauma or CPR; (3) severe hypertension; (4) suspected left heart thrombus; (5) subacute	**Contraindications**: recent (within past 2 months) cerebrovascular accident (CVA) or intracranial or intraspinal surgery, active internal bleeding, intracranial neoplasm. Pre-treatment monitoring: thrombin time, activated partial thromboplastin time, prothrombin time, hematocrit, platelet count; TT and APTT should be twice normal control values before starting streptokinase. Concomitant use of heparin or oral anticoagulants with IV streptokinase not generally recommended.

		bacterial endocarditis [SBE]; (6) hepatic or renal failure related coagulopathies; (7) pregnancy; (8) cerebrovascular disease; (9) diabetes retinopathy; (10) allergic reaction to streptokinase; (11) septic thrombophlebitis.	
Ticlopidine (Ticlid)	Tab: 250 mg	PO: 250 mg bid with food.	Used to reduce the risk of thrombotic stroke. Neutropenia/agranulocytosia may be life-threatening; therefore, use only in patients intolerant of aspirin therapy.
Urokinase (Abbokinase)	Vials: 250,000 IU/vial for IV only	**Pulmonary embolism:** 4400 IU/kg by IV infusion over 10 min initially, then 4400 IU/kg/h for 12 h. **Lysis of coronary artery thrombi:** 6000 IU/min for up to 2 h into thrombosed artery (after 2500-10,000 units IV heparin).	**Contraindications:** 1. Recent (within past 2 months) CVA or intracranial or intraspinal surgery. 2. Active internal bleeding. 3. Intracranial neoplasm (see Streptokinase for cautions).
Warfarin sodium (Coumadin, Panwarfin)	Tabs: 1, 2, 2.5, 5, 7.5, 10 mg	Initially 10 mg PO qd for 1-3 days, then 2-10 mg PO qd or qod. **Control of overcoumadinization:** 1. Discontinuation of Coumadin (slow control, days); 2. 2-5 mg vitamin K, PO, SC, or slow IV (control over 4-8 h); 3. 250-500 ml fresh frozen plasma (immediate effect). **Drug interactions:** *Decrease INR*: antacids,	Individualize dosage to maintain INR (international normalized ratio) between 2-3 for DVT/PE/MI and 3-4.5 for mechanical heart valve and cardiogenic embolus. INR should be monitored daily during initiation of therapy, then every 1-4 weeks thereafter.

(continued)

Anticoagulants and Thrombolytics—*(cont.)*

Drug	Supplied	Dose/Route	Remarks
		adrenocorticoteroids, steroids, antihistamines, barbiturates, carbamazepine, chlordiazepoxide, cholestogramine, ethclorvynol, estrogens, glutethidimide, griseofulvin, haloperidol, noreprobamate, oral contraceptives, paraldehyde, phenytoin, primidone, rifampin, vitamins C and K. *Increase INR*: allopurinol, aminosalicylic acid, anabolic steroids, antibiotics, bromelaine, chloramphenicol, chymotryprin, cimetidine, cinchophen, clofibrate, dextran, dextrothyroxine, diazoxide, disulfiram, ethacrynic acid, glucagon, indomethacin, MAO inhibitors, methyldopa, metronidazole, narcotics, phenytoin, quinidine, salicylates, sulfas, trimethoprim-sulfamethoxazole. *Increased anticonvulsant blood levels*: phenobarbital, phenytoin. *Increased hypoglycemic effect*: chlorpropamide, tolbutamide.	

Anti-Convulsants

Carbamazepine (Tegretol)	Tabs: 200 mg Chewable tabs: 100 mg Susp: 100 mg/5 ml	**ADULTS:** Oral: **Trigeminal neuralgia:** 100 mg PO bid; increase dose by 100 mg q 12 h (maximum: 1.2 g/24 h); once control of pain is achieved, dose may be reduced to 400-800 mg/day. **Seizures:** 200 mg PO bid; increase dose by 200 mg/day (maximum 2.4 g per 24 h); for high doses, administer in 3-4 divided doses to reduce side-effects. **CHILDREN:** Oral: [< 6 years old]: 5 mg/kg/day; increase dose by 10 mg/kg/day and 20 mg/kg/day every 5-7 days; [6-12 years old]: 100 mg PO bid; increase dose by 100 mg/day (maximum 1 g/24 h); [13-15 years old]: same as adult except maximum dose 1 g/day; [>15 years old]: same as adult except maximum dose 1.2 g/day.	Use in partial seizures with complex symptomatology (psychomotor or temporal lobe seizures), generalized tonic-clonic (grand mal) seizures, mixed seizure patterns, trigeminal neuralgia, and for control of pain and/or seizures in a variety of conditions. Adverse reactions include cardiovascular effects, GU and GI tract disturbances, and CNS disturbances. Administer with caution in patients with cardiovascular problems and patients with liver or renal problems. Carbamazepine may increase intraocular pressure. *Contraindications* include history of previous bone marrow depression and/or hypersensitivity to carbamazepine or tricyclic antidepressant agents. Carbamazepine may alter the metabolism of many drugs. Gradual tapering of the drug is necessary to avoid seizures. **Therapeutic concentration:** 3-14 μg/ml.

(continued)

Anti-Convulsants—*(cont.)*

Drug	Supplied	Dose/Route	Remarks
Clonazepam (Clonopin)	Tabs: 0.5,1,2 mg	**ADULTS:** Oral: 1.5 mg/day (3 divided doses); increase dose 0.5-1 mg q 3 days (maximum 20 mg per 24 h). **CHILDREN:** Oral: 0.05 mg/kg/day (2-3 divided doses); increase dose 0.5 mg q 3 days (maximum 0.2 mg/kg/24 h).	Use in Lennox-Gastant syndrome and other types of absence (petit mal) seizures. *Contraindications* include hypersensitivity to benzodiazepines, patients with liver disease and acute angle-closure glaucoma. Adverse reactions include CNS depression and behavioral disturbances in children. Doses should be tapered slowly to avoid seizures or withdrawal reactions. **Therapeutic concentration:** 20-80 μg/μλ.
Ethosuximide (Zarontin)	Caps: 250 mg Oral solution: 250 mg/5 ml	**ADULTS AND CHILDREN:** Oral: 3-6 years old: 250 mg PO qd; >6 years old: 500 mg PO daily (2 divided doses); increase dose 250 mg q 4-7 days. Usual dose 20 mg/kg/day. Maximum dose: 1.5 g/24 h; higher given under close supervision.	Use in absence (petit mal) seizures. Adverse reactions include GI tract disturbances and CNS disturbances. *Contraindications* include hypersensitivity to succinimides. Doses should be tapered slowly to avoid seizures. Use with caution in renal or hepatic disease. **Therapeutic concentration:** 40-100 μg/ml.
Gabapentin (Neurontin)	Caps: 100,300,400 mg	Effective dose is 900-1800 mg/day in divided doses (3 times/day). Titrate to effective dose over a few days. Dose may be increased up to 1800 mg/day in 300-400 mg increments.	Recommended for add-on therapy in patients >12 years of age in the treatment of partial seizures with and without secondary generalization. Time between doses should not be greater than 12 h. Dose must be

			adjusted in renal failure. Drug is removed in hemodialysis.
Lamotrigine (Lamictol)	Tabs: 25,100,150, 200 mg	**Dose**: 1) Lamotrigine + enzyme-inducing AEDs and no valproic acid: Weeks 1&2: 50 mg qd; Weeks 3&4: 100 mg (in divided doses). Usual maintenance dose: 300-500 mg/day in 2 divided doses. Escalate by 100 mg/day each week. 2) Lamotrigine + enzyme-inducing AED plus valproic acid: Weeks 1&2: 25 mg qod; Weeks 3&4: 25 mg qd. Usual maintenance dose: 100-150 mg/day in 2 divided doses. Escalate by 25-50 mg/day q 1-2 weeks.	10% of all individuals exposed to lamotrigine develop rash. Dizziness and headache are also major side-effects. Recommended as adjunctive therapy in the treatment of partial seizures in adults. Unlabled use: May be useful in adults with generalized tonic-clonic, atypical absence, and myoclonic seizures. May be useful in infants and children with Lennox-Gastant syndrome.
Phenobarbital sodium	Caps: 16 mg Extended release caps: 65 mg Elixir: 15,20 mg/5 ml Tabs: 8,15,16,30,32, 60, 65,100 mg Amps: 130 mg/ml Vials: 65,130 mg/ml Tubex: 30,60 mg/ml	**ADULTS:** Oral and Parenteral: **Sedation:** 30-120 mg PO/IV/SC/IM daily (2-3 divided doses). **Hypnosis:** 100-320 mg PO/IV/SC/IM daily (2-3 divided doses); not recommended for more than 2 weeks. **Epilepsy:** 100-300 mg PO daily at bedtime. **Status epilepticus:** 200-600 mg IV (maximum 20 mg/kg/24 h). **CHILDREN:** Oral and Parenteral: **Sedation:** 6 mg/kg/day PO (in 3 divided doses).	IV administration may cause respiratory depression if given too rapidly. *Contraindications* include hypersensitivity to barbiturates, patients with bronchopneumonia or other severe pulmonary deficit, and porphyria. Administer with caution in patients with renal disease. Reduce dose in liver disease. May cause psychic and physical dependency. Gradual tapering of the drug is necessary to avoid withdrawal reactions. Phenobarbital can alter the metabolism of many drugs including oral anticonvulsants.

(continued)

Anti-Convulsants—*(cont.)*

Drug	Supplied	Dose/Route	Remarks
		Epilepsy: 3-5 mg/kg/day PO at bedtime. **Status epilepticus:** 100-400 mg IV.	Adverse reactions include CNS depression and other CNS disturbances, hypersensitivity reactions in children and older patients, GI tract disturbances, and many types of hypersensitivity reactions. Maximum rate of IV administration should not exceed 60 mg/min to avoid respiratory depression. Decrease rate of administration in patients with pulmonary or cardiovascular disease. **Therapeutic concentration:** 15-40 µg/ml.
Phenytoin sodium (Dilantin)	Caps: 30,100 mg Oral susp: 30,125 mg/ 5 ml Chewable tabs: 50 mg Amps: 50 mg/ml	**ADULTS:** Oral: 300-600 mg PO per day (in 2-3 divided doses), or 6-7 mg/ kg/day; do not increase dose more than 100 mg q 2-4 weeks. Parenteral: **Status epilepticus:** loading dose 15 18 mg/kg IV at a rate of 25-50 mg/min. **Antiarrhythmic:** 100 mg IV q 5 min, repeat until arrhythmia is stopped or a total dose of 1 g, then 100 mg PO 2-4 times a day. **CHILDREN:** Oral: 4-8 mg/kg/day in 2-3 divided doses (maximum 300 mg per 24 h). Parenteral: **Status epilepticus:** loading dose 15-18 mg/kg at a rate of 25-50 mg/min.	*Contraindications* include hypersensitivity to phenytoin or other hydantoins. Adverse reactions associated with parenteral therapy include phlebitis, hypotension, cardiac arrhythmias, and cardiovascular collapse. In patients with a compromised cardiovascular system or on sympathomimetic amines, do not exceed a rate of 25 mg/min. Flush the line with normal saline or lactated Ringer's solution only. *Avoid* extravasation. Additional adverse reactions include GI tract disturbances, CNS changes, gingival hyperplasia, lymphadenopathy, hematologic toxicity, hepatotoxicity, osteomalacia, and

			dermatologic reactions. GI tract disturbances are associated with oral administration. May interfere with some of the thyroid function tests. Patients in renal failure may require lower doses. Saturation of metabolism may occur with high doses. **Therapeutic concentrations:** 10-20 μg/ml total phenytoin; 1-2 μg/ml free phenytoin.
Primidone (Mysoline)	Tabs: 50,250 mg Oral susp: 250 mg/ 5 ml	**ADULTS:** Oral: 100-125 mg PO qd, increase dose 100-125 mg every several days until 250 mg PO tid or qid (maximum 2 g/24 h). **CHILDREN** (< 8 years old): Oral: 50 mg PO qhs, increase dose 50 mg every several days until 125-150 mg tid; usual dose 10-25 mg/kg/day.	Use in partial (psychomotor) seizures, other partial seizures, akinetic seizures, and tonic-clonic (grand mal) seizures. Adverse reactions include CNS depression and GI tract disturbances. May cause psychic or physical dependency. Can cause hyperexcitability in children. *Contraindications* include hypersensitivity to primidone and barbiturates, and patients with porphyria. Reduce dose in liver or renal disease. **Therapeutic concentration:** 5-12 μg/ml (15-25% of the drug is metabolized to phenobarbital).

(continued)

Anti-Convulsants—*(cont.)*

Drug	Supplied	Dose/Route	Remarks
Valproate sodium (Depakene, Depakote)	**Depakene**: Caps: 250 mg Oral solution: 250 mg/5 ml **Depakote:** Tabs (delayed release): 125,250,500 mg Caps: 125 mg	**ADULTS AND CHILDREN:** Oral: 15 mg/kg/day (2-3 divided doses); increase dose by 5-10 mg/kg per day every 7 days (maximum 60 mg/kg/24 h). Rectal: **Status epilepticus** (refractory): 400-600 mg per enema q 6 h; consult reference.	Use in simple and complex absence (petit mal) seizures, status epilepticus and other types of epilepsy. Adverse reactions include GI tract disturbances, CNS depression and other disturbances, hepatotoxicity, acute pancreatitis, alterations in coagulation and cell counts. *Contraindications* include hypersensitivity to valproic acid. Administer with food to reduce GI tract disturbances. Enteric-coated tablets (Depakote) may decrease GI tract disturbances. Valproic acid may alter the metabolism of some drugs. **Therapeutic concentration:** 50-100 µg/ml.

Anti-Diarrheals

Drug	Supplied	Dose/Route	Remarks
Attapulgite (Advanced Formula Kaopectate)	Liquid: 600 mg/15 ml	**ADULTS:** 30 ml after each bowel movement, up to 7 doses/day.	Acts as adsorbent and protectant. *Contraindicated* in intestinal obstruction and undiagnosed abdominal pain.
Camphorated opium tincture (Paregoric)	Liquid: 0.04% morphine (2 mg/5 ml)	**ADULTS:** 5-10 ml po q 6 h prn	Contains 25 times less than the amount of morphine in tincture of opium (Do not confuse these preparations!). *Contraindicated* in hypersensitivity to morphine and in diarrhea caused by poisoning until toxic material has

			been removed by gastric lavage or cathartics. Contains camphor and benzoic acid.
Diphenoxylate atropine sulfate (Lomotil)	Tabs: diphenoxylate: 2.5 mg; atropine sulfate: 0.025 mg. Elixir: diphenoxylate: 2.5 mg/5 ml; atropine sulfate: 0.025 mg/5 ml	**ADULTS:** initially 2 tabs or 10 ml po q 6 h. Reduce dose as symptoms are controlled. Maintenance dose may be as low as 1 tab or 5 ml q 12 h prn.	*Contraindicated* in diphenoxylate, atropine, or meperidine hypersensitivity, jaundice, pseudomembranous enterocolitis, children less than 2 years old, acute ulcerative colitis, and use with MAO inhibitors. Diphenoxylate 2.5 mg is equivalent in anti-diarrheal efficacy to 5 ml of paregoric.
Kaolin and pectin	Liquid: Kaolin 20%, pectin 1%	60-120 ml after each loose bowel movement.	Act as adsorbants and protectants. *Contraindicated* in intestinal obstruction and undiagnosed abdominal pain.
Lactobacillus acidophilus (Bacid, Lactinex)	Caps: 100 mg Granules: 1 g packet	2 capsules or 4 tablets or 1 packet of granules 3-4 times daily.	A lactic acid-producing bacterium that inhibits the overgrowth of potentially pathogenic fungi and bacteria. Used for uncomplicated diarrhea caused by disruption of the intestinal flora by antibiotics.

(continued)

Anti-Diarrheals—*(cont.)*

Drug	Supplied	Dose/Route	Remarks
Loperamide (Imodium, Immodium A-D, Kaopectate II caplets, Maalox Antidiarrheal caplets, Pepto Diarrhea Control)	Caps & Tabs: 2 mg Solution: 1 mg/5 ml, 1 mg/ml	**Acute diarrhea:** Initially 4 mg, followed by 2 mg after each unformed stool. Maximum dose is 16 mg daily. **Chronic diarrhea:** 4-8 mg daily as a single dose or in divided doses. **OTC Acute Diarrhea** (Adults): Initially 4 mg, followed by 2 mg after each loose bowel movement. Maximum 8 mg/day for no more than 2 days.	Longer acting and 2-3 times more potent on a weight basis than diphenoxylate. As effective as diphenoxylate for control of acute diarrhea. *Contraindicated* in hypersensitivity to loperamide and in pseudomembranous enterocolitis. In acute diarrhea, if clinical improvement is not seen in 48 h, discontinue drug. May be useful for control of traveler's diarrhea and for reducing volume of discharge from ileostomies.

Anti-Emetics

Drug	Supplied	Dose/Route	Remarks
Benzquinamide (Emete-Con)	Vial: 50 mg	IM: 50 mg q 3-4 h prn.	Comparable antiemetic effects to those of perphenazine, prochlorperazine or thiethylperazine. May be more effective than trimethobenzamide. IV administration may result in sudden increases in blood pressure and transient cardiac arrhythmias.

Buclizine (Bucladin-S Softab)	Tabs: 50 mg	**Motion sickness:** PO: 50 mg 30 min before exposure to motion and q 4-6 h prn. **Nausea:** 50-150 mg/day. Usual maintenance dose 50 mg bid. Tablet can be taken without water; allow to dissolve in mouth or chew. May also be swallowed whole.	Used in the prevention and treatment of motion sickness and vertigo associated with diseases of the vestibular system. Less effective than the phenothiazines in controlling nausea and vomiting unrelated to vestibular stimulation.
Granisetron (Kytril)	Inj: 1 mg/ml	**ADULTS and CHILDREN (>2 yo)** 10 mg/kg infused IV over 5 min, 30 min prior to emetogenic chemotherapy *only* on days chemotherapy is given.	For prevention of nausea and vomiting associated with initial and repeat emetogenic cancer therapy. No dosage adjustment needed in elderly, or in renal or hepatic impairment.
Meclizine (Antivert, Bonine, Dramamine II)	Tabs: 12.5,25,50 mg Chewable Tabs: 25 mg Caps: 25,30 mg	**Motion sickness:** 25-50 mg, 1 h prior to travel. May repeat q 24 h for duration of journey. **Vertigo:** 25-100 mg daily in divided doses.	Anticholinergic, antihistamine useful for prevention and treatment of motion sickness. Possibly effective for vertigo. Less effective than phenothiazines for nausea and vomiting unrelated to vestibular stimulation. Not recommended for children under 12 years old. *Note*: Dramamine II is meclizine; Dramamine is dimenhydrinate.
Ondansetron (Zofran)	Inj: 2 mg/ml Tabs: 4, 8 mg	**Cancer chemotherapy** (Adults): 0.15 mg/kg x 3 doses: first dose infused over 15 min beginning 30 min before start of chemotherapy; 2nd and 3rd doses given 4 & 8 h after 1st dose, respectively. **Or** give 32 mg	For prevention of nausea and vomiting associated with initial and repeat courses of emetogenic cancer chemotherapy. Also for prevention of postoperative nausea and vomiting. Maximum daily 8 mg IV or PO dose

(continued)

Anti-Emetics—*(cont.)*

Drug	Supplied	Dose/Route	Remarks
		as single dose over 15 min 30 minutes prior to start of chemotherapy. **Prevention of postop nausea/vomiting:** 4 mg, undiluted, IV push over 2-5 min (not less than 30 sec) immediately prior to induction of anesthesia. **Treatment of postop nausea/vomiting refractory to phenothiazines, metoclopramide, etc.:** 4 mg IV push as above or IVPB. **Treatment of nausea/vomiting refractory to other therapies:** Continuous infusion of up to 1 mg/h for up to 24 h.	recommended in patients with hepatic impairment.
Prochlorperazine (Compazine)	Tabs: 5,10,25 mg Syrup: 5 mg/5 ml Supp: 2.5,5,25 mg Spans: 10,15,30 mg Amps: 5 mg/ml	PO: 5-10 mg tid/qid; PR: 25 mg bid; IM: 5-10 mg every 3-4 h prn (maximum 40 mg/day).	*Contraindicated* in phenothiazine hypersensitivity, CNS depression, bone marrow depression. Not effective in preventing vertigo or motion sickness.
Promethazine (Phenergan)	Tabs: 12.5,25,50 mg Amps: 25,50 mg/ml Syrup: 6.25 mg/5 ml, 25 mg/5 ml Supp: 12.5,25,50 mg	PO: 25-50 mg 3-4 times daily; PR: 25-50 mg 3-4 times daily; IM: 25-50 mg 3-4 times daily; IV: 12.5-25 mg 4-6 times daily.	*Contraindicated* in anti-dopaminergic phenothiazine sensitivity. Indicated for treatment and prophylaxis of motion sickness, and prevention and control of nausea and vomiting associated with surgery and

			anesthesia. Avoid intra-arterial injection: Can cause gangrene of affected extremity. Tissue necrosis may result from subcutaneous injection.
Scopolamine (Transderm-Scop)	Transdermal therapeutic system: 1.5 mg	One patch behind the ear every 3 days. Patch should be applied at least 4 h before antiemetic effect is required.	Anticholinergic for prevention of nausea and vomiting associated with motion sickness, in adults. *Contraindicated* in hypersensitivity to scopolamine, or glaucoma.
Thiethylperazine (Torecan)	Tabs: 10 mg Supp: 10 mg Vial: 5 mg/ml	PO: 10 mg 1-3 times daily; PR: 10 mg 1-3 times daily; IM: 10 mg 1-3 times daily.	Similar to other phenothiazines. *Contraindicated* in pregnancy. Do not use IV, as it may cause severe hypotension.
Trimethobenzamide hydrochloride (Tigan)	Caps: 100,250 mg Amps: 100 mg/ml Supp: 100,200 mg	PO: 250 mg 3-4 times daily; PR: 200 mg 3-4 times daily; IM: 200 mg 3-4 times daily.	Anticholinergic. Contraindicated in patients hypersensitive to trimethobenzamide, benzocaine, or similar local anesthetics. Less effective as an antiemetic than phenothiazines, but may be useful in patients allergic to phenothiazines.

(continued)

Anti-Fungal Agents

Drug	Supplied	Dose/Route	Remarks
Amphotericin B (Fungizone)	Parenteral: 50 mg Topical: Cream 3%, Lotion 3%, Ointment 3%.	Day 1: 5 mg in 500 ml D5W over 6-8 h Day 2: 10 mg . . . Day 3: 15 mg . . . Day 4: 20 mg . . . Day 5: 25 mg . . . Day 6: 30 mg . . . Increase dose by 5 mg increments to 50 mg/day, but do not exceed 1.5 mg/kg/day. Total dose up to 30 mg/kg. **Bladder irrigation:** 10 mg in 1 L sterile water. Instill 250 ml tid for 3-5 days. **Intrathecal:** Mix 0.25-0.5 mg amphotericin B in 5 ml D5W and 25 mg hydro cortisone. First inject 25 mg hydrocortisone into IP site, then inject the hyperbaric amphotericin solution. Place the patient in Trendelenburg position for 45 min.	Test dose not necessary. **Indications:** Candidiasis, cryptococcal infection, blastomycosis, coccidiomycosis, histoplasmosis, mucormycosis, sporotrichosis, aspergillosis. Precipitate in saline solutions. Monitor serum renal profile, CBC, and platelet counts closely. *Acute* adverse reactions: fever, nausea, vomiting, anorexia, headache, thrombophlebitis. Premedication with aspirin or acetaminophen, compazine, and diphenhydramine. 25 mg hydrocortisone may be added to infusion if needed. Chronic adverse reactions: anemia, hypokalemia, renal failure, hypomagnesemia. No dosage adjustment is necessary in patients with existing renal dysfunction. If renal function deteriorates, however, therapy should be withheld.

Clotrimazole (Lotrimin, Mycelex)	Troches: 10 mg Vaginal tabs:100,500 mg Cream: 1% Vaginal cream: 1% Lotion: 1% Solution: 1%	PO: Troche held in mouth 5 times daily. Vaginal: 1 tab per vagina q HS for 7 days.	**Indications:** *Candida* prophylaxis, skin infection with pathogenic dermatophytes, trichomoniasis in pregnancy. Systemic use is not recommended secondary to hallucinations and disorientation. Adverse reactions include cutaneous erythema, edema, GI disturbance.
Fluconazole (Diflucan)	Tabs: 50,100,200 mg Injection: 200 mg/100 ml, 400 mg/200 ml	PO/IV: 100-400 mg qd.	Alternative in patients with severely compromised renal function and in whom amphotericin is contraindicated. Minimal adverse effects. Dosage reduction in renal failure.
Flucytosine (Ancobon)	Caps: 250,500 mg	Dosage schedule depends on renal function.	Variable susceptibility of *Candida* or *Cryptococcus* strains. Adverse reactions: nausea, vomiting, diarrhea. Agranulocytosis and aplastic anemia may be dose-related. Hepatotoxicity is rare.
Griseofulvin [*Microsize*] (Grisactin, Grifulvin, Fulvicin)	Caps: 125,250 Susp: 125 mg/5 ml Tabs: 250,500 mg	PO: 500 mg - 1 g daily as a single dose.	Active against species of *Trichophyton*, *Microsporum*, and *Epidermophyton*. Absorption is variable (25-70%). Headache may be severe, but often disappears with continued therapy.
Griseofulvin [*Ultramicrosize*]	Tabs: 125,165,250, 330 mg	PO: 330-660 mg daily as a single dose.	Absorption is almost complete.

(continued)

Anti-Fungal Agents—*(cont.)*

Drug	Supplied	Dose/Route	Remarks
Itraconazole (Sporanox)	Caps: 100 mg	PO: 200 mg qd.	Give with food for maximal absorption. Tachyarrhythmias when taken with terfenadine and astemazole. Effective for blastomycosis, histoplasmosis, and aspergillus.
Ketoconazole (Nizoral)	Tabs: 200 mg	PO: 200 mg qd, usually for 10 days, up to 2 months for cutaneous infection; 400 mg qd for histoplasmosis and coccidiomycosis. Disseminated infections may require 800-1600 mg qd.	For mucocutaneous candidiasis, histoplasmosis, paracoccidiomycosis, pulmonary coccidiomycosis as alternative to amphotericin B. Adverse reactions include nausea and vomiting. Drug absorption is reduced when administered with meals. Reversible hepatitis that is not dose related has been observed. Adrenal suppression and gynecomastia have also been seen. Antacids and H_2 blockers can decrease absorption. In patients with achlorhydria, each tablet should be dissolved in 4 ml of 0.2N HCl and administered through a straw. Tachyarrhythmias when taken with terfenadine and astemazole.

Miconazole (Monistat)	Parenteral: 10 mg/ml (vehicle is poly-ethioxylated castor oil). Supp: 100,200 mg Cream: 2% Lotion: 2% Powder: 2%		IV form not recommended due to adverse effects.
Nystatin (Mycostatin, Nilstat)	Susp: 100,000 units/ml Tabs: 500,000 units Vaginal tabs: 100,000 units/tab Cream/ointment: 100,000 units/g Powder: multiple strength	PO: 500,000 - 1,000,000 units (tab); 500,000 units oral, swish & swallow tid.	For treatment of candidiasis. Adverse reactions are mild and rare, but can include nausea, vomiting, diarrhea. Irritation may occur with topical application.
Tolnaftate (Tinactin)	Topical aerosol: 1% Aerosol powder: 1% Cream: 1% Powder: 1% Solution: 1%	Topically: twice daily.	

(continued)

Anti-Lipemics

Drug	Supplied	Dose/Route	Remarks
Cholestyramine resin (Questran, Cuemid)	Powder: 9 g packet	PO: 4 g tid before meals; mixed with 60-180 ml of water, milk, or fruit juice.	Anion exchange resin produces an increased fecal bile acid excretion. May cause constipation (20%), vomiting, vitamin A, D, E, and K deficiencies. Give other oral meds 1 h before or 4-6 h after cholestyramine dose. Prolonged use may lead to hyperchloremic acidosis. May help as an adjunct to diet in type IIa and type IIb hypercholesterolemia. Also used in treatment of pruritis associated with partial cholestasis.
Clofibrate (Atromid-S)	Caps: 500 mg	PO: 500 mg qid.	For hypercholesterolemia and hypertriglyceridemia. May potentiate oral anticoagulants. *Contraindicated* in primary biliary cirrhosis, pregnancy, lactation, hepatic and renal failure. May cause an increased release of antidiuretic hormone (ADH).
Colestipol (Colestid)	Susp: 5 g packet	PO: 15-30 g daily in 2-4 divided doses; mixed with 90 ml of a liquid. Do *not* give in dry form.	Anion-exchange resin that binds bile acids in the intestine which is then excreted in feces. May cause constipation (10%), vitamin A, D, E, and K deficiencies. Give other oral meds 1 h before or 4-6 h after cholestyramine dose.

Fluvastatin (Lescol)	Caps: 20, 40 mg	20-40 mg daily.	Competitively inhibits HMG-CoA reductase. Appropriate when a 15-25% reduction in LDL-C is desired.
Gemfibrozil (Lopid)	Caps: 300,600 mg	PO: 300 mg bid, 30 min before meals.	May increase cholesterol excretion in bile and cause cholelithiasis.
Lovastatin (Mevacor)	Tabs: 10,20,40 mg	20-80 mg/day in single or divided dose.	Competitively inhibits HMG-CoA reductase. Elevated serum transaminases have occurred. May increase effects of warfarin. Appropriate when a desired reduction of LDL-C exceeds 25%.
Niacin	Tabs: 100,250,500 mg Solution: 50 mg/5 ml	PO: 1.5-6 g daily in 2-4 divided doses with meals.	Mechanism of action in the decrease of elevated serum cholesterol is independent of the drug's role as a vitamin. GI upset, facial flushing, and skin burning are common. Pretreatment with a prostaglandin inhibitor (e.g., aspirin) may reduce flushing.
Pravastatin (Pravachol)	Tabs: 10,20 mg	10-40 mg mg qd at bedtime.	Competitively inhibits HMG-CoA reductase. Elevated serum transaminases have occurred. May increase effects of warfarin. Appropriate when a desired reduction of LDL-C exceeds 25%.
Probucol (Lorelco)	Tabs: 250 mg	PO: 500 mg bid with meals.	Diarrhea can occur in about 10% of patients.

(continued)

Anti-Lipemics—*(cont.)*

Drug	Supplied	Dose/Route	Remarks
Simvastatin (Zocor)	Tabs: 5,10,20,40 mg	5-40 mg/day as single dose.	Competitively inhibits HMG-CoA reductase. Elevated serum transaminases have occurred. May increase effects of warfarin. Appropriate when a desired reduction of LDL-C exceeds 25%.

Anti-Virals

Drug	Supplied	Dose/Route	Remarks
Acyclovir (Zovirax)	Ointment: 5% Parenteral: 500 mg, 1 g Caps: 200 mg Susp: 200 mg/5 ml	PO: CrCl >10—200 mg q 4 h; CrCl 0-10—200 mg q 12 h. IV: CrCl >50—5 mg/kg q 8 h; CrCl 25-50—5 mg/kg q 12 h; CrCl 10-25—5 mg/kg q 24 h; CrCl 0-10—2.5 mg/kg q 24 h.	Anti-viral activity against herpes simplex virus types 1 and 2 (HSV-1, HSV-2), varicella-zoster virus, Epstein-Barr virus, herpes virus simiae (B virus), and cytomegalovirus. Impaired renal function occurs in 10% of patients who receive acyclovir by rapid IV injection and 5% of patients who receive it by slow IV infusion (over 1 h), a result of precipitation of drug in the renal tubules.
Amantadine (Symmetrel)	Caps: 100 mg Solution: 50 mg/5 ml	PO: 100-200 mg daily as a single dose or in 2 divided doses.	Used for the prophylaxis and symptomatic treatment of respiratory infections caused by influenza A virus strains. CNS disturbances (nervousness, psychosis, inability to concentrate), livedo reticularis, and seizures are common.

Didanosine [*Dideoxyinosine, DDI*] (Videx)	Tabs (chewable): 25,50,100,150 mg Powder for oral solution: 100,167,250,365 mg	Patient Weight >75 kg: 300 mg bid; 50-74 kg: 200 mg bid; 35-49 kg: 125 mg bid. Administer on an empty stomach.	Treatment of HIV infection. 9% incidence of pancreatitis and 34% incidence of peripheral neuropathy. Used in patients who are intolerant to zidovudine.
Famciclovir (Famvir)	Tabs: 500 mg	500 mg q 8 h for 7 days	Management of acute herpes zoster (shingles). Dosage reduction in renal failure.
Foscarnet (Foscavir)	Injection: 24 mg/ml	IV: Induction 60 mg/kg over 1 h q 8 h for 2-3 wks. Maintenance 90-120 mg/kg/day over 2 h.	Treatment of CMV retinitis in patients with AIDS. Infusion device must be used to control rate of infusion, as toxicity (renal failure, hypocalcemia, hypomagnesemia, hypokalemia, hypophosphatemia, seizures) can be increased as a result of excessive plasma levels. Dosage adjustment in renal failure is mandatory.
Ganciclovir [*DHPG*] (Cytoxene)	Powder for injection: 500 mg/vial	**CrCl** (ml/min/1.73 m^2) 780: 5.0 mg/kg q 12 h; 50-79: 2.5 mg/kg q 12 h; 25-49: 2.5 mg/kg q 24 h; 0-25: 1.25 mg/kg q 24 h.	Treatment of CMV retinitis in immuno-compromised patients including those with AIDS. 20% incidence of thrombocytopenia and 40% incidence of granulocytopenia.
Stavudine (d4T) (Zerit)	Caps: 15,20,30,40 mg	$\geq$ 60 kg: 40 mg bid < 60 kg: 30 mg bid	Indicated for advanced HIV infection in patients who are intolerant or unresponsive to approved therapies. Major clinical toxicity is peripheral neuropathy (dose related).
Valacyclovir (Valtrex)	Caps: 500 mg	1 g tid for 7 days.	Treatment of herpes zoster (shingles) in immunocompetent adults.

(continued)

Anti-Virals—*(cont.)*

Drug	Supplied	Dose/Route	Remarks
Vidarabine (Vira-A)	Parenteral: 200 mg/ml	**Herpes simplex encephalitis:** IV: 15 mg/kg daily for 10 days. **Herpes zoster:** IV: 10 mg/kg daily for 5 days.	Not to be administered IM or SQ. Administered over 12-24 h using an in-line membrane filter with a pore size of 0.45 µm or smaller. Appears to be less effective than acyclovir in the treatment of herpes simplex encephalitis. Nausea, vomiting, diarrhea, malaise, muscle weakness, and psychosis occur infrequently.
Zalcitabine [*Dideoxycytidine, DDC*] (Hivid)	Tabs: 0.375, 0.75 mg	PO: 0.75 mg q 8 h concomitantly with 200 mg zidovudine q 8 h.	Combination of zalcitabine and zidovudine is indicated in patients with advanced HIV infection (CD4 cell count ≤ $300/mm^3$). Peripheral neuropathy is common (17-31%).
Zidovudine [*Azidothymidine, AZT*] *(Retrovir)*	Caps: 100 mg Syrup: 50 mg/5 ml Injection: 10 mg/ml	PO: Symptomatic: 200 mg q 4 h. Asymptomatic: 100 mg q 4 h. IV: 1-2 mg/kg over 1 h q 4 h.	Treatment of patients with HIV infection and CD4 cell count ≤ $500/\ mm^3$. Monitor hematologic indices every 2 weeks for anemia or granulocytopenia.

Benzodiazepines

Drug	Supplied	Dose/Route	Remarks
Alprazolam (Xanax)	Tabs: 0.25,0.5,1,2 mg	**ADULTS** (Oral—PO/SL): **Sedation:** 0.25-0.5 mg PO tid; increase dose gradually up to 4 mg daily. **Panic disorders:** 0.5 mg 3x daily. Dose range: 1-10 mg.	Caution: Paradoxical reactions have occurred in psychiatric patients. Geriatric patients may require lower doses. See diazepam for additional comments.

Chlordiazepoxide (Librium, Libritabs)	Caps: 5,10,25 mg Tabs: 5,10,25 mg Amps: 100 mg powder injection (supplied with 2 ml amp of IM diluent)	**ADULTS** (Oral and Parenteral): **Sedation:** 5-25 mg PO/IV tid or qid. **Alcohol withdrawal:** 50-100 mg PO/IV; repeat as necessary (600- 800 mg daily is not uncommon); reduce dose gradually.	Rate of administration for IV use should not exceed 12.5 mg/min. IM administration is reserved for cases in which oral or IV administration is not possible. Special IM diluent provided—do not use IM diluent for IV administration. Keep refrigerated. See diazepam for additional comments.
Clonazepam (Klonopin)	Tabs: 0.5,1,2 mg	**ADULTS** (Oral): **Seizures:** Initial 1.5 mg/day in 3 divided doses. Increase 0.5-1 mg q 3 days. Maximum dose 20 mg/day. **INFANTS and CHILDREN** (up to 10 years old or 30 kg): Oral: Initial dose 0.01-0.03 mg/kg; dose not to exceed 0.05 mg/kg/day in 2 or 3 divided doses. Maximum dose 0.1-0.2 mg/kg in 3 divided doses.	Used in petit mal seizures. Abrupt withdrawal may precipitate status epilepticus. Exercise caution in renal failure, chronic respiratory disease. May increase or precipitate the onset of grand mal seizures in patients who have several types of seizure disorders.
Clorazepate dipotassium (Tranxene)	Caps: 3.75,7.5,15 mg Tabs: 3.75,7.5,11.25, 15,22.5 mg	**ADULTS** (Oral): **Sedation:** 15 mg PO bid; increase dose gradually up to 60 mg daily. **Adjunctive therapy, prophylaxis of epileptic seizures:** 7.5 mg tid increased gradually to 90 mg/day.	See diazepam.

(continued)

Benzodiazepines—*(cont.)*

Drug	Supplied	Dose/Route	Remarks
Diazepam (Valium, Valrelease)	Caps (extended release): 15 mg Tabs: 2,5,10 mg Amps: 5 mg/ml Vials: 5 mg/ml Solution: 5 mg/5 ml Intensol: 5 mg/ml	**ADULTS**: Oral and Parenteral: **Anxiety, muscle spasm, prophylaxis of epileptic seizure:** 2-10 mg PO/IV tid or qid. Pre-op: 10 mg IM 1-2 h prior to surgery. **Alcohol withdrawal:** 10 mg PO tid or qid x 24 h, then 5 mg PO tid or qid, or 10 mg IV; repeat every 20-30 min. **Status epilepticus:** 5-10 mg IV; repeat in 10-15 min. **CHILDREN:** Oral: 0.12-0.8 mg/kg/day divided in 3-4 doses. Parenteral: 0.04-0.6 mg/kg per dose q 2-8 h.	Rate of administration for IV use should not exceed 2.5 mg/min. Geriatric or debilitated patients require lower doses. May cause psychic and physical dependency. Adverse reactions include CNS depression and other disturbances; paradoxical CNS stimulation; GI tract disturbances; GU disturbances; visual disturbances. Respiratory depression, hypotension, bradycardia and cardiac arrest have been associated with rapid IV administration. Use with caution in hepatic or renal disease. *Contraindications* include patients with acute alcohol intoxication with depressed vital signs and patients with hypersensitivity to the drugs. Absorption is slow and erratic with IM administration. Cimetidine and ranitidine may increase the half-life of diazepam. In chronic therapy, discontinue drug gradually to avoid withdrawal reactions.
Estazolam (ProSom)	Tabs: 1,2 mg	**ADULTS** (Oral): **Hypnotic:** 1-2 mg at bedtime.	See diazepam.

Flurazepam hydrochloride (Dalmane)	Caps: 15,30 mg	**ADULTS** (Oral): **Hypnotic:** 15-30 mg PO at bedtime.	See diazepam.
Halazepam (Paxipam)	Tabs: 20,40 mg	**ADULTS** (Oral): **Sedation:** 20-40 mg PO tid or qid; increase dose gradually up to 160 mg daily.	See diazepam.
Lorazepam (Ativan)	Tabs: 0.5,1,2 mg Vials: 2,4 mg/ml Tubex: 2,4 mg/ml	**ADULTS** (Oral and Parenteral): **Sedation:** 1-2 mg PO/IV/IM bid or tid; increase dose gradually up to 10 mg daily. **Hypnosis:** 2-4 mg PO at bedtime. **Pre-op:** 0.05 mg/kg deep IM 2 h prior to surgery (up to 4 mg). **Status epilepticus:** 2-15 mg IVP; may repeat dose or 2 mg/min IV infusion. **Chemotherapy-induced nausea and vomiting:** 1-2 mg q 4 h prn.	Lorazepam and oxazepam are recommended in liver disease (little or no change in dosage is necessary). Lorazepam is absorbed more predictably from IM administration than are diazepam and chlordiazepoxide. Lorazepam has been used in the treatment of alcohol withdrawal. May be used as IV infusion for sedation in ICU setting. See diazepam for additional comments.
Midazolam hydrochloride (Versed)	Vials: 1,5 mg/ml Disposable syringe: 5 mg/ml	**ADULTS** (Parenteral): **Pre-op:** 0.07-0.08 mg/kg IM. **Endoscopic or cardiovascular procedures:** 0.1-0.2 mg/kg IV. **Induction of anesthesia:** 0.3-0.35 mg/kg IV.	Short-acting water-soluble benzodiazepine. Give slow IVP. Midazolam has been used in the treatment of alcohol withdrawal. May be used as IV infusion for sedation (ICU setting). May cause respiratory depression. See diazepam for additional comments.
Oxazepam (Serax)	Caps: 10,15,30 mg Tabs: 15 mg	**ADULTS** (Oral): **Sedation:** 10-30 mg PO tid or qid.	See diazepam and lorazepam.

(continued)

Benzodiazepines—*(cont.)*

Drug	Supplied	Dose/Route	Remarks
Prazepam (Centrax)	Caps: 5,10,20 mg Tabs: 10 mg	**ADULTS** (Oral): **Sedation:** 30 mg PO daily (one or two divided doses); increase dose gradually up to 60 mg daily.	See diazepam.
Quazepam (Doral)	Tabs: 7.5,15 mg	**ADULTS** (Oral): **Hypnotic:** Initiate 15 mg at h. May decrease to 7.5 mg after 1st or 2nd day of therapy.	See diazepam.
Temazepam (Restoril)	Caps: 15,30 mg	**ADULTS** (Oral): **Hypnotic:** 15-30 mg PO at bedtime.	See diazepam.
Triazolam (Halcion)	Tabs: 0.125,0.25 mg	**ADULTS** (Oral): **Hypnotic:** 0.125-0.5 mg PO at bedtime.	Short-acting benzodiazepine. Caution: Advise patients not to take when a full night's sleep and clearance of the drug from the body are not possible before they would again need to be active and functional. Decrease in elderly. See diazepam for additional comments.

Benzodiazepine Antagonists

Flumazenil (Mazicon)	Injection: 0.1 mg/ml vials	**Reversal of conscious sedation or in general anesthesia:** Initial dose 0.2 mg (0.2 ml). Wait 45-60 sec and re-dose if necessary, up to 4 additional times to maximum dose of 1 mg. **Suspected benzodiazepine overdosage:** Initial dose 0.2 mg (0.2 ml). Administer IV over 30 sec. If needed after 30 sec, a further dose of 0.3 mg administered over 30 sec. Further doses of 0.5 mg over 30 sec at 1-min intervals up to cumulative dose of 5 mg. If no response after 5 mg, major cause of sedation is not likely due to benzodiazepines.	Individualize dosage. The serious adverse side-effects are related to the reversal of benzodiazepine effects. Use *caution* in patients who are physically dependent on benzodiazepines because of risk of precipitating seizures or benzodiazepine withdrawal symptoms. Also use caution in mixed drug overdose, especially with cyclic antidepressants. Administer as a series of small injections. Do not rush administration of flumazenil in overdose. Patient should have secure airway and IV access. In the event of resedation, repeated doses can be given at 20 minute intervals.

Beta-Blockers

Acebutolol (Sectral)	Caps: 200,400 mg	PO: 200-1200 mg/day	Used to treat hypertension.
Atenolol (Tenormin)	Tabs: 25,50,100 mg Injection: 5 mg/10 ml	PO: 50-100 mg qd IV (**MI**): 5 mg IV over 5 min followed by 5 mg 10 min later, then 50-100 mg qd	Hypertension, angina, myocardial infarction.
Betaxolol (Kerlone)	Tabs: 10,20 mg	PO: 10-20 mg qd	Hypertension.

(continued)

Beta-Blockers—*(cont.)*

Drug	Supplied	Dose/Route	Remarks
Bisoprolol (Zebeta)	Tabs: 5,10 mg	PO: 5-10 mg qd	Hypertension.
Carteolol (Cartrol)	Tabs: 2.5, 5 mg	PO: 2.5-10 mg qd	Hypertension.
Esmolol (Brevibloc)	(see Anti-Arrhythmics)	(see Anti-Arrhythmics)	Supraventricular tachycardia.
Labetalol HCl (Trandate, Normodyne)	(see Vasodilators)	(see Vasodilators)	Hypertension (see Vasodilators).
Metoprolol (Lopressor)	Tabs: 50 mg Injection: 1 mg/5 ml (5 ml amp)	PO: 100-400 mg/day IV (**MI**): 5 mg IV x 3 at 2-min intervals, then 50 mg PO q 6 h x 48 h 15 min after test IV dose; then 100 mg bid PO.	Hypertension, angina, myocardial infarction.
Nadolol (Corgard)	Tabs: 20,40,80,120, 160 mg	PO: 40-80 mg qd (usual dose)	Hypertension, angina.
Penbutolol (Lexatol)	Tabs: 20 mg	PO: 20 mg qd	Hypertension.
Pindolol (Visken)	Tabs: 5,10 mg	PO: 30 mg bid	Hypertension.
Propranolol HCl (Inderal)	(see Anti-Arrhythmics)	(see Anti-Arrhythmics)	Migraine, hypertension, pheochromocytoma, angina, supraventricular tachycardia, myocardial infarction.

Timolol (Blocadren)	Tabs: 5,10,20 mg	PO: 10-20 mg bid **MI**: 10 mg bid	Hypertension, myocardial infarction, migraine.

Biologicals

Epoetin Alfa [*Erythropoetin Human Glycoform α-Recombinant*] (Epogen, Procrit)	Injection: 2000, 3000, 4000, 10,000 U	SQ or IV: 50-100 U/kg 3 x/week initially, then decrease dose by 25 U/kg, titrating to hematocrit level.	Use for anemia associated with chronic renal failure, bone marrow transplant, antineoplastic drug treatment, and HIV-infection. Adverse effects include hypertension, thrombotic complications, seizures, nausea, vomiting, and diarrhea.
Granulocyte-colony stimulating factor, recombinant (G-CSF) (Filgrastim, Neupogen)	Injection: 300 μg/ml, 480 μg/1.6 ml	SQ or IV: **Post-myelosupprssive chemotherapy:** 5 μg/kg/day as a single dose until absolute neutrophil count (ANC) >10,000/mm^3 after expected chemotherapy-induced nadir. **Bone marrow transplantation:** 10 μg/kg/day up to a maximum of 60 μg/kg/day until ANC >1000/mm^3 for 3 consecutive days or absolute granulocyte count (AGC) >2500/mm^3 for 3 consecutive days.	Indicated for neutropenia after myelo-suppressive chemotherapy or bone marrow transplantation.

(continued)

Biologicals—*(cont.)*

Drug	Supplied	Dose/Route	Remarks
Granulocyte macrophage-colony stimulating factor, recombinant (GM-CSF) (Sargramostim, Leukine)	Injection: 250,500 μg/vial	250 μg/m^2/day for 21 days until ANC ≥ 20,000 cells/mm^3	Indicated for patients with non-myeloid malignancies undergoing autologous bone marrow transplantation who are expected to experience prolonged periods of neutropenia.

Diuretics

Drug	Supplied	Dose/Route	Remarks
Bumetanide (Bumex)	Tabs: 0.5, 1, 2 mg Amps: 0.5 mg/2 ml	**Edema:** Oral: 0.5-2 mg/day given in a single dose; if necessary, give 1 or 2 more doses qd but not more than 10 mg/day with a 4-5 h interval between doses. Parenteral: 0.5-1 mg slow IV push initially, then 1 or 2 more doses up to 10 mg/day with a 2-3 h interval between doses.	Use with caution in hepatic coma, anuria, or severe electrolyte depletion. *Contraindicated* in patients with a history of hypersensitivity to the drug. Onset of diuresis after IV administration is 5-10 min with a duration of 2-4 h. After oral administration, diuresis occurs within 30 to 60 minutes with a duration of 6-8 h. One mg of bumetanide has a diuretic potency equivalent to about 40 mg of furosemide. Less ototoxic than furosemide.

Chlorothiazide (Diuril)	Tabs: 250, 500 mg Oral suspension: 250 mg/5 ml Injection: 500 mg vial	**Edema and HTN:** Oral and IV: 500 mg 2 g/day in single or 2 divided doses.	IV route should only be used if patient is unable to take drug orally or in emergency situations. Injection must not be given SQ or IM.
Ethacrynic acid (Edecrin)	Tabs: 25,50 mg Parenteral: 50 mg/vial	Oral: Usual initial dose is 50 mg given as a single dose after a meal. Doses as high as 200 mg per day, given in divided doses after meal, may be required in some patients. Parenteral: 0.5 to 1 mg/kg as an initial dose. Single doses generally should not exceed 100 mg.	Use with caution in hepatic coma, anuria, and severe electrolyte depletion. Ototoxicity is associated with rapid IVP administration.
Furosemide (Lasix)	Tabs: 20,40,80 mg Oral solution: 10 mg/ml Amps: 10 mg/ml	**Edema** (oral): 20-80 mg PO initially, then increments of 20-40 mg PO q 6-8 h up to 600 mg/day. **Edema** (parenteral): 20-40 mg slow IV push initially, then increments of 20 mg q 2 h until adequate diuresis ensues. **Hypertension:** 40 mg PO bid; adjust dosage to patient response up to 480 mg/day. **Acute pulmonary edema:** 40-100 mg slow IV push.	Use with caution in hepatic coma, anuria, or severe electrolyte depletion. *Contraindicated* in patients with a history of hypersensitivity to the drug. Onset of diuresis after IV administration is 5-10 min with a duration of action of 2-4 h. After oral administration, diuresis begins within 30 to 60 minutes with a duration of 6-8 h.
Hydrochlorothiazide (Esidrix, Hydrodiuril, Oretic)	Tabs: 25,50,100 mg Oral solution: 50 mg/5 ml, 100 mg/ml	**Edema:** 25-200 mg/day PO in single or 2 divided doses. **HTN:** 25 mg PO qd; may increase to 50 mg/day in single or 2 divided doses.	Use with caution in patients with severe renal disease. Electrolyte disturbances may occur during thiazide therapy. *Contraindicated* in patients allergic to any thiazides or other

(continued)

Diuretics—*(cont.)*

Drug	Supplied	Dose/Route	Remarks
			sulfonamide derivatives. Routine use *contraindicated* in pregnancy.
Mannitol	Parenteral: 5%, 10%, 15%, 20%, and 25% injection	**Reduction of elevated intracranial pressure (ICP):** 1-2 g/kg IV as a 20% solution over 30-60 min. Repeat dose q 4-6 h prn. **Prevention of oliguria or acute renal failure:** 50-100 g IV.	Patients with questionable renal function should receive 12.5 g infused over a 3-5 min period as a test dose. A response is considered adequate if at least 30-50 ml of urine per h is excreted over the next 2-3 h. If an adequate response is not attained, a second test dose may be given. Fluid and electrolyte imbalances may occur.
Metolazone (Mykrox, Zaroxolyn)	Tabs (Mykrox): 0.5 mg Tabs (Zaroxolyn): 2.5, 5, 10 mg	Mykrox: **HTN:** 0.5-1 mg QD. Zaroxolyn: **Edema:** 5-10 mg daily as a single dose. Up to 20 mg per day may be required for edema associated with renal disease. **HTN:** 1.25-5 mg QD.	May be used concomitantly with furosemide to induce diuresis in patients who did not respond to either diuretic alone. Electrolyte disturbances may occur. Severe volume and electrolyte depletion may occur when used concurrently with furosemide. *Contraindicated* in patients allergic to any thiazides or other sulfonamide derivative. Mykrox has better and more rapid absorption than Zaroxolyn; therefore, dosing is not the same—do not interchange.

Spironolactone (Aldactone)	Tabs: 25,50,100 mg	**Edema:** 25-200 mg/day in single or divided doses. **HTN:** 50-100 mg/day in single or divided doses.	May be used for the treatment of diuretic-induced hypokalemia when oral potassium supplements are considered inappropriate. Severe hyperkalemia may occur in patients receiving potassium supplements concomitantly and in patients with renal insufficiency. Effective in ascites of liver cirrhosis.

Gastrointestinal

HISTAMINE H_2-RECEPTOR ANTAGONISTS:

Cimetidine (Tagamet, Tagamet HB)	Tabs: 100, 200 ,300, 400 mg Vial: 150 mg/ml Syrup: 300 mg/5 ml	**Duodenal ulcer:** 800 mg PO qhs for 4-6 weeks; also may give 300 mg qid with meals and at bedtime or 400 mg bid. Maintenance: 400 mg PO qhs. **Active benign gastric ulcer:** 800 mg PO qhs or 300 mg qid with meals and at bedtime. **Erosive gastroesophageal reflux disease:** 800 mg PO bid or 400 mg qid for 12 weeks. **Pathological hypersecretory conditions:** 300 mg PO qid with meals and at bedtime; may give 300 mg doses more often—do not exceed 2400 mg/day. **Heartburn, acid indigestion, sour stomach (OTC only):** 200 mg PO as symptoms occur	Reduces hepatic metabolism of drugs metabolized via cytochrome P-450 pathway, causing increased levels (benzodiazepines, calcium channel blockers, beta blockers, phenytoin, quinidine, sulfonylureas, theophylline, TCAs, valproic acid, warfarin). Antacids may interfere with absorption of cimetidine—stagger doses. Mental confusion may occur, especially in elderly patients with renal insufficiency. In prophylaxis of stress ulceration, doses greater than 300 mg qid may be necessary to maintain adequate gastric pH. Reduce dose in renal impairment. See ranitidine for additional comments.

(continued)

Drug	Supplied	Dose/Route	Remarks
HISTAMINE H_2-RECEPTOR ANTAGONISTS—*(cont.)*			
		up to bid for up to 2 weeks. Parenteral: 300 mg IM/IV q 6-8 h; may give additional 300 mg doses if necessary, up to 2400 mg/day. Continuous infusion: 37.5 mg/h (900 mg/day). **Prevention of upper GI bleeding:** continuous IV infusion at 50 mg/h.	
Famotidine (Pepcid)	Tabs: 20, 40 mg Vial: 20 mg Susp: 40 mg/5 ml	**Duodenal ulcer:** 40 mg PO qhs or 20 mg PO bid for up to 8 weeks. Maintenance therapy: 20 mg PO qhs. IV dose: 20 mg q 12 h. **Gastric ulcer:** 40 mg PO qhs for up to 8 weeks. **Gastroesophageal reflux:** 20 mg PO bid for up to 6 weeks. May increase dose to 40 mg PO bid x 12 weeks for esophagitis associated with reflux. **Pathological GI hypersecretory conditions:** 20 mg PO/IV q 6 h; higher doses may be necessary, up to 160 mg PO/IV q 6 h.	Comparable to cimetidine or ranitidine in healing duodenal ulcers and preventing recurrence. No anti-androgenic activity (which can occur with cimetidine). Does not interfere with hepatic metabolism. Reduce dose in renal impairment. See ranitidine for additional comments.

Nizatidine (Axid)	Caps: 150,300 mg	**Active duodenal ulcer:** 300 mg PO qhs or 150 mg PO bid. Maintenance 150 mg PO qhs. **GERD:** 150 mg PO bid.	Comparable to other H_2 blockers in healing rates of duodenal ulcers. Does not interfere with hepatic metabolism. Reduce dose in renal impairment. See ranitidine for additional comments.
Ranitidine hydrochloride (Zantac)	Caps: 150,300 mg Tabs: 150,300 mg Vial: 25 mg/ml Oral solution: 75 mg/5 ml Effervescent granules: 150 mg Effervescent tabs: 150 mg	**Duodenal ulcer:** 150 mg PO bid or 300 mg PO qhs for up to 8 weeks. Maintenance therapy: 150 mg PO qhs. **Gastric ulcer:** 150 mg PO bid for up to 6 weeks. **Gastroesophageal reflux:** 150 mg PO bid for up to 6 weeks. **Erosive esophagitis:** 150 mg PO qid. **Pathologic GI hypersecretory conditions:** 150 mg PO bid; may be given more frequently—titrate to response. Parenteral: 50 mg IM/IV q 6-8 h up to 400 mg daily; may be given as a continuous IV infusion of 150 mg over 24 h (6.25 mg/h). **Hypersecretory conditions:** 1 mg/kg/h; titrate in increments of 0.5 mg/kg to gastric pH.	Does not interfere with hepatic metabolism. May need doses up to 6 g/day in divided doses in pathologic hypersecretory conditions such as Zollinger-Ellison syndrome and systemic mastocytosis. Antacids may interfere with absorption (stagger doses). Reduce dose in renal insufficiency. Adverse reactions include CNS (headache, dizziness, somnolence, insomnia, mental confusion, hallucinations), GI (nausea and vomiting, abdominal discomfort), rash, hematologic (leukopenia, thrombocytopenia, granulocytopenia).

(continued)

Gastrointestinal—*(cont.)*

Drug	Supplied	Dose/Route	Remarks
MISCELLANEOUS:			
Mesalamine [5-ASA] (Asacol, Pentasa, Rowasa)	Tabs: 400 mg (delayed release); Supp: 500 mg; Rectal Susp: 4 g/60 ml enema Caps: 250 mg (controlled release).	Tabs: 800 mg tid. Supp: 500 mg bid. Susp: 4 g (60 ml) qd, preferably at HS; retain for 8 h; continue for 3-6 weeks. Caps: 1 g PO qid for up to 8 weeks.	Management of ulcerative colitis. *Contraindicated* in salicylate allergy.
Misoprostol (Cytotec)	Tabs: 100,200 µg	**NSAID induced ulcer prevention:** PO: 200 µg qid.	Synthetic analog of prostaglandin E_1. Gastric anti-secretory agent; protective effects in gastroduodenal mucosa. Diarrhea is common side-effect, dose-related. *Contraindicated* in pregnant women.
Octreotide acetate (Sandostatin)	Injectable: 0.05 mg, 0.1 mg, 0.5 mg, 1 mg	**Initial dosage:** 50 µg IV/SC 1-3 x/day. **Carcinoid tumors:** 100-600 µg/day in 2-4 doses during first 2 weeks. Median daily dosage is 450 µg/day for maintenance therapy. **VIPomas:** 200-300 µg/day in 2-4 doses during first 2 weeks to control symptoms. **Esophageal varices:** Bolus: 250 µg. Infusion: 250 µg/h.	Mimics action of natural hormone somatostatin. Suppresses secretion of serotonin, gastrin, vasoactive intestinal peptide, insulin, glucagon, secretin, motilin, pancreatic polypeptide. Use in management of GI fistulas under investigation. Therapy may be associated with cholelithiasis. Initial therapy occasionally associated with hypo- or hyperglycemia. Nausea, diarrhea, abdominal pain, loose stools, pain at injection site may

			occur. Reduce dose in the elderly and in renal failure.
Omeprazole (Prilosec)	Caps (sustained release): 10, 20 mg	**ADULTS:** **Active duodenal ulcer:** 200 mg PO qd for 4-8 weeks. **Severe erosive esophagitis or poorly responsive gastroesophageal reflux (GER):** 20 mg PO daily for 4-8 weeks. **Hypersecretory conditions:** Initial adult dose 60 mg PO qd. Individualize dosage. Doses of 120 mg tid have been used. Dosages in excess of 80 mg should be given in divided doses. Do not open capsules. Do not crush contents of capsules.	Benzimidazole compound suppresses gastric acid secretion inhibition of H^+/K^+ ATPase system ("acid proton pump"). Causes increase in serum gastrin levels. Effective in treatment of severe GER in terms of healing and symptom control. Use in hypersecretory condition (i.e., Zollinger-Ellison syndrome). Inhibits gastric acid secretion and controls symptoms of diarrhea, pain and anorexia. Well tolerated in Zollinger-Ellison patients with up to 5 years of therapy. Potential interactions with drugs metabolized by cytochrome P-450 system. No dosage adjustment necessary for patients with renal or hepatic dysfunction or in the elderly.
Sucralfate (Carafate)	Tabs: 1 g	**Active duodenal ulcer:** 1 g 1 h before each meal and at bedtime. Maintenance: 1 g PO bid.	Does not affect gastric acid output or concentration. Binds to gastroduodenal mucosa and acts as a barrier to gastric acid. Do not give antacids within 30 minutes of sucralfate dose. Use with caution in renal failure. May decrease therapeutic effects of warfarin, digoxin, phenytoin, ketoconozole, quinidine, quinolones; do not give sucralfate within 2 h of these drugs.

(continued)

Gastrointestinal—*(cont.)*

Drug	Supplied	Dose/Route	Remarks
PROMOTILITY:			
Cisapride (Propulsio)	Tabs: 10,20 mg	**Nocturnal heartburn due to gastroesophageal reflux disease:** 10 mg PO qid at least 15 min before meals and at bedtime. May increase to 20 mg qid.	Most common adverse effects involve GI tract and CNS. Rare cases of cardial arrhythmias, including ventricular arrhythmias and torsades de pointes associated with QT prolongation, have occurred, most often in patients taking drugs which inhibit the cytochrome P-450 enzyme system. *Contraindicated* with ketoconozole, fluconazole, itralonazole, miconazole, troleandomycin, clarithromycin, erythromycin, cimetidine.
Metoclopramide hydrochloride (Maxolon, Octamide, Reglan)	Tabs: 10,25 mg Syrup: 5 mg/5 ml Amps: 5 mg/ml	**Intubation of small intestine:** 10 mg IVP. **Gastric stasis:** PO/IV/IM 10 mg qid, 30 min before meals and hs. **Chemotherapy-induced emesis:** 2 mg/kg IVPB 30 min before chemotherapy and repeated twice at 2 h intervals following initial dose. **Gastroesophageal reflux:** 10-15 mg PO up to qid 30 min before meals and at HS for up to 12 weeks. May give 20 mg intermittent doses prior to provoking situation. **Prevention of post-op nausea and vomiting:** 10-20 mg IM/IV q 4-6 h prn.	Useful in gastric stasis, gastroesophageal reflux, and prevention of cancer chemotherapy-induced emesis. *Contraindicated* in GI bleeding, bowel obstruction, epilepsy, pheochromocytoma, hypersensitivity to metoclopramide, and drugs with extra-pyramidal reaction side-effects. Most common side-effects include CNS (insomnia, drowsiness, dizziness, headache, extra-pyramidal and Parkinsonian symptoms, Tardive dyskinesia). Reduce dose in renal impairment.

Hypoglycemics

Drug	How Supplied	Dosage	Remarks
Acetohexamide (Dymelor)	Tabs: 250,500 mg	**ADULTS:** Oral: 250 mg PO QAM with breakfast, increase dose by 250-500 mg/day every 5-7 days. Doses may be divided in two (Maximum: 1.5 g in 24 h). Monitor urine sugar/acetone and/or blood sugar.	First-generation sulfonylurea. Elderly patients and severely compromised patients may have exaggerated hypoglycemic response (Monitor carefully during first 24 h). Adverse reactions include GI tract disturbances, cholestatic and mixed hepatic jaundice, and hematologic toxicities. *Contraindications* include type I diabetes mellitus, uncontrolled diabetes mellitus, diabetes mellitus secondary to renal dysfunction, patients with major surgery, severe infection, and severe trauma. Use with caution in patients with porphyria and in patients with cardiovascular disease. *Not* recommended in patients with renal or hepatic disease. Monitor for many potential drug interactions. Tolerance may develop. *Contraindicated* during pregnancy.
Chlorpropamide (Diabenese)	Tabs: 100,250 mg (scored)	**ADULTS:** Oral: 250 mg PO QAM with breakfast; increase dose by 50-125 mg/day every 3-5 days. **Geriatric patients:** 100-125 mg PO QAM initial dose.	First-generation oral hypoglycemic agent. Adverse reactions include hypersensitivity and idiosyncratic reactions. Disulfiram-like reactions in patients ingesting alcohol may occur. Can cause SIADH secretion, primarily in

(continued)

Hypoglycemics—*(cont.)*

Drug	Supplied	Dose/Route	Remarks
		Doses may be divided in two (Maximum 750 mg in 24 h). Monitor urine sugar/acetone and/or blood sugar.	elderly patients. See acetohexamide for additional comments.
Glipizide (Glucotrol, Glucotrol XL)	Tabs: 5,10 mg (scored) Extended release tabs: 5,10 mg	**ADULTS:** Oral: 5 mg PO QAM 30 min before breakfast; increase dose by 2.5-5 mg/day every 3-7 days. **Geriatric patients and hepatic disease:** 2.5 mg PO QAM initial dose. Doses may be divided in 2-3. Maximum single dose 15 mg (Maximum daily dose 40 mg/24 h). Monitor urine sugar/acetone and/or blood sugar.	Second-generation sulfonylurea. See acetohexamide for additional comments.
Glucagon hydrochloride	Vials: 1 unit plus 1 ml diluent; 10 units plus 10 ml diluent.	**ADULTS:** Parenteral: **Hypoglycemia:** 0.5-1 unit SC/IM/IV; may repeat dose in 5-20 min. **GI tract radiographic exam:** 0.25-2 units IV or 1-2 units IM.	Adverse reactions include nausea and vomiting. Use with caution in patients with insulinoma and pheochromocytoma. Supplemental carbohydrate source should be administered to patients with hypoglycemia. Short duration of action. Glucagon 1 unit = 1 mg.

Glyburide (Diabeta, Glynase Prestab, Micronase)	Tabs: 1.25, 2.5, 5 mg (scored) Micronized tabs: 1.5, 3, 6 mg	**ADULTS:** Oral: 2.5-5 mg PO QAM with breakfast; increase dose by 2.5 mg/day every 7 days. **Geriatric patients:** 1.25 mg PO QAM initial dose. Doses may be divided in 2 (Maximum: 20 mg in 24 h). Monitor urine sugar/acetone and/or blood sugar. **Glynase**: 1.5-3 mg/day with breakfast; increase dose in 1.5 mg increments every 7 days. May give in single or divided doses. Maximum dose 12 mg/day. **Geriatric patients:** 0.75 mg/day initially.	Second generation sulfonylurea. See acetohexamide for additional comments.
Metformin HCl (Glucophage)	Tabs: 500,850 mg	**500 mg tabs** (Oral): Initial dose 500 mg bid with morning & evening meals; increase dose in 500 mg increments every week up to a maximum of 2500 mg/day. Doses up to 2000 mg/day may be given twice a day, while 2500 mg/day may be better tolerated in 3 divided doses with meals. **850 mg tabs:** Initial dose 850 mg qd with morning meal. Increase dose in increments of 850 mg every other week, in divided doses, up to maximum of 2550 mg/day. Usual maintenance dose 850 mg bid with	Oral hypoglycemic agent unrelated to sulfonylureas. Adverse reactions include GI symptoms (nausea/vomiting, diarrhea, bloating), metallic taste, decreased vitamin B12 levels. Most serious side-effect is lactic acidosis (rare, but fatal in ~50% of cases), which occurs from drug accumulation. *Contraindicated* in renal/hepatic impairment, acute or chronic metabolic acidosis, hypersensitivity. Use with caution in the elderly. Withhold therapy in patients to receive iodinated contrast materials 48 h before and

(continued)

Hypoglycemics—*(cont.)*

Drug	Supplied	Dose/Route	Remarks
		meals. Give 2550 mg/day in 3 divided doses with meals.	after due to risk of acute renal failure. Transfer from other oral antidiabetic agents: Usually no transition period is necessary. Use caution when transferring patients from chlorpropamide to avoid possible hypoglycemia due to its prolonged retention. Cimetidine increases metformin levels by 60%.
Tolazamide (Tolinase)	Tabs: 100,250,500 mg (scored)	**ADULTS:** Oral: 100-250 mg PO QAM with breakfast; increase dose by 100-250 mg/day every 7 days. **Geriatric patients:** 100 mg QAM initially; adjust dose by 50-125 mg/day at weekly intervals. Maximum: 1 g in 24 h. Monitor urine sugar/acetone and/or blood sugar. Divide doses >500 mg/day.	First-generation sulfonylurea. See acetohexamide for additional comments.
Tolbutamide (Orinase)	Tabs: 250,500 mg (scored)	**ADULTS:** Oral: Usual initial dose 1-2 g/day (range: 250 mg - 3 g/day). May be given as a single daily dose in the morning, but is preferably given in divided doses after meals. Increase dose by 250 mg/day every several days. **Geriatric patients:** may require lower doses.	First-generation sulfonylurea. See acetohexamide for additional comments.

		Maximum: 3 g in 24 h. Monitor urine sugar/acetone and/or blood sugar.	

Inotropes

Amrinone (Inocor)	Vial: 5 mg/ml	**Loading dose:** 0.75 mg/kg IVP over 2-3 min. **Maintenance:** 5-10 µg/kg/min.	Activity is secondary to inotropic and/or vasodilatory properties. Reversible thrombocytopenia may occur in < 5% of patients. Comparable inotropic activity to that of dobutamine.
Dobutamine (Dobutrex)	Vial: 200 mg/5 ml	**Initial dose:** 2.5-15 µg/kg/min.	More potent inotropic agent than dopamine. Not a mesenteric or renal vasodilator; little peripheral vasoconstriction. Predominant β-adrenergic effects (β_1 and β_2). May induce tachycardia.
Dopamine (Intropin)	Amps: 200 mg/5 ml Vials: 200,400,800 mg/5 ml	1. Predominant dopaminergic effects: 1-2 µg/kg/min. 2. Predominant β-adrenergic effects: 2-10 µg/kg/min. 3. Predominant α-adrenergic effects: >10 µg/kg/min. **Initial dose:** 2-5 µg/kg/min; then titrate to desired response.	Stimulates αand β-receptors (β_1 and β_2) and dopaminergic receptors. Supports circulation in a variety of low-output states. In low doses, augments renal blood flow and promotes diuresis. At infusions over 20 µg/kg/min, α-activity predominates and antagonizes dopaminergic effects and increases ventricular afterload; therefore, avoid this agent at this dosage in myocardial ischemia. *Contraindicated* in pheochromocytoma. May

(continued)

Inotropes—*(cont.)*

Drug	Supplied	Dose/Route	Remarks
			induce tachycardia, requiring a reduction in or discontinuation of dose.
Epinephrine (Adrenalin)	Amp: 1 mg/ml Vial: 30 mg/30 ml Mix 1 mg in 100-250 cc D5W	**IV infusions:** 1. β-effects: 0.5-1.5 mg/min. 2. α and β-effects: >1.5 μg/min. **Intracardiac:** 0.5 mg SC or IM: 0.2-0.5 mg q 10 min prn. **Prolongation of action of local anesthetics:** 0.1-0.2 mg added to local anesthetic solution to a final concentration of 1:100,000 to 1:20,000.	α (α_1 and α_2) and β (β_1 and β_2) agonist. Useful in profound hypotension to maintain organ perfusion. Can support myocardial contractility and heart rate. Stimulates respiration and is potent bronchodilator in low doses. Useful in SC administration in asthma. Used to treat anaphylactic reactions. High doses may elevate myocardial oxygen consumption. *Contraindicated* in narrow-angle glaucoma, coronary insufficiency, labor, cyclopropane and halogenated hydrocarbons, local anesthesia of fingers and toes.
Flosequinan (Manoplax)	Tabs: 50,75,100 mg	50-100 mg qd	Fluoroquinolone vasodilator (preload and afterload) with mild inotropic/chronotropic effects used for management of congestive heart failure in patients not responding to diuretics (with or without digitalis) who cannot tolerate an angiotensin-converting enzyme (ACE)-inhibitor, or who have not responded to an ACE-inhibitor. Hypokalemia is common.

Isoproterenol (Isuprel)	Vial: 0.2 mg/ml, 1 mg/ 5 ml	**Initial dose:** 2-10 μg/min IV infusion. Rates greater than 30 μg/ min may be used in advanced stages of shock.	β-adrenergic (β_1 and β_2) agonist with chronotopic and inotropic properties. Used for inotropic support, especially when myocardial O_2 supply is not compromised. Can serve as a temporary acceleration of heart rate in heart block. *Contraindicated* with development of tachyarrhythmia and ventricular irritability. Muscle bed vasodilation can unmask relative hypovolemia and produce hypotension. *Avoid* in myocardial ischemia.
Milrinone (Primacor)	Vial: 1 mg/ml	**IV infusion:** LD: 50 μg/kg over 10 min. MD: 0.375-0.75 μg/kg/min.	Similar to amrinone. Ventricular arrhythmias 12%.

(continued)

Insulin

Drug	Supplied	Dose/Route	Remarks
Insulin (*regular* insulin, crystalline zinc insulin)	Vials: Single peak (pork) 100 U/ml Single peak (beef and pork) 100 U/ml Purified (beef) 100 U/ml Purified (pork) 100,500 U/ml Combination purified (pork) 30 U/ml plus Isophane 70 U/ml (NPH)	**ADULTS:** Parenteral: 5-10 U SC 15-30 min before meals and at bedtime. Doses should be individualized according to urine & blood sucrose. **Diabetic ketoacidosis:** Low dose: initial dose 2.4-7.2 U, then 2.4-7.2 U/h as an infusion. **CHILDREN:** Parenteral: 2-4 U SC 15-30 min before meals and at bedtime. Individualized dosing is essential. **Diabetic ketoacidosis:** Initial dose 1-2 U/kg in two divided doses (one IV, one SC), then 0.5-1 U/kg q 1-2 h.	Regular insulin can be given SC, IM, or IV infusion. Short-acting insulin. Adverse reactions include hypoglycemic reactions, atrophy or hypertrophy of subcutaneous fat tissue, mental status changes, insulin resistance and allergy. Rotate injection sites to avoid atrophy or hypertrophy. Decrease dose by 20% when converting from single-peak insulin to purified insulin. Any changes in insulin preparation or dosage regimen should be made carefully. Purified insulin may be less immunogenic than single-peak insulin. Pure pork insulin may be less immunogenic than mixed or beef insulin.

Insulin human (Humulin, Novolin), **recombinant DNA and semisynthetic**	Vials: Regular 100 U/ml; Zinc 100 U/ml (Lente); Zinc, extended (Ultralente): 100 U/ml; Isophane 100 U/ml (NPH); Combination: Regular 30 U/ml plus Isophane 70 U/ml. Insulin zinc extended: 100 U/ml.	**ADULTS AND CHILDREN:** Parenteral: doses should be individualized according to urine and blood glucose.	Regular human insulin can be given SC, IM, or IV. Zinc and Isophane human insulin must *not* be given IV. Human insulin may be less immunogenic than purified insulin. See Insulin (Regular) for additional comments.
Insulin, Isophane (Neutral Protamine Hagedorn, NPH Insulin)	Vials: Single peak (beef) 100 U/ml Single peak (beef and pork) 100 U/ml Purified (beef) 100 U/ml Purified (pork) 100 U/ml Purified combination (pork) 70 U/ml + regular 30 U/ml	**ADULTS:** Parenteral: 7-26 U SC QAM 30-60 min before breakfast. Some patients may require a smaller dose with supper or at bedtime. Increase dose by 2-10 U/day every few days. Doses should be individualized according to urine and blood glucose.	Isophane insulin must be given SC only. Intermediate-acting insulin. Equivalent doses can be used when changing from zinc to isophane insulins. See Insulin (Regular) for additional comments.

(continued)

Insulin—*(cont.)*

Drug	Supplied	Dose/Route	Remarks
Insulin zinc (Lente)	Vials: Single peak (beef) 100 U/ml Single peak (beef and pork) 100 U/ml Purified (beef) 100 U/ml Purified (pork) 100 U/ml	**ADULTS:** Parenteral: 7-26 U SC QAM 30-60 min before breakfast. Some patients may require a smaller dose with supper or at bedtime. Increase dose by 2-10 U/day every few days. Doses should be individualized according to urine and blood glucose.	Zinc insulin must be given SC only. Intermediate-acting insulin. Equivalent doses can be used when changing from isophane to zinc insulin. See Insulin (Regular) for additional comments.
Insulin zinc, extended (UltraLente)	Vials: Single peak (beef) 100 U/ml Single peak (beef and pork) 100 U/ml Purified (beef) 100 U/ml	**ADULTS:** Parenteral: 7-26 U SC QAM 30-60 min before breakfast. Doses should be individualized according to urine and blood glucose.	Extended zinc insulin must be given SC only. Long-acting insulin. Decrease dose by 1/3 when changing from regular insulin to extended zinc insulin. See Insulin (Regular) for additional comments.
Insulin zinc, prompt (SemiLente)	Vials: Single peak (beef) 100 U/ml Single peak (beef and pork) 100 U/ml Purified (pork) 100 U/ml	**ADULTS:** Parenteral: 10-20 U SC QAM 30 min before breakfast and 2-3 more times/day usually before meals. Doses should be individualized according to urine and blood glucose.	Prompt zinc insulin must be given SC only. Short-acting insulin. See Insulin (Regular) for additional comments.

Narcotic Agonist / Antagonist Analgesics

Buprenorphine hydrochloride (Buprenex)	Amps: 0.3 mg/ml	**ADULTS and CHILDREN** (>13 years): Parenteral: 0.3-0.6 mg IM or slow IV q 4-6 h prn. **ADULTS:** IV Infusion: 25-260 µg/h. Epidural: **Post-op pain:** Single doses of 60 µg up to total dose of 180 µg over 48 h. **Severe chronic pain:** 0.15-0.3 mg q 6 h, up to total daily dose of 0.86 mg (range 0.15-7.2 mg).	Narcotic agonist/antagonist. May precipitate withdrawal reactions in patients with narcotic addiction. Low physical dependence liability. May cause psychic dependency. *Contraindications* include hypersensitivity to buprenorphine. Side-effects include sedation, nausea, vertigo, dizziness, vomiting, hypotension, and respiratory depression. *Not* recommended in patients with increased intracranial pressure. High doses of naloxone may be required to reverse respiratory depression.
Butorphanol tartrate (Stadol)	Vials: 1,2 mg/ml Nasal spray: 10 mg/ml	**ADULTS: Analgesia:** Parenteral: 1-4 mg IM *or* 0.5-2 mg IV q 3-4 h prn. Nasal: 1 mg (1 spray in one nostril), may repeat after 60-90 min. In severe pain, may use initial 2 mg dose (1 spray in each nostril). Repeat q 3-4 h prn.	Narcotic agonist/antagonist. May precipitate withdrawal reaction in patients with narcotic addiction. *Contraindications* include hypersensitivity to butorphanol. Adverse reactions include sedation, nausea, vomiting, respiratory depression and blood pressure changes. *Not* recommended in patients with increased intracranial pressure. Low psychic and physical dependence liability. Reduce dose in hepatic disease. *Not* recommended in children <18 years old. Administer naloxone (see morphine sulfate) for respiratory

(continued)

Narcotic Agonist / Antagonist Analgesics—*(cont.)*

Drug	Supplied	Dose/Route	Remarks
			depression and overdoses. Causes less respiratory depression than morphine sulfate. Respiratory depression in healthy adults plateaus with 30-60 µg/kg dose (IV), but the duration of the effect increases with higher doses.
Nalbuphine (Nubain)	Vials and Amps: 10, 20 mg/ml Disposable syringe: 20 mg/ml	**ADULTS: Analgesia:** Parenteral: 10-20 mg SC/IM/IV q 3-6 h prn (maximum 160 mg per 24 h). Adults who have been on chronic opiate agonist therapy: 25% of usual nalbuphine dose. Observe for withdrawal symptoms; if none, continue with normal dosing. **ADULTS: Anesthesia:** Induction: 0.3-3 mg/kg IV over 10-15 min; Maintenance: 0.25-0.5 mg/kg IV prn.	Narcotic agonist/antagonist (less antagonist action than butorphanol). May precipitate withdrawal symptoms in patients with narcotic addiction. *Contraindications* include hypersensitivity to nalbuphine. Adverse reactions include sedation, nausea, vomiting, respiratory depression, cardiovascular changes, and mental status changes. Low psychic and physical dependence liability. *Not* recommended in patients with increased intracranial pressure. May cause biliary tract spasm. Reduce dose in hepatic or renal disease. *Not* recommended in children <18 years old. Administer naloxone (see morphine sulfate) for respiratory depression and overdoses. Respiratory depression is equal to morphine, but nalbuphrine exhibits a ceiling effect.

Narcotic Analgesics

Codeine sulfate or phosphate and combination products (Tylenol with Codeine 2,3,4)	Tabs: 15,30,60 mg Vials: 30,60 mg/ml Disposable syringe: 30,60 mg/ml **Combination products:** Tabs: 300 mg acetaminophen + 15, 30, 60 mg codeine; Oral liquid: 120 mg acetaminophen + 12 mg codeine/5 ml	**ADULTS: Antitussive:** Oral: 10-20 mg PO q 4-6 h (maximum 120 mg in 24 h). **Analgesic:** Oral and parenteral: 15-60 mg PO/IM/SC/IV q 4-6 h (maximum 360 mg in 24 h). **CHILDREN: Antitussive:** Oral [2-6 years]: 2.5-5 mg q 4-6 h (maximum 30 mg in 24 h). [6-12 years]: 5-10 mg PO q 4-6 h (maximum 60 mg in 24 h). **Analgesic** [>1 year]: Oral and parenteral: 0.5 mg/kg (15 mg/m^2) PO/IM/SC q 4-6 h.	*Contraindications* include hypersensitivity to codeine. May cause psychic and physical dependency. Adverse reactions include sedation, dizziness, nausea, vomiting, and respiratory depression. Administer naloxone (see morphine sulfate) for respiratory depression and overdoses. **DO NOT ADMINISTER IV IN CHILDREN!**
Fentanyl citrate (Sublimaze) **and combination product** (Innovar) (*Duragesic transdermal system*) (Fentanyl Oralet)	Amps: 0.05 mg/ml (50 µg/ml). Combination product: fentanyl 0.05 mg/ml + droperidol 2.5 mg/ml. Transdermal system: 25, 50, 75, 100 µg/h. Transmucosal system (Lozenges): 200,300, 400 µg.	**ADULTS:** Parenteral: Post-op pain 50-100 µg IV/IM, may repeat in 1-2 h; pre-op 0.05-0.1 mg IM 30-60 min before surgery. Transdermal: Initial dose 25 µg patch every 48-72 h, unless opiate tolerant. Epidural Infusion: 20-150 µg/h, as continuous infusion. Transmucosal (indicated only for use in-hospital in monitored anesthesia care setting): **Adults:** 5 µg/kg. **Children:** 5-15 µg/kg. Maximum dose in both: 400 µg.	Shorter acting, with less emetic effect, less sedation, and less histamine release than other narcotic analgesics. *Contraindications* include hypersensitivity and monoamine oxidase therapy. Adverse reactions include respiratory depression, muscular rigidity, bradycardia. Administer naloxone (see morphine sulfate) for respiratory depression and overdoses.

(continued)

Narcotic Analgesics—*(cont.)*

Drug	Supplied	Dose/Route	Remarks
Fioricet®with Codeine capsules (acetaminophen, butalbital, caffeine, and codeine)	Caps: acetaminophen 325 mg, butalbital 50 mg, caffeine 40 mg, codeine 30 g.	**ADULTS:** 1-2 capsules q 4 h prn (maximum 6 capsules/day).	*Contraindicated* in porphyria, hypersensitivity to acetaminophen, caffeine, barbiturates, or codeine.
Fiorinal®(aspirin, butalbital, and caffeine)	Caps: aspirin 325 mg, butalbital 50 mg, caffeine 40 mg. Tabs: same	**ADULTS:** Oral: 1-2 caps PO q 3-6 h.	*Contraindicated* in porphyria, hypersensitivity to aspirin, caffeine or barbiturate. Can cause psychic or physical dependence. Can raise prothrombin time. May be beneficial in vascular headaches. Other combination products available.
Hydromorphone hydrochloride (Dilaudid) **and combination product**	Tabs: 1,2,3,4 mg Amps: 1,2,3,4,10 mg/ml Vials: 2, 10 mg/ml Syringe: 1,2,3,4 mg/ml Supp: 3 mg Combination product syrup: hydromorphone 1 mg/5 ml + guaifenesin 100 mg/5 ml	**Analgesic—ADULTS:** Oral: 2 mg PO q 4-6 h prn. For severe pain 4 mg PO q 4-6 h prn. Parenteral: 1-2 mg SC/IM q 4-6 h prn (IV administration over 2-3 min). For severe pain 3-4 mg q 4-6 h. Rectal: 3 mg PR q 6-8 h prn. **Antitussive:** Oral: adults and children >12 years: 1 mg PO q 3-4 h prn; children 6-12 years: 0.5 mg PO q 3-4 h prn.	*Contraindications* include hypersensitivity and in patients with increased intracranial pressure. May cause psychic or physical dependence. Adverse reactions include CNS depression, nausea, vomiting, hypotension, and respiratory depression. Administer naloxone (see morphine sulfate) for respiratory depression and overdoses.

		Epidural Infusion: 0.15-0.3 mg/h, as continuous infusion.	
Meperidine hydrochloride (Demerol)	Tabs: 50,100 mg Syrup: 50 mg/5 ml Amps: 25,50,75,100 mg/dose Vials: 25,50,75,100 mg/dose Disposable syringe: 25,50,75,100 mg/dose	**ADULTS:** Oral: 50-150 mg PO q 3-4 h prn. Parenteral: 50-150 mg SC/IM q 3-4 h prn (or slow IV administration). IV infusion: 15-35 mg/h. **CHILDREN:** Oral: 1.1-1.8 mg/kg PO q 3-4 h prn. Parenteral: 1.1-1.8 mg/kg IM/SC q 3-4 h prn; pre-op 1-2 mg/kg IM/SC. Epidural Infusion: 5-20 mg/h, as continuous infusion.	Drug is least effective when given orally. IM route is preferred over SC route when repeated doses are needed. *Contraindications* include hypersensitivity, monoamine oxidase inhibition therapy, and lactation. May cause psychic or physical dependence. Adverse reactions include CNS alterations, nausea, vomiting, constipation, respiratory depression, cardiac arrhythmias, and hypotension. Patient with renal dysfunction may accumulate normoperidine (metabolite), causing seizures. Administer naloxone (see morphine sulfate) for respiratory depression and overdoses.
Methadone hydrochloride (Dolophine)	Oral solution: 5, 10 mg/5 ml; 10 mg/10 ml; 10 mg/ml (concentrated). Tabs: 5, 10 mg Tabs (dispersible): 40 mg Vials &Amps: 10 mg/ml	**ADULTS:** **Analgesic:** Oral and parenteral: 2.5-10 mg PO/SC/IM q 6 h prn. (In severe chronic pain in cancer patients, 5-20 mg PO/SC/IM q 6 h.) **Detoxification and maintenance of narcotic addicts:** Oral: various dose ranges may be necessary depending on the patient.	Used in severe pain and in detoxification and maintenance of narcotic addicts. *Contraindications* include hypersenstivity to methadone. May cause psychic and/or physical dependency. Side-effects include nausea, vomiting, biliary tract spasm, urinary retention, respiratory depression, cardiovascular changes, constipation, confusion, and sweating. Administer naloxone (see morphine sulfate) for respiratory

(continued)

Narcotic Analgesics—*(cont.)*

Drug	Supplied	Dose/Route	Remarks
			depression and overdoses (may require repeated doses of naloxone because of the long half-life). NOT RECOMMENDED FOR USE IN CHILDREN.
Morphine sulfate	Oral solution: 10, 20 mg/5 ml; 20 mg/ml. Amps: 0.5, 1, 8, 10, 15 mg/ml; Vials: 0.5, 1, 2, 3, 5, 8, 10, 15 mg/ml. Prefilled syringes: 2, 4, 8, 15 mg/ml. Soluble tablets: 10, 15, 30 mg. Tablets (immediate release): 15, 30 mg. Tablets (continuous release): 30, 60 mg. Rectal suppositories: 5, 10, 20, 30 mg	**ADULTS:** Oral solution: 10-30 mg PO q 4 h prn or as directed. Extended-release tabs: 30 mg PO q 8-12 h prn. Parenteral: SC/IM (Adults): 10 mg 5-20 mg)/70 kg q 4 h prn; IV: 2.5-15 mg/70 kg over 4-5 min q 4 h prn. IV infusion: start at 1-10 mg/h, titrate to 20-150 mg/h (for severe chronic pain associated with cancer). Epidural infusion: 0.2-1.5 mg/hr as continuous infusion. Rectal: 10-20 mg PR q 4 h prn. **CHILDREN:** Parenteral: 0.1-0.2 mg/kg up to 15 mg SC/IM 4 h prn.	For use as a pre-operative medication or in severe pain. *Contraindicated* with known hypersensitivity. May cause psychic or physical dependence. Adverse reactions include nausea, vomiting, biliary tract spasm, urinary retention, hypotension, respiratory depression, apnea, cardiac arrest. Administer naloxone for respiratory depression and overdoses.

Oxycodone hydrochloride and combination products (Percocet, Tylox, Percodan)	Tabs: 5 mg Oral solution: 5 mg/5 ml, 20 mg/ml **Combination products:** Tabs: 5 mg oxycodone HCl + 325 mg acetaminophen (Percocet); 5 mg oxycodone HCl + 500 mg acetaminophen (Tylox); 4.5 mg oxycodone HCl + 0.38 mg oxycodone terephthalate + 325 mg aspirin (Percodan); Oral solution: 5 mg oxycodone + 325 mg acetaminophen	**ADULTS:** Oral: 1-2 tabs PO q 4-6 h prn. **CHILDREN:** ≥ 12 years: 1/2 tab q 6 h prn; 6-12 years: 1/4 tab q 6 h prn.	*Contraindications* include hypersensitivity to oxycodone, acetaminophen, or aspirin (depending on the product). May cause psychic or physical dependency. Adverse reactions include light-headedness, sedation, nausea, and vomiting. Administer naloxone (see morphine sulfate) for respiratory depression or overdoses (in addition to appropriate therapy for aspirin or acetaminophen overdose if combination product).

(continued)

Narcotic Analgesics—*(cont.)*

Drug	Supplied	Dose/Route	Remarks
Pentazocine lactate or hydrochloride (Talwin, Talwin NX) **and combination products**	Tabs: 50 mg pentazocine + 0.5 mg naloxone. Amps: 30 mg/ml Vials: 30 mg/ml Disposable syringe: 30 mg/ml **Combination products:** Caplets: pentazocine 12.5 mg + aspirin 325 mg (Talwin compound); pentazocine 25 mg + acetaminophen 650 mg (Talacen)	**ADULTS:** Oral: 50-100 mg PO q 3-4 h prn (maximum 600 mg in 24 h). Parenteral: 30-60 mg IM/SC/IV q 3-4 h prn (maximum 360 mg in 24 h). Combination products: 2 Talwin compound caplets or 1 Talacen caplet q 4 h prn.	Narcotic agonist/antagonist. May precipitate withdrawal reactions in patients with narcotic addiction. May cause psychic or physical dependency. *Contraindications* include hypersensitivity to pentazocine. Adverse reactions include nausea, vomiting, dizziness, sedation, cardiovascular changes, and respiratory depression. *Not* recommended in patients with increased intracranial pressure. May increase biliary tract pressure. May cause skin and soft-tissue changes. Rotate injection sites. IM route is preferred over SC route. Dosage and/or frequency (especially oral forms) may need to be decreased with hepatic impairment. *Not* recommended in children under 12 years of age. Administer naloxone (see morphine sulfate) for respiratory depression and overdoses.

Propoxyphene hydrochloride (Darvon) **or napsylate** (Darvon-N) **or combination product** (Darvocet-N)	Caps: 32,65 mg propoxyphene (Darvon). Tabs: 100 mg propoxyphene napsylate (Darvon-N). Susp: 10 mg/ml propoxyphene naypsylate (Darvon-N). **Combination product:** Tabs: 50,100 mg propoxyphene napsylate + 325,650 mg acetaminophen (Darvocet-N).	**ADULTS:** Oral: 65 mg propoxyphene HCl PO q 4 h prn (maximum 390 mg in 24 h); 100 mg propoxyphene napsylate PO q 4 h prn (maximum 600 mg in 24 h).	*Contraindications* include hypersensitivity to propoxyphene, acetaminophen, or aspirin (depending on the product). May cause psychic and/or physical dependency. Adverse reactions include dizziness, sedation, nausea, and vomiting. Administer naloxone (see morphine sulfate) for respiratory depression and overdoses (may require repeated doses of naloxone because of the long half-life). NOT RECOMMENDED FOR USE IN CHILDREN.
Sufentanil citrate (Sufenta)	Amps: 50 μg/ml	**ADULTS:** Parenteral: **Single-Agent Anesthesia:** Initially 8-30 μg/kg IV, followed by 25-50 μg doses as needed. **CHILDREN** (2-12 years old): Parenteral: **Single-Agent Anesthesia:** Initially 10-25 μg/kg IV, followed by 25-50 mg doses as needed.	Respiratory depression and skeletal muscle rigidity are most common adverse reactions associated with sufentanil. Other side-effects include cardiovascular changes, nausea, vomiting. Patients on β-blocker therapy require lower doses. Administer with *caution* in patients with liver and renal disease. Administer naloxone (see morphine sulfate) for respiratory depression and overdoses.

(continued)

Narcotic Antagonists

Drug	Supplied	Dose/Route	Remarks
Nalmefene HCl (Revex)	Amps: 100 µg/ml (blue label for post-op use); 1000 µg/ml (green label for management of overdose)	**Reversal of post-op opioid depression:** IV: Use 100 µg/ml strength. Initial: 0.25 µg/kg. May be repeated at 2-5 min intervals until desired effect is achieved. **Management of opioid overdose:** IV: Use 1000 µg (1 mg) strength. Initial: 0.5 mg/70 kg. If needed, may follow with 1 mg/70 kg dose in 2-5 minutes. If no clinical response is seen with total dose of 1.5 mg/70 kg, further doses are not likely to help. If there is reason to suspect opioid dependency, give challenge dose of 0.1 mg/70 kg. If no evidence of withdrawal in 2 min, proceed as above.	Long-acting (half-life 10.8 h) opioid antagonist indicated for reversal of natural or synthetic opioids. May not completely reverse buprenorphine. May precipitate withdrawal in patients physically dependent on opioids. Doses should be administered over at least 60 sec in renal failure patients to minimize hypertension and dizziness. Use smaller incremental doses for reversal of post-op opioid depression (0.1 µg/kg). Solution may be diluted 1:1 with saline or sterile water.

Naloxone (Narcan and Narcan Neonatal)	Vials and Amps: 0.4, 1 mg/ml; Neonatal 0.02 mg/ml (amps, vials, and disposable syringes)	**ADULTS:** Parenteral: post-op 0.1-0.2 mg IV/SC/IM q 2-3 min until response, additional doses q 1-2 h; opiate overdose 0.4-2 mg IV/SC/IM q 2-3 min up to 10 mg. Infusion: 0.4 mg/h. **CHILDREN:** Parenteral: post-op IV 0.005-0.01 mg q 2-3 min until response, additional doses q 1-2 h; opiate overdoses 0.01 mg/kg IV/SC/IM. Infusion: 0.024-0.16 mg/kg/h.	Adverse reactions include nausea, vomiting, sweating, tachycardia. *Contraindications* include hypersensitivity to naloxone. Use with *caution* in patients with preexisting cardiovascular disease. May precipitate narcotic withdrawal reaction. IV administration is preferred in acute situations. In some narcotic overdoses, repeated doses or IV infusion may be necessary (some narcotics may have longer duration of action than naloxone). Naloxone is currently under investigation for many other purposes besides reversal of narcotic actions.

(continued)

Non-Narcotic Analgesics

Drug	Supplied	Dose/Route	Remarks
Acetaminophen (Tylenol, Panadol, Datril, and others)	Caps: 325, 500 mg Tabs:160,325,500, 650 mg Liquid: 120,160 mg/5 ml, 500 mg/15 ml Granules: 80 mg Chewable tabs: 80 mg Elixir: 120, 130, 160,325 mg per 5 ml Oral solution: 100 mg/ml, 120 mg per 2.5 ml Supp: 120,125,325,650 mg	**ADULTS and CHILDREN** (>11 years): Oral or rectal: 325-650 mg PO/PR q 4-6 h prn (maximum: short-term 4 g/day, long-term 2.6 g per 24 h).	*Contraindications* include hypersensitivity to acetaminophen; overdosage presents early as nausea, vomiting, and malaise, and presents late as clinical and laboratory evidence of hepatotoxicity. Do not use charcoal to treat overdoses. Acetylcysteine (Muco-Myst) may be administered depending on the time after ingestion and the acetaminophen blood levels present.
Methotrimeprazine HCl (Levoprome)	Vials: 20 mg/ml (for deep IM injection only)	**ADULTS:** **Analgesia:** 5-40 mg IM q 1-24 h prn. **Pre-op:** 2-20 mg IM 45 min to 3 h preop. **Post-op:** 2.5-7.5 mg q 4-6 h prn.	May be useful in pain complicated by a strong emotional component. Possible alternative to opiate agonists in patients with decreased lower GI motility. May produce too much sedation for use in chronic (except terminal) pain. Do not administer longer than 30 days except in terminal cases or when opiates are contraindicated. *Contraindicated* in patients

			who are hypersensitive to phenothiazines, or with severe renal, cardiac, or hepatic disease or a history of convulsive disorders. Adverse effects include orthostatic hypotension, nausea, vomiting, hematologic and hepatic effects with long-term use of high doses, neurologic reactions, cardiovascular effects, dermatologic and ocular disorders. See phenothiazines for additional comments.
Tramadol HCl (Ultram)	Tabs: 50 mg	**Analgesia:** 50-100 mg q 4-6 h prn up to 400 mg/day. Reduce dose in renal function impairment to 12 h dosing interval with maximum 200 mg/day. **Hepatic function impairment:** 50 mg q 12 h.	Centrally-acting analgesic used in acute and chronic pain. Low abuse/dependence potential compared with morphine and related centrally-acting analgesics. Causes significantly less respiratory depression than morphine. Most common adverse effects include dizziness, somnolence, headache, seizures, CNS stimulation, nausea/vomiting, constipation. Reduce dose in the elderly. Safe use in pregnancy has not been established. Patients receiving carbamazepine chronically may require up to twice the recommended dose. Use with caution in patients taking CNS depressants or MAO inhibitors.

(continued)

Non-Steroidal Anti-Inflammatory Agents

Drug	Supplied	Dose/Route	Remarks
Aspirin (ASA, acetylsalicylic acid)	Tabs: 325,500,650 mg Tabs (enteric coated): 81,165,325,500,650, 975 mg Tabs (chewable): 75, 81 mg Tabs (extended-release): 650,800 mg Tabs (film coated): 325,500 mg Supp: 60,120,125,200, 300,325,600,650 mg. Aspirin with buffers also available.	**ADULTS** (Oral or Rectal): **Pain and fever:** 325-650 mg PO/PR q 4 h prn. Maximum 4 g in 24 h. **Inflammatory diseases:** Initial: 2.4-3.6 g per day (divided doses); Maintenance: 3.6-5.4 g per day (divided doses). **Thrombosis: TIAs and stroke:** 1.3 g/day in 2-4 divided doses. **Myocardial infarction:** 160-325 mg once daily.	*Caution* in peptic ulcer disease, platelet disorders, anticoagulant therapy (Coumadin), hypoprothrombinemia, and asthma. *Contraindications* include hypersensitivity to salicylates and in patients with bleeding disorders. Cross-sensitivity may exist with other NSAIDS or tartazine dye. Adverse reactions include GI disturbances, GI bleeding, tinnitus and hearing loss, hepatotoxicity, renal dysfunction. *Contraindicated* in children or teenagers with Varicella or influenza and during presumed outbreaks of these diseases. *Contraindicated* in pregnancy.

Choline and magnesium salicylate (Trilisate)	Tabs: 500, 750, 1000 (expressed as mg of salicylate) Solution: Choline salicylate: 293 mg/5 ml Magnesium salicylate: 362 mg/5 ml (each 5 ml; of solution is equivalent to one Trilisate-500 tablet)	**ADULTS** (Oral): **Anti-inflammatory:** Initial: 1.5-2.5 g of salicylate daily as single dose or in 2-3 divided doses, with food or fluids. Maintenance: 1-4.5 g salicylate daily.	Anti-inflammatory, analgesic, and anti-pyretic effects probably comparable to ASA (500 mg salicylate is equivalent to 650 mg ASA). Does not inhibit platelet aggregation (cannot be used for prophylaxis of thrombosis). See aspirin for additional comments.
Diclofenac potassium (Cataflam)	Tabs: 50 mg	**Osteo- and rhemuatoid arthritis:** same as sodium salt. **Analgesia and primary dysmenorrhea** (potassium salt only): 50 mg tid (initial dose may be 100 mg). Maximum dose 150 mg/day (200 mg on 1st day).	See ibuprofen for additional comments.
Diclofenac sodium (Voltaren)	Tabs (enteric coated): 25, 50, 75 mg	**ADULTS** (Oral with food or milk): **Osteoarthritis:** 100-150 mg/day in divided doses. **Rheumatoid arthritis:** 150-200 mg/ day in divided doses. **Ankylosing spondylitis:** 25 mg qid.	See ibuprofen for additional comments.

(continued)

Non-Steroidal Anti-Inflammatory Agents—*(cont.)*

Drug	Supplied	Dose/Route	Remarks
Diflunisal (Dolobid)	Tabs: 250, 500 mg	**ADULTS** (Oral): **Anti-inflammatory:** 250-500 mg q 12 h with meals or milk. Maximum 1.5 g/day. **Analgesia:** 500-1000 mg PO, then 250-500 mg q 8-12 h with meals or milk. Maximum: 1.5 g in 24 h. **Do not chew or crush tablets.**	Non-steroidal anti-inflammatory agent. See ibuprofen for additional comments.
Etodolac (Lodine)	Caps: 200, 300 mg Tabs: 400 mg	**ADULTS** (Oral): **Osteoarthritis:** Initial 800-1200 mg/day in divided doses with food or milk. (Maximum 1200 mg/day.) **Analgesia:** 200-400 mg q 6-8 h prn. (Maximum 1200 mg/day.) Patients <60 kg: maximum 20 mg/kg/day.	See ibuprofen for additional comments.
Fenoprofen (Nalfon)	Caps: 200,300 mg Tabs: 600 mg (scored)	**ADULTS** (Oral): **Anti-inflammatory**: 300-600 mg tid or qid with meals or milk; increase dose depending on patient response. Maximum: 3.2 g in 24 h. **Analgesia:** 200-400 mg q 4-6 h prn with meals or milk.	*Contraindicated* in pre-existing renal disease. See ibuprofen for additional comments.

Flurbiprofen (ANSAID)	Tabs: 50, 100 mg	**ADULTS** (Oral): **Anti-inflammatory:** Initial: 200-300 mg daily in 2, 3, or 4 divided doses, with food or milk. (Maximum 300 mg/day with 100 mg maximum single dose.)	See ibuprofen for additional comments.
Ibuprofen (Motrin, Advil, Nuprin, Rufen)	Tabs: 200, 300, 400, 600, 800 mg Oral susp: 100 mg/5 ml	**ADULTS** (Oral): **Anti-inflammatory:** 400-800 mg tid or qid with meals or milk (maximum 3.2 g in 24 h). **Antipyretic, analgesia and dysmenorrhea:** 200-400 mg q 4-6 h.	*Adverse reactions* include GI tract disturbances (including ulcers and bleeding), CNS changes, hepatotoxicity, hematologic toxicity, renal toxicity, and edema. Use with *caution* in patients with peptic ulcer disease, bleeding abnormalities, renal dysfunction, hypertension, and cardiac dysfunction. *Contraindication* include hypersensitivity to ibuprofen and in patients in whom asthma, rhinitis, or urticaria is precipitated by aspirin or other NSAIAs. May inhibit platelet aggregation. May increase prothrombin time in patients receiving oral anticoagulants. Exercise caution if used concurrently with methotrexate or cyclosporin. Avoid concurrent use with salicylates. Avoid use during pregnancy.

(continued)

Non-Steroidal Anti-Inflammatory Agents—*(cont.)*

Drug	Supplied	Dose/Route	Remarks
Indomethacin (Indocin, Indocin SR, Indocin-IV)	Caps: 25, 50 mg; Caps, extended release: 75 mg; Oral susp: 25 mg/5 ml; Supp: 50 mg.	**ADULTS** (Oral or rectal): **Anti-inflammatory:** 25 mg PO/PR bid or tid; increase dose 25-50 mg/day q 7 days. Maximum 150-200 mg/day. **Rheumatoid arthritis, osteoarthritis, ankylosing spondylitis, acute painful shoulder:** 75-150 mg/day in 3-4 divided doses x 7-14 days. **Acute gouty arthritis:** 50 mg tid until pain is tolerable, then rapidly decrease dose; swelling disappears in 3-5 days. Extended-release cap (do not use in acute gouty arthritis): 75 mg PO QD as alternative to 25 mg cap tid; 75 mg bid as alternative to 50 mg cap tid.	Ocular and otic reactions may occur. CNS effects include headache, dizziness, aggravation of depression or other psychological disturbances, epilepsy, and parkinsonism. *Not* recommended for use as a simple analgesic due to toxicity. See ibuprofen for additional comments.
Ketoprofen (Orudis, Oruvail Extended-Release Caps)	Caps: 25,50,75 mg Caps (extended release): 200 mg	**ADULTS and CHILDREN** (>12 years): **Anti-inflammatory** (Oral): Initial: 75 mg tid or 50 mg qid with food or milk. Maintenance: 150-300 mg daily in 3-4 divided doses. **Pain, Dysmenorrhea:** 25-50 mg q 6-8 h prn; maximum 300 mg/day. **Extended-release cap (chronic treatment):** 200 mg qd.	Reduce dose by 33-50% in impaired renal function, impaired hepatic function, and/or geriatric patients. See ibuprofen for additional comments.

Ketorolac tromethamine (Toradol)	Disposable syringe: 15, 30 mg/ml Tabs: 10 mg	**ADULTS** (Parenteral): Single dose: < 65 yo: 60 mg IM or 30 mg IVP; ≥ 65 yo, renal impairment, or weight < 50 kg: 30 mg IM or 15 mg IVP. Multiple dose: < 65 yo: 30 mg IM/IVP q 6 h (maximum 120 mg/day); ≥ 65 yo, renal impairment, or weight < 50 kg: 15 mg IM/IVP q 6 h (maximum 60 mg/day). **ADULTS** (transition from IM/IV to oral): < 65 yo: 20 mg PO as 1st oral dose, then 10 mg PO q 4-6 h up to maximum of 40 mg/day; ≥ 65 yo, renal impairment, or weight < 50 kg: 10 mg PO as 1st oral dose, then 10 mg PO q 4-6 h up to maximum of 40 mg/day.	Indicated for short-term management of moderately severe acute pain that requires analgesia at the opioid level (not indicated for minor or chronic pain) due to risk of adverse effects. Combined duration of parenteral and oral therapy not to exceed 5 days. Oral therapy is indicated only as continuation therapy to IM/IV. Do not increase dose or frequency for breakthrough pain—may supplement with low-dose opioids. *Contraindicated* as prophylactic analgesia prior to or during major surgery. *Contraindicated* in obstetric patients in labor and delivery, patients with advanced renal impairment (or at high risk), and patients with history of peptic ulcer disease or GI bleeding. See ibuprofen for additional comments.
Meclofenamate sodium (Meclomen)	Caps: 50,100 mg	**ADULTS** (Oral): **Anti-inflammatory:** 200-400 mg daily in 3-4 divided doses with meals or milk. Maximum: 400 mg in 24 h. **Idiopathic excessive menstrual blood loss and primary dysmenorrhea:** 100 mg tid for up to 6 days starting at onset of menstruation.	See ibuprofen for additional comments.

(continued)

Non-Steroidal Anti-Inflammatory Agents—*(cont.)*

Drug	Supplied	Dose/Route	Remarks
Mefenamic acid (Ponstel)	Caps: 250 mg	**ADULTS: Analgesia or dysmenorrhea:** 500 mg PO, then 250 mg PO q 6 h with meals, up to 7 days (3 days for dysmenorrhea).	*Contraindicated* in pre-existing renal disease. May cause photosensitivity reaction. See ibuprofen for additional comments.
Nabumetone (Relafen)	Tabs: 500, 750 mg	**Osteoarthritis and rheumatoid arthritis (acute/chronic treatment):** 1000 mg qd with or without food, up to 2000 mg/day (may be given once or twice daily).	Use with caution in impaired hepatic function.
Naproxen (Naprosyn) **Naproxen enteric-coated** (Naprosyn) **Naproxen sodium** (Aleve, Anaprox)	Tabs: 250, 375, 500 mg (Naprosyn); 275, 550 mg (Anaprox); 220 mg (Aleve). Enteric-coated tabs: 375, 500 mg. Oral susp: 125 mg/5 ml	**ADULTS** (Oral): **Rheumatoid arthritis, osteoarthritis, ankylosing spondylitis:** 250-500 mg bid (275-550 mg Anaprox) up to 1.5 g/day (1.65 g Anaprox); Enteric-coated tabs (Naprosyn): 375-500 mg bid. **Acute gouty arthritis:** 750 mg PO, then 250 mg q 8 h until attack subsides (875 mg PO, then 275 mg q 8 h—Anaprox). Analgesia, primary dysmenorrhea, acute tendinitis and bursitis: 500 mg PO, then 250 mg q 6-8 h (550 mg PO, then 275 mg q 6-8 h—Anaprox). Maximum 1.25 g (1.375 g Anaprox) per day. OTC Recommendations (Aleve):	Dose may need to be reduced in cirrhotic liver patients. Enteric-coated tabs not recommended for acute pain or gout due to delay in absorption. See ibuprofen for additional comments.

		Analgesia, antipyretic: 200 mg q 8-12 h (initial dose may be 400 mg, then 200 mg 12 h later). Maximum 660 mg/day. Reduce dose to 220 mg q 12 h in patients >65 yo.	
Oxaprozin (Daypro)	Caplets: 600 mg	**ADULTS** (Oral): **Osteoarthritis and rheumatoid arthritis:** 1200 mg qd. May reduce dose in patients with low body weight. Maximum 1800 mg/day (or 26 mg/kg, whichever is lower) in divided doses. Reduce dose in renal impairment to 600 mg qd.	Use with caution in severe hepatic impairment. See ibuprofen for additional comments.
Piroxicam (Feldene)	Caps: 10,20 mg	**ADULTS** (Oral): **Osteoarthritis and rheumatoid arthritis:** 0 mg PO QD with meal or milk. May give in divided doses.	See ibuprofen for additional comments.
Sulindac (Clinoril)	Tabs: 150,200 mg (scored)	**ADULTS** (Oral): **Osteoarthritis, rheumatoid arthritis, ankylosing spondylitis:** 150 mg PO bid with meals or milk; increase dose depending on patient response. Maximum: 400 mg in 24 h. **Acute painful shoulder (bursitis and/or tendinitis) or acute gouty arthritis:** 200 mg bid x 7-14 days. Maximum 400 mg in 24 h.	Dose may need to be reduced in cirrhotic liver patients. See ibuprofen for additional comments.

(continued)

Non-Steroidal Anti-Inflammatory Agents—*(cont.)*

Drug	Supplied	Dose/Route	Remarks
Tolmetin sodium (Tolectin, Tolectin DS)	Caps: 400 mg (DS) Tabs: 200, 600 mg	**ADULTS** (Oral): **Rheumatoid and osteoarthritis:** 400 mg PO tid with meals or milk; increase dose depending on patient response. Maximum: 1800 mg in 24 h.	See ibuprofen for additional comments.

Potassium-Removing Resins

Drug	Supplied	Dose/Route	Remarks
Sodium polystyrene sulfonate (Kayexalate)	Susp: 15 g with 21.5 ml sorbitol and 65 mEq Na per 60 ml	Oral: 15-60 g 1-4 times per day. Enema: 30-50 g q 6 h.	Treatment of hyperkalemia. The exchange capacity *in vivo* is approximiately 1 mEq potassium per gram. However, there is a large range of response. Watch serum sodium.

Pulmonary

Drug	Supplied	Dose/Route	Remarks
Acetazolamide (Diamox)	Vial: 500 mg Tabs: 125,250 mg Caps (sustained release): 500 mg	250-500 mg IV q 6 h prn, or 125-250 mg PO q 6 h prn.	Treatment of metabolic alkalosis. Used when arterial pH exceeds 7.45, serum bicarbonate exceeds 29 mEq/dl, and serum K^+ is normal.
Albuterol (Proventil, Ventolin)	Oral solution: 2 mg/5 ml Tabs: 2, 4 mg Metered dose inhaler: 90 µg/spray	2-4 mg PO tid or 2 inhalations q 4-6 h	β_2 agonist. Use with caution in cardiac disease because it can cause systemic vasodilation and tachycardia.

Bitolterol (Tornalate)	Metered dose inhaler: 370 mg/spray	2 inhalations q 4-6 h	See albuterol.
Ipratropium (Atrovent)	Metered dose inhaler: 18 mg/spray	2 inhalations q 6 h	Synthetic quaternary ammonium compound chemically related to atropine. Achieves bronchodilation in patients with COPD including bronchitis and emphysema.
Metaproterenol (Alupent, Metaprel)	Oral solution: 10 mg/5 ml Metered dose inhaler: 0.65 mg/spray Solution for nebulization: 0.6%, 5%	20 mg PO q 6 or 8 h; or 2-3 inhalations by metered dose inhaler, 2.5 ml of the 0.6% solution *or* 0.2-0.3 ml of the 5% solution in 2.5 ml NS by hand-held nebulizer q 4-6 h.	β_2 agonist. Use with caution in cardiac disease because it can cause systemic vasodilation and tachycardia.
Pirbuterol (Maxair)	Metered dose inhaler: 200 mg/spray	2 inhalations q 4-6 h	See albuterol.
Salmeterol (Serevent)	Metered dose inhaler: 25 µg/spray	Inhalation bid.	Long-acting agent requiring only twice-daily dosing.
Terbutaline (Brethine, Bricanyl)	Tabs: 2.5, 5.0 mg Vial: 1 mg/ml Metered dose inhaler: 200 µg/spray	2.5 to 5 mg PO tid, or 0.25 mg SC q 4-6 h, or 2 inhalations q 4-6 h.	β_2 agonist. Use with caution in cardiac disease because it can cause systemic vasodilation and tachycardia.

(continued)

Pulmonary—*(cont.)*

Drug	Supplied	Dose/Route	Remarks
THEOPHYLLINES:			
1 Aminophylline (85% theophylline)	**Short action** (q 6 h doses): Tabs: 100,200 mg Liquid: 105 mg/5 ml **Sustained release:** Phyllocontin: Tab: 225 mg **Parenteral:** Available for dilution in common IV solutions.	IV: Loading dose of 3-6 mg of aminophylline over 20 mg, then maintenance infusion of 0.1 to 0.5 mg/kg/h. PO: Maintenance dose of 500-1100 mg/day in divided doses.	Maintenance dose is adjusted to maintain serum theophylline levels between 10-20 µg/ml. Lower maintenance dose should be used in patients with congestive heart failure or liver failure. Nausea, vomiting, and cardiac dysrhythmias can occur more frequently when levels exceed 20 µg/ml. Seizures may occur when serum levels exceed 30 µg/ml. Diarrhea may occur with use of liquid.

2 Theophylline	**Short action** (q 6 h doses): 1. Elixophyllin: Liquid: 27 mg/5 ml 2. Slo-Phyllin: Liquid: 27 mg/5 ml Tabs: 100,200 mg 3. Theolair: Liquid: 27 mg/5 ml Tabs: 125,250 mg **Sustained release** (q 8-12 h doses): 1. Theodur: Tabs: 100,200,300 mg 2. Uniphyl: Tabs: 200,400 mg **Parenteral:** 0.4-4 mg/ml in 5% dextrose	IV: Loading dose of 2.5-5 mg/kg of theophylline over 20 min, then maintenance infusion of 0.08 to 0.39 mg/kg/h. PO: Maintenance dose of 400-900 mg/day in divided doses.	Maintenance dose is adjusted to maintain serum theophylline levels between 10-20 μg/ml. Lower maintenance dose should be used in patients with congestive heart failure or liver failure. Nausea, vomiting, and cardiac dysrhythmias can occur more frequently when levels exceed 20 μg/ml. Seizures may occur when serum levels exceed 30 μg/ml. After dosage adjustment is made, wait at least 24 h before obtaining repeat theophylline level.

Sedatives

Buspirone hydrochloride (Buspar)	Tabs: 5,10 mg	**ADULTS:** Oral: **Sedation:** Initial 5 mg tid; increase 5 mg/day at 2-3 day intervals, up to 60 mg/day. Common dosage is 20-30 mg/day in divided doses.	Do *not* use in severe hepatic/renal impairment. *Caution* in pregnancy.

(continued)

Sedatives—*(cont.)*

Drug	Supplied	Dose/Route	Remarks
Chloral hydrate	Caps: 250,500 mg Oral solution: 250,500 mg/5 ml Supp: 325,500,650 mg	**ADULTS :** Oral and Rectal: **Sedation:** 250 mg PO/PR tid. **Hypnotic:** 500-1000 mg PO/PR at bedtime; increase dose gradually up to 2 g per dose. **CHILDREN:** Oral and Rectal: **Sedation:** 8.3 mg/kg PO/PR tid (up to 500 mg tid). **Hypnotic:** 50 mg/kg PO/PR (up to 1 g dose).	Adverse reactions include GI tract disturbances, CNS disturbances. *Contraindications* include patients with marked hepatic or renal disease and patients with hypersensitivity or idiosyncratic reactions to chloral hydrate. Use with caution in patients on warfarin therapy. May interfere with some urine glucose tests.
Diphenhydramine hydrochloride (Benadryl)	Caps: 25,50 mg Oral elixir: 12.5 mg/5 ml Oral solution: 12.5 mg/5 ml Tabs: 25,50 mg Vials: 10,50 mg/ml Topical cream: 1%,2% Topical lotion: 1% Topical spray: 1%, 2%	**ADULTS:** Oral and Parenteral: 25-50 mg PO/IM/IV q 6 h. Topical: 1-2% applied to area tid or qid. **CHILDREN:** Oral and Parenteral: 5 mg/kg daily in 3 or 4 divided doses.	Adverse reactions include CNS depression and other CNS disturbances, CNS tract disturbances. Use with caution in patients with angle-closure glaucoma, prostatic hypertrophy, stenosing peptic ulcer, pyloroduodenal obstruction or bladder neck obstruction, asthma, COPD, increased intraocular pressure, hyperthyroidism, cardiovascular disease, and hypertension. *Contraindications* include patients with acute asthma attacks and hypersensitivity to drug. May cause CNS stimulant effect, especially in children.

Hydroxyzine hydrochloride and pamoate (Vistaril, Atarax)	Caps: 25,50,100 mg Tabs: 10,25,50,100 mg Tabs (film-coated): 10,25,50,100 mg Oral solution: 10 mg/5 ml Oral susp: 25 mg/5 ml Vials: 25,50 mg/ml	**ADULTS:** Oral: **Pruritis:** 25-50 mg PO qid. **Sedation:** 50-100 mg PO qid. Parenteral (IM only): 25-100 mg qid. **CHILDREN:** Oral: **Pruritis and sedation:** < 6 years old: 50 mg daily; > 6 years old: 50-100 mg daily in divided doses. Parenteral (IM only): **Pre-op:** 0.6 mg/kg.	Use Z-track technique for IM administration. Do *not* give IV. Adverse reactions include CNS depression and other CNS disturbances, local discomfort, and sterile abscesses with IM injections.
Pentobarbital (Nembutal)	Caps: 50,100 mg Oral elixir: 18.2 mg/5 ml Vials: 50 mg/ml Supp: 30,60,120, 200 mg	**ADULTS** (Oral, Parenteral, Rectal): **Sedation:** 20-40 mg PO/IV/IM/PR bid or qid. **Hypnotic:** 100-200 mg PO/IV/IM/PR at bedtime. **CHILDREN** (Oral, Parenteral, Rectal): **Sedation:** 2-6 mg/kg daily in 3 divided doses (up to 100 mg daily).	Rate of IV administration should not exceed 50 mg/min. Gradual withdrawal of pentobarbital is recommended after prolonged use. Do *not* administer more than 250 mg or 5 ml at any given site. See phenobarbital for additional comments.
Zolpidem (Ambien)	Tabs: 5,10 mg	5-10 mg qhs.	Non-benzodiazepine sedative/hypnotic for sleep.

(continued)

Serums

Drug	Supplied	Dose/Route	Remarks
Cytomegalovirus Immune Globulin Intravenous (CMV-IGIV)	Powder for injection: 2500 mg ± 250 mg^2	**Time** / **Dose** Within 2 h of transplant: 150 mg/kg; 2 weeks post-transplant: 100 mg/kg; 4 weeks post-transplant: 100 mg/kg; 6 weeks post-transplant: 100 mg/kg; 8 weeks post-transplant:: 100 mg/kg; 12 weeks post-transplant: 50 mg/kg; 16 weeks post-transplant: 50 mg/kg.	Attenuation of pulmonary CMV disease associated with kidney transplant. For transplant recipients who are seronegative for CMV and who receive a kidney from a seropositive CMV donor.
Hepatitis B immune globulin (H-BIG, Hep-B-Gammagee, HyperHep)	Vial: 5 ml	0.06 ml/kg IM within 24-48 h of exposure, and also 1 month later.	Post-exposure prophylaxis is recommended following either needlestick or direct mucous membrane inoculation or oral ingestion involving HB_SAg-positive materials such as blood, plasma, serum. Confirmation of HB_SAg in the donor is *essential* and anti-HB_S screening of potential recipient is desirable prior to receipt of HBIG.

Immune Globulin (IG) for Hepatitis A (Gammar, Gamastan)	IM Vial: 5 ml	IM: **Pre-exposure:** Travelers to endemic areas: Residence for <3 months: 0.02 ml/kg IM one-time dose. Residence for >3 months: 0.06 ml/kg IM q 5 months. **Post-exposure**—*close* contact: 0.02 ml/kg IM one-time dose. *In cases of common source exposure, IG is *not* recommended once cases have begun to occur.	
Immune Globulin Intravenous (IGIV) (Gamimmune N, Gammagard, Gammar IV, Iveegam, Sandoglobulin Venoglobulin-1)		IV: 200-400 mg/kg. First dose must be infused slowly to avoid a precipitous fall in blood pressure and the clinical picture of anaphylaxis. Consult pharmacy for rate of administration of the various products.	Indicated for immunodeficiency syndrome and idiopathic thrombocytopenia purpura (ITP).
Lymphocyte Immune Globulin, Anti-Thymocyte Globulin (Atgam)	Injection: 50 mg/ml	IV: 10-30 mg/kg day **Test dose**: Intradermal 0.1 ml of a 1:1000 dilution.	Only physicians experienced in immunosuppressive therapy should use this product. Used for management of allograft rejection in renal transplant patients.

(continued)

Serums—*(cont.)*

Drug	Supplied	Dose/Route	Remarks
Tetanus Antitoxin	Injection: Not less than 400 units/ml	IM: **Prophylaxis:** Patients ≤ 30 kg—1500 units Patients >30 kg—3000-5000 units **Treatment:** 50,000-100,000 units	For prevention of tetanus when tetanus immune globulin is not available.
Tetanus Immune Globulin (Hyper-Tet)	Injection: 250 units	IM only: 250 units.	For passive immunization against tetanus.
Varicella-Zoster Immune Globulin (VZIG)	Injection: 125 units	Deep IM only in a large muscle mass; 125 units per 10 kg up to a maximum of 625 units. Do *not* give fractional doses.	Administer as soon as possible after presumed exposure.

Skeletal Muscle Relaxants

[General Information for Neuromuscular Blockers: To minimize the possibility of overdosage and prolonged paralyzation, use a peripheral nerve stimulation to monitor muscle twitch response (Train of Four). Neuromuscular blockers have no effect on sensorium or pain threshold. Therefore, paralyzation must be accompanied by continuous sedation and, if indicated, analgesia.]

Drug	Supplied	Dose/Route	Remarks
Atracurium besylate (Tracrium)	Vials: 10 mg/ml	**ADULTS AND CHILDREN** (>2 years old): Parenteral (IV push): Initial dose: 0.4-0.5 mg/kg IV for intubation. **To facilitate mechanical ventilation:** Loading dose: 0.4-0.5 mg/kg; Infusion: 0.5-1 mg/kg/h.	Non-depolarizing neuromuscular blocking agent. Adverse reactions include histamine release effects and cardiovascular changes. Use with *extreme caution* in myasthenia gravis. Useful in impaired hepatic function due to lack of dependence on biliary excretion. *Contraindications* include hypersensitivity to

			atracurium. Doses may be reduced depending on anesthetic agent used. Burn patients may need substantially larger doses.
Doxacurium (Nuromax)	Vials: 1 mg/ml	Parenteral: 0.05 mg/kg **To facilitate mechanical ventilation:** 0.03 mg/kg bolus followed by 0.01-0.03 mg/kg/h.	Intermediate-acting agent.
Mivacurium (Mivacron)	Vials: 2 mg/ml Premixed infusion in D5W 50 ml: 0.5 mg/ml	**ADULTS** Parenteral: Initial dose: 0.15 mg/kg for intubation. Maintenance dose: 0.1 mg/kg at 15-minute intervals. Continuous infusion: After early evidence of spontaneous recovery from initial dose, start infusion at 9-10 μg/kg/min. If the infusion is started at the same time as the initial dose, use 4 μg/kg/min. **CHILDREN** (2-12 years): Initial dose: 0.2 mg/kg over 5-15 sec. Maintenance doses are usually required more frequently than in adults. Continuous infusion: Average 14 μg/kg/min (range 5-31 μg/kg/min).	Non-depolarizing agent with a very short half-life as compared to other agents. Onset of maximum blockade is approximately 2 minutes (intermediate). Contraindicated in allergic hypersensitivity to mivacurium. Multiple dose vial contains benzyl alcohol. Decreased clearance in renal failure and hepatic failure.

(continued)

Skeletal Muscle Relaxants—*(cont.)*

Drug	Supplied	Dose/Route	Remarks
Pancuronium bromide (Pavulon)	Amps: 2 mg/ml Vials: 1 mg/ml	**ADULTS AND CHILDREN** (>1 month old): Parenteral: 0.04-0.1 mg/kg IV; additional doses of 0.01 mg/kg may be administered at 25 and 60 min intervals. **To facilitate mechanical ventilation:** Loading dose: 0.03-0.1 mg/kg; Infusion: 0.06-0.1 mg/kg/h.	Non-depolarizing neuromuscular blocking agent. Adverse reactions include tachycardia, increase in blood pressure. Use with *caution* in renal disease. *Contraindications* include hypersensitivity to pancuronium and/or bromides. Doses may be reduced depending on anesthetic agent used. Causes minimal histamine release and no ganglionic blockade (does not cause bronchospasm or hypotension).
Pipecuronium bromide (Ardvan)	Powder for injection: 10 mg/vial	**ADULTS: Endotracheal intubation under balanced anesthesia, halothane, isoflurane, or enflurane.** Initial dose in non-obese patients with normal renal function: 0.07-0.085 mg/kg. Maintenance: 0.01-0.015 mg/kg. When administered at 25% of control T, provides ~50 min duration. **CHILDREN (under balanced anesthesia or halothane):** 0.04 mg/kg in infants (3 mo - 1 yr); 0.57 mg/kg in children (1-14 yrs).	Long-acting non-depolarizing neuromuscular blocker to provide skeletal muscle relaxation during general anesthesia and during endotracheal intubation. Only recommended for procedures lasting at least 90 minutes. Adjust dose based on creatinine clearance and ideal body weight. Not recommended for use in ICU patients requiring prolonged mechanical ventilation. Adverse effects include hypotension and bradycardia.

Rocuronium (Zemuron)	Vials: 10 mg/ml	Parenteral: 0.6 mg/kg	Similar to vecuronium except for a faster onset of action.
Succinylcholine chloride	Amps: 50 mg/ml Vials: 20,100 mg/ml Powder for injection: 100 mg per vial. Powder for infusion: 500 mg or 1 g per vial.	**ADULTS:** Parenteral: **Test dose:** 0.1 mg/kg IV. **Short procedures:** 0.6 mg/kg IV over 10-30 sec (0.3-1.1 mg/kg). **Prolonged procedures:** 2.5 mg/min IV infusion (0.5-10 mg/min) or 2.5-4 mg/kg IM (up to 150 mg). **CHILDREN:** Parenteral: 1-2 mg/kg IV or 2.5-4 mg/kg IM. Continuous IV infusion unsafe due to risk of malignant hyperthermia.	Ultra-short-acting depolarizing neuromuscular blocking agent. Doses may be reduced depending on anesthetic agent used. Adverse reactions include bradycardia, hypotension, and cardiac arrhythmias. Use with *extreme caution* in patients recovering from severe trauma, patients with electrolyte imbalances, patients on quinidine or digitalis, patients with pre-existing hyperkalemia, paraplegia, extensive or severe burns, extensive denervation of skeletal muscle, head trauma, degenerative or dystrophic neuromuscular disease, during ocular surgery, and glaucoma. *Contraindications* include hypersensitivity to succinylcholine, genetically determined disorders of plasma pseudocholinesterase, history of malignant hyperthermia, myopathies associated with elevated serum creatine kinase values, angle-closure glaucoma, or penetrating eye injuries.

(continued)

Skeletal Muscle Relaxants—*(cont.)*

Drug	Supplied	Dose/Route	Remarks
Vecuronium bromide (Norcuron)	Vials: 10 mg for reconstitution	Intubation: 0.08-0.1 mg/kg IV. Maintenance: **Balanced anesthesia:** 0.01-0.015 mg/kg IV; **Inhalation anesthesia:** 0.008- 0.012 mg/kg IV. **CHILDREN** (<10 years old): 1-9 years old: may require higher initial doses than adults; <1 year old: more sensitive to the drug. **To facilitate mechanical ventilation:** Loading dose: 0.1 mg/kg; Infusion: 0.05-0.1 mg/kg/h.	Non-depolarizing neuromuscular blocking agent. Adverse reactions include cardiovascular changes which are usually minimal and transient. Use with *caution* in liver dysfunction and in patients with myasthenia gravis. *Contraindications* include hypersensitivity to vecuronium. Doses may be reduced depending on anesthetic agent used. Burn patients may require substantially higher doses. Not recommended for children under 7 weeks old. May accumulate, causing prolonged paralyzation, if used as a continuous infusion in severe renal failure (CrCl <30 ml/min).

Steroids—Clinical Uses (see also "Preoperative Preparation")

Equivalents: Methylprednisolone 4 mg = Prednisone 5 mg = Hydrocortisone 20 mg.

1. Physiological replacement.
   a.
      1) Hydrocortisone: 12.5 mg/M2/day IM or IV, qd; 25.0 mg/M2/day PO in 3 divided doses.
      2) Cortisone acetate: 15-16 mg/M2/day IM or IV, qd; 30-32 mg/M2/day PO in 3 divided doses.

   b. Mineralocorticoid.
      1) Deoxycorticosterone acetate (DOCA): 1.0-2.0 mg/day IM (in oil), single dose.
      2) 9-alpha-fluorocortisol (Florinef): 0.05-0.15 mg/day PO.
2. Acute adrenal insufficiency—Hydrocortisone: 100 mg IV push loading dose, then 100 mg IVPB q 8 h.

3. Chronic adrenal insufficiency—Hydrocortisone: 30 mg qd PO in divided doses (20 mg PO a.m., 10 mg PO p.m.).
4. Cerebral edema—Dexamethasone: 10 mg IV loading dose, then 4 mg IV q 4-6 h for 36-72 h.
5. Sarcoidosis—Prednisone: 40 mg PO qd.
6. Acute polyneuritis—Prednisone: 40 mg PO qd.
7. Polymyositis and dermatomyositis—Prednisone: 40-60 mg PO qd.
8. Anti-inflammatory.
   a. Prednisone: less than 100 mg/day.
   b. Dexamethasone: 3-6 mg/kg IV bolus, then 3-6 mg/kg IVPB q 2 h until positive response, or up to 3 doses.
9. Idiopathic thrombocytopenia—Prednisone: 1.0-2.0 mg/kg/day PO.
10. Periarteritis nodosa—Prednisone: 40-60 mg PO qd.
11. Wegener's granulomatosis—Prednisone: 60 mg PO qd.
12. Systemic lupus erythematosis—Prednisone: 40-60 mg PO qd.
13. Pemphigus vulgaris—Prednisone: 80-300 mg PO qd.
14. Keloids, intra-articular administration.
   a. Dexamethasone suspension (8 mg/ml vial).
      1) Large joints: 2-4 mg.
      2) Small joints: 0.8-1.0 mg.
      3) Soft tissue infiltration: 2-6 mg.
      4) Ganglia: 1-2 mg.
      5) Tendon sheaths: 0.4-1.0 mg.
   b. Triamcinolone hexacetonide (Aristospan): 5 mg or 20 mg/ml, or triamcinolone acetonide (Kenalog).
      1) Soft-tissue infiltration up to 0.5 mg/in^2.
      2) Intraarticular 2-20 mg (depending on joint size and degree of inflammation) q 3-4 weeks.
      3) Up to 1 ml of 1% lidocaine may be administered simultaneously to promote immediate relief.
15. Spinal cord injury—Methylprednisolone: 30 mg/kg IV bolus over 1 h, then 5.4 mg/kg/h for 23 h.

(continued)

Topicals, Antiseptics, Disinfectants

Drug	Supplied	Dose/Route	Remarks
Bacitracin preparations 1. Bacitracin zinc 400 units/g plus Neomycin sulfate 0.5% plus Polymyxin B sulfate 5000 units/g (Neosporin, Triple Antibiotic ointment) 2. Hydrocortisone 1.0% plus all the medications in #2 above (Cortisporin ointment). 3. Bacitracin zinc 500 units/g plus Polymyxin B sulfate 10,000 units/g (Polysporin ointment [PSO]).	Ointment: 500 units/g	Topical application qd to tid	For the treatment of superficial skin infections. May lead to fungal overgrowth, especially *Candida*. Bacitracin is active against many gram-positives. Bactericidal and bacteriostatic. Not absorbed in any appreciable amount from skin, denuded skin, wounds, or mucous membranes. Low toxicity topically, but anaphylactoid reactions have occurred. Local irritation, itching, or burning should lead to discontinuation of the preparation.

Chlorhexidine gluconate (Exidine-2, Hibiclens, Hibistat)	Exidine-2 scrub: 2% solution with 4% isopropyl alcohol Hibiclens: 4% in base. Hibistat: 0.5% weight/weight chlorhexidine in 70% isopropanol with emollients.	Topical	For wound antisepsis, general skin cleansing, and surgical scrubs. pH range 5-8. Effective against gram-positives (10 μg/ml), gram-negatives (50 μg/ml), and fungi (200 μg/ml). Rapid acting, considerable residual activity, low potential for contact- and photosensitivity; is poorly absorbed. No plasmid-mediated resistance.
Dakin's Solution	0.5% sodium hypochlorite adjusted to neutral pH with $NaHCO_3$	Topical	Use 1/4 (0.125%) to 1/2 (0.25%) strength solution in treatment of suppurative wounds; solvent action in debridement of wounds. Active against vegetative bacteria and viruses, spores, and fungi. Avoid contact with healthy skin and eyes.
Gamma benzene (Kwell, Lindane)	Cream: 1% Lotion: 1% Shampoo: 1%	Topical: 1 oz lotion or 60 g cream.	For scabies, lice, crabs, gnats. *Contraindicated* in patients with known seizure disorders and in premature neonates due to CNS toxicity from cutaneous absorption. Use cautiously in children. Do not use prophylactically. Treat no more than twice during pregnancy. Do not apply to face or mucous membranes. Carefully follow instructions with product.

(continued)

Topicals, Antiseptics, Disinfectants—*(cont.)*

Drug	Supplied	Dose/Route	Remarks
Hexachlorophene (Phisohex, Septisol)	Solution (Phisohex): 3% Foam (Septisol): 0.23%	Topical	Bacteriostatic against gram-positive organisms. Systemic toxicity under conditions permitting absorption (e.g., skin of premature infants).
Hydrogen peroxide (H202)	Solution: 3%	Topical	When H_2O_2 comes in contact with catalase, it rapidly decomposes into H_2O and O_2 in wounds and on mucous membranes, loosening and debriding infectious detritus. Solutions diluted with mouthwash are used for stomatitis and gingivitis. *Never* use H_2O_2 in closed body cavities or abscesses—gas cannot escape.
Isopropyl alcohol	Liquid: 70% solution	Topical	Disinfectant. Avoid contact with eyes and mucous membranes.
Mafenide acetate (Sulfamylon)	Cream: 8.5%	Topical: qd to bid	Owing to superior wound penetration, it is drug of choice for established burn wound infections. When used over large areas for prolonged periods, may cause systemic toxicity, especially metabolic acidosis. *Contraindicated* in sulfa allergy. Painful on application. Not inhibited by purulent discharge. Bacteriostatic against most gram-positives, especially *Clostridia*, and

			gram-negatives, especially pseudomonas. Good anaerobic activity. Very little effect on MRSA or fungi.
Mupirocin (Bactroban)	Ointment: 2%	Topical: tid	Structurally unrelated to other available anti-infectives. Primary activity is against gram-positive aerobes, especially staphylococci (including MRSA) and streptococci species, but not enterococci. Not effective against fungi, anaerobes, or most *Enterobacteriaceae*. Used for topical treatment of impetigo and other superficial skin infections. Also used intranasally to temporarily eliminate nasal carriage of *S. aureus*.
Neomycin	Cream or ointment: 0.5% (as sulfate)	Apply qd to tid topically. Apply to soak gauze dressings bid to tid.	Aminoglycoside; bactericidal. Active against aerobic gram-negatives and some aerobic gram-positives. Inactive against viruses, fungi and most anaerobes, *E. coli*, *H. influenza*, *Proteus* sp., *Staph* sp., and *Serratis*. Minimally active against *Strep* sp.; no activity against *Pseudomonas*. Not absorbed from intact skin, but readily absorbed from denuded areas. Can be a contact sensitizer in 5-15% of patients treated. Hypersensitivity reactions dermatitis and urticaria. Cross allergenicity has been observed with other aminoglycosides.

(continued)

Topicals, Antiseptics, Disinfectants—*(cont.)*

Drug	Supplied	Dose/Route	Remarks
			Ototoxicity, nephrotoxicity, and neuromuscular blockade have been seen following topical application to large areas of altered skin integrity (e.g., burns).
Nitrofurazone (Furacin)	Cream: 0.2% Ointment: 0.2% Solution: 0.2%	Topical	Used as topical agent for skin infections and burn wounds. Bactericidal for many gram-positive and gram-negative organisms, but most *Pseudomonae* and fungi are resistant. *Avoid* in renal failure. Can cause GI disturbances, rash, pruritus; occasionally causes drug fever and neuropathy.
Podophyllin resin [*Keratolytic agent*] (Podocon-25)	Solution: 25%	Topical: applied and washed off within 1-4 h (not longer than 4-6 h); repeat weekly for up to 4 applications.	For condylomata acuminata; if no regression after 4 weekly applications, use alternative treatment such as cryo-, electro-, or laser therapy. Avoid contact with eyes and healthy tissue. Do not use on pregnant patients or patients who plan to become pregnant. Use of large amounts for widespread lesions can cause significant neuropathy and death. To be applied by physician only. Do not dispense to patient.

Povidone-iodine (Betadine, Pharmadine)	10% ointment, solution, and numerous other forms.	Topical	Bactericidal, antifungal, antiviral. Can facilitate debridement of contaminated wounds. Metabolic acidosis; some absorption. *Avoid* in iodine allergics. May be inactivated by wound exudate.
Silver nitrate	Ophthalmic solution: 1%	2 drops in each eye.	Prophylaxis of gonococcal ophthalmia neonatorum. Not effective for prevention of neonatal chlamydial conjunctivitis. *Avoid* repeated applications since cauterization of the cornea, and blindness, may result.
Silver sulfadiazine (Silvadene)	Cream: 1%	Topical to burn wounds, with dressing changes qd or bid.	Drug of choice for prophylaxis of infection in deep partial-thickness and full-thickness burns. Poorly absorbed, so not useful for most established infections. May cause transient leukopenia which is normally not clinically significant. Broad spectrum, easy to apply, minimal pain, relatively inexpensive. *Contraindicated* in sulfa allergies.
Tincture of iodine	2-7% solution of I_2 in aqueous alcohol	Topical	Bactericidal (see Povidone-iodine). Highly toxic if ingested. Do not use occlusive dressing.

(continued)

Vaccines

Drug	Supplied	Dose/Route	Remarks
Hemophilus b conjugate vaccine (HibTITER PedVaxHIB, ProHIBIT)	Vial: Powder for injection Inj: 0.5 ml	Single 0.5 ml IM dose (ProHIBIT)	Immunization of children 24 months to 6 years of age against diseases caused by *Hemophilus influenza* b.
Hepatitis B virus vaccine inactivated (Heptavax-B)	Vial: 20 µg/ml	20 µg IM in 3 doses; first 2 doses are spaced 1 month apart, and 3rd dose at 6 months.	High-risk populations: 1. Medical and lab personnel who have frequent contact with hepatitis B-positive blood or blood products. 2. Hemodialysis patients. 3. Male homosexuals. 4. Neonates of chronic HB_SAg carriers. Anti-HB_s or anti-HB_c screening tests should be done on all potential recipients of the vaccine who are at high risk prior to administration. Cost of vaccine approximately $100 for 3 doses.
Influenza virus vaccine	Vial: 5 ml	0.5 ml IM as a single dose	Formulated annually based on specifications of the U.S. Public Health Service. High-risk populations: 1. Geriatric patients. 2. Adults and children with chronic disorders of the cardiovascular, pulmonary, and/or renal systems, metabolic diseases, severe anemia,

			and/or compromised immune function. 3. Medical personnel who have extensive contact with high-risk patients. 4. Residents of chronic-care facilities. Subvirion vaccine should be used in children 12 years or younger; whole virion vaccine should be used in adults.
Measles (Rubella) virus vaccine (Attenuvax)	Inj: vial	Total volume of 1 vial SC	Measles vaccine.
Pneumococcal vaccine, polyvalent (Pneumovax 23)	Vial: 0.5 ml Syringe: 0.5 ml	0.5 ml IM/SC as a single dose	Current vaccine contains 23 capsular polysaccharide types of *Streptococcus* pneumonia. Recommended in (1) Adults with chronic disease (cardiovascular & pulmonary) who present with increased morbidity with respiratory infections; (2) Adults with increased risk for pneumococcal disease (i.e., splenic dysfunction or anatomic asplenia). Booster doses *not* recommended.
Varicella virus vaccine (Varivax)	Powder for injection: 1350 PFU of varicella virus	**CHILDREN (1-12 years):** 0.5 ml SQ **ADULTS (>13 years):** Two 0.5 ml SQ at 8 weeks apart.	

(continued)

Vasoconstrictors

Drug	Supplied	Dose/Route	Remarks
Ephedrine (Ephedrine Sulfate)	Caps: 25,50 mg Inj: 5,25,50 mg/ml	**Bronchospasm:** Acute: 12.5-25 mg IVP. Chronic: 25-50 mg PO q 4 h prn. **Hypotension:** 10-25 mg IVP slowly.	Agonist for both α- and β-adrenergic receptors. Used to treat bronchospasm as well as hypotension primarily during anesthesia. CNS effects include agitation, anxiety, tremor. Do not use in hypovolemic patients.
Norepinephrine (Levophed)	Amp: 4 mg/4 ml	**Initial IV dose:** 1-4 μg/min up to 8-12 μg/min or more as needed to maintain a low-normal blood pressure (80-100 mm Hg systolic)	Predominant α-agonist; some β-adrenergic (β_1) activity. Powerful peripheral vasoconstrictor. Also causes visceral, renal and mesenteric vasoconstriction. *Contraindicated* in hypovolemia and with cyclopropane and halothane. Extravasation can lead to tissue sloughing.
Phenylephrine HCl (Neo-synephrine)	Amp: 10 mg/ml	**Initial dose:** 0.01 mg/min; dose is highly variable—titrate to effect.	Stimulates primarily α-receptors; powerful peripheral vasoconstriction. Deleterious if vasoconstriction already present. *Contraindicated* in severe hypertension, hypovolemia, ventricular tachycardia, and hypersensitivity.

Vasopressin (Pitressin)	Vials: 20 units/ml (Vasopressin) Susp: 5 units/ml (Vasopressin tannate)	**GI hemorrhage** (Vasopressin): Initial IV dose (same as intra-arterial dose): 0.2 units/min, then up to maximum safe dose of 0.6 units/min. **Diabetes insipidus** (Vasopressin): 5-10 units IM/SQ 2-4 times daily as needed, or as infusion 0.1-0.2 units/min.	Portal pressure can be reduced by giving either systemically or with selective superior mesenteric artery (SMA) infusions in patients with GI hemorrhage. If bleeding is well-controlled by peripheral infusion, the infusion rate should be left at the controlling dose for 12 h, then tapered every 8-12 h. Also used in the treatment of diabetes insipidus.

Vasodilators

Alpha methyldopa (Aldomet)	Vial: 250 mg/5 ml Tabs: 125,250,500 mg Susp: 250 mg/5 ml	250-500 mg IV or PO q 6 h. **Initial adult PO:** 250 mg bid/tid 2x/day, then increase or decrease until adequate response achieved. **Maintenance adult PO:** 500-2000 mg/day given in 2-4 divided doses.	Stimulates central α-adrenergic receptors. Often requires 24-48 h to achieve its effect. *Contraindicated* in active hepatic disease and hypersensitivity to methyldopa. Drowsiness is fairly common.
Amlodipine (Norvase)	Tabs: 2.5,5,10 mg	**PO:** 5-10 mg qd.	Calcium channel blocker for hypertension and angina.
Bepridil (Vascor)	Tabs: 200,300,400 mg	**PO:** Initial dose 200 mg qd; usual dose 200-400 mg qd.	Calcium channel blocker. Used for chronic stable angina. Ventricular arrhythmias and agranulocytosis are common. Therefore, measure use for patients refractory to other agents.

(continued)

Vasodilators—*(cont.)*

Drug	Supplied	Dose/Route	Remarks
Clonidine (Catapres)	Tabs: 0.1,0.2,0.3 mg Transdermal: TTS-1 (0.1 mg/24 h); TTS-2 (0.2 mg/24 h); TTS-3 (0.3 mg/24 h)	PO: 0.1-0.4 bid. SL: 0.1-0.4 bid. Transdermal: every week.	Hypertension.
Diltiazem HCl (Cardizem)	Tabs: 30,60 mg	PO: 30 mg 4 times/day and increased at 1-2 day intervals as needed.	Slows sinoatrial and atrioventricular nodal conduction. Used in management of Prinzmetal's variant angina and chronic stable angina pectoris. May increase digoxin plasma concentrations.
Felodipine (Plendil)	Tabs (extended release): 5,10 mg	PO: Initial dose 5 mg qid; usual dose 5-10 mg qid.	Treatment of hypertension alone or concurrently with other antihypertensives.
Hydralazine (Apresoline)	Amp: 20 mg/ml Tabs: 10,25,50,100 mg	Initially: PO: 10 mg 4 times/day for 2-4 days, then prn increase to 25-50 mg 4 times/day. IV: 10-20 mg and repeated prn in severe hypertension or hypertensive emergencies.	Vascular smooth muscle relaxant, primarily arterioles. Potent antihypertensive; reduces systemic vascular resistance in congestive heart failure. *Contraindicated* in hypovolemia. Can lead to tachycardia. Has been associated with rheumatoid states and systemic lupus erythematosis (SLE) in high doses. Can cause increased pulmonary artery pressure in mitral valve disease. 75-100 mg PO hydralazine is equivalent to 20-25 mg IV hydralazine.

Isradipine (DynaCirc)	Caps: 2.5, 5 mg	**PO:** Initial dose 2.5 mg bid to a maximum of 10 mg bid	Calcium channel blocker. Used for hypertension alone or concurrently with Ureazide-type diuretics.
Labetalol HCl (Trandate, Normodyne)	Tabs: 100,200,300 mg Vial: 5 mg/ml	Oral: initially 100 mg PO bid, adjusted in 100 mg 2/day q 2-3 days until optimal blood pressure achieved. Usual dose is 200-400 mg PO bid. Parenteral: Initially 20 mg IV push, then 20-80 mg IV push q 10 min until desired effect is achieved (up to 300 mg total), or continuous infusion at initial rate of 2 mg/min; adjust rate according to blood pressure response.	Non-selective β-adrenergic blocker and selective α_1-adrenergic blocker. β-blocker: α-blocker activity is 3:1 (oral) and 7:1 (IV). Decrease in heart rate is minimal secondary to α-blockade. IV administration requires patients to be kept supine to avoid a substantial fall in blood pressure. Useful in treatment of coexisting systemic and intracranial hypertension.
Nicardipine (Cardene)	Caps: 20,30 mg Tabs (sustained release): 20,30 mg	PO: 20-40 mg tid. SR: 30 mg bid.	Chronic stable angina and essential hypertension. Use lower doses with renal/hepatic failure.
Nifedipine (Procardia, Adalat, Procardia XL)	Caps: 10, 20 mg Tabs (sustained release): 30,60,90 mg Amps: 2.5 mg/ml	PO: 10 mg 3 times/day; usual maintenance dose is 30-60 mg given in 3 divided doses. SR: 30 mg qd. IV: 5-15 mg/h.	Used in the management of Prinzmetal's variant angina and chronic stable angina pectoris. No effect on sinoatrial and atrioventricular nodal conduction. Principal effect is vasodilation of main coronary and systemic arteries. Monitor blood pressure initially. Sustained release preparation for hypertension.

(continued)

Vasodilators—*(cont.)*

Drug	Supplied	Dose/Route	Remarks
Nimodipine (Nimotop)	Caps: 30 mg	PO: 60 mg q 4 h for 21 days. Begin therapy within 96 hrs of subarachnoid hemorrhage.	Useful in treatment of cerebral artery spasm following subarachnoid hemorrhage from ruptured congenital intracranial aneurysms.
Nitroglycerin	Cutaneous paste 2% Sublingual tabs: 0.15, 0.3, 0.4, 0.6 mg Vial: 0.5 mg/ml (5 mg) Transdermal system: 2.5 μg; 5, 7.5, 10, 15 mg	**Initial IV dose:** 10 μg/min; titrate to response. Sublingual tabs: variable dosing. Topical: variable dosing.	Vascular smooth muscle relaxant with predominant venous capacitance activity. Can antagonize coronary artery spasm and increase coronary blood flow. Reduce LV end-diastolic pressure by reducing preload. Alleviates myocardial ischemia induced by coronary spasm or subendocardial ischemia seen with an elevation of LV end-diastolic pressure. Can reduce blood pressure. *Contraindicated* in hypovolemia.
Phentolamine (Regitine)	Vial: 5 mg	**Diagnosis of pheochromocytoma**: IVP or IM: 5 mg **Hypertension in pheochromocytoma:** 5 mg IM/IV q 1-2 h. **Extravasation:** 5-10 mg in 10 ml 0.9% NaCl infiltrated into the affected area.	Competitively blocks α-adrenergic receptors. However, activity is relatively transient. Minimal β-adrenergic receptor activity. Used primarily in diagnosis of pheochromocytoma and immediately prior to or during adrenalectomy to improve or control paroxysmal hypertension. Also used to prevent dermal necrosis following IV extravasation of norepinephrine and dopamine.

Sodium nitroprusside (Nipride)	Vial: 50 mg	**Initial dose:** 0.5-10 µg/kg/min. Solution must be protected from light.	Direct venous and arterial vascular smooth muscle relaxant resulting in peripheral vasodilation. Useful in cardiogenic shock, post open-heart surgery, control of peripheral vascular resistance in low-flow states, hypertensive crisis, mitral regurgitation, reduction of pulmonary vascular resistance, induced hypotension. Use with continuous arterial blood pressure monitoring. *Contraindicated* in hypovolemia and acute myocardial ischemia. Must monitor cyanide levels, especially when used in high doses for prolonged periods of time. Signs of cyanide toxicity include progressive acidosis, tachyphylaxis, resistance to nitroprusside, and hypotension.

PART V

Reference Data

Normal Lab Values at the University of Cincinnati Medical Center

Test	Units	Specimen Type	Norms
5-Nucleotidase	MIU/ML	Blood	3.0-11.0
Acid Phosphatase, Total	MIU/ML	Blood	0.0-6.0
Albumin	GM/D/L	Blood	3.5-5.0
Alkaline Phosphatase	MIU/ML	Blood	35-95
Alpha-1-Antitrypsin	MG/DL	Blood	85-213
Alpha-Feto Protein	NG/ML	Blood	<10
Ammonia	MCMOL/L	Blood	6-48
Amylase, Serum	MIU/ML	Blood	0-88
Amylase, Urine, Fluid	U/TVOL	Urine	0-400
APTT	SEC	Blood	22-32
Bilirubin, Direct	MG/DL	Blood	0.0-0.4
Bilirubin, Total	MG/DL	Blood	0.1-1.1
Bleeding Time	MIN		≤9.5
BUN	MG/DL	Blood	5.0-20.0
CA-125	U/ML	Blood	0-35
C-Peptide	NG/ML	Blood	0.5-3.0
Calcitonin	PG/ML	Blood	Male 4.4-31.6 Female 3.0-14.8
Calcium, Fluid	MG/TVOL	Urine	100-250
Calcium, Ionized	MG/DL	Blood	4.5-5.3
Calcium, Serum	MG/DL	Blood	8.5-10.5
Carbamazepine	MCG/ML	Blood	4.0-12.0
Carboxyhemoglobin	%	Blood	0-2% (Non-Smoker) 0-8% (Smoker)
Carcinoembryonic Antigen	NG/ML	Blood	0-3 (Non-Smoker) 0-5 (Smoker)
Chloride	MEQ/ML	Blood	95-110
Cholesterol	MIU/ML	Blood	<200
Chromium, Serum	MCG/L	Blood	0.0-5.0
CO2, Total	MEQ/L	Blood	21-33
CPK	MIU/ML	Blood	<250
CPK-MB%	%	Blood	0.0-5.0
Creatinine	MG/DL	Blood	0.7-1.4
Creatinine, Urine, Fluid	GM/VOL	Urine	1.0-1.8
CSF Glucose	MG/DL	CSF	40-70
CSF Protein	MG/DL	CSF	15-45
Cyanide	MCG/ML	Blood	<0.1
Digoxin	NG/ML	Blood	0.5-2.2
Eosinophil Count, Blood	CUMM	Blood	0.0-450.0
Erythrocyte Sedimentation Rate	SEC	Blood	<20
Ethanol	MG/DL	Blood	<100
Fecal Fat	GM/72 HR	Stool	<15.0

(*continued*)

Lab Values (*Cont.*)

Test	Units	Specimen Type	Norms
Ferritin, Serum	NG/ML	Blood	30-300
Fibrin Degradation	PMCG/ML	Blood	<16
Fibrinogen	MG/DL	Blood	150-400
Folate Level, Serum	NG/ML	Blood	>3.0
Gamma GT	MIU/ML	Blood	8.0-40.0
Gastrin Level, Serum	PG/ML	Blood	<97.0 (fasting)
Glucose	MG/DL	Blood	60-100
Glycohemoglobin	%	Blood	4-8
Haptoglobin	MG/DL	Blood	27.0-139.0
Hematocrit	%	Blood	Adult: Male: 47 ± 7; Female: 42 ± 5
Hemoglobin	GM/DL	Blood	Adult: Male: 16.0 ± 2.0; Female: 14.0 ± 2.0
IgA	MG/DL	Blood	48-348
IgD	MG/DL	Blood	0.0-14.0
IgE, Total	IU/ML	Blood	<150
IgG	MG/DL	Blood	627-1465
IgM	MG/DL	Blood	66-277
IgM Neonatal	MG/DL	Blood	<23
Lactic Acid	MEQ/L	Blood	0.0-2.0
Lactate Dehydrogenase (LDH)	MU/ML	Blood	55-200
Lidocaine	MCG/ML	Blood	1.2-5.0
Lipase, Serum	U/L	Blood	25-170
Lithium	MEQ/L	Blood	0.7-1.4
Magnesium, Serum	MG/DL	Blood	1.5-2.5
N-Acetylprocainamide (NAPA)	MCG/ML	Blood	<30
Osmolality, Serum	MOSM/L	Blood	280-305
Osmolality, Urine	MOSM/L	Urine	50-1200
Phenobarbital	MCG/ML	Blood	15-40
Phenytoin	MCG/ML	Blood	10-20
Phosphate, Urine, Fluid	MG/TVOL	Urine	0.0-1600.0
Phosphorus, Serum	MG/DL	Blood	2.5-4.5
Platelet Count	THOUS/CU	Blood	100-375
Porphobilinogen Quantitative	MG/24 HR	Urine	0.0-2.0
Potassium	MEQ/L	Blood	3.5-5.0
Potassium, Urine, Fluid	MEQ/TVOL	Urine	25-125
Procainamide	MCG/ML	Stool	4.0-8.0
Prolactin	NG/ML	Blood	<20
Protein, Total	GM/DL	Blood	6.0-8.0
Protein, Urine, 24 Hours	MG/TVOL	Urine	0.0-150
Prothrombin Time	SEC	Blood	11.0-13.6
PTH Mid-Molecule	NG/ML	Blood	0.3-1.08

(continued)

Lab Values ***(Cont.)***

Test	Units	Specimen Type	Norms
PTH, Intact	MCLEQ/ML	Blood	6.6-55.8
Reticulocyte Count	%	Blood	0.2-2.0
Retinol Binding Protein	MG/DL	Blood	3.0-6.0
SGOT	MIU/ML	Blood	10.0-30.0
SGPT	MIU/ML	Blood	7.0-35.0
Sodium	MEQ/L	Blood	133-145
Sodium, Urine, Fluid	MEQ/TVOL	Urine	40-220
T3 Resin Uptake	%	Blood	84-117
T3, Reverse	PG/ML	Blood	100-500
T4	MCG/DL	Blood	4.5-11.5
Theophylline	MCG/ML	Blood	10.0-20.0
Thyroglobulin	NG/ML	Blood	<18
Thyroxine Binding Globulin	MCG T4/DL	Blood	11.0-27.0
Tocainide	MCG/ML	Blood	4.0-10.0
Transferrin	MG/DL	Blood	155-355
TSH	MCIU/ML	Blood	0.5-6.0
Urea, Urine or Fluid	GM/VOL	Urine	7.0-16.0
Uric Acid	MG/DL	Blood	4.0-8.0
Urine Free Cortisol	MCG/24 HR	Urine	29-140
Valproic Acid	MCGM/L	Blood	5-120
Vitamin B-12 Level	PG/ML	Blood	180-900
Vitamin B1	MCG/ML	Blood	1.6-4.0
Vitamin B6	NG/ML	Blood	3.6-18.0
Vitamin D (25-OH)	NG/DL	Blood	12-68
Vitamin E	MG/DL	Blood	0.5-2.5
Zinc, Serum	MCG/L	Blood	700-1100

Conversion Data

Pounds to Kilograms
(1 kg = 2.2 lb; 1 lb = 0.45 kg)

Feet and Inches to Centimeters
(1 cm = 0.39 in; 1 in = 2.54 cm)

Fahrenheit/Celsius Temperature Conversion
(F = 9/5 C + 32; C = 5/9 [F − 32])

F		C	F		C	F		C
90	=	32.2	97	=	36.1	104	=	40.0
91	=	32.8	98	=	36.7	105	=	40.6
92	=	33.3	99	=	37.2	106	=	41.1
93	=	33.9	100	=	37.8	107	=	41.7
94	=	34.4	101	=	38.3	108	=	42.2
95	=	35.0	102	=	38.9	109	=	42.8
96	=	35.6	103	=	39.4			

Metric System Prefixes
(Small Measurement)

k	kilo-	10^{3}	n	nano-	10^{-9}
c	centi-	10^{-2}	p	pico-	10^{-12}
m	milli-	10^{-3}	f	fento-	10^{-15}
μ	micro-	10^{-6}	a	atto-	10^{-18}

Nomogram for the Determination of Body Surface Area of Children and Adults

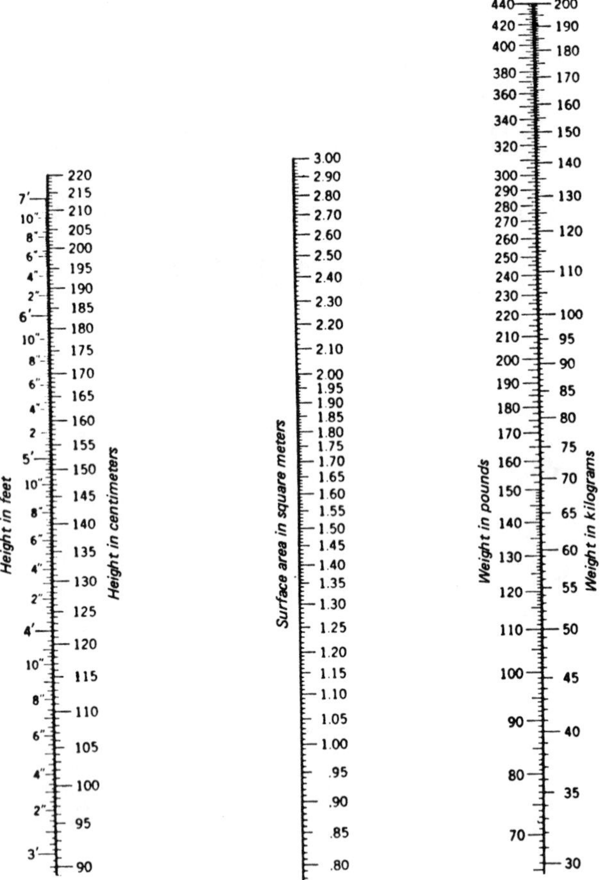

From Way LW (ed): *Current Surgical Diagnosis and Treatment,* 7th ed. Lange Medical Publications, Los Altos, CA, 1985, p. 1188, with permission.

Oxyhemoglobin Dissociation Curves for Whole Blood

$$\text{Hb saturation} = \frac{\text{Total blood } O_2 \text{ content (ml/100 ml)} - \text{Physically dissolved } O_2}{O_2 \text{ capacity of blood (ml/100 ml)} - \text{Physically dissolved } O_2}$$

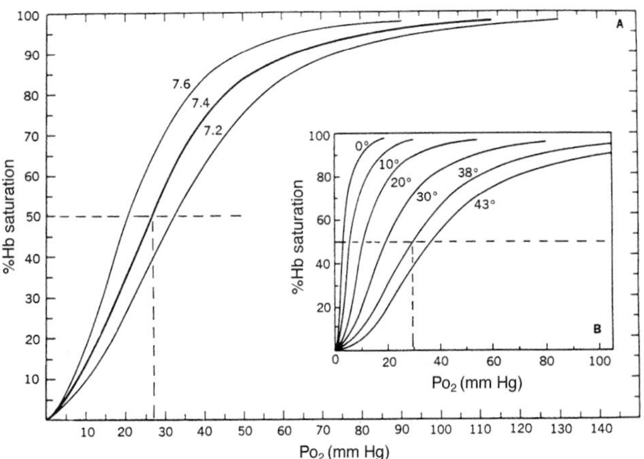

Large diagram indicates influence of change in acidity of blood on affinity of blood for O_2. Curves are based on studies by Dill and by Bock et al. on blood of one man (A.V. Bock). At a particular PO_2 (e.g., 40 mm Hg), acidification of blood results in release of O_2. Action of changes in PCO_2 appear due in part to their effect on pH and in part to formation of carbamino compounds, displacing 2,3-DPG from Hb. *Inset* shows, for blood of sheep, influence of temperature change on PO_2-% HbO_2 relationships; an increase in temperature (as in working muscle) aids in "unloading" O_2 from HbO_2; during hypothermia, hemoglobin has increased affinity for O_2.

Reproduced by permission from C.J. Lambertsen, "Transport of oxygen, carbon dioxide, and inert gases by the blood," in *Medical Physiology,* 14th ed., V.B. Mountcastle, ed. St. Louis, MO, 1980, The C.V. Mosby Co., p. 1725.

INDEX

Note that page numbers in *italic* designate figures; those followed by "t" designate tables.

A

B

D

E

I

N

O

P

Q

R

T